Surgery of Exotic Animals

Surgery of Exotic Animals

Edited by

R. Avery Bennett, DVM, MS, DACVS
Department of Small Animal Clinical Services Louisiana State University
School of Veterinary Medicine
Baton Rouge, LA, USA

Geoffrey W. Pye, BVSc, MSc, DACZM
Disney's Animals, Science, and Environment Team
Disney's Animal Kingdom
Bay Lake, FL, USA

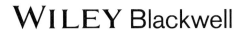

Registered Office
John Wiley & Sons, Inc., 111 River Street, Hoboken, NJ 07030, USA

Editorial Office
111 River Street, Hoboken, NJ 07030, USA

For details of our global editorial offices, customer services, and more information about Wiley products visit us at www.wiley.com.

Wiley also publishes its books in a variety of electronic formats and by print-on-demand. Some content that appears in standard print versions of this book may not be available in other formats.

Library of Congress Cataloging-in-Publication Data

Names: Bennett, R. Avery, editor. | Pye, Geoffrey W., editor.
Title: Surgery of exotic animals / edited by R. Avery Bennett, Geoffrey W.
   Pye.
Description: First edition. | Hoboken, NJ : Wiley-Blackwell, 2022. |
   Includes bibliographical references and index.
Identifiers: LCCN 2021028715 (print) | LCCN 2021028716 (ebook) |
   ISBN 9781119139584 (hardback) | ISBN 9781119139591 (adobe pdf) |
   ISBN 9781119139607 (epub)
Subjects: MESH: Animals, Exotic | Surgery, Veterinary–methods
Classification: LCC SF997.5.E95 (print) | LCC SF997.5.E95 (ebook) | NLM
   SF 997.5.E95 | DDC 636.089/7–dc23
LC record available at https://lccn.loc.gov/2021028715
LC ebook record available at https://lccn.loc.gov/2021028716

Cover Design: Wiley
Cover Image: © Kerri A. D'Ancicco, Michael Karlin, Geoffrey W. Pye, R. Avery Bennett

Set in 9.5/12.5pt STIXTwoText by Straive, Pondicherry, India

Printed in Singapore
M005567_250923

Avery

Since childhood I have been fascinated with veterinary medicine and the diversity of species. Because of various events I abandoned my dream of becoming a veterinarian and obtained a Bachelor of Science degree in Secondary Education. After being a teacher for three years, I joined the Peace Corps and served in Belize. It was while serving, I decided to try again to complete my preveterinary sciences to be eligible to apply. During Veterinary School, my interests were surgery and zoological medicine. While I applied for residencies in both, I was granted a residency in Small Animal Surgery. After graduation, I went into my Rotating Internship at Texas A&M University where I met Elizabeth A. Russo, DVM, MS, DACVIM. Liz was my first mentor in zoological medicine. She had done a residency in Zoological Medicine at the Bronx Zoo, but I remember her telling me she felt she had not learned medicine. So, she completed at residency in Small Animal Medicine and Surgery and became a Diplomate of the American College of Veterinary Internal Medicine. Her goal was to apply the principles she had learned in her training to become a board certified specialist in Internal Medicine to exotic animal species. While she passed away before I finished my training in Veterinary Surgery, I modeled my career after her, applying the principles and techniques I learned in my training becoming a boarded Veterinary Surgeon to exotic animals. I dedicate this book to Claudio Ribeiro da Silva, my husband and life partner; and to Elizabeth A Russo, DVM, MS, DACVIM for inspiring me to advance the field of surgery in exotic animals. For many years Geoff has pushed me to write this book and, in all honesty, without him this book would never have come to be. All my thanks to you, Geoff!

Geoff

There are always pivotal moments and people that change the trajectory of life. For me, I have been lucky to have both hugely influence my life and career. I dedicate this book to my parents, Cath and Bill, who instilled in me a love for nature, and to my family, Dodi, Hannah, and Zach, who instill in me a love for life and have been immensely supportive in this endeavor. I wish to recognize Drs. Jim Carpenter, Pat Morris, Don Janssen, and Scott Terrell who took leaps of faith based on what they saw I could be rather than who I was and have provided me with so many opportunities and learnings that have helped me grow my career and as a person. Finally I would like to thank Avery for being a patient and amazing mentor and encouraging my passion for surgery. "May I make a suggestion?," as I incorrectly held an instrument, chose an inappropriate suture, planned to cut in the wrong place/grab the wrong tissue, or looked to create too much surgical trauma, lives fondly in my many memories of Avery. Thank you sir.

Contents

List of Contributors

R. Avery Bennett, DVM, MS, DACVS
Adjunct Professor of Companion Animal Surgery
Department of Small Animal Clinical Services
School of Veterinary Medicine, Louisiana State
University
Baton Rouge, LA, USA

Elizabeth Bicknese, DVM, MPVM, cVMA
Senior Veterinarian, Veterinary Services, San Diego
Zoo Wildlife Alliance
San Diego, CA, USA

Estella Böhmer, DVM, Dr. med vet
Clinic of Small Animal Surgery and Reproduction,
Center of Veterinary Clinical Medicine
Ludwig-Maximilians-University Veterinärstr
Munich, Germany

Carmen M. H. Colitz, DVM, PhD, MBA, DACVO, DCLOVE (hon)
All Animal Eye Care in Jupiter Pet Emergency and
Specialty Center
Jupiter, FL, USA

Brett Darrow, DVM, DACVS, CCRP
Staff Veterinary Surgeon
Capital Veterinary Specialists
Department of Veterinary Surgery
Jacksonville, FL, USA

Daniel J. Duffy BVM&S(Hons.), MS, FHEA, MRCVS, DACVS-SA, DECVS
Assistant Professor Orthopaedic Surgery
North Carolina State University College of Veterinary
Medicine
Department of Clinical Sciences
Raleigh, NC, USA

David A. Fagan, DDS
Executive Director
The Colyer Institute
San Diego, CA, USA

Dean A. Hendrickson, DVM, MS, DACVS
Professor of Equine Surgery
Colorado State University College of Veterinary
Medicine and Biomedical Sciences
Department of Clinical Sciences, Veterinary Teaching
Hospital
Fort Collins, CO, USA

Jennifer L. Higgins, DVM, PhD
Colorado State University College of Veterinary Medicine
and Biomedical Sciences
Department of Clinical Sciences, Veterinary Teaching
Hospital
Fort Collins, CO, USA

Gregory A. Lewbart VMD, MS, DACZM, DECZM (ZHM)
Professor of Aquatic, Wildlife, and Zoological
Medicine
North Carolina State University
College of Veterinary Medicine
Department of Clinical Sciences
Raleigh, NC, USA

Catriona MacPhail, DVM, PhD
Professor of Small Animal Surgery
Colorado State University
Department of Clinical Sciences
Fort Collins, CO, USA

Elizabeth A. Maxwell, DVM, MS, DACVS-SA, CVPP
Clinical Assistant Professor, Surgical Oncology
University of Florida
Department of Small Animal Clinical Sciences
College of Veterinary Medicine
Gainesville, FL, USA

Michael S. McFadden, MS, DVM, DACVS-SA
Owner, Houston Mobile Veterinary Surgery
Magnolia, TX, USA

Stephen J. Mehler, DVM, DACVS-SA
Chief Medical Officer
Veterinarian Recommended Solutions
Blue Bell, PA, USA
Co-Founder
Main Line Veterinary Specialists
Devon, PA, USA

Michael B. Mison, DVM , DACVS-SA
Professor of Clinical Surgery
University of Pennsylvania School of Veterinary Medicine
Department of Clinical Sciences and Advanced Medicine
Philadelphia, PA, USA

James E. Oosterhuis, DVM
Principal Veterinarian
San Diego Zoo Safari Park
Escondido, CA, USA
Director of Research and Medical Care
The Colyer Institute
San Diego, CA, USA

Heidi Phillips, DVM, DACVS-SA
Associate Professor, Small Animal Surgery
University of Illinois College of Veterinary Medicine
Department of Veterinary Clinical Medicine
Urbana, IL, USA

Geoffrey W. Pye, BVSc, MS, DACZM
Animal Health Director
Disney's Animals, Science, and Environment Team
Disney's Animal Kingdom, Bay Lake, FL, USA

Mark Stetter, DVM, DACZM
Dean & Professor
Colorado State University
Department of Clinical Sciences
College of Veterinary Medicine & Biomedical Sciences
Fort Collins, CO, USA

Claire Vergneau-Grosset, DVM, IPSAV, CES, DACZM
Assistant Professor – Zoological Medicine Service,
Veterinarian of the Aquarium du Québec
Faculté de médecine vétérinaire, Université de Montréal
Saint-Hyacinthe, QC, Canada

Celia R. Valverde, DVM, DACVS
SAGE Veterinary Referral Centers-Dublin
Dublin, CA, USA

E. Scott Weber, III, MSc., VMD, Dipl ACVPM, CertAqVet
White Marsh Hollow
Conestoga, PA, USA

Allison D. Woody, DVM, DAVDC
Clinical Veterinarian
The Colyer Institute
San Diego, CA, USA
San Diego Animal Dentistry
San Diego, CA, USA

Preface

We have two main goals with the "Surgery of Exotic Animals": (i) collate surgical information on exotic species into one book rather than have it scattered throughout the literature and (ii) ensure that every chapter is written and/or edited by a surgery specialist. Exotic animal surgery developed along a different pathway compared to domestic species because surgery specialists have felt out of depth with species with which they had no familiarity. Consequently, surgical techniques were developed by veterinarians with a special interest in exotics, but no specialized training in surgery. Principles instilled during a formal training program in surgery apply across species, including humans, but are only touched on during veterinary school. Veterinary surgeons are able to perform the procedures; however, they feel uncomfortable with the husbandry, anesthesia, and preoperative and postoperative patient care. Occasionally, a specialist surgeon is found with a special interest in exotic species. For the majority of this book, it is these rare individuals that have written chapters using sound surgical principles paired with knowledge of exotic species. An exotic specialist with a special interest in surgery or the pairing of a surgery specialist with an exotic animal specialist is used for some chapters. The latter was also used for editing the book to ensure both aspects were considered in every chapter. These partnerships should be encouraged as it can be hugely beneficial for the animal as each person will bring their skillset to the table. The surgeon can bring strong surgical principles and the exotic animal specialist can help them extrapolate those to the unique anatomy of and what may or may not work for the exotic species. Diplomates of the American College of Veterinary Surgeons, Diplomates of the American Veterinary Dental College, and specialist surgeons from the human medicine field are great resources for exotic animal veterinarians and are at the cutting edge of new techniques, equipment, and products that could be used in exotic patients. These specialists need to be encouraged to take the leap into the unknown that exotic animal veterinarians take on a routine basis. Solid surgical principles used in domestic species and humans can be readily extrapolated for use in exotic animals in most cases.

Avery and Geoff
FL, USA
2020

About the Editors

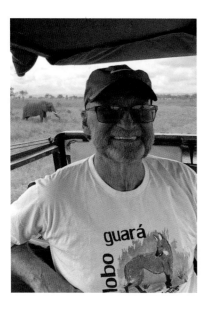

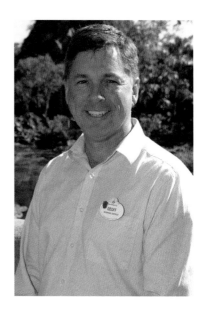

Dr. R. Avery Bennett recently retired from Louisiana State University where he served for four years as professor of Companion Animal Surgery and now remains as an adjunct professor. He has served in senior positions in academia and the public sector in both surgical and exotic animal fields at the University of Florida, University of Pennsylvania, University of Illinois, Animal Medical Center – New York, San Francisco Zoo, and private surgical referral practices in California and Florida. Avery earned his doctorate of Veterinary Medicine with high honors from Michigan State University (1983). He completed a rotating internship in small animal medicine and surgery at Texas A&M University (1984) and a small animal surgery residency at Colorado State University along with a master's degree in veterinary clinical sciences (1987). Avery is a Diplomate of the American College of Veterinary Surgeons (1988). While Avery is competent in both soft tissue and orthopedic surgery, his areas of interest include surgery of exotic animals, minimally invasive surgery – laparoscopic and thoracoscopic surgery, oncologic surgery, and microsurgery.

Dr. Geoffrey W. Pye serves Disney's Animals, Science, and Environment team as the Animal Health Director and joined the team in 2014 to lead the animal health and animal nutrition teams at Disney's Animal Kingdom, the Seas with Nemo and Friends at Epcot, the TriCircle D Ranch, Castaway Cay, and the Aulani Resort. He has also served a senior veterinarian for the San Diego Zoo, Werribee Open Range Zoo, and Currumbin Sanctuary. Geoff completed his bachelor of veterinary science at the University of Melbourne (1988) and earned a master of science in wild animal health from the University of London in association with the London Zoo (1995). He completed an internship in zoological medicine at Kansas State University (1998) and a residency in zoological medicine at the University of Florida (2001). Geoff is a Diplomate of the American College of Zoological Medicine (2001).

1

General Principles, Instruments, and Equipment

R. Avery Bennett

Introduction

Many surgeries in exotic animal are analogous to those performed in other species. The size of some patients makes surgery more challenging. Appropriate preoperative work up, patient preparation, surgeon preparation, perioperative antibiotic therapy, thermal support, and hemostasis are essential for a successful outcome. Preemptive, multimodal analgesia has long been known to improve recovery from surgery and is especially important with wildlife and exotic prey species. Additionally, in recent years, patients' anxiety has become an important consideration when these patients have to be hospitalized. Use medications evaluated for the species having surgery to develop a preemptive analgesic and antianxiety treatment plan. When prey species experience anxiety, stress, fear, and pain, they often die for no apparent reason. Alternatively, they may recover from the surgical event only to die a day or two later, likely from these stresses. In pet species, it appears that if they are accustomed to being handled by humans they are more likely to survive the perioperative period. If multiple procedures need to be accomplished, as a general rule, it is better to perform multiple short anesthetic events and surgeries than to try to do everything under one long anesthetic event. This is especially true when imaging is needed for surgical planning. It is best to anesthetize the patient for imaging, then recover it and evaluate the study. Once a diagnosis is made and a plan developed, anesthetize the patient the next day for the surgical procedure.

It is important that patients resume eating for nutritional support as soon as possible after surgery. Many small patients are not able to undergo long periods of anorexia because they do not have the energy stores to support themselves because in their natural environment they are constantly eating. The nutritional needs of the patient must be addressed and supplemented as needed either per os, using a feeding tube, or intravenously.

Presurgical Considerations

Prior to performing surgery, it is vital to evaluate the patient and address any abnormalities. In many situations, fasting is recommended; however, sometimes it is not necessary. Hemodynamic support is important for all but the shortest surgical procedures. Patient and surgeon aseptic techniques should be followed for all surgeries regardless of size and species. Perioperative or therapeutic antibiotic therapy needs to be considered. Because small patients become hypothermic quickly, thermal support is essential even for diagnostic procedures done under anesthesia.

Patient Support

Small exotic animals are especially prone to developing perioperative complications such as hypovolemia from blood loss, hypothermia, and renal and respiratory compromise. It is important to evaluate the patient systemically prior to anesthesia and surgery and to address any abnormalities preoperatively. During anesthesia and surgery, provide fluid therapy to support the cardiovascular system. Monitor body temperature and take measures to minimize hypothermia. Take appropriate steps to minimize blood loss and take precautions to minimize the risk of surgical site infections.

Data Base

The ideal preoperative data base includes a complete blood count, serum or plasma biochemistry panel, and a urinalysis. Additional diagnostics may be indicated based on the species and the medical problem being addressed. For example, mice and rats are prone to mycoplasmosis pneumonia, and preoperative chest radiographs are indicated prior to anesthesia in these species. While it may be difficult to obtain a urine sample from a small rodent, they are prone to developing renal insufficiency later in life, so it is important to evaluate urine specific gravity and a dipstick for proteinuria. These can be done with two drops of urine

Surgery of Exotic Animals, First Edition. Edited by R. Avery Bennett and Geoffrey W. Pye.
© 2022 John Wiley & Sons, Inc. Published 2022 by John Wiley & Sons, Inc.

that can be obtained by placing the patient in a plastic or glass container for several minutes. In ferrets, it is important to determine the blood glucose level prior to anesthesia because they are prone to forming insulinomas. In very small patients, it may not be feasible to take enough blood for all of the abovementioned diagnostics. At a minimum determine a hematocrit, total protein, blood urea nitrogen (azotemia test strip), glucose, and urine specific gravity.

Preoperative Fasting

Various species such as equids, rabbits, and rodents are not able to vomit for physiologic reason, so fasting to prevent aspiration pneumonia is not necessary. Additionally, if attempting to decrease gastrointestinal contents for a surgery, it can take days to make a difference because the majority of ingesta is within the hindgut. A short fast is recommended to allow these species to swallow any food material to reduce the risk of food entering the trachea during intubation. A prolonged fast in small mammals can result in a negative energy balance which increases their risk for developing complications after surgery (Jenkins 2000). Many small patients have low hepatic glycogen stores and may develop hypoglycemia during a prolonged fast (Harkness 1993; Redrobe 2002). Administer fluids containing dextrose subcutaneously (SC), intravenously (IV), or intraosseously (IOs) in patients prone to developing hypoglycemia. The gastrointestinal transit time in ferrets is rapid, and a prolonged fast is not recommended. An hour fast in ferrets is long enough for the stomach to empty minimizing the risk of developing aspiration pneumonia. On the other end of the spectrum, some reptiles may only eat once a week or even less often so there is no need for a fast.

Hemodynamic Support

Small patients have a small total blood volume and what may appear to be minimal hemorrhage can be life-threatening. If the patient is anemic and surgery can be postponed, it should be postponed until the hematocrit is into the normal range. It would be a rare event that surgery made a hematocrit increase, typically the opposite is the norm. Consider a blood transfusion from a conspecific, if more than minimal hemorrhage is anticipated or if the patient is anemic preoperatively. Strict attention to intraoperative hemostasis is essential when performing surgery on any small patient.

In patients experiencing serious blood loss during surgery, crystalloid or colloid fluid therapy should be administered as quickly as possible for cardiovascular support. More ideal, blood from a conspecific should be used, but often this is not available. Preplanning by having a conspecific blood donor available can be life-saving. In ferrets, there are no blood types and no reports of transfusion reactions. It is safe to use any ferret as a blood donor. In many species, blood typing may not be known. If it is unknown whether a species has blood types, a crossmatch should be performed prior to administering a blood transfusion.

Anesthesia results in loss of fluids because of dry gases making parenteral fluid administration vital for most surgical procedures. It can be difficult to achieve vascular access in small patients. Vascular access provides a route for the administration of fluids during anesthesia at the standard rate of 10 ml/kg/hr and, maybe more importantly, provides a route for administration of emergency drugs in the event of a crisis. An IOs catheter can be placed relatively easily in most species even in small patients. SC administration of fluids is much less effective than IV or IOs and is an ineffective route for administration of emergency drugs. A single dose of 10 ml/kg SC of 4% dextrose has been recommended for short procedures in healthy small exotic mammals (Redrobe 2002). Fluids administered subcutaneously or intraperitoneally are slowly absorbed and not appropriate for treatment of severely ill, dehydrated, or shocky patients.

Maintain vascular access in the postoperative period if at all possible. Continue to administer fluid at least at a maintenance rate until the patient has completely recovered and is eating and drinking well.

Perioperative Antibiotic Therapy

The aim in administering perioperative antibiotics is that the blood level of antibiotic will be effective in preventing incision site infection from target organisms. In most cases, the target organisms are normal skin flora that cannot be completely eliminated during patient skin preparation. The antibiotic should be administered prior to making an incision, which is when the first exposure occurs and should continue until the surgery is complete so any blood clots that form will have therapeutic levels of antibiotic. If the patient is already receiving antibiotics for treatment of an infection and has therapeutic circulating levels of antibiotics effective against the target organisms, additional IV perioperative antibiotic is not needed. If the therapeutic antibiotic is not expected to be effective against the surgical target organisms, perioperative antibiotic administration of an antibiotic expected to be effective against the surgical target organisms should be administered perioperatively. For example, if a patient is receiving cephalexin for a skin infection, but the surgery is in the perineal area where fecal contamination is a concern, adding a perioperative antibiotic against which fecal flora are likely to be sensitive is appropriate. There is no evidence that continuing to administer a perioperative antibiotic for a brief period of time postoperatively is beneficial for preventing surgical site infections (SSIs) and may select for resistant organisms.

Surgeon Aseptic Preparation

The goal of surgeon aseptic preparation is to reduce the incidence of SSI. In human medicine, SSI has been shown to delay wound healing, increase antibiotic use, increase hospital stay, and increase costs, and can result in fatal consequences. Minimizing the risk of SSI in exotic animals is essential for many reasons. Surgeons should wear a cap, mask, gloves, surgical gown, and shoe covers for all surgical procedures (Figure 1.1). Procedures should be done in the cleanest environment possible. A dedicated operating room is ideal, but avoid doing surgery in rooms where abscesses are treated, dirty procedures are performed, or there is fecal contamination.

In one study, glove perforation occurred in 67% of surgeries underscoring the need for hand antisepsis to reduce skin flora before gloving (Verwilghen et al. 2011). Scrubbing is *not* recommended because it removes protective mechanisms on the skin surface and exposes more potentially pathogenic bacteria. Additionally, it causes small abrasions and excoriations damaging the surgeon's skin and increasing the risk of colonization by pathogenic organisms.

Alcohol-based hand rubs are recommended because they have rapid action, are faster to use, and cause less skin damage compared with antiseptic soaps. Alcohol-based hand rubs do not require water. It has been estimated that on average 20l of water are used per hand when using antiseptic soaps. Additionally, many water faucets and municipal water sources are contaminated with *Pseudomonas* sp. and other Gram negative organisms that can recontaminate the hands. There is no reason to do a one-minute hand wash with a neutral soap before applying the hand treatment, and it has been shown that omitting hand washing prior to applying Sterilium® (Medline Industries, www.medline.com) increases its efficacy (Verwilghen et al. 2011). The World Health Organization recommends alcohol-based hand rubs over antiseptic soaps because of their superior efficacy both *in vitro* and *in vivo*, better skin tolerance, lower environmental impact, and no risk of recontamination from rinsing with contaminated water.

Patient Preparation

Regardless of the patient size or species, standard aseptic technique is essential for reducing the risk of SSI. Commonly, exotic animals are more likely to develop SSI than domestic animals because their housing often require them to be in proximity to their urine and feces. Prepare an appropriate area around the proposed surgical incision. Some species like chinchillas and rabbits have fragile skin

Figure 1.1 The surgeon must adhere to proper aseptic technique wearing clean scrubs (a). A cap, mask, and shoe covers, and sterile gown and gloves are proper attire regardless of the size and species of the patient (b).

(a)

(b)

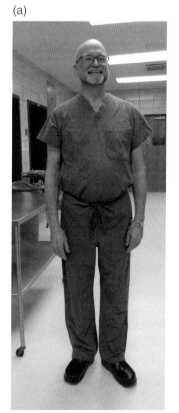
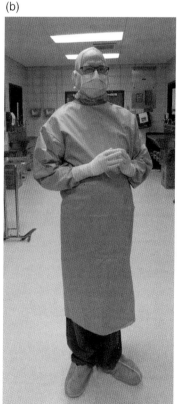

that can easily be damaged during clipping for surgery. For most mammals, a No. 40 clipper blade is used; however, in patients with very fine fur a No. 50 clipper blade (Oster Professional Products, McMinnville, TN) is better suited. The teeth of the No. 50 blade are closer together than those of the No. 40, making it more difficult for the patient's skin to get caught between the teeth and be cut. Move slowly over the skin and keep the skin in front of the clipper blade flattened. Clean and lubricate the blade frequently to help decrease the risk of damaging the skin.

In birds, it is best to pluck feathers which then regrow rapidly; however, it is best not to pluck primary flight and tail feathers as this can damage the follicle resulting in abnormal feather growth. Some birds, such as penguins, have very small dense feathers that are very difficult to pluck. Use a No. 10 clipper blade for these birds. The No. 10 blade teeth are farther apart and clip the feathers at the base. Cut or clipped feathers will not be replaced until the shaft is molted and replaced naturally.

For many years, it has been suggested that alcohol be avoided for skin preparation of small patients because evaporative cooling might cause clinically important hypothermia. A study in mice compared the effect of skin preparation on hypothermia (Skorupski et al. 2017). They compared alcohol alone, povidone iodine alone, povidone iodine alternating with alcohol or saline or warmed saline. Alcohol alone or alternating with povidone iodine caused a dramatic drop in surface and core temperatures, but it rebounded quickly. When alcohol was used alone, the these temperatures returned to nearly the level of the control animals within minutes; however, when alternating with povidone iodine, this was not observed to occur. The authors theorized that the alcohol evaporates very quickly and the cooling stops, whereas povidone iodine and saline evaporate over a longer period of time resulting in more profound hypothermia. Using warmed saline did not modify this effect. The coldest core temperatures were observed in all povidone iodine treatment groups, and this hypothermia persisted. The authors suggested the povidone iodine takes longer to evaporate than saline, resulting in these low body temperatures. The authors concluded that using alcohol for rodent aseptic preparation causes less hypothermia and should be encouraged.

In that study, three applications alternating povidone iodine with either saline or alcohol was used. In veterinary, surgery tradition has been to apply alternating patient skin preparation solutions such as povidone iodine or chlorhexidine alternating with alcohol or saline. The author has been unable to find any scientific evidence for this protocol. It is not applied to humans where a single application of a skin preparation solution is applied prior to making an incision. In fact, the instructions for use on the stock bottle of chlorhexidine indicate to apply the solution and allow it to remain in place for two minutes, then wipe it off and be done.

In another study, an alcohol-based skin preparation was compared to chlorhexidine for reducing skin surface bacteria (Maxwell et al. 2018). The alcohol-based skin preparation sprayed onto the surgical site and allowed to dry was equally as effective as chlorhexidine used according to manufacturer instructions. Make sure the alcohol has completely evaporated prior to using electrosurgery or a CO_2 laser that can ignite the alcohol.

It is not necessary to scrub the patient's skin and actually may be contraindicated. Scrubbing not only irritates the skin, but it also exposes deeper and more pathogenic bacteria to the skin surface potentially contaminating the deeper tissues when the incision is made. A study in horses comparing mechanical and nonmechanical sterile preoperative skin preparation with chlorhexidine gluconate showed there was no difference between a five-minute mechanical scrub and a five-minute application with no scrubbing (Davids et al. 2015). The manufacturer's instructions for using chlorhexidine direct that it be applied to the site and allowed to remain for two minutes before wiping it off. Wiping it off with either saline or alcohol may remove the chlorhexidine negating its residual activity and should, therefore, not be done. A need for alternating between a preparation solution and saline or alcohol has never been established in any species. A newer skin preparation product, ChloraPrep™ One Step (BD Medical, www.bd.com) is applied to the skin for 30 seconds and left to dry for 30 seconds after which the skin is ready for incision. The World Health Organization Global Guidelines for Prevention of Surgical Site Infections states "The panel recommends alcohol-based antiseptic solutions based on chlorhexidine gluconate for surgical skin preparation in patients undergoing surgical procedures" (www.who.int/gpsc/ssi-guidelines/en/).

Patient Draping

Proper aseptic technique is indicated for all surgical patients regardless of size and species. Place quarter drapes around the surgical site and then cover with a patient drape with a fenestration around the site. Currently, disposable paper drapes are commonly used for both quarter drapes and patient drapes. Avoid the tendency to make a small sterile field as it is then easy to contaminate yourself by accidentally touching objects on the table outside the sterile field. Create a sterile field of the entire table top and take appropriate action to reestablish a sterile field if contamination occurs (Figure 1.2). When working with very small patients, it may be beneficial to use a clear plastic drape over the patient to allow respiration to be monitored; however, other respiratory monitoring devices such as end-tidal CO_2 monitors allow monitoring of respiration more accurately and do not require the ability to visualize the patient.

(a)

(c)

(b)

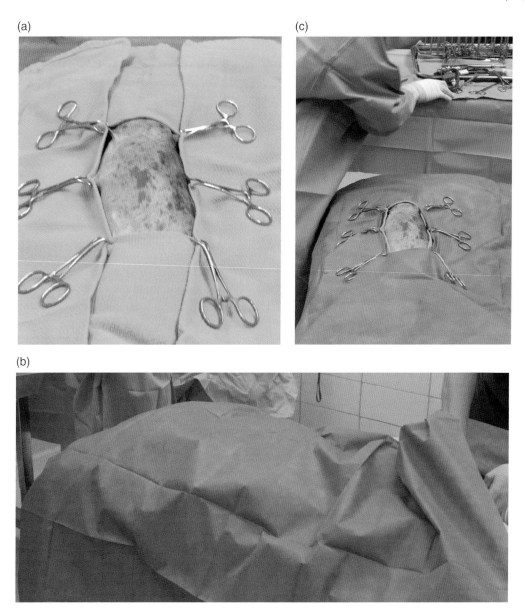

Figure 1.2 This 1.2 kg patient is being draped for a thoracotomy. First quarter drapes of Huck towels are placed to isolate the surgical field (a). Then the patient is covered with a patient drape large enough to create a sterile field of the entire table (b). The instruments are on the back table, and this is pulled up to the patient drape to complete the sterile field (c).

Thermal Support

Hypothermia during anesthesia is a major concern for many reasons including decreased metabolic functions and excretion of anesthetic agents. Many small exotic animals have a large body surface area/volume ratio predisposing them to developing hypothermia during anesthesia. The body temperature of a rat can drop 18 °F (10 °C) after 20 minutes of anesthesia (Harkness et al. 2010). Use an esophageal or rectal temperature probe to continuously monitor the patient's body temperature. The normal temperature for a given species may not be known; however, once the patient is anesthetized insert a temperature probe to determine its body

temperature. Then monitor the temperature and how much it drops during anesthesia. Even in poikilotherms, this is very helpful and can help make decisions about the need to provide additional thermal support.

A short anesthesia and operative time accomplished by having all the necessary equipment ready and accessible will help to minimize hypothermia. It is best to use patient warming devices with temperature control such as forced warm air and warm water blankets. It can be difficult to place a warm air blanket around a small patient. These devices blow warm dry air, so pay particular attention to keeping the cornea lubricated to reduce the risk of creating corneal ulcers. This is especially important with small patients where the head is hard to visualize under the blanket. It is considered beneficial to use more than one patient warming device. For example combine a circulating warm water blanket under the patient and a forced warm air device around and over the patient where possible. For most small exotic animals set the circulating warm water blanket and forced warm air device at 104 °F (40 °C) because these patients have a high body temperature. Drape the patient as quickly as possible to help hold heat in under the drapes.

Use warm (101–103 °F; 39–40 °C) saline for abdominal and thoracic lavage. Fill the body cavity with the warm saline and do not immediately remove it. Allow it to dwell within the body for several minutes. Repeat this process until the body temperature begins to rise. Once the downward trend in body temperature reverses and the body cavity has been closed, in most cases, the temperature will continue to rise assuming other patient warming devices are in place. For most species, if the body temperature drops below 96 °F (35.5 °C) during the surgery, stop the procedure and instill warm saline into the body cavity before continuing the procedure. Repeat the process before closing.

Instrumentation and Equipment

Hemostatic Aids

The average cotton-tipped applicator (CTA) holds approximately 0.1 ml of blood when completely soaked and a 4×4 gauze sponge holds 10 ± 2 ml (Hughes et al. 2007). The total blood volume of small mammals is 57 ml/kg of body weight (Jenkins 2000; Bennett 2009). If a patient loses 10–15% of total blood volume (approximately 1% of body weight), it is generally considered safe. Most mammals experience hypovolemic shock and release large amounts of catecholamines with loss of 15–20% of the total blood volume. Loss of 20–30% of the total blood volume can have life-threatening consequences (Jenkins 2000; Bennett 2009). As an example, if a 50 g mouse loses more than five CTAs full of blood, it is equivalent to more than 20% of the blood volume (Harkness 1993). Table 1.1 shows approximately 20% of the blood volume of common rodent pets.

Magnification is an aid for hemostasis (see Chapter 3). What would seem a small amount of blood to the naked eye observer appears to be major blood loss when magnified drawing the surgeon's attention to the hemorrhage and the need to arrest it. Additionally, small vessels can be identified and controlled more easily when working under magnification.

Hemostatic clips are available in various sizes including microclips. These are very useful for controlling hemorrhage in small patients, where it is difficult to accurately place a ligature. Additionally, they can be applied in deep,

Table 1.1 Loss of approximately 20% of total blood volume results in cardiovascular compromise with potentially life-threatening consequences.

Species	20% of blood volume (ml)
Gerbil	1.2
Hamster	1.4
Rat	4.0
Guinea pig	4.5

Twenty percent of the approximate blood volume of rodents.
Source: Harkness (1993), Jenkins (2000), Harkness et al. (2010).

hard-to-reach locations. With some types of hemostatic clips, both straight and right-angled appliers are also available (Figure 1.3). This applier makes it easier to get under a hemostat to apply a clip to a severed vessel.

Sterile CTAs are useful for atraumatic tissue dissection and manipulation. They can be used to apply pressure to damaged vessels allowing a clot to form. Use moistened CTAs when using them for tissue manipulation and dissection and dry ones to absorb fluids.

Absorbable gelatin sponge is made from treated purified gelatin solution. It is capable of absorbing many times its weight in blood and also provides a scaffolding for clot formation. It is completely absorbed in 4–6 weeks. Surgicel (Ethicon, Inc., Sommerville, NJ) is oxidized regenerated cellulose resembling cloth. It is a hemostatic aid that adheres nicely to moist tissues, but is not capable of absorbing much fluid and does not adhere well to dry tissue. Gelatin sponges are thick and absorb more fluid than oxidized regenerated cellulose but are prone to becoming dislodged from the tissue.

Topical thrombin is commercially available and when applied uses the patient's fibrinogen to form a fibrin clot. It is most useful for oozing and minor bleeding from capillaries and venules where standard surgical techniques are ineffective at halting the hemorrhage. It can be applied directly to the source of hemorrhage or can be applied onto gelatin sponge that is then placed over the site of hemorrhage. A hemostatic "taco" can be made of gelatin sponge wrapped in oxidized regenerated cellulose and soaked in topical thrombin and is very effective for controlling hemorrhage (Figure 1.4).

Electronic Hemostatic Devices

Electrocautery

Electrocautery uses direct current electricity to heat metal until it is red hot. The red hot tip is applied to the source of hemorrhage to heat and coagulate tissues. Electrocautery causes heat damage to adjacent tissues that then undergo necrosis minimizing its value in many situations. Cautery pens (Convenient

(a)

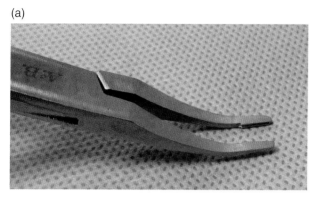

(b)

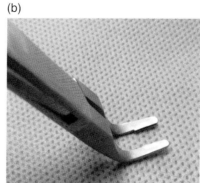

Figure 1.3 Straight and right-angled hemostatic clip appliers are available. Compared with the standard applier (a), the right-angled appliers (b) can be inserted into a small body cavity to place a hemostatic clip at nearly a right angle, while the standard applier requires the handles to be almost perpendicular to the vessel, making it difficult to place through a small approach into a body cavity.

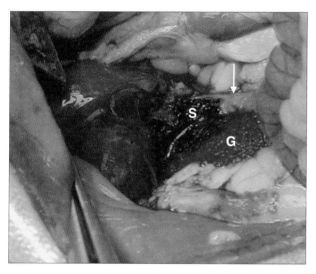

Figure 1.4 A "hemostatic taco" made of gelatin sponge (G) wrapped in oxidized, regenerated cellulose (S) and soaked in topical thrombin has been applied to the caudal vena cava (arrow) after right adrenalectomy.

Cautery Kit; Jorgensen Labs; www.jorvet.com) may be useful to cauterize small vessels in small exotic mammals if electrosurgery is not available. They have a fine wire tip and are battery-operated. Keep in mind that the longer the heat is applied to the tissue, the more thermal necrosis occurs.

Electrosurgery

Electrosurgery uses high-frequency alternating current to generate energy. There is an active electrode and an indifferent electrode or ground. With monopolar electrosurgery the current exits the generator, passes to the active electrode, and concentrates at the tip which contacts the patient. After creating a thermal event at the tip, the current disperses throughout the patient's body, exits through the ground plate, and is carried back to the generator to complete the electrical circuit. Therefore, the patient is within the electrical circuit. If the ground plate only contacts a small area of

the patient's skin burns and subsequent necrosis can result because the current concentrates where it exits the patient. The Surgitron® Dual Frequency 120 (Ellman International, Inc., Hewlett, NY) generates 4.0 MHz current which is in the radio frequency wavelength. Current is received by the indifferent electrode acting as an antenna. Because the current is in the radio frequency, the area of contact between the patient and the ground plate is irrelevant and thermal injury should not occur. This is helpful with small patients where it might be difficult to disperse the current exiting the patient adequately.

The bipolar electrosurgical forceps are primarily used for hemostasis, but can also be used for tissue dissection resulting in minimal hemorrhage. The same generator is used, but the patient is not within the electrical circuit so the current only affects tissue within the tips of the forceps. Bipolar forceps are most useful near structures that would be adversely affected by the current such as the heart, brain, spinal cord, etc., or for hemostasis deep within body cavities. When using bipolar to dissect or cut tissue, grasp the tissue in the forceps and activate the current while pulling the forceps. The tissue within the tips will be affected by the current providing hemostasis for small vessels within the tissue grasped. In birds, this technique is useful for making a skin incision. Grasp the skin with the forceps and activate the current to create a small defect in the skin. Then insert one limb of the forceps under the skin for 1–2 cm, oppose the other limb of the forceps, activate the current, and withdraw the forceps, thus cutting the skin. Bipolar mode is available on most electrosurgical units including the Surgitron®.

Vessel Sealing Devices

LigaSure™ (Medtronic, Minneaplis, MN) is a vessel/tissue sealing system that is commonly used in veterinary surgery. The ForceTriad™ (Medtronics, Minneapolis, MN) combines the LigaSure technology with monopolar and bipolar electrosurgery. While the specific technology is proprietary, LigaSure™ is a type of bipolar electrosurgery. The generator senses the electrical impedance of the tissues within the tips and delivers the amount of current needed to melt the elastin and collagen; it then allows the elastin and collagen to re-form, creating a permanent seal in a single application. It generates less than 1 mm of heat lateral to the seal and is Food and Drug Administration (FDA)-approved to seal vessels up to 7 mm diameter. A wide range of handpieces are available for open surgical procedures and for minimally invasive surgeries.

Harmonic Scalpel

Ethicon® Harmonic Scalpel (Ethicon US, LLC, www.ethicon. com/na) is an ultrasonically activated cutting instrument that converts electrical energy to mechanical energy. The blade vibrates at 55,500 Hz creating heat that coagulates vessels and cuts tissue. Hand pieces are available in various sizes and types for both open surgical procedures and minimally invasive surgery. It is FDA-approved to seal vessels up to 5 mm diameter and does not create smoke. The tissue is compressed between a Teflon anvil and the vibrating blade. There are two settings, one to seal the tissue and another to cut through the tissue.

Carbon Dioxide Laser

The carbon dioxide (CO_2) laser (Aesculight; LuxarCare LLC, Bothell, WA) gained popularity in veterinary surgery in the 1990s and continues to be in common use today. CO_2 lasers produce a beam of intense light at a wavelength that is highly absorbed by water molecules. It cuts tissue when the beam is very focused and coagulates for hemostasis when it is more diffused. The CO_2 laser seals vessels <0.6 mm, so most skin incisions are bloodless with minimal or no bruising. It also seals lymphatic vessels and nerves so there is less swelling and reportedly less pain associated with incisions compared with those made using a scalpel. When used with correct technique, the amount of lateral heat damage is minimal (Harkness et al. 2010); however, when used incorrectly, lasers can cause significant thermal damage.

In addition to being able to incise skin and other tissues, CO_2 lasers can also be used to fulgurate or destroy tissue, such as a tumor or the tissue bed after a tumor has been removed in an effort to eliminate residual microscopic disease. Use a high-power setting and keep the tip as close to the tissue as possible when cutting tissue. Do not touch the tip to the tissue. If there is hemorrhage, move the tip farther from the tissue, which will diffuse the beam and coagulate vessels. Use a smaller tip to create a small spot of light which will then cut better with less collateral heat. A wider tip will not cut as well and will cause more heat damage, but will also control hemorrhage better by coagulating vessels. Proper safety training for all personnel is important when using surgical lasers.

Magnification

Magnification is a vital part of efficiently performing surgery on small exotic animals, but it is also useful for delicate procedures in any size animal (see Chapter 3).

Focal Light

Overhead surgery lights are not adequate for surgery in small exotic animals and are becoming obsolete being replaced by head-mounted focal light sources that illuminate whereever the surgeon is looking, including deep into body cavities. These lights illuminate a smaller area allowing better visualization of the tissues. Inexpensive head-mounted cool focal lights are available with or without magnifying loupes from many sources (LED Headlight; MDS, Inc., Brandon, FL). SurgiTel loupes (General Scientific Corporation, Inc., Ann Arbor, MI) are available with different light options that mount onto the frame to illuminate the surgeon's field of view.

General Scientific Corporation, Inc., also offers SurgiCam HD, a head-mounted digital video camera with 3× magnification. The procedure can be viewed on a monitor, and images, and videos can be captured onto a computer.

Retractors

In the past, spring-loaded eyelid retractors have been recommended for abdominal wall retractors in small patients. The tension cannot be adjusted and is often too much for small patients. Heiss and Alm Self-Retaining Retractors work well as abdominal and tissue retractors in companion exotic animals (Figure 1.5). The Lone Star™ Retractor (Veterinary Specialty Products, Inc., Mission, KS) consists of a plastic frame and silastic bands with tissue hooks on the ends (stays) (Figure 1.6). Be sure to look for the models with all components that are fully autoclavable. Place the stay hooks in the tissue and using an appropriate amount of tension, pull and insert the silastic bands into the notches of the frame to retract tissue. These retractors are very versatile and have a wide range of applications.

Instrumentation

In the past, many surgeons have turned to using ophthalmic instruments for surgery in small exotic animals; however, they are not well suited for this purpose. Being made for surgery on a superficial structure, the eye, they are short making them more difficult to control and to manipulate tissues deep in a body cavity. Microsurgical instruments are manufactured so they are of a standard length and only the tips are miniaturized (Bennett 2009) (see Chapter 3). They are long enough for the instrument to

(a)

(b)

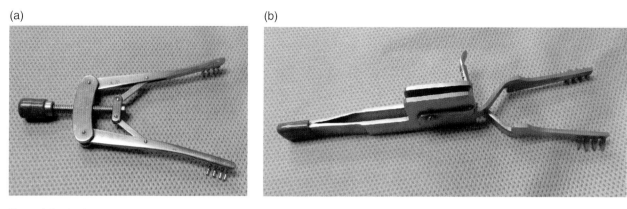

Figure 1.5 An Alm retractor (a) uses a thumb screw to open the jaws, while the Heiss retractor (b) has a quick release ratchet mechanism.

(a)

(b)

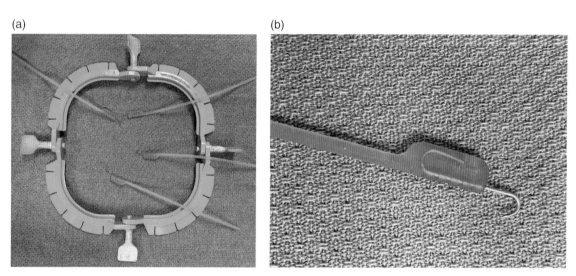

Figure 1.6 The Lone Star retractor system consists of a plastic ring with notches around the perimeter (a) and silastic bands with tissue hooks that are placed in the tissue to be retracted (b). Insert the bands into the notches in the ring to maintain tissue retraction.

balance in the hand while the tips extend beyond the surgeon's hand into the patient's body cavity (Figure 1.7). They should be counterbalanced to minimize hand fatigue. Round handles are recommended because the instruments should be rolled between the thumb and first two fingers rather than using wrist action. Having round handles is most important for needle holders because the curved needle has to be passed through the tissue using this rolling action between the thumb and fingers. Even with scissors and forceps, it is easier to roll them if the handles are round. Many surgeons prefer needle holders without box lock for delicate tissue because when the lock is set, the needle can jump and tear tissues. Hold a microsurgical instrument as if you were holding a pen (Figure 1.8a). An across-the-palm grip is inappropriate (Figure 1.8b). As a starting point, a microsurgical pack should contain a microsurgical needle holder, a microsurgical scissors, and microsurgical thumb forceps (Figure 1.9). Add other microsurgical instruments to the pack with increasing experience.

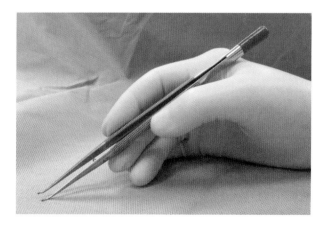

Figure 1.7 Microsurgical instruments should be a standard length with miniaturized tips that extend beyond the hand into the tissue and should be counterbalanced to minimize hand fatigue.

Suction and Irrigation

Ophthalmic bulb syringes work well for tissue irrigation in small exotic animals (Figure 1.10). Alternatively, use a

(a)   (b)

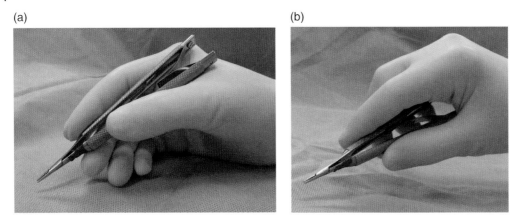

Figure 1.8   Hold the instruments like a pen (a) and not across the palm (b) for better control and the ability to roll the instrument.

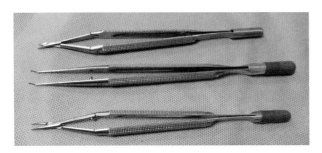

Figure 1.9   The basic microsurgical pack should consist of a needle holder, scissors, and forceps.

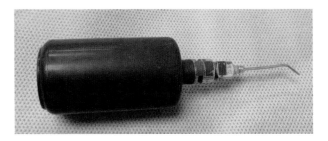

Figure 1.10   Ophthalmic bulb syringe is useful for irrigation in small patients.

syringe with a needle attached and bend the needle at the hub repeatedly until it breaks off to minimize the risk damaging tissue with the needle. Fine Barron suction tips have a release hole providing two degrees of suction; stronger suction with the hole covered and more delicate suction with the hole open. If tissues suck up against the tip, place the corner of a gauze over the end of the suction tip so it is not able to suck up tissue.

References

Bennett, R.A. (2009). Rodents: soft tissue surgery. In: *BSAVA Manual of Rodents and Ferrets* (eds. E. Keeble and A. Meredith), 73–79. Gloucester: British Small Animal Veterinary Association.

Davids, B.I., Davidson, M.J., Tenbroeck, S.H. et al. (2015). Efficacy of mechanical versus non-mechanical sterile preoperative skin preparation with chlorhexidine gluconate 4% solution. *Veterinary Surgery* **44** (5): 648–652.

Harkness, J.E. (1993). Anesthesia, surgery. In: *A Practitioner's Guide to Domestic Rodents* (ed. J.E. Harkness), 37–50. Denver, CO: American Animal Hospital Association.

Harkness, J.E., Turner, P.V., VandeWoude, S., and Wheeler, C. (2010). *Harkness and Wagner's Biology and Medicine of Rabbits and Rodents*, 5e. Ames, IA: Wiley-Blackwell.

Hughes, K., Chang, Y.C., Sedrak, J., and Torres, A. (2007). A clinically practical way to estimate surgical blood loss. *Dermatology Online Journal* **13** (4): 17.

Jenkins, J.R. (2000). Surgical sterilization in small mammals. Spay and castration. *Veterinary Clinics of North America: Exotic Animal Practice* 3: 617–627.

Maxwell, E.A., Bennett, R.A., and Mitchell, M.A. (2018). Efficacy of application of an alcohol-based antiseptic hand rub or a 2% chlorhexidine gluconate scrub for immediate reduction in the bacterial population on the skin of dogs. *American Journal of Veterinary Research* **79** (9): 1001–1007.

Redrobe, S. (2002). Soft tissue surgery of rabbits and rodents. *Seminars in Avian and Exotic Pet Medicine* **11**: 231–245.

Skorupski, A.M., Zhang, J., Ferguson, D. et al. (2017). Quantification of induced hypothermia from aseptic scrub applications during rodent surgery preparation. *Journal of the American Association for Laboratory Animal Science* **56** (5): 562–569.

Verwilghen, D., Grulke, S., and Kampf, G. (2011). Presurgical hand antisepsis: concepts and current habits of veterinary surgeons. *Veterinary Surgery* **40**: 515–521.

2

Suture Materials

Michael S. McFadden

Introduction

Suture materials play an important role in veterinary surgery, but many veterinarians overlook important details and try to use one suture material for too many applications. Most veterinarians with no postgraduate training in surgery select suture materials based on hospital policy or cost, whereas veterinarians with postgraduate training in surgery select suture material based on a more complete understanding of suture materials and indications. The ideal suture would be in place only as long as needed and would then immediately disappear. Tissues heal at different rates, so materials that are more slowly absorbed are best used only in tissues that take a long time to heal. Suture should cause minimal tissue reaction, and the surgeon should attempt to minimize the amount of suture buried because all suture is foreign material. The amount of inflammation caused by different suture materials is illustrated in Figure 2.1. With the exception of rodents and rabbits, there are relatively few studies specifically examining suture materials in exotic animals.

Suture Materials

The role of sutures is to maintain incised or injured tissue in apposition to allow the tissue to heal (Bellenger 1982; van Rijssel et al. 1989; Roush 2003). The ideal suture material would provide high tensile strength for a sufficient time to allow the tissue to heal, have good knot security, resist infection, and cause no inflammatory, immunogenic, or carcinogenic reactions. The reaction of tissue to sutures depends on several variables such as the type, quantity, and duration of suture implantation as well as the tissues into which suture is implanted.

Surgeons must be familiar with different suture materials in order to make the most appropriate choice for specific clinical situations (Ratner et al. 1994). It is important to have a thorough understanding of the tissues, healing time required, the time the suture retains sufficient tensile strength to support the tissues as they heal, and time to complete absorption. The suture that is chosen may affect wound healing, functional outcome, and cosmetics. The number of suture types available has increased dramatically, and each suture type has specific physical, handling, and tissue reaction characteristics. Sutures are classified in many ways based on their ability to be absorbed and whether they are single, stranded, or braided. Different suture properties can also affect the knot security which must also be considered when choosing suture materials (Marturello et al. 2014).

Absorbable Suture Materials

Absorbable suture materials are defined as materials that lose their tensile strength within 60 days of implantation (Tan et al. 2003). These sutures are either composed of different synthetic polymers or are of biologic origin. Absorbable sutures that are biologic in origin are broken down by phagocytosis, while synthetic polymers are absorbed by hydrolysis. Hydrolysis involves breaking down polymers into monomers by direct water cleavage, and the monomers are then absorbed and metabolized by the body (Tan et al. 2003). Common absorbable sutures include chromic gut, polydioxanone (PDS™, Ethicon Inc., Cincinnati, OH), poliglecaprone 25 (Monocryl™, Ethicon Inc., Cincinnati, OH), polyglactin 910 (Vicryl™, Ethicon Inc., Cincinnati, OH), polyglyconate (Maxon™, Covidien, Medtronics, Minneapolis, MN), synthetic polyester called Glycomer™ 631 (Covidien, Medtronics, Minneapolis, MN) comprised of glycolide (60%), dioxanone (14%), and trimethyelene carbonate (14%) (Biosyn™,

Surgery of Exotic Animals, First Edition. Edited by R. Avery Bennett and Geoffrey W. Pye.
© 2022 John Wiley & Sons, Inc. Published 2022 by John Wiley & Sons, Inc.

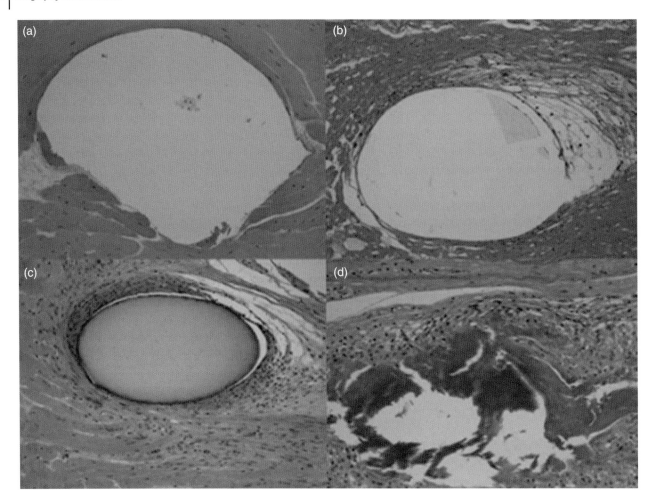

Figure 2.1 Inflammatory reactions after implantation of different suture materials to demonstrate variation in inflammatory reactions. Samples were chosen as representative examples of zero (a), mild (b), moderate (c), and severe (d) inflammatory responses. Suture material was lost in (a) and (b) during processing, but surrounding inflammatory reaction is intact. Images are 20× magnification.

Covidien, Medtronics, Minneapolis, MN), polyglycolic acid (Dexon™, Covidien, Medtronics, Minneapolis, MN), polyglytone 6211 (Caprosyn™, Covidien, Medtronics, Minneapolis, MN), and synthetic polyester called Lactomer™ comprised of a copolymer of glycolide and lactide (Polysorb™, Covidien, Medtronics, Minneapolis, MN).

Various companies manufacture generic versions of most of these suture materials. In one study comparing the same material made by two different companies (Ethicon, Inc., and Hyaiyin Medical Instruments Co. Ltd.), the materials had significantly different tensile strength and stiffness (De La Puerta et al. 2011). In some comparisons, the generic outperformed the brand name materials. Most studies of suture materials are conducted using brand name materials. Based on this study, direct comparisons between brand names and generic materials cannot be made.

Biologic Absorbable Suture Material

Chromic Gut

Chromic gut is a monofilament absorbable suture composed of purified connective tissue (mostly collagen) derived from either bovine or ovine intestine and is absorbed by phagocytosis and enzymatic digestion by macrophages (Bellenger 1982; Roush 2003). Chromic salts are used to coat the suture to help delay absorption, increase tensile strength, and decrease tissue reactivity. Chromic gut is rapidly absorbed in mammals, is completely absorbed in approximately 60–90 days, and only maintains tensile strength for 7–10 days (Ratner et al. 1994). Chromic gut has a tendency to cause increased inflammatory response compared to other absorbable sutures which makes it less desirable.

Synthetic Absorbable Suture Materials

Synthetic absorbable sutures are all composed of different monomers or polymers. Each monomer affects the resultant strength, flexibility, and speed at which the suture is absorbed. Monomers used in most currently available sutures include glycolide, lactide, *p*-dioxanone, ε-caprolactone, and trimethylene carbonate. Glycolide and lactide contribute to the resulting strength of the suture, while ε-caprolactone and trimethylene carbonate contribute to increased flexibility. *p*-Dioxanone contributes moderate strength and moderate flexibility. Combinations of these monomers in different proportions are used to obtain desired properties for different applications.

Polydioxanone

Polydioxanone is a monofilament absorbable suture that elicits minimal reaction, is slowly absorbed, and maintains tensile strength for extended periods. It maintains 70% of its tensile strength at 2 weeks, 50% at 4 weeks, and 25% at 6 weeks with complete absorption in approximately 180 days (Bellenger 1982; Ratner et al. 1994; Roush 2003). Initial tensile strength for polydioxanone is greater than surgical gut, polyglycolic acid, or polyglactin 910, but it has the poorest knot security of the synthetic absorbable sutures (Boothe 1998). It is useful when prolonged support of healing tissue is desired (Tan et al. 2003).

Poliglecaprone 25

Poliglecaprone 25 is a monofilament absorbable suture composed of segmented block copolymers of ε-caprolactone and glycolide (Bezwada et al. 1995). Soft segments of ε-caprolactone and glycolide contribute to favorable handling characteristics and hard segments of polyglycolide contribute to tensile strength. Poliglecaprone 25 is one of the strongest absorbable sutures, although it rapidly weakens after implantation (Tan et al. 2003). Tensile strength of 20–30% is maintained at 2 weeks and complete absorption occurs between 90 and 100 days (Bezwada et al. 1995; Roush 2003).

Polyglactin 910

Polyglactin 910 is a multifilament suture composed of a copolymer of lactic and glycolic acids that are coated with calcium stearate and a second copolymer of glycolide and lactide. The braided nature of this suture not only results in good handling properties but also increases tissue drag (Ratner et al. 1994). Tensile strength is approximately 60% at 2 weeks and only 30% at 3 weeks with complete absorption in approximately 60 days (Bellenger 1982; Ratner et al. 1994; Fossum 2002; Roush 2003). Vicryl Rapide™ (polyglactin 910) has 66% of the initial tensile strength and loses tensile strength faster compared to regular polyglactin 910 (Tan et al. 2003). It is designed for rapidly healing tissues where long-term support is not required.

Polyglyconate

Polyglyconate is a monofilament suture composed of copolymers of glycolide and trimethylene carbonate. Tensile strength is approximately 80% at 1 week, 75% at 2 weeks, 50% at 4 weeks, and 25% at 6 weeks with complete absorption at 180 days (Tan et al. 2003).

Glycomer™ 631

Glycomer 631 is a monofilament suture composed of synthetic polyesters and alternating segments of glycolide and dioxanone with segments of trimethylene carbonate and dioxanone. It retains 75% of its tensile strength at 2 weeks and 40% at 3 weeks. Complete absorption occurs between 90 and 110 days.

Polyglycolic Acid

Polyglycolic acid is a braided suture composed of the homopolymer of glycolic acid and coated with polycaprolate (Tan et al. 2003). Polycaprolate is a copolymer of glycolide and ε-caprolactone. Polyglycolic acid is rapidly absorbed and quickly loses tensile strength. Fourteen days following implantation, polyglycolic acid only has 20% of its initial tensile strength and is completely absorbed in 60 days.

Polyglytone 6211

Polyglytone 6211 is a newer monofilament absorbable suture composed of synthetic polyester of glycolide, caprolactone, trimethylene carbonate, and lactide (Pineros-Fernandez et al. 2004). It provides short-term tensile strength combined with the benefits of rapid absorption losing 70–80% of its tensile strength in 10 days and being completely absorbed in 56 days (van Heerden 2005).

Lactomer™

Lactomer is a braided suture composed of polymers of glycolide and lactide. It is coated with ε-caprolactone glycolide and calcium stearoyl lactylate to improve handling properties. Lactomer retains 80% of its tensile strength at 2 weeks and 30% at 3 weeks with complete absorption between 56 and 70 days.

Nonabsorbable Suture Materials

Nonabsorbable suture materials do not undergo significant degradation after implantation. These sutures are used where extended wound support is required or in areas where suture removal is expected (skin closure). Nonabsorbable sutures, like absorbable sutures, are composed of natural or synthetic fibers. Natural fibers tend to invoke significant inflammatory reactions; thus, there may be a preference for synthetic nonabsorbable sutures depending on the application. Nonabsorbable suture materials commonly used in veterinary surgery include silk, nylon (Ethilon™, Ethicon Inc., Cincinnati, OH; Monosof™, Covidien, Medtronics, Minneapolis, MN; Nurolon™, Ethicon Inc., Cincinnati, OH; Supramid™, S. Jackson, Inc., Alexandria, VA), polypropylene (Prolene™, Ethicon Inc., Cincinnati, OH; Surgipro™, Covidien, Medtronics, Minneapolis, MN), and stainless steel.

Biologic Nonabsorbable Suture Materials

Silk

Silk is the most commonly used organic nonabsorbable suture material (Fossum 2002; Roush 2003; Tan et al. 2003). It is a braided suture with excellent handling properties and knot security. Silk loses a significant amount of its tensile strength after extended implantation but is considered nonabsorbable because the material remains in the tissues for a significant amount of time. There is a 30% loss of tensile strength at 14 days and 50% loss at 1 year. Time for complete absorption is greater than 2 years. Silk leads to significant reaction in tissues, and the presence of silk suture can reduce the number of bacteria needed to induce an infection from 10^6 to 10^3 (Fossum 2002).

Nylon

Nylon is a synthetic nonabsorbable suture that is available as a monofilament or braided suture (Ratner et al. 1994; Fossum 2002; Roush 2003; Tan et al. 2003). Nylon maintains a high level of elasticity, but undergoes little to no plastic deformation prior to breakage and monofilament nylon is relatively stiff. Overall, it has moderate handling characteristics and knot security with minimal tissue response. Multifilament nylon has improved handling characteristics, but increased capillarity. Although it is nonabsorbable, monofilament nylon loses 30% of its tensile strength after two years and braided nylon loses 75–100% of its tensile strength at 6 months.

Polypropylene

Polypropylene is a synthetic monofilament nonabsorbable suture material composed of stereoisomers of polypropylene (Tan et al. 2003). It has the greatest strength of the synthetic nonabsorbable sutures and has no appreciable loss of tensile strength after implantation (Tan et al. 2003); however, evaluation of polypropylene sutures over 2 and 5 year periods show some fragmentation (Postlethwait 1970, 1979). Polypropylene has a very smooth surface and has minimal tissue drag, but this property can also lead to slippage and poor knot security (Ratner et al. 1994). Other disadvantages are the handling properties and memory.

Stainless Steel

Stainless steel is an alloy of chromium, nickel, and molybdenum and is available as a monofilament or braided suture (Fossum 2002; Tan et al. 2003). It is biologically inert and has the greatest strength of all suture materials. Stainless steel sutures are extremely stiff and tend to cut through tissues or cause necrosis when there is tissue movement over buried knots.

Barbed and Antibacterial-Coated Suture

Barbed sutures have been used for a variety of human surgical procedures. The suture barbs are arranged in order to prevent pull out and eliminate the need for a knot at the end of the suture line. There are a few studies in the veterinary literature regarding barbed sutures, but their use is not widespread.

Triclosan is a broad spectrum antibacterial agent that has been added to many suture materials. Triclosan-coated sutures inhibit growth of common skin flora and some methicillin-resistant strains of *Staphylococcus in vitro*. Triclosan-coated sutures are available for use in veterinary surgery; however, their efficacy in reducing surgical site infections is unclear and current studies have varying results (Rothenburger et al. 2002; Storch et al. 2004; Etter et al. 2013). Triclosan-coated sutures were studied in ball pythons and no difference was seen in inflammatory response or surgical site infections (McFadden et al. 2011).

In addition to triclosan, chlorhexidine-coated sutures are also available. Chlorhexidine diacetate is a biguanide antiseptic that exhibits a broad range of antimicrobial activity intended to inhibit the growth of Gram-negative and Gram-positive bacteria. Studies assessing the effectiveness of chlorhexidine are limited (Onesti et al. 2018), and at the time of this chapter preparation, no veterinary specific studies have been published.

Tissue Healing

In addition to understanding specific characteristics of available suture materials, it is important to understand tissue healing. Although tissues heal through the same basic phases of wound healing, there are significant differences in the healing times. This affects the amount of time the sutures are required to support the tissue during the healing process. Table 2.1 summarizes tissue healing times and suture absorption profiles.

Compared with other tissues, the bladder heals very quickly and regains normal tensile strength in 14–21 days (Cornell 2012). When choosing a suture material to use for bladder repair, Monocryl, Biosyn, Dexon, or Vicryl may be recommended based on the amount of time these suture materials retain sufficient tensile strength, thus allowing the bladder tissue to heal. Longer-lasting absorbable sutures such as Maxon or PDS are probably not appropriate for bladder surgery unless delayed healing is anticipated. Nonabsorbable sutures may promote calculus formation. Conversely, sutures that are absorbed very rapidly (e.g. Caprosyn, Vicryl Rapide) probably do not retain sufficient tensile strength long enough and may increase the risk of dehiscence.

The gastrointestinal tract also heals at a relatively rapid rate, with the strength of the repair site approximating the original tissue strength in 10–17 days for the small intestine and up to 30 days for the large intestine (Durdey and Bucknall 1984; Hedlund 2002). The maturation phase in gastrointestinal tract healing occurs between 10 and 180 days after surgery. Polydioxanone, Monocryl, Biosyn, or Maxon provide sufficient tissue support for the gastrointestinal tract to allow for adequate healing.

Healing time for fascia is longer than for the gastrointestinal tract or urinary tract; therefore, fascia requires prolonged tissue support. Twenty days after surgery, the body wall has only regained 20% of its original tensile strength (Cornell 2012). Because fascia has a slower healing time, suture materials that will provide longer support of the tissues (e.g. PDS, Maxon) are recommended. Tissues such as tendons can take six weeks to a year to completely heal and require long-term support with orthopedic implants or external coaptation in addition to sutures (Montgomery and Fitch 2003). When repairing tissues that take an extended period of time to heal, longer-lasting sutures such as PDS or Maxon, or nonabsorbable sutures like Prolene or nylon should be used.

In many cases, tissue-healing times were determined using animal models to assess healing in mammalian tissues. Studies have shown differences in healing times between mammalian species (Cornell 2012), and these will

Table 2.1 Percentage of retained tensile strength following implantation and number of days required for complete absorption for commonly available suture materials.

Suture material	7 d	14 d	21 d	28 d	42 d	Complete absorption (d)
Chromic gut				0		60–90
Polydioxanone (PDS)		70		50	25	180–210
Polyglyconate (Maxon)	80	75	65	50	25	180
Glycomer 631 (Biosyn)		75	40			90–110
Polyglecaprone 25 (Monocryl)	60–70	30–40				90–120
Polyglycolic acid (Dexon)		20				60
Polyglactin 910 (Vicryl)		75	50	25		56–70
Lactomer (Polysorb)		80	30			56–70
Polyglytone 6211 (Caprosyn)	50–60	20–30	0			56
Polyglactin 910 (Vicryl Rapide)	50	0				42
Oral mucosa	X----X					
Skin	X------------X					
Subcutaneous tissue	X------------X					
Bladder	X-----------X					
Gastrointestinal tract	X----------X (SI)					
	X----------------------------------X (LI)					
Fascia	X--X					

Ranges in healing times are shown for different tissues. SI, small intestine; LI, large intestine.

vary significantly from reptile or amphibian tissues. The healing times presented here are to demonstrate the relationship between loss of tensile strength, time to complete absorption, and tissue healing. Veterinarians must consider the specifics of the species and tissues they are operating on to determine the best suture choice.

Sutures in Exotic Animals

Rodents

Due to extensive use of rodents in research, suture reaction in rodents has been studied extensively with studies evaluating many suture types in specific applications. Rats have been used extensively to compare suture materials in the body wall, subcutaneous tissues, skin, urogenital tract, gastrointestinal tract, and oral cavity.

Several studies have compared suture materials in the body wall, subcutaneous tissues, and skin using rodent models. A study evaluating polyglyconate, polyglactin 910, chromic gut, and polydioxanone in the body wall of rats showed that polyglyconate and polydioxanone caused significantly less inflammation 28 days following implantation (Sanz et al. 1988). When polyglytone 6211 was compared to poliglecaprone 25 in the body wall of rats, there was no significant difference in the inflammatory response 2 or 10 days following implantation (van Heerden 2005). Comparison of poliglecaprone 25, polyglactin 910, and polytetrafluoroethylene (Teflon) in subcutaneous tissues showed that poliglecaprone 25 caused significantly less inflammation 48 hours after implantation and polytetra-fluoroethylene sutures caused significantly more inflammation and fibrosis 7, 14, and 21 days following implantation (Nary-Filho et al. 2002). A study comparing polyglactin 910, catgut, silk, and polypropylene in the skin showed that polyglactin 910 caused significantly less inflammation over a period of 7 days (Yaltirik et al. 2003). Comparison of polydioxanone, poliglecaprone 25, and Glycomer 631 in rat skin showed that poliglecaprone 25 and Glycomer 631 were less reactive than polydioxanone, but all three were acceptable due to extremely low reaction scores (Molea et al. 2000). When polyglytone 6211 was compared to chromic gut for skin closure in rats, polyglytone 6211 had significantly less tissue drag and less potentiation for infection when surgical wounds were inoculated with *Staphylococcus aureus* (Pineros-Fernandez et al. 2004).

Several studies have been performed comparing suture materials in the urogenital tracts of rats with the aim to evaluate inflammation, fibrosis, and adhesion formation. A comparison of polyglactin 910 and polyglycolic acid in uterine tissue showed that there was significantly less inflammation

and fibrosis with polyglactin 910 90 days following implantation (Riddick et al. 1977). Another study evaluating suture material in uterine tissues compared polyglycolic acid, polyglactin 910, polydioxanone, silk, and polypropylene. The results showed that polydioxanone caused the lowest reaction scores and polypropylene lead to the highest rate of granuloma formation (Quesada et al. 1995). Evaluation of inflammatory reactions to polypropylene, polyglactin 910, and catgut and their role in adhesion formation showed that polypropylene had the lowest inflammatory score followed by polyglactin 910 and catgut, but no correlation to adhesion formation was found (Bakkum et al. 1995).

Suture reaction in bladder tissue has been evaluated to determine differences in inflammation and calculogenic potential. An early study showed that there was no difference in calcification around polyglycolic acid or chromic gut sutures in sterile or infected rat urine. The presence of infection did decrease the time that the suture remained within the bladder wall (Millroy 1976). When polydioxanone, polyglactin 910, and chromic gut were compared in bladder tissue, polydioxanone had the greatest initial inflammatory response, but there was no difference among groups at later time points. There was no difference in calculogenic potential between suture types over a 6 months period (Stewart et al. 1990). A similar study compared polydioxanone, polyglactin 910, and chromic gut and found that inflammation and stone formation were greater for chromic gut and polyglactin 910 compared to polydioxanone (Kosan et al. 2008).

Studies comparing suture materials in the gastrointestinal tract have also been performed. Using polyglycolic acid and catgut was compared in rat colonic anastomoses and found no difference in the degree of inflammation or strength of the anastomotic site (Munday and McGinn 1976). Another study comparing polyglactin 910 and polydioxanone in colonic anastomoses did not show any significant differences despite the belief that the multifilament nature of the polyglactin 910 in contaminated tissue could lead to more inflammation or abscess formation (Andersen et al. 1989). A third study evaluated polyglycolic acid, silk, polyglactin 910, chromic gut, polypropylene, and polydioxanone in wounds inoculated with bacteria commonly found in the colon. This study determined that monofilament absorbable sutures, with the exception of polydioxanone, lose strength too quickly and are not recommended for colonic surgery. In addition, braided materials led to prolonged inflammation and harbored bacteria (Durdey and Bucknall 1984).

Rabbits

Like rats, rabbits have been used as a model to evaluate biomaterials and techniques for use in human surgery. Several studies comparing suture materials in the rabbit urogenital tract have been performed. Comparison of polyglactin 910, polyethylene, and nylon in rabbit uteri showed that polyglactin 910 had a lower inflammation score at 24 days, and 80% of samples were absorbed by 80 days with little residual inflammation. The nonabsorbable sutures were present at 80 days and caused a persistent inflammatory response (Gomel et al. 1980). A similar study comparing polyglactin 910, polyglycolic acid, polypropylene, nylon, and chromic gut in rabbit uterine tissue found that polyglactin 910 had the lowest short-term (16 days) and long-term (42 days) tissue reaction. Like other studies, the nonabsorbable sutures remained in the tissues and caused a persistent inflammatory response (Beauchamp et al. 1988). Another study showed that there was no difference in histologic reaction or pregnancy rates between polyglactin 910 and polypropylene in microsurgical anastomoses in rabbit oviducts (Scheidel et al. 1986). Comparison of chromic gut, polyglactin 910, polydioxanone, and polyglyconate in rabbit pyeloureterotomies show that chromic gut caused the most severe inflammatory reaction. The reactions of the synthetic absorbable sutures were similar, but there was persistence of suture in 50% and 100% of pyeloureterotomies closed with polydioxanone and polyglyconate 12 weeks following implantation (Wainstein et al. 1997).

A study comparing gut, chromic gut, polyglactin 910, and polypropylene in rabbit bladder tissue found that the gut and chromic gut had the highest inflammation scores followed by polyglactin 910 and polypropylene. Fifteen weeks following implantation, the gut sutures and polyglactin 910 were almost completely absorbed with little residual inflammation compared to polypropylene (Hanke et al. 1994). Another study evaluating suture material in rabbit bladders compared chromic gut, polydioxanone, and polypropylene. Bladders were evaluated for calculi at 15, 30, 60, and 90 days and calculi formed on all sutures. The persistence of the calculi was dependent on the longevity of the suture material (Morris et al. 1986).

The studies performed in rodents and rabbits show that in most cases, chromic gut is more reactive than synthetic absorbable sutures. Nonabsorbable suture materials tend to cause chronic inflammatory responses where absorbable suture materials leave little residual inflammation after they are broken down. These studies and others on domestic species demonstrate the importance of choosing suture material that will retain tensile strength only long enough for the tissues to heal. Any suture that remains after the tissue has healed can lead to granulomas, calculi, or possibly malignant transformation of the tissues.

Ferrets

A single case report exists pertaining to suture material use in ferrets (Petterino et al. 2010). An intraabdominal malignant mesenchymoma was removed from a 6 year old spayed female ferret. The mass originated at the area of the previous ovariectomy performed five years previously. Histopathologic examination showed a mixed population of neoplastic cells, and nonabsorbable suture material was admixed with the neoplastic tissue. A chronic inflammatory reaction to the suture may have played a role in tumor development. Unfortunately, the type of suture implanted was not determined.

Birds

Despite their popularity and the increasing frequency for which veterinary care is pursued (Shepherd 2008), only a single study exists evaluating suture materials in birds. In this study, histologic reaction to five suture materials (chromic gut, polydioxanone, polyglactin 910, monofilament nylon, and stainless steel) was evaluated in the body wall of rock doves (*Columba livia*) over a period of 120 days (Bennett et al. 1997). Polyglactin 910 caused an early and intense inflammatory response and had higher inflammation scores than all other suture types. Chromic gut also caused an early and sustained inflammatory response. Initially, polydioxanone caused minimal reaction, but there was an increase in inflammation between 60 and 90 days. Steel and monofilament nylon stimulated minimal inflammatory reaction, but lead to hematomas, seromas, and caseogranulomas. Based on this study, polydioxanone is the optimal suture for closing the body wall due to the minimal inflammatory response and lack of complications seen with stiff nonabsorbable sutures. Interestingly, the lead author of that study prefers polyglactin 910 for skin closure in birds because the soft suture is less irritating (R. Avery Bennett, personal communication).

Reptiles and Amphibians

A few studies have evaluated sutures in reptiles and a single study evaluated suture materials in amphibians (Tuttle et al. 2006). Five suture materials (silk, monofilament nylon, polydioxanone, polyglactin 910, and chromic gut) were evaluated in African clawed frogs (*Xenopus laevis*) to determine which suture material elicited the fewest inflammatory changes in amphibian skin over 14 days. All sutures caused significantly more inflammation than a stab incision that was left to heal by second intention. Chromic gut and silk caused significantly more inflammation than all other sutures and 67% of incisions closed with silk sutures dehisced. Polydioxanone and polyglactin 910 caused significantly more inflammation than monofilament nylon. There were no significant differences in scores between 7 and 14 days. Based on these results, chromic gut and silk are not recommended and monofilament nylon may be the most appropriate suture in amphibian skin.

Using absorbable suture may result in premature suture material dissolution and wound dehiscence in aquatic amphibians (Baitchman and Herman 2015). Alternatively, cyanoacrylate tissue adhesive has been used for skin closure both in terrestrial and aquatic amphibians because it is waterproof. Studies are needed to compare cutaneous healing following suture or cyanoacrylate tissue adhesive application in amphibians. The use of polydioxanone has been reported anecdotally for amphibian internal organs (Green 2010; Norton et al. 2014).

Early studies on wound healing in reptiles compared sutured and unsutured wounds in garter snakes (Smith et al. 1988). Paired 1 cm incisions were either sutured with 5-0 polypropylene or left to heal by second intention. They showed that unsutured wounds had significantly less disruption of scale pattern and overlap of wound margins, and less-intense inflammatory infiltrates.

Four different suture materials (chromic gut, polyglyconate, polyglactin 910, and poliglecaprone 25) were evaluated histologically 7 days following laparoscopic sex determination (Govett et al. 2004). Results indicate that poliglecaprone 25 and polyglyconate caused the least tissue reaction of the four suture types examined. These synthetic monofilament absorbable suture materials caused significantly less crust formation and panniculus inflammation than chromic gut and polyglactin 910.

A study evaluated eight suture materials (polydioxanone, polydioxanone/triclosan, poliglecaprone 25, poliglecaprone 25/triclosan, polyglactin 910, chromic gut, monofilament nylon, and surgical steel) and cyanoacrylate tissue adhesive in hatchling ball pythons over a period of 90 days (McFadden et al. 2011). Samples were evaluated histologically at 3, 7, 14, 30, 60, and 90 days following implantation. Over all time points, all suture types caused significantly more inflammation compared to the negative control. Cyanoacrylate tissue adhesive did not cause significantly more inflammation than the negative control at any time point suggesting that small superficial skin incisions or lacerations can be closed with cyanoacrylate tissue adhesive. All suture materials caused chronic inflammatory responses that were significantly higher than the negative control 90 days following suture implantation. No sutures were completely absorbed by the end of the study period suggesting that absorption times are prolonged compared to mammals. Despite previous reports that reptiles are

unable to breakdown chromic gut (Jacobson et al. 1985; Bennett 1989), there was histologic evidence of fragmentation of these sutures. Interestingly, there was also evidence that prolonged absorption may lead to suture extrusion prior to complete absorption.

Based on these studies, monofilament synthetic rapidly absorbed suture material such as poliglecaprone 25 should be used in reptiles. Unfortunately, glycomer 631 and polyglytone 6211 have not been compared to poliglecaprone 25 in reptiles.

Fish

Of all exotic species commonly kept as pets, fish represent the largest group with over 75 million fish kept in nearly 8% of US households (Shepherd 2008). Despite their popularity, veterinarians play a limited role in health care, and few studies exist examining tissue reaction to suture materials in fish (Gilliland 1994; Hurty et al. 2002; Deters et al. 2009).

A single study evaluated the histopathological reaction to different suture materials (Hurty et al. 2002). Five different suture materials (silk, monofilament nylon, polyglyconate, polyglactin 910, and chromic gut) were placed in the skin and body wall of koi (*Cyprinus carpio*). Biopsies of the sutured tissues were taken 7 and 14 days following implantation and evaluated for inflammation. Silk caused an inflammatory response that increased from 7 to 14 days and was the suture with the highest inflammation score at 14 days. The synthetic sutures induced a moderate inflammatory response at 7 days with a decrease in inflammation at 14 days. Polyglactin 910 caused a higher inflammation score at 7 days compared to polyglyconate. Monofilament nylon produced a moderate, sustained inflammatory response over the study period. Chromic gut produced a significant inflammatory response at 7 days and all sutures had been extruded out by 14 days.

Other studies evaluating suture material in fish used gross inflammation and suture retention to evaluate suture materials (Gilliland 1994; Deters et al. 2009). Healing response and suture absorption using four suture materials (gut, chromic gut, polyglactin 910, and polydioxanone) were evaluated in largemouth bass for 8 weeks following surgery to obtain liver biopsies (Gilliland 1994). Gut sutures were completely absorbed at 5 weeks, and incisions were healed at 6 weeks. Polyglactin 910 sutures were completely absorbed by 7 weeks and incisions were healed by 8 weeks. All polydioxanone sutures were intact at the end of the evaluation period, and all incisions in this group were healed at 3 weeks.

Seven suture materials (monofilament nylon, poligle-caprone 25, braided nylon, polyglactin 910, coated polyglactin 910 [Vicryl Rapide, Ethicon Inc., Cincinnati, OH], polyglactin 910/triclosan, and silk) were evaluated in Chinook salmon (*Oncorhynchus tshawytscha*) (Deters et al. 2009). Functional suture retention was assessed for all fish and was defined as suture that was present in the fish, remained knotted, and did not tear through the body wall of the fish. Poliglecaprone 25 exhibited greater suture retention than all other suture types and braided nylon had significantly lower retention than all other suture types at 7 days following implantation. Monofilament sutures had better retention than all braided sutures at 14 days. Inflammation scores were lower for monofilament nylon, braided nylon, and poliglecaprone 25 than all other suture types at 7 and 14 days following implantation.

In Siberian sturgeon (*Acipenser baerii*), antibacterial poliglecaprone 25, poliglecaprone 25, polyglactin 910, and polypropylene were evaluated for celiotomy closure (Boone et al. 2010). Polypropylene exhibited expected retention, but polyglactin 910 also exhibited suture retention up to 12 weeks. Polyglactin 910 caused higher rates of suture loss and dehiscence throughout the initial eight weeks. It was concluded that antibacterial poliglecaprone 25 or poliglecaprone 25 appear more appropriate for celiotomy closure in Siberian sturgeon.

Based on these studies, synthetic monofilament absorbable sutures appear to be the optimal suture material in fish. Unfortunately, there were no direct comparisons made between polyglyconate, polydioxanone, and poliglecaprone 25 in each study to determine which is best suited in teleost fish.

Three different suture patterns (simple interrupted, interrupted horizontal mattress, and subcuticular) were used to close full thickness coelomic incisions (skin and body wall) in goldfish (*Carassius auratus*) (Nematollahi et al. 2010). The interrupted horizontal mattress induced a moderately severe to severe inflammatory response and necrosis, but the subcuticular suture induced a very mild to mild inflammatory response. The simple interrupted suture induced a moderate to moderately severe inflammatory response. It was concluded that a subcuticular suture is the most appropriate to use in the closure of a full thickness body wall incision in goldfish.

Nylon suture has been recommended to close the shark coelomic cavity (Lloyd and Lloyd 2011).

Invertebrates

Anderson et al. (2010) examined five different suture materials in the skin of the sea hare (*Aplysia californica*). They found that braided silk produced the least amount of granuloma formation but aside from that, monofilament nylon, poliglecaprone, polydioxanone, and polyglactin 910 all had similar overall histology scores calculated on edema, inflammation, and granuloma formation.

A recent study described the tissue reactions in common earthworms (*Lumbricus terrestris*) to five different suture materials: chromic gut, monofilament nylon, polydioxanone, polyglactin 910, and silk. There was mild to moderate tissue reaction to all five suture materials and the results indicated polyglactin 910 was best with regards to tissue security and minimal reaction (Salgado et al. 2014).

While there would likely be few applications for the use of sutures in horseshoe crabs (*Limulus polyphemus*), one study found that polydioxanone produced the least amount of tissue reaction compared to nylon, poliglecaprone, polyglycolic 910, and silk (Krasner et al., unpublished data).

Conclusion

This chapter emphasizes the need to have an in depth understanding of available suture materials and knowledge of tissues and their healing times in order to select the best suture for each patient and procedure. Articles describing or comparing tissue reactions to suture can aid in selection, but these studies vary in the methods used to evaluate the reaction, time periods that reactions are evaluated, and types and numbers of sutures evaluated with no single standard for grading such evaluations (Sanz et al. 1988). To cause more confusion, similar studies may have varied or contradictory results. Some believe that these types of studies fail to evaluate acute reactions over the first 7–14 days when surgical trauma and inflammation from the surgical procedure nullifies the possible differences in reaction to the suture materials. In many cases (particularly when healing occurs quickly), long-term results are not clinically relevant (Smit et al. 1991). Further studies evaluating loss in tensile strength and time to complete absorption in exotics species (especially nonmammalian) and studies evaluating healing times of different tissues can help veterinarians determine the optimal suture.

Acknowledgments

The editors would like to thank the authors of the Invertebrate (Lewbart, G. A.) and Fish and Amphibian (Vergneau-Grosset, C. and Weber, S.) chapters for their contributions to this chapter.

References

Andersen, E., Sondenaa, K., and Holter, J. (1989). A comparative study of polydioxanone (PDS) and polyglactin 910 (Vicryl) in colonic anastomoses in rats. *International Journal of Colorectal Disease* 4: 251–254.

Anderson, E.T., Davis, A.S., Law, J.M. et al. (2010). Gross and histological evaluation of five suture materials in the skin and subcutaneous tissue of the California sea hare (*Aplysia californica*). *Journal of the American Association for Laboratory Animal Science* 49: 1–5.

Baitchman, E.J. and Herman, T.A. (2015). Caudata (Urodela). In: Fowler's Zoo and Wild Animal Medicine, vol. 8 (eds. R.E. Miller and M.E. Fowler), 13–20. St. Louis, MO: Elsevier Saunders.

Bakkum, E.A., Dalmeijer, R.A.J., Verdel, M.J.C. et al. (1995). Quantatative analysis of the inflammatory reaction surrounding sutures commonly used in operative procedures and the realation to post surgical adhesion formation. *Biomaterials* 16: 1283–1289.

Beauchamp, P.J., Guzick, D.S., Held, B. et al. (1988). Histologic response to microsuture materials. *Journal of Reproductive Medicine* 33: 615–623.

Bellenger, C. (1982). Sutures Part I: The purpose of sutures and available suture materials. *Compendium* 4: 507–515.

Bennett, R.A. (1989). Reptilian surgery part I: Basic principles. *Compendium* 11: 10–20.

Bennett, R.A., Yaeger, M.J., Trapp, A. et al. (1997). Histologic evaluation of the tissue reaction to five suture materials in the body wall of rock doves (*Columba livia*). *Journal of Avian Medicine and Surgery* 11: 175–182.

Bezwada, R.S., Jamiolkowski, D.D., Lee, I.Y. et al. (1995). Monocryl suture, a new ultra-pliableabsorbable monofilament suture. *Biomaterials* 16: 1141–1148.

Boone, S., Divers, S.J., and Hernandez, S.M. (2010). Evaluation of surgical techniques and internal sonic transmitter implantation in sturgeon (Acipenseridae). *Proceedings American Association of Zoo Veterinarians and American Association Wildlife Veterinarians Joint Conference*, pp. 199–200.

Boothe, H. (1998). Selecting suture materials for small animal surgery. *Compendium* 20: 155–163.

Cornell, K. (2012). Wound healing. In: Veterinary Surgery: Small Animal, 2e (eds. S.A. Johnston and K.M. Tobias), 125–134. St. Louis, MO: Eselvier.

De La Puerta, B., Parsons, K.J., Draper, E.R.C. et al. (2011). in vitro comparison of mechanical and degradation properties of equivalent absorbable suture materials from two different manufacturers. *Veterinary Surgery* 40: 223–227.

Deters, K., Brown, R., Carter, K. et al. (2009). Performance assessment of suture type, water temperature, and surgeon skill in juvenile chinook salmon surgically implanted with acoustic transmitters. *Transactions of the American Fisheries Society* 139: 888–899.

Durdey, P. and Bucknall, T.E. (1984). Assessment of sutures for use in colonic surgery: an experimental study. *Journal of the Royal Society of Medicine* 77: 472–477.

Etter, S.W., Ragetly, G.R., Bennett, R.A., and Schaeffer, D.J. (2013). Effect of using triclosan-impregnated suture for incisional closure on surgical site infection and inflammation following tibial plateau leveling osteotomy in dogs. *Journal of the American Veterinary Medical Association* 242: 355–358.

Fossum, T.W. (2002). Biomaterials, suturing, and hemostasis. In: Small Animal Surgery, 2e (ed. T.W. Fossum), 43–59. St. Louis, MO: Mosby.

Gilliland, E. (1994). Comparison of absorbable sutures used in largemouth bass liver biopsy surgery. *The Progressive Fish Culturist* 56: 60–61.

Gomel, V., McComb, P., and Boer-Meisel, M. (1980). Histologic reactions to polyglactin 910, polyethylene, and nylon microsuture. *Journal of Reproductive Medicine* 25: 56–59.

Govett, P.D., Harms, C.A., Linder, K.E. et al. (2004). Effects of four different suture materials on the surgical wound healing of loggerhead sea turtles, *Caretta caretta*. *Journal of Herpetological Medicine and Surgery* 14: 6–10.

Green, S.L. (2010). The Laboratory Xenopus sp. Boca Raton, FL: CRC Press.

Hanke, P.R., Timm, P., Falk, G. et al. (1994). Behavior of different suture materials in the urinary bladder of the rabbit with special reference to wound healing, epithelization and crystallization. *Urologia Internationalis* 52: 26–33.

van Heerden, J. (2005). Comparison of inflammatory response to polyglytone 6211 and polyglecaprone 25 in a rat model. *South African Medical Journal* 95: 972–974.

Hurty, C.A., Brazik, D.C., Law, J.M. et al. (2002). Evaluation of the tissue reactions in the skin and body wall of koi (*Cyprinus carpio*) to five suture materials. *The Veterinary Record* 151: 324–328.

Jacobson, E.R., Millichamp, N.J., and Gaskin, J.M. (1985). Use of a polyvalent autogenous bacterin for treatment of mixed gram-negative bacterial osteomyelitis in a rhinoceros viper. *Journal of the American Veterinary Medical Association* 187: 1224–1225.

Kosan, M., Gonulalan, U., Ozturk, B. et al. (2008). Tissue reactions of suture materials (polyglactine 910, chromed catgut and polydioxanone) on rat bladder wall and their role in bladder stone formation. *Urological Research* 36: 43–49.

Lloyd, R. and Lloyd, C. (2011). Surgical removal of a gastric foreign body in a sand tiger shark, *Carcharias taurus* Rafinesque. *Journal of Fish Diseases* 34: 951–953.

MacPhail, C.M. (2019). Biomaterials, suturing, and hemostasis. In: Small Animal Surgery, 5e (ed. T.W. Fossum), 60–78. St. Louis, MO: Mosby.

Marturello, D.M., McFadden, M.S., Bennett, R.A. et al. (2014). Knot security and tensile strength of suture materials. *Veterinary Surgery* 43: 73–79.

McFadden, M., Bennett, R.A., Kinsel, M. et al. (2011). Evaluation of the histologic reactions to commonly used suture materials in the skin and musculature of ball pythons (*Python regius*). *American Journal of Veterinary Research* 72: 1397–1406.

Millroy, E. (1976). An experimental study of the calcification and absorption of polyglycolic acid and catgut sutures within the urinary tract. *Investigative Urology* 14: 141–142.

Molea, G., Schonauer, F., Bifulco, G. et al. (2000). Comparative study on biocompatibility and absorption times of three absorbable monofilament suture materials (ploydioxanone, poliglecaprone 25, and glycomer 631). *British Journal of Plastic Surgery* 53: 137–141.

Montgomery, R. and Fitch, R. (2003). Muscle and tendon disorders. In: Textbook of Small Animal Surgery, 3e (ed. D. Slatter), 2264–2271. Philadelphia, PA: W.B. Saunders.

Morris, M.C., Baquero, A., Redovan, E. et al. (1986). Urolithiasis on absorbable and nonabsorbable suture materials in the rabbit bladder. *Journal of Urology* 153: 602–603.

Munday, C. and McGinn, F.P. (1976). A comparison of polyglycolic acid and catgut sutures in rat colonic anastomoses. *British Journal of Surgery* 63: 870–872.

Nary-Filho, H., Matsumoto, M.A., Batista, A.C. et al. (2002). Comparative study of tissue response to polyglecaprone 25, polyglactin 910, and polytetrefuorethylene suture material in rats. *Brazilian Dental Journal* 13: 86–91.

Nematollahi, A., Bigham, A.S., Karimi, I., and Abbasi, F. (2010). Reactions of goldfish (*Carassius auratus*) to three suture patterns following full thickness skin incisions. *Research in Veterinary Science* 89: 451–454.

Norton, T.M., Andres, K., and Li, S. (2014). Techniques for working with wild reptiles. In: Current Therapy in Reptile Medicine and Surgery (eds. D. Mader and S. Divers), 310–340. St Louis, MO: Elsevier Saunders.

Onesti, M.G., Carella, S., and Scuderi, N. (2018). Effectiveness of antimicrobial-coated sutures for the prevention of surgical site infection: a review of the literature. *European Review for Medical and Pharmacological Sciences* 22: 5729–5739.

Petterino, C., Bedin, M., Vascellari, M. et al. (2010). An intra-abdominal malignant mesenchymoma associated with nonabsorbable sutures in a ferret (*Mustela putorius furo*). *Journal of Veterinary Diagnostic Investigation* 22: 327–331.

Pineros-Fernandez, A., Drake, D.B., Rodeheaver, P.A. et al. (2004). Caprosyn, another major advance in synthetic monofilament absorbable suture. *Journal of Long-Term Effects of Medical Implants* 14: 359–368.

Postlethwait, R.W. (1970). Long term comparative study of nonabsorbable suture. *Annals of Surgery* 171: 892.

Postlethwait, R.W. (1979). Five year study of tissue reaction to synthetic sutures. *Annals of Surgery* 190: 54–57.

Quesada, G., Diago, V., Redondo, L. et al. (1995). Histologic effects of different suture materials in microsurgical anastomosis of the rat uterine horn. *The Journal of Reproductive Medicine* 40: 579–584.

Ratner, D., Nelson, B., and Johnson, T. (1994). Basic suture materials and suturing techniques. *Seminars in Dermatology* 13: 20–26.

Riddick, D.H., De Grazia, C.T., and Maenza, R.M. (1977). Comparison of polyglactic and polyglycolic acid sutures in reproductive tissue. *Fertility and Sterility* 28: 1220–1225.

van Rijssel, E.J.C., Brand, R., Admiraal, C. et al. (1989). Tissue reaction and surgical knots: the effect of suture size, knot configuration, and knot volume. *Obstetrics and Gynecology* 74: 64–68.

Rothenburger, S., Spangler, D., Bhende, S. et al. (2002). *in vitro* evaluation of coated VICRYL™ plus antibacterial suture (coated ployglaction 910-with triclosan) using zone of inhibiton assays. *Surgical Infections (Larchmt)* 3 (Suppl. 1): S79–S87.

Roush, J.K. (2003). Biomaterials and surgical implants. In: Textbook of Small Animal Surgery, 3e (ed. D. Slatter), 141–148. Philadelphia, PA: W.B. Saunders.

Salgado, M.A., Lewbart, G.A., Christian, L.S. et al. (2014). Evaluation of five different suture materials in the skin of the earthworm (*Lumbricus terrestris*). *Springerplus* 3: 423. https://doi.org/10.1186/2193-1801-3-423.

Sanz, L.E., Patterson, J.A., Kamath, R. et al. (1988). Comparison of Maxon suture with Vicryl, chromic catgut, and PDS sutures in fascial closure in rats. *Obstetrics and Gynecology* 71: 418–422.

Scheidel, P.H., Wallwiener, D.R., Hollander, D. et al. (1986). Absorbable or nonabsorbable suture material for microsurgical tubal anastomosis: Randomized experimental study in rabbits. *Gynecolic and Obstetric Investigation* 21: 96–102.

Shepherd, A. (2008). Results of the 2007 AVMA survey of US pet-owning households regarding use of veterinary services and expenditures. *Journal of the American Veterinary Medical Association* 233: 727–728.

Smit, I.B., Witte, E., Brand, R. et al. (1991). Tissue reaction to suture materials revisited: Is there argument to change our views? *European Surgical Research* 23: 347–354.

Smith, D.A., Barker, I.K., and Allen, B. (1988). The effect of ambient temperature and type of wound on healing of cutaneous wounds in the common garter snake (*Thamnophis sirtalis*). *Canadian Journal of Veterinary Research* 52: 120–128.

Stewart, D.W., Buffington, P.J., and Wacksman, J. (1990). Suture material in bladder surgery: a comparison of polydioxanone, polyglactin, and chromic catgut. *Journal of Urology* 143: 1261–1263.

Storch, M.L., Rothernburger, S.J., and Jacinto, G. (2004). Experimental efficacy study of coated VICRYL plus antibacterial suture in guinea pigs challenged with *Staphylococcus aureus. Surgical Infections (Larchmt)* 5: 281–288.

Tan, R., Bell, R., Dowling, B. et al. (2003). Suture materials: composition and applications in veterinary wound repair. *Australian Veterinary Journal* 81: 140–145.

Tuttle, A.D., Law, J.M., Harms, C.A. et al. (2006). Evaluation of the gross and histologic reactions to five commonly used suture materials in the skin of the African clawed frog (*Xenopus laevis*). *Journal of the American Association for Laboratory Animal Science* 45: 22–26.

Wainstein, M., Anderson, J., and Elder, J.S. (1997). Comparison of effects of suture materials on wound healing in a rabbit pyeloplasty model. *Urology* 49: 261–264.

Yaltirik, M., Dedeoglu, K., Bilgic, B. et al. (2003). Comparison of four different suture materials in soft tissues of rats. *Oral Diseases* 9: 284–286.

3

Magnification Surgery

Heidi Phillips

Introduction

Surgery of exotic animals frequently involves small anatomic structures and the need for consistent and reliable exposure, illumination, precision, and clear focus while operating in a confined space. Using some form of magnification is recommended for most surgeries of small exotic animals (Beeber 2000; Bennett 2000b; Bennett and Lock 2000; Jenkins 2000b; Lock 2000; Mullen 2000; Mullen and Beeber 2000; Samour 2010). Technological advances in magnification surgery and refinement of microinstruments and microsuture enable the exotic animal surgeon to successfully perform technically demanding surgical procedures (Jarrett 2004; Bohan et al. 2010; Carr and Castellucci 2010). Magnification surgery enables visualization of detail and differences of anatomy, pathology, and tissue color and character not otherwise discernible (Jarrett 2004; Mungadi 2010; Al-Benna 2011; Stanbury and Elfar 2011). Small, bleeding vessels are more readily identified for coagulation, minimizing hemorrhage, and improving outcome for many procedures (Bennett 2000b; Mungadi 2010).

Optics and Principles of Magnification

Resolution is the ability of an optical system to discern detail in an object or distinguish two separate objects. The human eye is the limiting factor of many optical systems, its ocular resolution being 0.2 mm (Carr and Castellucci 2010). This means that people who observe two points closer together than 0.2 mm will see only one point.

Magnification of an image is increased most easily by decreasing the distance between the eye and the object being imaged. The resolution limit of the unaided eye can be increased by close proximity to objects (Chang 2013). This is not always achievable in surgery as decreasing the distance between the surgeon and patient may not permit safe, aseptic manipulation of instruments and tissues or an ergonomic,

comfortable, and sustainable posture for the surgeon (Bennett 2000a). Moreover, the healthiest human eye cannot refocus an image at distances closer than 10–12 cm (Carr and Castellucci 2010). Optical aids such as operating microscopes and surgical loupes can improve resolution by many orders of magnitude (Carr and Castellucci 2010). Optical aids permit safe magnification of tissues by increasing the size of the image of the object that is projected to the surgeon's retina.

Operating microscopes and commonly used surgical loupes achieve magnification using a two-lens system: the objective lens and eyepiece lens (Figure 3.1). The objective lens, which is nearest the object being imaged, focuses light rays from the object to generate a real, inverted image. The eyepiece lens transforms this image to the magnified, virtual image seen by the surgeon (Carr and Castellucci 2010; Cordero 2014). Total magnification of the system is the product of the magnification afforded by both the objective and eyepiece lenses (Carr and Castellucci 2010).

Although operating microscopes and surgical loupes utilize similar optical principles, they differ in how magnification is defined. The distance between the objective lens of operating microscopes and the objects to be operated is fixed, and all users achieve the same magnified image. The distance between the objective lens of a surgical loupe and object to be operated varies according to the surgeon's stature and posture; not all users achieve the same magnified image with the same loupe. As the working distance increases, the magnification power decreases. Loupe models are named according to magnification power, but specified magnification power can be achieved only at a specified distance. Users with longer working distances require higher-power loupes than users with shorter working distances to achieve the same level of magnification (Chang 2014a).

To effectively utilize optical aids in surgery, the exotic animal surgeon must understand the principles of magnification, including focal length, depth of focus, working distance, and field of view particular to the optical aid (Pieptu and Luchian 2003). A surgeon must properly

Surgery of Exotic Animals, First Edition. Edited by R. Avery Bennett and Geoffrey W. Pye.
© 2022 John Wiley & Sons, Inc. Published 2022 by John Wiley & Sons, Inc.

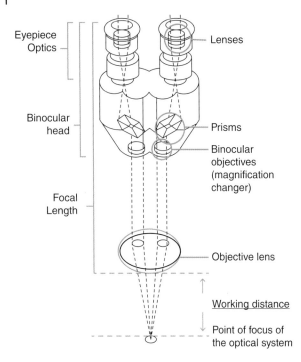

Figure 3.1 Optics of magnification aids that use a two-lens system. Note the focal length and working distance. *Source:* Pieptu and Luchian (2003) and Cordero (2014).

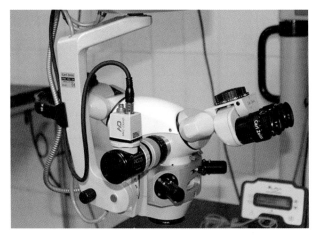

Figure 3.2 Binocular head–body of the operating microscope. Contains the eyepieces, lenses and prisms, and magnification changer.

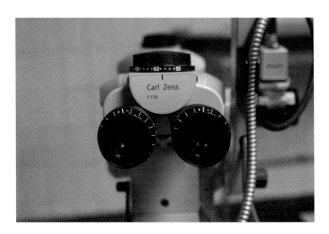

Figure 3.3 Eyepieces contribute to the total magnification of an operating microscope. Note the rubber cups and diopter settings adjustable to an individual surgeon.

manipulate the components of the optical system and surgical instruments ergonomically and in an ergonomic posture. (Carr and Castellucci 2010; Eivazi et al. 2015). The fundamental principles of optical magnification and components of the most commonly used optical systems are defined below:

Stereopsis: Perception of depth and three-dimensional structure obtained by processing visual information delivered through the eyepieces to the surgeon's eyes. Stereopsis is achieved using an operating microscope or surgical loupe by manipulation of the eyepieces to accommodate the surgeon's interpupillary distance and visual deficits, also termed stereoscopy (Carr and Castellucci 2010; Socea et al. 2015).

Binocular head: Body of an operating microscope. Contains the eyepieces, lenses and/or prisms, and magnification changer (Figure 3.2). The binocular head may be straight, inclined, or inclinable (Carr and Castellucci 2010). Inclinable binoculars are adjustable through a wide range of angles to allow the surgeon comfortable head and neck posture and working position.

Eyepieces: Eyepieces contain the binocular lenses and/or prisms necessary for magnification. Eyepieces of operating microscopes are available in powers of 10× and 12.5× most commonly and contribute to total magnification achieved by the optical aid (Carr and Castellucci 2010). Eyepieces have rubber cups adjustable in height to accommodate surgeons wearing corrective eyeglasses and have diopter settings adjustable for each surgeon's vision deficits (Figure 3.3).

Focal length: A measure of how strongly a lens converges or diverges light. The distance from the center of the lens to the area on the lens where light rays originating from a point on the focused object converge (Pieptu and Luchian 2003; Cordero 2014) (Figure 3.1).

Interpupillary distance: The distance between the centers of the surgeon's pupils. Eyepieces of an operating microscope or surgical loupe are adjustable or customized to accommodate the interpupillary distance of the individual surgeon (Carr and Castellucci 2010; Mungadi 2010) (Figure 3.4).

Focal depth (*depth of focus*): Range of object position through which the object may be viewed at a set magnification level and remain in focus (Pieptu and Luchian 2003).

Working distance: The distance from the objective lens to the object. Working distance is dependent on the focal length of the lenses and ranges from 22 to 50 cm (Pieptu and Luchian 2003; Carr and Castellucci 2010; Cordero 2014) (Figure 3.1).

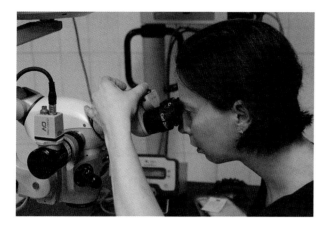

Figure 3.4 Eyepieces of an operating microscope are adjustable to accommodate the interpupillary distance of the individual surgeon.

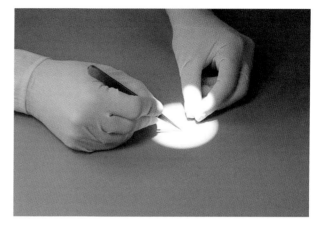

Figure 3.5 Field of view is the extent of the operating field seen in focus through the optical system. Here, the field of view is contained within the lighted circle as seen external to the microscope.

Field of view: Extent of the operating field seen in focus through the optical system (Figure 3.5). Field of view changes with magnification level according to the formula: field of view diameter = 200/total magnification factor (Pieptu and Luchian 2003). The diameter of the field of view is inversely proportional to the level of magnification; the higher the magnification, the smaller the field of view (Carr and Castellucci 2010). In exotic animal surgery, it is possible at times to fit the entire patient into the field of view (Bennett 2000a).

Magnification changer of operating microscopes: A system of lenses between the objective and eyepiece lenses that allows for changing magnification manually by 3–6 steps at a time or for continuous adjustment of magnification (power zoom) (Carr and Castellucci 2010; Cordero 2014).

Magnification changer of surgical loupes: Interchangeable working distance optics available with some loupes can increase magnification power for special procedures (Chang 2015).

The Operating Microscope

The surgical microscope is considered by many surgeons to be the gold standard of operative optical aids, a mandatory instrument for performing many technically demanding procedures and an indispensible teaching tool (McManamny 1983; Pieptu and Luchian 2003; Al-Benna 2011). A standard operating microscope is capable of magnifying an image from 6 to 40×, enabling many procedures that would otherwise be impossible to perform (Mungadi 2010; Stanbury and Elfar 2011). With the size amplification afforded by the microscope, visualization of tissue anatomy, pathology, color, and character is enhanced; suture and instrument placement is more precise; and small, bleeding vessels and other abnormalities are more readily appreciated (Bennett 2000b;

Mungadi 2010). Although the degree of precise manipulation and dexterity possible with magnification is far superior to that achieved with the unaided eye, performing accurate surgical maneuvers with extensive magnification requires practice (Carr and Castellucci 2010; Eivazi et al. 2015). Operating microscopes are expensive and can be cumbersome requiring intimate familiarity with their precision parts to permit proper and efficient use during surgery (McManamny 1983; Mungadi 2010).

The optical system of an operating microscope consists of a binocular head containing the eyepieces, lenses, prisms, and magnification changer; the objective lens; an illumination source; a suspension system; and a foot pedal or handpiece for controlling magnification, focus, and *x*–*y* position of the objective lens (Carr and Castellucci 2010; Cordero 2014). During surgery, a skilled surgeon must adjust the level of magnification frequently as tissues are manipulated and sutures are passed and tied (Eivazi et al. 2015). For this reason, the author prefers a foot pedal to a handpiece for manipulation of magnification and *x*–*y* settings (Figure 3.6). Using a foot pedal permits the surgeon to maintain a desired position with instruments in both hands without disrupting the flow of surgery (Carr and Castellucci 2010).

Preoperative Preparation of the Microscope and Operating Room

When planning a procedure using the operating microscope, preoperative preparation is essential. The surgeon must consider the interaction of numerous variables including the position and posture of the surgeon; positions of the patient, microscope, and instrument table; operating table and stool height; basic functions of the microscope and illumination system; and gross and fine focus of the microscope (Carr and Castellucci 2010; Socea et al. 2015).

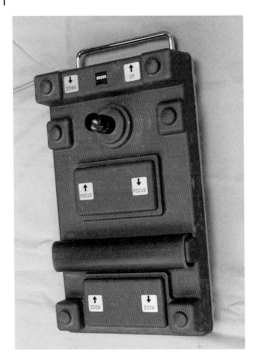

Figure 3.6 Operating microscope foot pedal displaying the joystick for adjustment in an *x−y* plane and buttons for adjustment of level of magnification (zoom) and focus.

In most operative procedures of exotic animals, the surgeon and assistant surgeon sit in a face-to-face configuration perpendicular to the long axis of the operating table and patient. Position the operating microscope such that the stand does not interfere with normal personnel flow and allows easy manipulation of its suspension arms in and out of the surgical field (Carr and Castellucci 2010). To begin, situate the stool and operating table height with the surgeon's feet flat on the floor, knees flexed below the hips, hips slightly extended, elbows flexed 90° to the shoulders, and elbows and antebrachii resting on the operating table (Valachi and Valachi 2003; Bohan et al. 2010; Carr and Castellucci 2010; Socea et al. 2015). In such a position, the surgeon's feet and seat create three points of contact with the floor, a very stable position that minimizes strain on the lower back during surgery (Figure 3.7). Also, resting the elbows and antebrachii on the surgical table minimizes physiologic tremor due to muscle fatigue (Figure 3.8). Next, adjust the inclinable binocular head up or down to permit the eyepieces to meet the surgeon's eyes while the surgeon maintains an erect posture with minimal slouching.

Once the table and stool height and surgeon's posture have been properly adjusted, the microscope must be

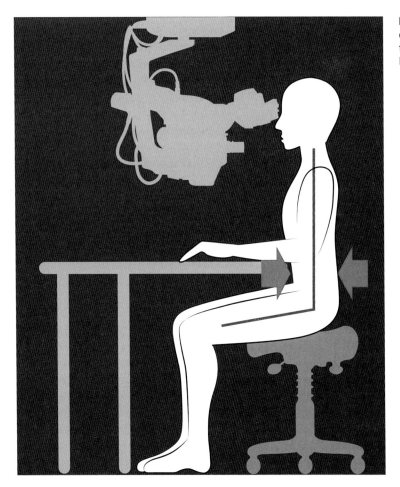

Figure 3.7 The surgeon should sit at the operating table with hips slightly extended and feet flat on the floor with the knees flexed slightly below the hips.

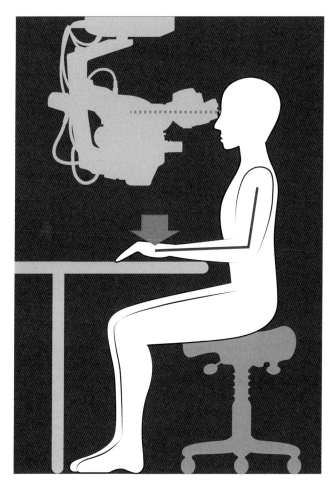

Figure 3.8 Resting the elbows and antebrachii on the surgical table at 90° to the shoulders minimizes physiologic tremor due to muscle fatigue.

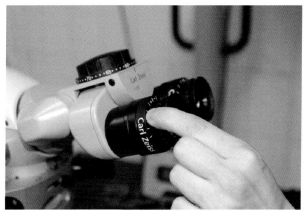

Figure 3.9 Adjust the diopter settings for each eye, one eye at a time, to ensure that both eyes see a clear image.

both eyes see a clear image (Carr and Castellucci 2010) (Figure 3.9). Surgeons with perfect vision or those wearing corrective lenses should maintain the eyepiece diopter settings at "0." Finally, the assistant surgeon should adjust the diopter settings on the assistant binocular. Following these manipulations, the scope should be returned to the lowest magnification level (zoomed all the way out) and should remain in focus throughout all levels of magnification. The microscope is now par focaled and ready for surgery (Carr and Castellucci 2010; Socea et al. 2015).

Surgical Loupes

Operating loupes are magnifying lenses worn by a surgeon to enhance visualization during surgery. Commercially available surgical loupes provide magnification of an image 2.5–8× the size seen by the unaided surgeon's eye (Ross et al. 2003; Carr and Castellucci 2010; Stanbury and Elfar 2011). Shortening the working distance increases magnification. Loupes are classified according to the optical system by which they provide magnification (Carr and Castellucci 2010).

Simple loupes are analogous to reading glasses and used by jewelers evaluating gems and by hobbyists. One pair of positive meniscus lenses comprises the optical system of simple loupes (Stanbury and Elfar 2011). Although inexpensive, the poor quality of the image produced by simple loupes precludes their use in exotic animal surgery. Additionally, spherical aberrations and purple or green color-fringing along the margin of the image are serious disadvantages of this optical system (Carr and Castellucci 2010; Stanbury and Elfar 2011).

Compound loupes, also known as Galilean loupes, are the most commonly used loupes and composed of two pair of magnification lenses separated by a layer of air. Chromatic anomalies are not observed with this system, but spherical aberrations may be seen at magnification

focused (Socea et al. 2015). Adjustment of the microscope to maintain focus through all levels of magnification is termed "par focaling" of the microscope and *must* be performed prior to surgery. To par focal the scope, first adjust the eyepieces to accommodate the surgeon's individual interpupillary distance to achieve stereopsis. Next, be sure the microscope is set to the lowest level of magnification (zoomed all the way out) and the fine focus is set to midrange (Carr and Castellucci 2010). Manually move the binocular head and objective lens up or down to rest a distance from the patient equal to the working distance of the microscope (Carr and Castellucci 2010). For example, if the working distance of the microscope is 200 mm, the part of the objective lens closest to the patient should be positioned 200 mm (8 in.) from the area of the patient to be operated. Following this step, reassess the inclination of the binocular head to be certain it does not require readjustment. Next, turn the magnification level to the highest setting (zoomed all the way in) and adjust the fine focus until the image is most clear. At this time, the surgeon should adjust the diopter settings for each eye, one eye at a time, to ensure that levels greater than 2.5× (Carr and Castellucci 2010; Stanbury and Elfar 2011). Compound loupes are less expensive than prismatic loupes and are widely available from numerous medical optics vendors.

Prismatic loupes, also known as Kelperian loupes, provide image amplification using Schmidt prisms. These prisms fold and lengthen paths of light through the loupes, yielding improved magnification, expanded field of view, deeper depth of focus, and longer working distance than other optical systems (Carr and Castellucci 2010; Stanbury and Elfar 2011). Although prismatic loupes are traditionally very heavy and much more expensive than compound loupes, recent innovations have permitted the development of prismatic loupes that are lighter weight and more comfortable (Chang 2014b).

Choosing Surgical Loupes

When choosing surgical loupes, exotic animal surgeons should consider numerous factors; the quality of stereopsis, level of magnification, depth of field, working distance, fit and comfort, ergonomics, and cost (Pieptu and Luchian 2003; Hart and Hall 2007). Loupes differ by level of magnification provided, declination angle, type of fixation of the lenses, addition of a headlamp or video camera, and type of frame or headband. Compound loupes provide magnification from 2.5 to 3.5× and are available with frames for front-lens-mounted (FLM) or through-the-lens mounted (TTL) magnifying lenses or with an adjustable headband configuration (Pieptu and Luchian 2003; Chang 2014b). TTL loupes are configured with the magnifying lenses permanently mounted to the eyeglass lenses, customized to the exact interpupillary distance of the wearer (Figure 3.10). FLM loupes have the advantage of being repeatedly adjustable to the needs of different wearers and can be shared by several associates of a practice. FLM loupes can be adjusted by turning a dial to match the wearer's interpupillary distance and permit individualized stereopsis. Front-mounted lenses can be flipped out of the surgeon's line of sight to permit using magnification only when desired. This "flip-up" ability discourages loupes wearers from looking over the top of lenses and promotes good posture and surgical ergonomics.

Prismatic loupes provide magnification from 3.5 to 8× and are available with FLM or TTL frames. Although higher magnification levels often results in smaller fields of view, technological advances have permitted development of high magnification prismatic loupes with expanded fields of view (Chang 2014a).

Ergonomics and surgeon fatigue are important considerations when purchasing and wearing surgical loupes. Loupe customizations that greatly affect ergonomics include working distance and declination angle (Chang 2014a). Determining the best working distance and declination angle of surgical loupes requires custom measurements of the surgeon positioned for work in the operating arena. Studies in clinical ergonomics have identified a number of distance and angle measurements important in selection and building of customized and adjustable loupes (Chang 2014a). All measurements are taken from a lateral view of the surgeon and operating field. First, the *reference line* is the line connecting the tops of the surgeon's ears with the corners of the eyes. The *reference line angle* (RLA) is the angle between this line and the optical axis of the eyes or loupes. The *operating hand position* (OHP) is the most comfortable and balanced position of the hands when standing or sitting to operate on the patient (Chang 2014a). This position will vary greatly in veterinary surgery, but the most balanced and relaxed position of the hands should be used for measurement. The *body posture angle* (BPA) is the angle between the vertical axis and line of sight of the eyes or loupes to the OHP. When operating ergonomically, the *head tilt angle* (HTA) is the angle from the horizontal axis to the reference line and should be no greater than 20°. When the head is erect with the eyes looking forward, the HTA is zero (Chang 2014a). The BPA decreases as the HTA increases, but increases in HTA should be minimized to avoid neck and shoulder strain and long-term injury. The maximum and minimum rotation angles of the eyes should also be calculated. The rotation angle of the eyes is the angle between the reference line and the OHP. When the head is in an erect position, the rotation angle of the eyes will be greatest – the *maximum rotation angle*. When the head is tilted downward no more than the maximum amount of tilt without producing strain (HTA less than 20°), the rotation angle of the eyes will be least – the *minimum rotation angle*. The maximum rotation angle = 90° – BPA–RLA. The minimum rotation angle = 90° – BPA–RLA – HTA (Chang 2014a).

Once these values are known, the optimal declination angle for customized TTL loupes or adjustable FLM loupes can be determined. The optimal declination angle is *between* the minimum and maximum rotation angles of the eyes (Chang 2014a). The author prefers loupes with a large declination angle to minimize HTA. A loupe declination angle of 45° facilitates a small HTA of only 9–10° and an erect, ergonomic posture (Chang 2014a) (Figure 3.10).

Historically, wearing less optimized loupes with shorter working distances and smaller declination angles necessitated the surgeon adopt a larger HTA and slouching posture to maintain the operated tissue in focus. A shorter working distance also corresponded to a narrower field of view, and neck and back strain induced by slouching were detrimental to the surgeon. Recent innovations result in

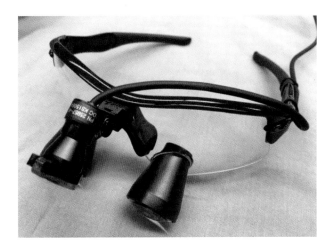

Figure 3.10 The author's through-the-lens (TTL) mounted loupes. Note the steep angle of declination and LED headlamp.

loupes with longer working distances (40–55 cm), wider fields of view, and lenses mounted at larger declination angles that permit the surgeon to adopt an erect posture and smaller HTA (<20°) (Chang 2014a).

First-time wearers of loupes should adopt several practices to facilitate and encourage proper and consistent use. Begin by wearing loupes for only 1–2 hours/day the first 1–2 weeks of use, using the loupes during simple procedures in the morning that do not require exhaustive concentration. Gradually work up to longer and more complex procedures performed over the entire day during the third to fourth and subsequent weeks of use. Always adopt an erect posture during surgery, drawing the shoulder blades medially and downward, and maintaining a small HTA (<20°). Do not bend the neck to look over the lenses, but diligently look through the magnification oculars when wearing loupes or flip the lenses of FLM loupes out of the line of sight when not in use.

Do not wear loupes on the tip of the nose as this decreases field of view. Conversely, do not wear loupes too close to the eyes as this permits fogging of the lenses. Practice using loupes at the measured working distance, bringing instruments and suture into the field of view slowly at first, and gradually introduce faster movements as dexterity improves. Proper use of surgical loupes and careful observation of ergonomic principles will optimize the practice of exotic animal surgery.

Comparing the Operating Microscope and Surgical Loupes

Whether the operating microscope or surgical loupe represents the optimal magnification aid for a particular type of surgery is often debated. To date, the choice seems to be one of surgeon preference, as study findings conflict and both

pieces of equipment have advantages and disadvantages (McManamny 1983; Ross et al. 2003: Eivazi et al. 2015; Al-Benna 2011; Stanbury and Elfar 2011). The operating microscope offers greater magnification than surgical loupes, is considered the gold standard in microsurgery, and is a superior teaching tool (McManamny 1983; Pieptu and Luchian 2003; Al-Benna 2011). However, loupe magnification has been found to achieve comparable clinical outcomes, and in some studies, resulted in shorter operative times (Ross et al. 2003; Jarrett 2004; Al-Benna 2011). Some propose of the operating microscope always be chosen by less-experienced microsurgeons and when operating tubular structures less than 3–4 mm in diameter (Pieptu and Luchian 2003; Ross et al. 2003; Jarrett 2004; Al-Benna 2011; Stanbury and Elfar 2011). Others suggest that so-called "macro-microsurgical procedures," those involving structures >1.5 mm in diameter, may be safely performed with loupes (Pieptu and Luchian 2003; Mungadi 2010; Stanbury and Elfar 2011). Although the operating microscope can be moved through six degrees of freedom, loupes offer the convenience of being able to change field of view simply by turning one's head (Ross et al. 2003; Stanbury and Elfar 2011; Eivazi et al. 2015). The operating microscope offers the advantage of being able to change level of magnification from low to high and high to low, a maneuver often necessary when passing the needle and tying sutures (Eivazi et al. 2015). While surgical loupes allow the surgeon and assistant surgeon to view the surgery from individual and rapidly dynamic vantage points, the operating microscope requires the surgeon and assistant to view the surgery from relatively fixed positions (Ross et al. 2003; Jarrett 2004). Whereas the operating microscope should be moved only short distances and with great caution to avoid damaging the intricate lenses and prisms within, loupes offer the advantage of portability (Jarrett 2004; Hart and Hall 2007; Stanbury and Elfar 2011). Some of the mobility issues associated with the operating microscope can be overcome by using a foot pedal programmed to permit movement of the scope in the x–y planes and by changing level of magnification and focus. Operating microscopes may offer superior illumination from halogen and xenon light sources, but the addition of LED coaxial headlamps to surgical loupes has greatly improved loupe illumination capabilities (Pieptu and Luchian 2003). Although the use of loupes has been reported to result in operator fatigue, discomfort, and limited fields of view due to inappropriate working distance, poor optics, and diminished depth of focus, technological advances in loupe magnification and use of carefully obtained measurements to guide customization of loupes have diminished the impact of these limitations (Ross et al. 2003; Jarrett 2004; Hart and Hall 2007; Chang 2014b). Loupes are also significantly less expensive than operating microscopes (Pieptu and Luchian 2003; Jarrett 2004; Stanbury and Elfar 2011).

Illumination

Properly adjusted and color-balanced illumination increases apparent resolution, enhancing the surgeon's ability to discern tissue color, depth, and dimension and more readily distinguish anatomic structures in the patient (Carr and Castellucci 2010). Standard overhead surgical lights, including LED lights, are often too far to provide adequate illumination of structures in small or deep body cavities of exotic animals. Both operating microscopes and surgical loupes are equipped with coaxial light sources that illuminate a path parallel to the line of sight and reduce the potential for shadows and other visual obstructions (Carr and Castellucci 2010; Cordero 2014). Both the xenon light source of an operating microscope and the LED lights of surgical loupes illuminate without the risk of added warmth and tissue desiccation (Carr and Castellucci 2010; Cordero 2014) (Figure 3.10).

Instrumentation

Fine, delicate instruments are of great utility when operating on small exotic animals. Such instruments are designed to exert minimal pressure while maintaining a firm hold on tissues. Microsurgical forceps and needle holders eliminate or discourage wide, erratic, or irregular movements when opening and closing the instrument. Observation of such movements is greatly exaggerated with magnification and damage to delicate tissues may be substantial.

Microsurgical Instrumentation

Along with basic instrumentation required for soft tissue procedures, exotic animal surgeons benefit from using a number of additional microsurgical instruments (Bennett 2000b; Hernandez-Divers 2008; Alworth et al. 2011; Capello 2011) (Figure 3.11). A fine-pointed, diamond-jawed needle holder, vascular forceps such as DeBakey forceps, curved and straight microsurgical dissecting scissors, adventitia scissors and small Metzenbaum scissors, atraumatic vascular clamps, and a right-angled dissecting forceps such as a small, blunt-tipped mixter are recommended.

Many microsurgical instruments are manufactured with ergonomic qualities that offer advantages in delicate procedures (Bennett 2000b; Hart and Hall 2007). Nearly all instruments are manufactured in a variety of lengths to accommodate a range of hand sizes. Lengths of 4–6 in. are used most commonly. Detailed operations in small spaces

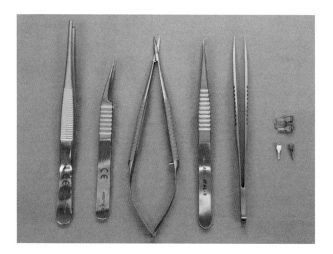

Figure 3.11 Small collection of microsurgical instruments. From right to left: microsurgical clamp applier, vessel dilator, straight microvascular scissor, curved jeweler's forceps, straight jeweler's forceps, and single and double Acland microvascular clamps mounted on a frame.

benefit from fine and smooth movements, and precise movements are most readily accomplished by rolling the instrument (Bennett 2000b). Choose needle holders and tissue forceps with rounded handles to permit rolling between the thumb and index finger. Another quality of microsurgical instruments that enables smooth and precise movements is *counterbalancing*. Counterbalanced instruments are notched and weighted at the nonoperative end to encourage stability of the instrument in the groove between the surgeon's thumb and index finger (Bennett 2000b) (Figure 3.12). Finally, choose microsurgical instruments without locking mechanisms. A needle holder that automatically locks or ratchets closed requires added exertion and excessive force to open. Such force may cause irreparable and unnecessary damage to tissues.

Castroviejo and Vannas needle holders maintain a precise and fine grip on tiny needles. The author prefers small, curved, or straight jeweler's forceps with 0.2–0.3 mm tips for use as needle holders, and frequently maintains a jeweler's forceps in each hand when suturing. One jeweler's forceps acts as a needle holder, and the other is used to manipulate tissue or suture ends when knot tying. A curved jeweler's forceps as a needle holder can be used to readily grasp a suture tag by lightly turning in any direction and is preferred by some microsurgeons. The author, however, prefers a straight jeweler's forceps with a tying platform as a needle holder and a fine jeweler's forceps or vessel dilator for tissue manipulation. A tying platform extends the grasping area of the forceps, and a vessel dilator has fine tips (0.1–0.2 mm) for grasping very thin or delicate tissue. Take care when using a vessel dilator as tissue

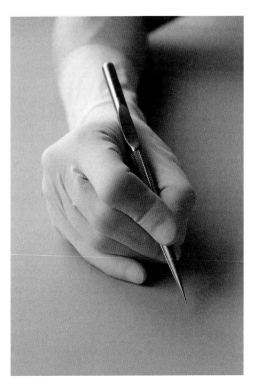

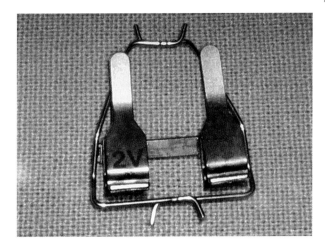

Figure 3.13 Double Acland microvascular clamps on an approximating frame. The frame facilitates sliding of the clamps closer together or further apart as needed to maintain approximation of vessel or intestinal ends. Note the U-shaped hooks at each end meant for tethering of stay sutures.

Figure 3.12 A stable hand position with fingers stacked on one another holding a round-handled, counterbalanced jeweler's forceps. Counterbalanced instruments are notched and weighted at the nonoperative end to encourage stability of the instrument in the groove between the surgeon's thumb and index finger.

forceps as the tips, though accurate, are thinner than the tips of jeweler's forceps and may cause trauma.

Atraumatic vascular clamps, such as Satinsky, Cooley, and Codman clamps, come in a variety of sizes and configurations, and pediatric sizes are available for vascular use in small exotic animals, as in adrenalectomy in ferrets. Acland-style microvascular approximating clamps are very helpful as atraumatic gastrointestinal clamps, serving as Doyen clamps would to prevent accidental spillage of ingesta during enterotomy and resection and anastomosis procedures (Jenkins 2000a). Acland microvascular clamps come in arterial and venous patterns and several sizes, designed to exert specific degrees of closing pressure on vessels in a range of sizes. The clamps exert a pressure of $5\,\text{g/mm}^2$ when used on the largest structure in the size range, and $15\,\text{g/mm}^2$ when used on the smallest structure in the recommended size range (Jenkins 2000a). The approximating frame facilitates sliding of the clamps closer together or further apart as needed to maintain approximation of vessel or intestinal ends. U-shaped hooks at each end of the approximating frame are meant for tethering of stay sutures that facilitate maintenance of tension on the anastomotic line, improving visualization, and suture placement (Figure 3.13).

Care and Handling of Instruments

Microsurgical instruments are highly refined to permit accurate and precise use, and are very fragile and prone to damage. Storage trays for microsurgical instruments are lined with rubber pads with finger-like projections that softly and securely grip instruments for safe placement and storage or are equipped with slots for each instrument. Storage trays are sterilizable. Be sure to return instruments to the protective pad of the storage tray even during surgery when they are not in immediate use. Use microsurgical instruments appropriately and as indicated and not for grasping or cutting thick or tough tissues, needles, or suture larger than 5-0 USP.

When cleaning instruments, pick up microsurgical instruments one at a time. Rinse instruments with distilled water or according to manufacturer's instructions, and gently remove organic debris with a microsurgical brush. Place instruments in a single layer in an ultrasonic cleaner with enzymatic detergent after each use. Never allow instruments to soak overnight in water or the ultrasonic cleaner. Always remove them promptly after the cycle is finished and allow them to air-dry on an absorbent drying pad in an open position to prevent rusting of the joints and box-lock mechanisms. Once the instruments are dry, carefully return them to the storage tray. Wrap the tray for steam sterilization in an autoclave. Most manufacturers do not recommend sterilization in a plasma sterilizer.

Assess instruments for damage before each use. Check with magnification to be certain the tips of needle holders and forceps and blades of scissors meet exactly. Never attempt to operate with a misshapen or damaged instrument. Return broken instruments to the manufacturer or to a service professional for repair or discard them. Use caution and care when using instruments as dropping a microsurgical instrument on its tip from a height as little as 2–3 cm can damage the instrument irrevocably and result in costly losses. Although microsurgical instruments can be expensive, proper care and use will ensure these instruments are an integral part of your exotic animal surgical equipment for many years.

Microsuture

The ideal suture for delicate surgery in small exotic animals should have excellent knot-holding capability and ease of handling, and should elicit a minimal inflammatory reaction (Phillips and Aronson 2012). Microsuture is swaged onto a 1/2 or 3/8 circle needle with a round taper-point or micropoint spatula-shaped needle tip. Surgical Specialties Corporation (Wyomissing, PA) uses specialized needle geometry in the manufacture of Sharppoint™ microsutures to flatten the middle ⅓ of the needle for secure grasping while maintaining a pointed microsurgical needle tip.

Sizes of suture for microsurgical procedures range from 4-0 to 11-0, progressing from less to more delicate work. Although monofilament sutures such as nylon, polypropylene, or polydioxanone are preferred for strength, durability, and inciting minimal inflammation, multifilament sutures have excellent knot-holding ability. When passed though bone wax, braided multifilament sutures have improved handling and less drag through tissues. Multifilament sutures should be used with caution in infected tissues as the braided configuration may provide a nidus for bacterial growth and proliferation (Phillips and Aronson 2012).

Principles of Microsurgical Techniques

Magnification surgery requires concentration, patience, and physical and mental endurance. To accurately and efficiently perform microsurgery, the surgeon must be properly prepared. Thorough preparation of the operating arena, magnification aids, instruments and suture as described in this chapter will help to ensure smooth flow of microsurgical operations and prevent physical and mental disruptions during a procedure. However, the surgeon should attend to his or her own physical and mental needs prior to a procedure.

Posture

Instructions and guidelines regarding the organization of the operating arena and customization and adjustment of magnification aids are offered elsewhere in this chapter. It is important to note here that maintaining ergonomic and appropriate posture is an extremely important principle of microsurgery that permits the performance of lengthy and difficult procedures with minimal fatigue and tremor.

Preparation and Mindset

Learning and mastering any new skill can be frustrating and test patience and resolve. The merits of developing microsurgical skills are numerous and efforts spent mastering magnification surgery are worthwhile.

Be certain to approach procedures and practice time well rested and free of any significant physical, mental, or emotional burden. Ensuring the operating arena is equipped; the surgical table and stools are properly adjusted; and the operating microscope or surgical loupes are properly functioning, ergonomic, and customized will help to limit physical burden during surgery. Avoid strenuous exercise, including isometric exercises and lifting heavy objects prior to performing or practicing microsurgical procedures. Strenuous exercise, especially of the forearms, brachial area, and shoulders, predisposes to exaggerated physiologic tremor. If possible, avoid alcoholic beverages and the excessive use of stimulants including nicotine and caffeine the day before a procedure. It is important to consider what the surgeon's normal intake of stimulants such as caffeine is and to limit intake to only the amount normally consumed – no more or less – as withdrawal from caffeine and other stimulants can also predispose to tremor.

To prevent mental burden, deal with telephone calls, messages, e-mails, and other correspondence prior to the procedure as much as possible, and assign personnel to limit interruptions in the operating arena to only those that are most emergent.

Hand Position

Proper hand position is critical to placement of microsutures and accurate use of microsurgical instruments in small spaces and helps to limit fatigue and tremor during procedures.

Hands should be placed properly relative to the surgeon's ideal OHP as discussed earlier. This position is relaxed and balanced during the operative procedure. The OHP may be used to adjust the table height and stool height when using an operating microscope and to determine the ideal working distance when using surgical loupes.

Hands should be positioned properly relative to the surgical table. The surgeon's elbows and forearms should rest on the surgical table at an approximate angle of 90° from the shoulders. This can prove difficult when the patient is placed on the table and a sterile drape is applied to the patient but is critical for ergonomics and endurance. Tremor can persist if the surgeon's hands remain elevated from the table. An elevated hand position induces contraction of

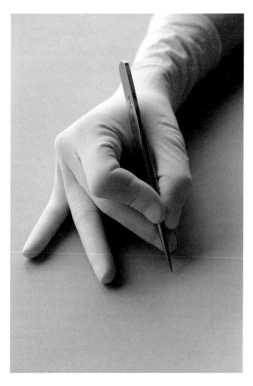

Figure 3.14 Alternate stable hand position with fingers splayed instead of stacked on one another.

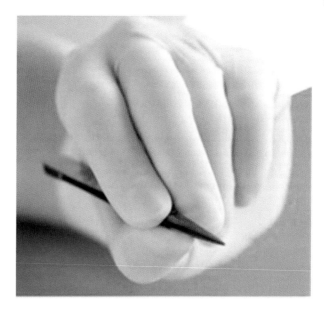

Figure 3.15 The surgeon's thumb and first two fingers should surround the instrument in a three-point pencil hold, and the thumb and each digit should touch each other.

antebrachial musculature and eventual muscle fatigue and tremor despite a resting antebrachial and elbow position. To achieve the greatest stability and reduction of tremor, the surgeon's wrists and fifth digits of each hand should also rest on the surgical table or patient, and the fingers should be stacked on top of each other or splayed (Figures 3.12 and 3.14). If it is not possible for the wrists and fifth digits to rest on the table or patient, sterilizable hand rests may permit resting the entire hand.

Lastly, hands should be positioned properly relative to the surgical instruments. When holding a microsurgical needle driver, forceps, or scissor, the surgeon's thumb and first two fingers should surround the instrument in a three-point pencil hold, and the thumb and each digit should touch each other (Figure 3.15). By touching each other, the thumb and digits serve to stabilize one another. The thumb and digits should grasp the instrument about 2–3 cm from the tip of the instrument. This allows enough instrument to protrude from the hold for the instrument to be seen sufficiently in the field of view and provides stability to the end of the instrument, reducing tremor while permitting extension into the small body cavity of a bird, reptile, or fish.

References

Al-Benna, S. (2011). The use of intraoperative magnification equipment by surgical residents. *European Journal of Plastic Surgery* **34**: 475–478.

Alworth, L.C., Hernandez, S.M., and Divers, S.J. (2011). Laboratory reptile surgery: principles and techniques. *Journal of the American Association of Laboratory Animal Science* **50**: 11–26.

Beeber, N.L. (2000). Abdominal surgery in ferrets. In: *Veterinary Clinics of North America Exotic Animal Practice: Soft Tissue Surgery*, vol. 3 (eds. R.A. Bennett and A.B. Rupley), 617–628. Philadelphia, PA: W.B. Saunders Company.

Bennett, R.A. (2000a). Nonreproductive surgery in reptiles. In: *Veterinary Clinics of North America Exotic Animal Practice: Soft Tissue Surgery*, vol. 3 (eds. R.A. Bennett and A.B. Rupley), 715–732. Philadelphia, PA: W.B. Saunders Company.

Bennett, R.A. (2000b). Preparation and equipment useful for surgery in small exotic pets. In: *Veterinary Clinics of North America Exotic Animal Practice: Soft Tissue Surgery*, vol. 3 (eds. R.A. Bennett and A.B. Rupley), 563–586. Philadelphia, PA: W.B. Saunders Company.

Bohan, M., McConnell, D.S., Chaparro, A. et al. (2010). The effects of visual magnification and physical movement scale on the manipulation of a tool with indirect vision. *Journal of Experimental Psychology: Applied* **16**: 33–44.

Capello, V. (2011). Common surgical procedures in pet rodents. *Journal of Exotic Pet Medicine* **20**: 294–307.

Carr, G.B. and Castellucci, A. (2010). The use of the operating microscope in endodontics. *Dental Clinics of North America* **54**: 191–214.

Chang, B.J. (2013). Are you using the right magnification loupes?. http://archive.constantcontact.com/fs113/1113715421610/archive/1116449819730.html (accessed September 2013).

Chang, B.J. (2014a). Declination angle as the key ergonomic factor - Key factors for ordering custom loupes: Part 1. http://archive.constantcontact.com/fs113/1113715421610/archive/1117208896207.html (April 2014).

Chang, B.J. (2014b). Key factors for ordering custom loupes: Part 2: Magnification power as the key vision factor. http://archive.constantcontact.com/fs113/1113715421610/archive/1117451356844.html (May 2014).

Chang, B.J. (2015). Demystifying magnification power of loupes: 7 questions and answers. http://archive.constantcontact.com/fs113/1113715421610/archive/1120530386901.html (May 2015).

Cordero, I. (2014). Understanding and caring for an operating microscope. *Community Eye Health Journal* **27**: 17.

Eivazi, S., Afkari, H., Bednarik, R. et al. (2015). Analysis of disruptive events and precarious situations caused by interaction with neurosurgical microscope. *Acta Neurochirurgica* **157**: 1147–1154.

Hart, R.G. and Hall, J. (2007). The value of loupe magnification: an underused tool in emergency medicine. *American Journal of Emergency Medicine* **25**: 704–707.

Hernandez-Divers, S.J. (2008). Clinical technique: dental endoscopy of rabbits and rodents. *Journal of Exotic Pet Medicine* **17**: 87–92.

Jarrett, P.M. (2004). Intraoperative magnification: who uses it? *Microsurgery* **24**: 420–422.

Jenkins, J.R. (2000a). Surgery of the avian reproductive and gastrointestinal systems. In: *Veterinary Clinics of North America Exotic Animal Practice: Soft Tissue Surgery*, vol. 3 (eds. R.A. Bennett and A.B. Rupley), 673–692. Philadelphia, PA: W.B. Saunders Company.

Jenkins, J.R. (2000b). Surgical sterilization in small mammals. In: *Veterinary Clinics of North America Exotic Animal Practice: Soft Tissue Surgery*, vol. 3 (eds. R.A. Bennett and A.B. Rupley), 617–628. Philadelphia, PA: W.B. Saunders Company.

Lock, B.A. (2000). Reproductive surgery in reptiles. In: *Veterinary Clinics of North America Exotic Animal Practice: Soft Tissue Surgery*, vol. 3 (eds. R.A. Bennett and A.B. Rupley), 733–752. Philadelphia, PA: W.B. Saunders Company.

McManamny, D.S. (1983). Comparison of microscope and loupe magnification: assistance for the repair of median and ulnar nerves. *British Journal of Plastic Surgery* **36**: 367–372.

Mullen, H.S. (2000). Nonreproductive surgery in small mammals. In: *Veterinary Clinics of North America Exotic Animal Practice: Soft Tissue Surgery*, vol. 3 (eds. R.A. Bennett and A.B. Rupley), 629–646. Philadelphia, PA: W.B. Saunders Company.

Mullen, H.S. and Beeber, N.L. (2000). Miscellaneous surgeries in ferrets. In: *Veterinary Clinics of North America Exotic Animal Practice: Soft Tissue Surgery*, vol. 3 (eds. R.A. Bennett and A.B. Rupley), 663–672. Philadelphia, PA: W.B. Saunders Company.

Mungadi, I.A. (2010). Refinement on surgical technique: role of magnification. *Journal of Surgical Technique and Case Report* **2**: 1–2.

Phillips, H. and Aronson, L.R. (2012). Vascular surgery. In: *Veterinary Surgery Small Animal* (eds. K.M. Tobias and S.A. Johnston), 1854–1869. St. Louis, MO: Elsevier-Saunders.

Pieptu, D. and Luchian, S. (2003). Loupes-only microsurgery. *Microsurgery* **23**: 181–188.

Ross, D.A., Ariyan, S., Restifo, R. et al. (2003). Use of the operating microscope and loupes for head and neck microvascular tissue transfer. *Archives of Otolaryngology – Head & Neck Surgery* **129**: 189–193.

Samour, J. (2010). Vasectomy in birds: a review. *Journal of Avian Medicine and Surgery* **24**: 169–173.

Socea, S.D., Barak, Y., and Blumenthal, E.Z. (2015). Focusing the surgical microscope. *Survey of Ophthalmology* **60**: 373–377.

Stanbury, S.J. and Elfar, J. (2011). The use of surgical loupes in microsurgery. *The Journal of Hand Surgery* **36**: 154–156.

Valachi, B. and Valachi, K. (2003). Preventing musculoskeletal disorders in clinical dentistry: strategies to address the mechanisms leading to musculoskeletal disorders. *Journal of the American Dental Association* **134**: 1604–1612.

4

Invertebrate Surgery
Gregory A. Lewbart

Introduction

Invertebrates are a collection of animals unified by the lack of a vertebral column. While invertebrate animals comprise greater than 95% of the animal kingdom's species well over 95% of the literature pertaining to surgery deals with vertebrates.

This chapter covers the current state of surgery on the most prominent invertebrate groups (sponges, coelenterates, mollusks, crustaceans, insects, horseshoe crabs, spiders, echinoderms, and urochordates). Since various taxa are largely unrelated and possess specialized anatomic and physiologic features, each taxon is handled separately and specific procedures reviewed and addressed accordingly.

For reviews of anesthesia and analgesia please refer to Braun et al. (2006), Dombrowski and De Voe (2007), Cooper (2011), Andrews et al. (2013), Gunkel and Lewbart (2008), Mosley and Lewbart (2014), Fregin and Bickmeyer (2016), Butler-Struben et al. (2018), and Archibald et al. (2019).

Porifera (Sponges)

The phylum Porifera is a diverse group of primitive animals commonly referred to as sponges. Until the early 1800s, sponges were actually classified as plants. Sponges occur in fossil records back to the Precambrian Era (over 600 million years ago) and were the most important contributors to reefs during the Palaeozoic and Mesozoic Eras (Hooper and Van Soest 2002). All members lack defined organs; however, differentiated cells within connective tissue perform necessary biologic functions. Unique systems of water canals facilitate transport of food, waste products, and gametes. Most of the 5000-plus species are marine with just 3% of sponges occurring in freshwater environments.

Sponges are normally found on firm substrates in shallow water, although some occur on soft bottoms.

Sponges maintain a close association with a variety of bacterial genera. While some can be pathogenic, most form a symbiotic relationship with the sponge and provide nutrients. These symbionts are what impart the vast array of bright colors seen in some sponges.

Surgery on sponges is frequently employed to study regeneration and reproductive strategies (Korotkova 1970; Simpson 1984; Kuhns et al. 1997; Henry and Hart 2005). A recent study by Borisenko et al. (2015) examined regeneration in the sponge *Halisarca dujardini* (Figures 4.1 and 4.2). The authors were interested in healing at the cellular level and use microscopy to describe the production of a blastema, an accumulation of undifferentiated cells that will become a new tissue or organ (Carlson 2007). In the case of sponges, the blastema differentiates into new sponge tissue capable of nearly all biologic functions. In the Borisenko et al. (2015) study, the authors used Castroviejo scissors and microscalpels to perform the tissue excisions under a stereomicroscope.

Coelenterates

This large taxonomic grouping includes two phyla: the Ctenophora (comb jellies) and the Cnidaria (Hydrozoans [hydras, fire coral, Portuguese Man-O-War], Scyphozoans [jellyfishes], and Anthozoans [stony corals, soft corals, sea anemones]). This is an economically important group for research, environmental monitoring, public and private display, tourism, and to a lesser degree human food. Coral reefs collectively are one of the most beautiful, diverse, economically important, and fragile ecosystems on the planet. The most common surgery performed on coelenterates involves fracturing pieces of hard coral or cutting segments of soft coral for propagation. This surgical process is referred to as "fragging" in the hobby industry. The technique requires some creativity and foresight, but the procedures are easy to master. For hard coral fragging,

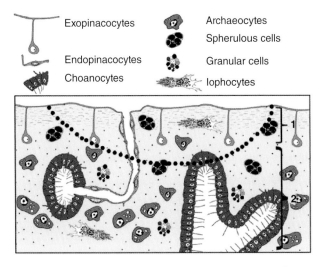

Exopinacocytes   Archaeocytes

   Spherulous cells

Endopinacocytes   Granular cells

Choanocytes   lophocytes

Figure 4.1 This schematic shows the cellular structure of a sponge (*Halisarca dujardini*). The dotted line represents an area of surgical excision. *Source*: Borisenko et al. (2015).

remove large "parent" corals from a system and fracture off small sections with a suitable instrument (e.g. rongeurs, bone cutters) and then secure carefully to a pedestal or other firm substrate with waterproof adhesive. Figure 4.3 shows a system full of "frags." For soft corals, use sharp scissors to sever a suitable fragment that can be attached to a substrate with monofilament suture.

Another process that is occasionally utilized with corals is transplantation. Much work has gone into the process with many species belonging to both invertebrate and vertebrate taxa. With coelenterates, autogenous grafts generally take well, but allografts and xenografts do not (Bigger and Hildemann 1982). In the case of corals, polyps from the same colony can be surgically removed and then attached to another area of the colony with good success as long as freshly cut polyps are placed adjacent to one another (Hildemann et al. 1974).

Coelenterates have an amazing ability to heal and regenerate. This has been know and studied for well over a century (Metchnikoff 1892; Bigger and Hildemann 1982). Amebocytes play an important role in the healing process and it appears that specialized "wound cells" are involved in the initial reaction and healing process, at least in anemones (Young 1974).

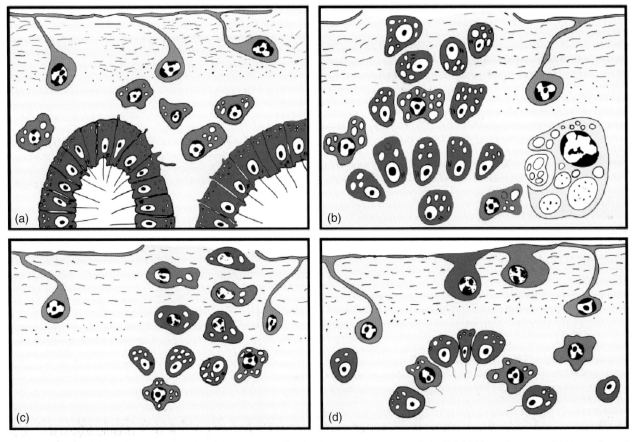

Figure 4.2 This schematic shows three stages of regeneration in the sponge, *Halisarca dujardini*. (a) Normal sponge. (b) Formation of a "regenerative plug" (Stage I). (c) Formation of a "blastema" (Stage II). (d) Ectosome and choanosome restoration (Stage III). Cell colors correspond to Figure 4.1. *Source*: Borisenko et al. (2015).

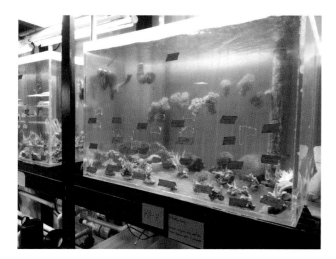

Figure 4.3 This aquarium is filled with coral "frags" representing a number of species and morphological types.

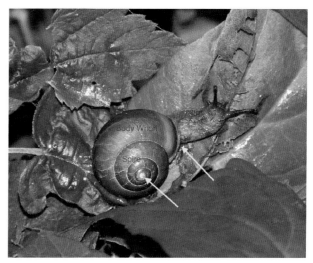

Figure 4.4 This image illustrates the major external anatomical features of a terrestrial shelled gastropod.

One can purchase commercial fragging kits from companies such as Tamsco (Bridgeview, IL), TB Aquatics (Flemington, NJ), and DR Instruments (Palos Hills, IL). Numerous demonstration videos can be found on "YouTube" that illustrate the process of fragging corals.

Gastropod Mollusks

The gastropods belong in the phylum Mollusca and include over 60,000 marine, fresh water, and terrestrial species. The group includes abalone, conchs, nudibranchs, sea hares, slipper shells, slugs, snails, and whelks, among many others. They account for approximately 80% of all mollusk species. Gastropods have a ventrally flattened foot that provides locomotion along the various surfaces of their habitats. They are important display, food, and research animals. Some species are successfully cultured although wild capture is the most common method of procurement. They can be quite large and many are long-lived. Investigators working on the sea hare, *Aplysia*, were awarded a Nobel Prize for medicine or physiology in 2000 for their work on neurophysiology, behavior, and learning. The Nobel Prize in Physiology or Medicine 2000. NobelPrize.org. Nobel Prize Outreach AB 2021 (https://www.nobelprize.org/prizes/medicine/2000/summary/ accessed Mon. 2 Aug 2021). These factors and others make them important animals for veterinary consideration.

There is very little in the literature on gastropod surgery. Much of what is published deals with the amputation of structures like eyes and tentacles, and the surgical compromise of neural tissue to study regeneration (Moffett 2000; Tartakovskaya et al. 2003; Matsuo et al. 2010a,b). These procedures generally do not require wound closure or postoperative therapy. Anderson et al. (2010) determined that silk, among the five suture materials (braided silk, monofilament

nylon, monofilament polylecaprone, polydioxanone, and polyglactin 910) tested in the skin of *Aplysia californica*, resulted in the least amount of granuloma formation. The amount of tissue reaction did not differ among the various sutures.

With regards to hard tissue surgery, there is a case report of shell repair in an apple snail, *Pomacea bridgesii* (Lewbart and Christian 2003). Apple snails are common in the pet trade and a number of species are maintained in aquariums globally. The shell of a typical gastropod contains the apex, spire (made up of whorls), and the body whorl, which terminates at the aperture (Figure 4.4). The head and foot of the snail protrude from the aperture. The oldest whorls are those closest to the apex of the shell. The gastropod shell is composed of four layers. The outer periostracum is composed of conchin, a horny protein, and the internal layers are composed of calcium carbonate and organic material (Ruppert and Barnes 1994). A mature female apple snail crawled out of its aquarium, fell to the floor, and fractured its shell. A depression fracture and a full-thickness "U-shaped" crack were noted on the body whorl (Figure 4.5).

The fractured shell and underlying tissues were flushed with sterile saline and an abrasive Dremel drill bit was used to roughen the surfaces on each side of the fracture. Epoxy (Epoxy Putty®, Oatey, Cleveland, OH) was used to construct a bridge that was attached with digital pressure (Figure 4.6). A section of transparent bandage (Tegaderm®, 3-M) was secured to the shell over the area of the depression fracture. Three months later the shell was stable, but the defects remained. Since mollusks lay down shell at the free edges of the mantle, they cannot regenerate or remodel shell in other areas. The stability of the shell was most likely due to soft tissue healing beneath the fracture sites.

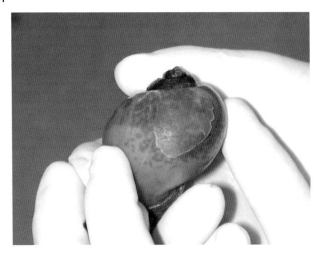

Figure 4.5 This apple snail (Ampullariidae) suffered a fractured shell after falling from its aquarium onto a firm substrate.

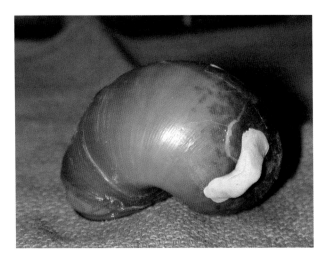

Figure 4.6 The same snail in Figure 4.5 after the application of an epoxy bridge and transparent bandage.

Cephalopod Mollusks

There are about 800 species of cephalopods; a group that includes the octopuses, squids, cuttlefish, and chambered nautiluses. This is an important group in that they serve as a food source for humans and other animals, are popular display animals, and are frequently employed in a variety of research applications. Their acute vision, dexterity, and intelligence make them fascinating animals to observe and study. In Great Britain an Institutional Animal Care and Use Committee (IACUC) application is required to perform research on cephalopods, largely due to their sentience (Mather and Anderson 2007). Unfortunately, most species are short-lived in the wild and captivity. Common problems in captivity include trauma, anorexia, microbial infections, and water quality challenges (Hanlon and Forsythe 1990; Sherrill et al. 2000; Scimeca 2012).

There is not a lot of published information on clinical cephalopod surgery. Harms et al. (2006) describe surgical excision of fungal granulomas from a cuttlefish (*Sepia officinalis*) mantle. They did not use any surgical scrub for fear of damaging the sensitive skin or inducing toxic effects on the circulating anesthesia water. A 5 mm diameter wound was closed with 4-0 polyglyconate on a taper needle using a simple continuous pattern. A larger (3 x 4 cm) wound was closed using the same suture and needle with an interrupted cruciate pattern.

A fairly large body of literature exists regarding research surgical procedures in cephalopods, particularly octopuses, but most of the surgeries are short and apply to amputation and destruction of organs and tissues in order to study behavior, regeneration, and behavioral and physiologic responses (Wells and Wells 1975; Wells 1980; Andrews et al. 1983; Sumbre et al. 2001; Fossati et al. 2013).

Annelids

The annelids are a large and diverse group of segmented vermiform animals that are divided into three main classes: the Polychaetes, Oligochaetes, and Hirudineans. All are characterized by regular segmentation of the trunk. It is believed this segmentation evolved as a means of burrowing via peristaltic contractions (Ruppert and Barnes 1994). Annelids have a coelomic cavity that is divided into segments by septa. The circulatory, excretory, and nervous systems are also segmented. A cuticle covers the animal and segmented setae occur in nearly all members of the phylum. The mouth is located cranially and the anus caudally with a straight gut between the two openings (Ruppert and Barnes 1994). Certain species such as tropical marine polychaetes like feather duster and Christmas tree worms are important and valuable display animals.

Some polychaetes and oligochaetes have the capacity to regenerate portions of their bodies (Ruppert and Barnes 1994). Park et al. (2013) reports on healing and blastema formation after tail amputation in earthworms. Like coelenterates and cephalopods, this has led to experimental amputations and bisections requiring nothing more than a scalpel or other sharp instrument (Bely and Wray 2001; Zattara and Bely 2011). In nearly every case, the details of the procedure are minimal (e.g. *a scalpel was used* or *amputated with a scalpel*). Much of the early research on tissue grafting and rejection was performed on earthworms (Cooper 1968, 1969a,b; Bailey et al. 1971; Cooper and Roch 1986). More recently, earthworms have been used as models for microsurgery training (Figure 4.7) since they resemble mammalian vessels and are superior to synthetic materials (Ramdhian et al. 2011; Leclère et al. 2012, 2013).

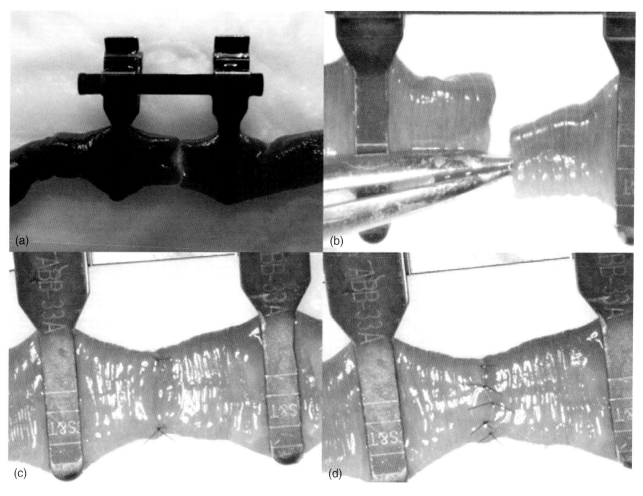

Figure 4.7 This series of images shows how earthworms can be a model for vascular surgery training (anastomosis). (a) Clamping the earthworm (*Lumbricus* sp.), (b) opening the body lumen, (c) two initial sutures, and (d) completed anastomosis. *Source*: LeClere et al. 2013.

Salgado et al. (2014) determined that polyglactin 910, among the five suture materials (braided silk, chromic gut, monofilament nylon, polydioxanone, and polyglactin 910) tested in the skin of Lumbricus terrestris, resulted in the most tissue holding security. Moderate tissue reaction was noted to all five suture materials. A study from the human medical literature focused on anchoring the medicinal leech (Hirudo medicinalis) to patients with superficial and deep tissue with braided silk found found no difference in survival among leech groups with deep and superficial braided silk versus control leeches without suture (Davila et al. 2009).

Crustaceans

The crustaceans are a highly successful class of the Phylum Arthropoda although the nomenclature ranking varies among scientists. This group includes lobsters, crabs, crayfish, shrimp, barnacles, and hermit crabs. Numerous other taxa belonging to this taxon include isopods, amphipods, and brine shrimp. Economically, this is one of the most important groups of invertebrates and its members are utilized for food, as display animals, and for research.

Like many of the preceding taxa, much of the surgery applied to crustaceans has been in research and not the clinical setting. Scientists implant electrodes to study physiology (Forgan et al. 2014), surgically remove eyestalks to impact reproductive behavior (Uawisetwathana et al. 2011), sever nerves to study blood pressure changes (Wilkens and Young 2006), ablate neurons to study regeneration of these structures (Harrison et al. 2003, 2004), and use fine forceps to remove the gonads of a pill bug-like isopod (Suzuki and Yamasaki 1991).

In a more ambitious technical work, Weissburg et al. (2001) transplanted fiddler crab (*Uca pugilator*) limbs in order to study the well-known differences between male and female behavior in this species and the neurosensory basis of these behaviors. Fiddler crabs will autotomize limbs when stressed or traumatized. The researchers would apply pressure to a portion (merus) of the feeding appendages in order to induce autotomy. The animals were then maintained through molting stages until a 2.0 mm limb bud appeared. At this time, the animals were placed in 25 ppt artificial seawater with 30 mg/L gentamicin and 4.0 ml/L Fungizone® for three days before surgery. Host crabs were similarly prepared and another surgeon-induced autotomy of the major claw, and a donor bud was secured to the empty socket with cyanoacrylate adhesive. Over a three-year period the authors transplanted over 680 claws with 101 developing into functioning feeding claws by the second postsurgical molt. For a thorough review of autotomy among the invertebrates, please refer to Fleming et al. (2007).

Arachnids

The Class Arachnida is a huge group of animals (over 100,000 species) that includes over 30,000 spiders, and less conspicuous groups such as the harvestmen, mites, ticks, and scorpions. Tarantulas (actually not true spiders) represent an important taxon of commonly kept arachnids that commonly require medical care. Scorpions also appear with some frequency in the pet trade and are common display animals in zoos and museums.

Surgical repair of the fractured exoskeleton can be accomplished with surgical adhesives like methylmethacrylate or cyanoacrylate (Wolff 1993). A fractured abdomen in a tarantula carries a grave prognosis, but if the hemolymph hemorrhage can be contained with the use of a topical adhesive, the animal can survive. Another common problem that may require intervention is dysecdysis (difficulty shedding). A tarantula or other arachnid that experiences this life-threatening problem can be either anesthetized or manually restrained while forceps or other appropriate instruments are used to gently extract the animal from the adhered exoskeleton (Figure 4.8).

Like many arthropods, scorpions can display autotomy (Pizzi 2002), but in the case of some species belonging to the genus *Ananteris*, they can autotomize their tail (metastoma), including a portion of the gastrointestinal (GI) tract, and survive for up to eight months (Mattoni et al. 2015). Virtually all other arthropods that practice autotomy drop (and can redevelop) limbs. In the case of the *Ananteris* scorpions, tail autotomy appears to be a defense or escape response practiced most commonly by males. While survivors can no longer defecate or sting, they can live long enough to consume small meals and mate (Mattoni et al. 2015). According to one study, sutures are of little use on spiders (Pizzi and Ezendam 2002). Autotomy can be induced in tarantulas by using forceps to grasp the injured appendage by the most proximal segment (femur) and quickly pulling upward (Zachariah and Mitchell 2008). Another small surgical

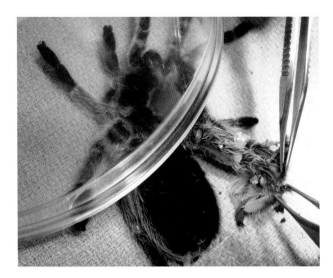

Figure 4.8 This image shows the careful removal of a retained exoskeleton from a tarantula. *Source:* Courtesy of Dan Johnson.

procedure involves inserting microchips (passive integrated transponder [PIT] tags) into manually restrained tarantulas. To do this, an area on the opisthosoma between the heart and intestines was prepared by gently removing the setae from a 1.5 × 1.5 mm area with a 20-gauge needle. The needle tip was then used like a scalpel to open the exoskeleton allowing for insertion of the PIT tag with fine sterile forceps. The wound was then dabbed dry and sealed with cyanoacrylate to minimize hemolymph loss (Reichling and Tabaka 2001).

Limulus

Limulus polyphemus, the American horseshoe crab, is actually not a crab at all but a member of the Class Merostomata in the Phylum Chelicerata. Horseshoe crabs are more closely related to arachnids than crustaceans. *Limulus* is a very important animal for biomedical research, is used as bait and fertilizer, and is an important display and "touch tank" animal in public aquaria (Smith and Berkson 2005; Smith 2012). The anatomy and physiology of these animals have been thoroughly researched, and they are easy to handle and work with. Investigators examining vision and communication of the numerous ommatidia in the *Limulus* lateral eye were awarded the Nobel Prize for medicine or physiology in 1967 (Hartline and Ratliff 1958).

Trauma to the exoskeleton can be stabilized using epoxy. In the case of a fractured carapace, prepare the exoskeletal area where the epoxy will be affixed with an abrasive material like sandpaper. Manually reduce the fracture and stabilize it with the epoxy using digital pressure (Figure 4.9). The epoxy braces can be left in place as long as needed, but healing should occur within three to four months (Smith 2012).

(a)

(b)

(c)

(d)

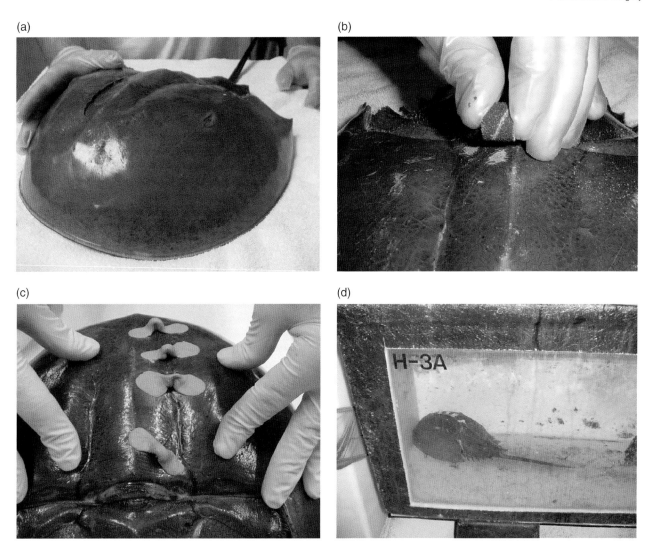

Figure 4.9 These images illustrate fracture repair of a horseshoe crab (*Limulus polyphemus*) prosoma caused by a fall from a raised, shallow tank. (a) The fracture is located on the animal's right side and extends from an area rostral and medial to the compound eye caudally through the arthrodial ligament. (b) A sandpaper wheel is used to freshen areas of the prosoma for better epoxy adherence. (c) The fracture was manually reduced and stabilized, while a suite of four epoxy bridges were placed. (d) The animal responded well to the procedure and can be seen in its tank several weeks later.

Healing is initiated by amoebocytes, which initially form a clot, and progresses to scab formation and tissue healing. There are several kinds of cells involved in the process (Bursey 1977; Clare et al. 1990). Pluripotent cells called plasmatocytes appear to be responsible for the regeneration of tissues, like telsons, in very young animals (Clare et al. 1990).

Krasner et al. examined various suture materials (nylon, polyglecaprone, polydioxanone, polyglycolic acid, and silk) in the telson ligament of horseshoe crabs and found that monofilament nylon produced the least amount of tissue reaction, but none of the materials were superior with regards to holding, and none of the wounds dehisced.

Insects

This is by far the largest group of invertebrates at nearly 1 million described species and possibly the most economically important. Insects are loved and despised worldwide and occupy nearly all niches, except the marine environment. They are important as a human food source in parts of the world and both sustain and destroy agricultural crops, depending on the species of insect and plant. For these reasons, they have been well studied with regards to diseases and pathology (Boucias and Pendland 1999; Cooper 2012). Probably no species has been more thoroughly studied than the domestic honeybee, *Apis mellifera* (Vidal-Naquet 2012, 2015). Despite this, virtually nothing traditionally considered surgery, has been published for insects. As with other invertebrates, a fair amount of literature exists describing techniques and procedures where insects are utilized for research and modeling purposes. A 1985 study (Endo et al. 1985) describes "etherized larvae fixed on wooden beds with threads" followed by bisection of the brain and removal of the right lobe. This technique was part of a photoperiod study.

For microsurgery, vibrating glass stylets have been used with insects (Gödde 1989). This technique is primarily used to produce very small lesions (to 0.1 μm) on various insect tissues.

Another area of increasing interest and work is hybrid insect robots (Sanchez et al. 2015). Researchers insert tiny electrodes into various neural ganglia in order to stimulate roach behaviors (Figure 4.10). While this is not veterinary surgery in the strictest sense, it does require skill, experience, and, in some cases, surgical dissection through tissue.

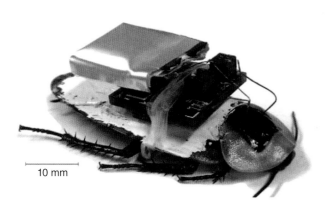

10 mm

Figure 4.10 This cockroach (*Blaberus discoidalis*) has been outfitted with a battery-powered pack and two electrodes entering its pronotal area and inserting into the prothoracic ganglion. This roach/robot hybrid could be controlled remotely to change direction. *Source*: Sanchez et al. 2015.

Echinoderms

This interesting and diverse group of about 7000 species includes the sea stars, brittle stars, sea cucumbers, sea urchins, sea biscuits, and crinoids. All are marine, and many are commonly displayed in aquaria and used in research. Humans do not consume most species, but the gonads of sea urchins are a popular food item in some sushi restaurants. This is the first group of invertebrates classified as deuterostomes (embryonically the anus is formed by the blastopore). In all of the previous taxa of this chapter, the blastopore forms the mouth. All chordates, including vertebrates, are deuterostomes (Ruppert et al. 2004). Some species have regenerative capabilities and generally heal well and quickly. Published surgical techniques focus on studies in regeneration and reviews of echinoderm regeneration adequately summarize the topic (Candia Carnevali and Bonasoro 2001; Candia Carnevali 2006). Candia Carnevali and Bonasoro (2001) introduce an entire journal issue (Microscopy Research and Technique) dedicated to the topic. Crinoids (feather stars) are particularly adept at regenerating arms and, in some cases, nearly the entire body (Candia Carnevali et al. 1996, 1998). Some sand dollars, sea cucumbers, and sea urchins are even able to clone themselves (Eaves and Palmer 2003).

Urochordates

This group of invertebrates is closely related to vertebrates in that members have a nerve cord during embryologic development (Ruppert et al. 2004). They are commonly known as sea squirts and can be found on pilings, dock supports, boat hulls, and the ocean floor. In a study examining regeneration in a colonial species, researchers used razor blades and needles to remove individual buds and zoids from the colony (Brown et al. 2009). The authors found that circulating stem cells are responsible for the complex multi-tissue zoid regeneration.

References

Anderson, E.T., Davis, A.S., Law, J.M. et al. (2010). Gross and histological evaluation of five suture materials in the skin and subcutaneous tissue of the California sea hare (*Aplysia californica*). *Journal of the American Association for Laboratory Animal Science* 49: 1–5.

Andrews, P.L.R., Messenger, J.B., and Tansey, E.M. (1983). The chromatic and motor effect of neurotransmitter injection in intact and brain-lesioned *Octopus. Journal of the Marine Biological Association of the United Kingdom* 63: 355–270.

Andrews, P.L.R., Darmaillacq, A.-S., Dennison, N. et al. (2013). The identification and management of pain, suffering and distress in cephalopods, including anaesthesia, analgesia and humane killing. *Journal of Experimental Marine Biology and Ecology* 447: 46–64.

Archibald, K.E., Scott, G.N., Bailey, K.M. et al. (2019). 2-phenoxyethanol (2-PE) and tricaine methanesulfonate (MS-222) immersion anesthesia of American horseshoe crabs (*Limulus polyphemus*). *Journal of Zoo and Wildlife Medicine* 50: 96–106.

Bailey, S., Miller, B.J., and Cooper, E.L. (1971). Transplantation immunity in annelids II. Adoptive transfer of the xenograft reaction. *Immunology* 21: 81–86.

Bely, A.E. and Wray, G.A. (2001). Evolution of regeneration and fission in annelids: insights from engrailed- and orthodenticle-class gene expression. *Development* 128: 2781–2791.

Bigger, C.H. & Hildemann, W.H. (1982) Cellular defense systems of the Coelenterata. In: *Phylogeny and Ontology* 3 (eds N. Cohen and M. Sigel) pp. 59–87. Plenum Press, New York.

Borisenko, I.E., Adamska, M., Tokina, D.B. et al. (2015). Transdifferentiation is a driving force of regeneration in *Halisarca dujardini* (Demospongiae, Porifera). *PeerJ* 3: e1211. https://doi.org/10.7717/peerj.1211.

Boucias, D.G. and Pendland, J.C. (1999). *Principles of Insect Pathology*. The Netherlands: Kluwer.

Braun, M.E., Heatley, J.J., and Chitty, J. (2006). Clinical techniques of invertebrates. *Veterinary Clinics of North America: Exotic Animal Practice* 9: 205–221.

Brown, F.D., Keeling, E.L., Le, A.D. et al. (2009). Whole body regeneration in a colonial ascidian, *Botrylloides violaceus*. *Journal of Experimental Zoology (Molecular and Developmental Evolution)* 312B: 885–900.

Bursey, C.R. (1977). Histological response to injury in the horseshoe crab, *Limulus polyphemus*. *Canadian Journal of Zoology* 55: 1158–1165.

Butler-Struben, H.M., Brophy, S.M., Johnson, N.A. et al. (2018). *in vivo* recording of neural and behavioral correlates of anesthesia induction, reversal, and euthanasia in cephalopod mollusks. *Frontiers in Physiology* 9: 109. https://doi.org/10.3389/phys.2018.00109.

Candia Carnevali, M.D. (2006). Regeneration in echinoderms: repair, regrowth, cloning. *Invertebrate Survival Journal* 3: 64–76.

Candia Carnevali, M.D. and Bonasoro, F. (2001). Introduction to the biology of regeneration in echinoderms. *Microscopy Research and Technique* 55: 365–369.

Candia Carnevali, M.D., Bonasoro, F., Invernizzi, R. et al. (1996). Tissue distribution of monoamine neurotransmitters in normal and regenerating arms of the feather star *Antedon mediterranea*. *Cell and Tissue Research* 285: 41–352.

Candia Carnevali, M.D., Bonasoro, F., Patruno, M. et al. (1998). Cellular and molecular mechanisms of arm regeneration in crinoid echinoderms: the potential of arm explants. *Development Genes and Evolution* 208: 421–430.

Carlson, R.B. (2007). Morphogenesis of regenerating structures. In: *Principles of Regenerative Biology*, 127–163. New York: Academic Press.

Clare, A.S., Lumb, G., Clare, P.A. et al. (1990). A morphological study of wound repair and telson regeneration in postlarval *Limulus polyphemus*. *Invertebrate Reproduction and Development* 17: 77–87.

Cooper, E.L. (1968). Transplantation immunity in annelids. I. Rejection of xenografts exchanged between *Lumbricus terrestris* and *Eisenia foetida*. *Transplantation* 6: 322–327.

Cooper, E.L. (1969a). Specific tissue graft rejection in earthworms. *Science* 166 (3911): 1414–1415.

Cooper, E.L. (1969b). Chronic allograft rejection in *Lumbricus terrestris*. *Journal of Experimental Zoology* 171: 69–74.

Cooper, J.E. (2011). Anesthesia, analgesia, and euthanasia of invertebrates. *ILAR Journal* 52: 196–204.

Cooper, J.E. (2012). Insects. In: *Invertebrate Medicine*, 2e (ed. G.A. Lewbart), 267–283. Oxford: Wiley-Blackwell Publishing.

Cooper, E.L. and Roch, P. (1986). Second-set allograft responses in the earthworm *Lumbricus terrestris*. *Transplantation* 41: 514–520.

Davila, V.J., Hoppe, I.C., Landi, R. et al. (2009). The effect of anchoring sutures on medicinal leech mortality. *Eplasty* 9: 278–281.

Dombrowski, D. and De Voe, R. (2007). Emergency care of invertebrates. *Veterinary Clinics of North America: Exotic Animal Practice* 10: 621–645.

Eaves, A.A. and Palmer, A.R. (2003). Widespread cloning in echinoderm larvae. *Nature* 425: 146.

Endo, K., Yamashita, I., and Chiba, Y. (1985). Effect of photoperiodic transfer and brain surgery on the photoperiodic control of pupal diapause and seasonal morphs in the swallowtail, *Papilio xuthus* L. (Lepidoptera: Papilionidae). *Applied Entomology and Zoology* 20: 470–478.

Fleming, P.A., Muller, D., and Bateman, P.W. (2007). Leave it all behind: a taxonomic perspective of autotomy in invertebrates. *Biological Reviews* 82: 481–510.

Forgan, L.G., Tuckey, N.P.L., Cook, D.G. et al. (2014). Temperature effects of metabolic rate and cardiorespiratory physiology of the spiny rock lobster (*Jasus edwardsii*) during rest, emersion and recovery. *Journal of Comparative Physiology B* 184: 437–447.

Fossati, S.M., Carella, F., De Vico, G. et al. (2013). Octopus arm regeneration: role of acetylcholinesterase during morphological modification. *Journal of Experimental Marine Biology and Ecology* 447: 93–99.

Fregin, T. and Bickmeyer, U. (2016). Electrophysiological investigation of different methods of anesthesia in lobster and crayfish. *PLoS One* https://doi.org/10.1371/journal.pone.0162894.

Gödde, J. (1989). Vibrating glass stylets: tools for precise microsurgery of cuticular structures. *Journal of Neuroscience Methods* 29: 77–83.

Gunkel, C. and Lewbart, G.A. (2008). Anesthesia and analgesia of invertebrates. In: *Anesthesia and Analgesia in Laboratory Animals*, 2e (eds. R. Fish, P. Danneman, M. Brown and A. Karas), 535–546. New York: Elsevier Publishing.

Hanlon, R.T. and Forsythe, J.W. (1990). Diseases of Mollusca: Cephalopoda 1.1 Diseases caused by microorganisms. In: *Diseases of Marine Animals*, vol. 3 (ed. O. Kinne), 23–46. Hamburg: Biologische Anstalt Helgoland.

Harms, C.A., Lewbart, G.A., McAlarney, R. et al. (2006). Surgical excision of mycotic (*Cladosporium* sp.) granulomas from the mantle of a cuttlefish (*Sepia officinalis*). *Journal of Zoo and Wildlife Medicine* 37: 524–530.

Harrison, P.J., Cate, H.S., Steullet, P. et al. (2003). Amputation-induced activity of progenitor cells leads to rapid regeneration of olfactory tissue in lobsters. *Journal of Neurobiology* 55: 97–114.

Harrison, P.J., Cate, H.S., and Derby, C.D. (2004). Localized ablation of olfactory receptor neurons induces both localized regeneration and widespread replacement of neurons in spiny lobsters. *Journal of Comparative Neurology* 471: 72–84.

Hartline, H.K. and Ratliff, F. (1958). Spatial summation of inhibitory influences in the eye of *Limulus*, and the mutual interaction of receptor units. *Journal of General Physiology* 41: 1049–1066.

Henry, L. and Hart, M. (2005). Regeneration from injury and resource allocation in sponges and corals – a review. *International Review of Hydrobiology* 90: 125–158.

Hildemann, W.H., Dix, T.G., and Collins, J.D. (1974). Tissue transplantation in diverse marine invertebrates. In: *Contemporary Topics in Invertebrate Immunobiology*, vol. 4 (ed. E.L. Cooper), 141–150. New York: Springer US/ Plenum Publishers.

Hooper, J.N.A. and Van Soest, R.W.M. (2002). *Systema Porifera: A Guide to the Classification of Sponges*, vols. 1 & 2. New York: Kluwer Academic/Plenum Publishers.

Korotkova, G.P. (1970). Regeneration and somatic embryogenesis in sponges. In: *The Biology of the Porifera*, Symposia of the Zoological Society of London (ed. W.G. Fry), 423–436. London: Academic Press.

Kuhns, W.J., Ho, M., Burger, M.M. et al. (1997). Apoptosis and tissue regression in the marine sponge *Microciona prolifera*. *Biological Bulletin* 193: 239–241.

Leclère, F.M., Lewbart, G.A., Rieben, R. et al. (2012). Microsurgery and liver research: *Lumbricus terrestris*, a reliable animal model for training? *Clinics and Research in Hepatology and Gastroenterology* 3: 166–170.

Leclère, F.M., Trelles, M., Lewbart, G.A. et al. (2013). Is there good simulation basic training for end-to-side vascular microanastomoses? *Aesthetic Plastic Surgery* https://doi.org/10.1007/s002266-012-0005-0.

Lewbart, G.A. and Christian, L. (2003). Repair of a fractured shell in an apple snail. *Exotic DVM Veterinary Magazine* 5: 8–9.

Mather, J.A. and Anderson, R.C. (2007). Ethics and invertebrates: a cephalopod perspective. *Diseases of Aquatic Organisms* 75: 119–129.

Matsuo, R., Kobayashi, S., Murakami, J. et al. (2010a). Spontaneous recover of the injured higher olfactory center in the terrestrial slug *Limax*. *PLoS One* 5 (2): e9054.

Matsuo, R., Kobayashi, S., Tanaka, Y. et al. (2010b). Effects of tentacle amputation and regeneration on the morphology and activity of the olfactory center of the terrestrial slug *Lomax valentines*. *Journal of Experimental Biology* 213: 3144–3149.

Mattoni, C.I., Garcia-Hernández, S., Botero-Trukillo, R. et al. (2015). Scorpion sheds "tail" to escape: consequences and implications of autotomy in scorpions (Buthidae:*Ananteris*). *PLoS One* https://doi.org/10.1371/journal.pone.0116639.

Metchnikoff, E. (1892). *Lecons sur la Pathologie Comparée de l'Inflammation, Masson*, Paris; reissued (1968) in English as Lectures on the Comparative Pathology of Inflammation. New York: Dover.

Moffett, S.B. (2000). Regeneration as an application of gastropod neural plasticity. *Microscopy Research and Technique* 49: 579–588.

Mosley, C.I. and Lewbart, G.A. (2014). Invertebrates. In: *Zoo Animal and Wildlife Immobilization and Anesthesia*, 2e (eds. G. West, D. Heard and N. Caulkett), 191–208. New York: Wiley.

Park, S.K., Cho, S.-J., and Park, S.C. (2013). Histological observations of blastema formation during earthworm tail regeneration. *Invertebrate Reproductive Development* 57: 165–169.

Pizzi, R. (2002). Induction of autotomy in Theraphosidae spiders as a surgical technique. *Veterinary Invertebrate Society Newsletter* 2: 2–6.

Pizzi, R. and Ezendam, T. (2002). So much for sutures. *The Forum Magazine of the American Tarantula Society* 11: 122–123.

Ramdhian, R.M., Bednar, M., Mantovani, G.R. et al. (2011). Microsurgery and telemicrosurgery training: a comparative study. *Journal of Reconstructive Microsurgery* 27: 537–542.

Reichling, S.B. and Tabaka, C. (2001). A technique for individually identifying tarantulas using passive integrated transponders. *Journal of Arachnology* 29: 117–118.

Ruppert, E.E. and Barnes, R.D. (1994). *Invertebrate Zoology*, 6e, 1056. Philadelphia, PA: Saunders College Publishing.

Ruppert, E.E., Fox, R.S., and Barnes, R.D. (2004). *Invertebrate Zoology: A Functional Evolutionary Approach*, 7e, 963. Belmont, CA: Thompson-Brooks/Cole.

Salgado, M.A., Lewbart, G.A., Christian, L.S. et al. (2014). Evaluation of five different suture materials in the skin of the earthworm (*Lumbricus terrestris*). *Springerplus* 3: 423. https://doi.org/10.1186/2193-1801-3-423.

Sanchez, C.J., Chie, C.-W., Zhou, Y. et al. (2015). Locomotion control of hybrid cockroach robots. *Journal of the Royal Society Interface* 12 https://doi.org/10.1098/rsif.2014.1363.

Scimeca, J. (2012). Cephalopods. In: *Invertebrate Medicine*, 2e (ed. G.A. Lewbart), 113–125. Oxford: Wiley-Blackwell Publishing.

Sherrill, J., Spelman, L.H., Reidel, C.L. et al. (2000). Common cuttlefish (*Sepia officianalis*) mortality at the National Zoological Park: Implications for clinical management. *Journal of Zoo and Wildlife Medicine* 31: 523–531.

Simpson, T.L. (1984). *The Cell Biology of Sponges*. New York: Springer-Verlag.

Smith, S.A. (2012). Horseshoe crabs. In: *Invertebrate Medicine*, 2e (ed. G.A. Lewbart), 173–185. Oxford: Wiley-Blackwell Publishing.

Smith, S.A. and Berkson, J.M. (2005). Laboratory culture and maintenance of the horseshoe crab (*Limulus polyphemus*). *Lab Animal* 34: 27–34.

Sumbre, G., Gutfreund, Y., Fiorito, G. et al. (2001). Control of octopus arm extension by a peripheral motor program. *Science* 293: 1845–1848.

Suzuki, S. and Yamasaki, K. (1991). Sex-reversal of male *Armadillidium vulgare* (Isopoda, Malacostraca, Crustacea) following andrectomy and partial gonadectomy. *General and Comparative Endocrinology* 83: 375–378.

Tartakovskaya, O.S., Borisenko, S.L., and Zhukov, V.V. (2003). Role of the age factor in eye regeneration in the gastropod *Achatina fulica*. *Biology Bulletin of the Russian Academy of Sciences* 30: 228–235.

Uawisetwathana, U., Leelatanawit, R., Klanchui, A. et al. (2011). Insights into eyestalk ablation mechanism to induce ovarian maturation in the black tiger shrimp. *PLoS One* 6 (9): e24427.

Vidal-Naquet, N. (2012). Honeybees. In: *Invertebrate Medicine*, 2e (ed. G.A. Lewbart), 285–321. Oxford: Wiley-Blackwell Publishing.

Vidal-Naquet, N. (2015). *Honeybee Veterinary Medicine*, 280. Sheffield: 5M Publishing/Benchmark House.

Weissburg, M.J., Derby, C.D., Johnson, O. et al. (2001). Transsexual limb transplants in fiddler crabs and expression of novel sensory capabilities. *Journal of Comparative Neurology* 440: 311–320.

Wells, M.J. (1980). Nervous control of the heartbeat in octopus. *Journal of Experimental Biology* 85: 111–128.

Wells, M.J. and Wells, J. (1975). Optic gland implants and their effects on the gonads of Octopus. *Journal of Experimental Biology* 62: 579–588.

Wilkens, J.L. and Young, R.E. (2006). Regulation of blood pressure in the land crab *Cardisoma guanhumi*. *Physiological and Biochemical Zoology* 79: 178–187.

Wolff, P.L. (1993). Achy breaky arachnids. *Proceedings of the American Association of Zoo Veterinarians*, Oakland, CA, pp. 113–119.

Young, J.A.C. (1974). The nature of tissue regeneration after wounding in the sea anemone *Calliactis parasitica* (Couch). *Journal of the Marine Biological Association of the United Kingdom* 54: 599–617.

Zachariah, T.T. and Mitchell, M.A. (2008). Invertebrate medicine and surgery. In: *Manual of Exotic Pet Practice* (eds. T.N. Tully and M.A. Mitchell), 11–38. St. Louis, MO: Saunders.

Zattara, E.E. and Bely, A.E. (2011). Evolution of a novel developmental trajectory: fission is distinct from regeneration in the annelid *Pristina leidyi*. *Evolution and Development* 13: 80–95.

5

Fish Surgery

Claire Vergneau-Grosset and E. Scott Weber, III

Surgeons working with fish should be familiar with their anatomy and physiology. Given that fish are the largest class of vertebrates, anatomic variability is common, and the surgeon should refer to species-specific information, remembering that while many references are not veterinary based, they still provide critical information about anatomy and physiology (Harder 1975). In addition, there are an increasing number of articles describing normal and abnormal anatomic structures obtained with ultrasonography (Walsh et al. 1993; Raidal et al. 2006; Grant et al. 2013; Jafarey et al. 2015), radiography (Love and Lewbart 1997; Bakal et al. 1998; Govett et al. 2004; Schwarz et al. 2002), computed tomography (CT) (Figure 5.1a,b) (Pees et al. 2010; Carr et al. 2014; Schwarz et al. 2002), and magnetic resonance imaging (MRI) (Chanet et al. 2009). Ultrasound, CT, and MRI images may be obtained with the fish remaining in water (Pees et al. 2010).

Perioperative and Postoperative Surgical Management

Water

Thermoregulation, osmoregulation, and other water quality parameters must be maintained throughout surgery. Postoperatively, to reduce osmotic stress, add salt to the water at a concentration of 3–5 ppt for freshwater species. Increasing the water temperature to the higher temperature range of the species can hasten incision healing. It may be important to isolate the patient for improved monitoring depending on logistical and behavioral constraints. Because of the lower environmental temperatures, absorbable suture material will remain for a long period. Suture removal is usually not performed before three to four weeks and may take months in cold-water species and careful examination of the wound margins to assess skin continuity is recommended prior to suture removal,

typically after four to eight weeks in temperate species (Sladky and Clarke 2016).

Analgesia, Anesthesia, and Fluids

Various models have been used to investigate nociception, and nociceptive receptors are present in fish, predicating the importance to minimize noxious stimulations associated with fish surgery (Weber 2011a). The use of a perioperative opioid drug is currently recommended. Morphine 5 mg/kg intramuscularly (IM) has been proposed in koi (*Cyprinus carpio*) (Baker et al. 2013). Morphine at this dose caused temporary bouts of excitability and, if used, owners should be made aware of potential adverse effects (Baker et al. 2013). The pharmacokinetics of morphine have also been reported in goldfish (*Carassius auratus*) and salmon (*Salmo salar*) administered, respectively, 40 and 100 mg/kg IM and mean elimination half-lives were 12.5–13.5 hours (Nordgreen et al. 2009). Nonsteroidal anti-inflammatory drugs are used as part of multimodal analgesia in fish. Ketoprofen (Harms et al. 2005; Davis et al. 2006; Ward et al. 2012), carprofen (Mettam et al. 2011), and meloxicam (Larouche 2018; Fredholm et al. 2016) have been evaluated in fish. Adverse effects of other non steroidal anti-inflammatory drugs have been reported and empirical use at high doses should be avoided (Schwaiger et al. 2004; Lovy et al. 2007). In-depth reviews of fish anesthesia are available (Stoskopf and Posner 2014; Whiteside 2014). Perioperative fluids are chosen based on the plasma osmolarity of the species, ranging between 900 and 1500 mOsm/l in elasmobranchs (Hadfield et al. 2010).

Antibiotics

Only a few antibiotics are approved for specific species use in aquaculture, and these vary by country (Health Canada 2010; Tell et al. 2012). A growing number of pharmacokinetic

(a)

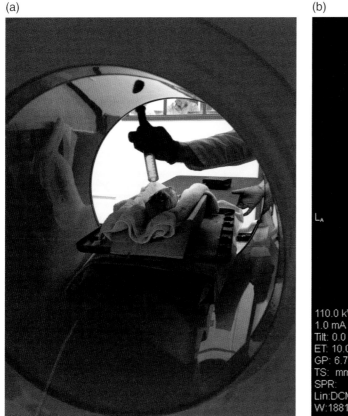

(b)

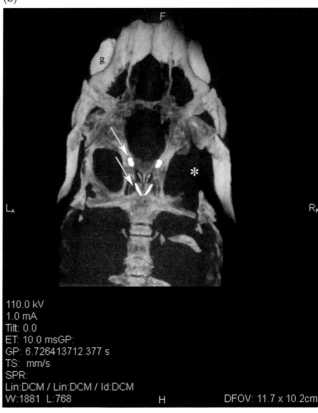

Figure 5.1 (a) Positioning for a CT-scan in an anesthetized koi (*Cyprinus carpio*) presented with an inability to close the mouth. The koi is kept anesthetized via a water-circulating system over the gills and irrigation of the skin is provided with a syringe just before a very quick image-acquisition period. Care should be taken to avoid any water leakage with the use of absorbing towels and foam. (b) Example of a CT-scan of a koi (*Cyprinus carpio*) patient that presented for an inability to close the mouth: longitudinal section showing the ossicles (arrows), the globes (g), and opercular cavity (*). *Source:* Photo courtesy: Companion Avian and Exotic Pet Medicine Service, University of California, Davis.

studies evaluate therapeutic antibiotic use in ornamental fish (Nouws et al. 1988; Grondel et al. 1986; Lewbart et al. 1997; Yanong et al. 2011; Grosset et al. 2015).

Surgical Table

Most fish surgeries are performed out of the water to facilitate visualization, tissue dissection, and suturing (Wildgoose 2000). Surgery tables adapted for fish should include a recirculating water system and a support element for the patient (Weber et al. 2009). The support element is typically made of nonabrasive material to preserve cutaneous mucus and should be permeable to allow water used for irrigation of the gills to return to a container placed underneath the table for recirculating systems (see Figure 5.2). For laterally compressed fish, a V-shaped foam tray is useful to keep the fish in dorsal recumbency. Irrigation of the gills is performed using a Y-shaped perforated tubing or two tubes connected to submersed pumps as previously described (Figure 5.2) (Weber et al. 2009; Mylniczenko et al. 2014). If an oral cavity procedure is

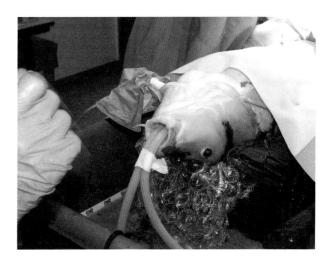

Figure 5.2 Anesthetic equipment used for a large 8 kg koi (*Cyprinus carpio*) anesthetized for a surgical procedure: a Doppler probe protected by a glove filled with conducting gel is placed in the left opercular chamber for heart rate monitoring and two tubes, each connected to a submersible pump are placed in each opercular cavity. *Source:* Photo courtesy: Companion Avian and Exotic Pet Medicine Service, University of California, Davis.

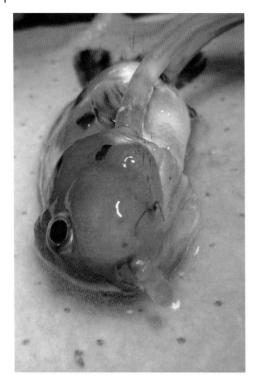

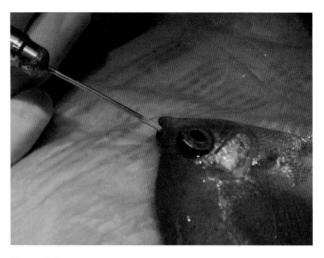

Figure 5.4 Use of adjunctive cryotherapy for excision of an odontoma in an angelfish (*Pterophyllum dumerilii*) presented for recurring maxillary masses. *Source:* Photo courtesy: Companion Avian and Exotic Pet Medicine Service, University of California, Davis.

Figure 5.3 Intervention in the oropharyngeal cavity of a Ranchu goldfish (*Carassius auratus*): a suture from a previous incisional biopsy is visible on the mass extending from the left commissure to left side of the face, ventral to the left eye. Irrigation of the gills is achieved with tubing placed caudally in each opercular cavity, which allows maintenance of anesthesia. *Source:* Photo courtesy: Companion Avian and Exotic Pet Medicine Service, University of California, Davis.

performed, the tubing may be placed with retrograde flow in each opercular cavity with water irrigating the gills from their caudal aspect (Figure 5.3) (Mylniczenko et al. 2014).

Surgical Modalities

Modalities such as cryosurgery and CO_2 laser have been used extensively in fish for mass ablation (Figure 5.4) (Francis-Floyd et al. 1993; Harms et al. 2008; Boylan et al. 2015). These modalities improve hemostasis but do not allow for histologic evaluation and no study has demonstrated superior results using these modalities in fish. Protocols are extrapolated from those used in mammals. Hand-held electrocautery can be used for hemostasis, but electrosurgery should not be used due to the omnipresence of conductive water (Figure 5.5).

Wounds

Wound healing has been studied extensively in zebrafish (*Danio rerio*) (Rapanan et al. 2015). Fish have exceptional regenerative capability (Ochandio et al. 2015). Fish skin

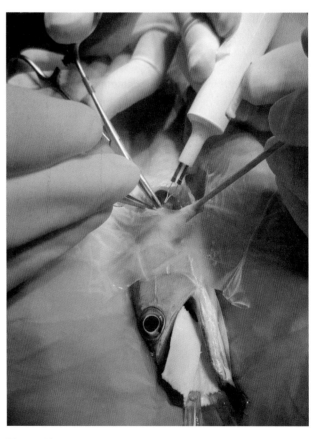

Figure 5.5 Use of a hand-held electrocautery during a lateral celiotomy in a silver arowana (*Osteoglossum bicirrhosum*). *Source:* Photo courtesy: Companion Avian and Exotic Pet Medicine Service, University of California, Davis.

has intrinsic healing properties, and products derived from fish skin are under investigation for xenografts (Baldursson et al. 2015). Healing time depends on environmental parameters such as water temperature, alkalinity, pH, salinity, and photoperiod (Andrews et al. 2015). Skin healing may take months in a cold-water species. Keeping the patient at the higher end of its temperature range hastens healing time (Andrews et al. 2015; Ang et al. 2021).

For wound debridement, follow the same principles as those used in mammals. Debride necrotic tissues and remove detached scales from the wound and surrounding damaged tissue (Wildgoose 2000). Repeated debridement may disrupt the apical epidermal cap and is not recommended as this delays wound healing (Harms and Wildgoose 2001). Appose large clean fresh traumatic wounds with suture (Wildgoose 2000).

As in mammals, in cases of external ulcerations, the etiology should be investigated to prevent recurrence (Figure 5.6). Improper life support system design, such as an over-sized pump, misplaced water inlets or outlets, or misaligned or improper filtration equipment can cause traumatic injuries to fish. Prolonged pond treatments, electrical currents, or chemicals in the water such as seen with an overdose of salt treatment for freshwater fish and/or copper intoxication may cause hyperexcitability leading to traumatic injuries. Predators such as piscivorous birds, river otters, and domestic or feral cats can kill small fish and injure larger animals. In cases of buoyancy problems, skin subjected to air exposure or rubbing against a tank substrate can cause ulcerations (Britt et al. 2002). Provide a

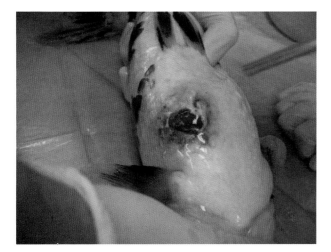

Figure 5.6 Large ulceration on the ventrum of a female koi (*Cyprinus carpio*) with coelomic distension due to egg retention. Treating the egg retention is important for skin healing in this case. *Source:* Photo courtesy: Companion Avian and Exotic Pet Medicine Service, University of California, Davis.

nonabrasive pond substrate during healing such as with the addition of a soft plastic lining at the bottom and sides of the pond.

The use of becaplermin (Regranex®, 0.01% gel, Ortho-McNeil Pharmaceutical Inc., Raritan, NJ, USA), a recombinant platelet-derived growth factor, improves skin healing after a single application (Boerner et al. 2003; Fleming et al. 2008). Apply becaplermin to the wound for 60 seconds every three weeks; this frequency is as efficient as more prolonged application (Fleming et al. 2008). Lavage the wound with sterile saline to loosen debris, gently debride necrotic tissues and exudates to create fresh vital tissue margins, rinse the wound again, and apply a thin layer of gel. After a contact time of 60–120 seconds, rinse the gel off or leave it on the wound. The use of topical manuka honey and aloe vera every four days with a three-minute contact time has been associated with accelerated wound healing in koi (Ang et al. 2021), while the use of a phenytoin and misoprostol powder or silver sulfadiazine gel has been associated with delayed wound healing (Coutant et al. 2019; Ang et al. 2021).

Skin Surgery

The indication for surgery should be confirmed before performing a procedure. Surgical excision of masses associated with lymphocystivirus or cyprinid herpesvirus 1 (CyHV1) infections is not recommended, as they will spontaneously regress (Weber 2013). Surgical preparation should not disrupt the natural mucus layer of the integument. Mucus is critical for innate immunity and protection (Benhamed et al. 2014; Guardiola et al. 2014). Scale removal is recommended to facilitate skin closure and healing (Wildgoose 2000). Gently extract the scales with a pair of forceps along the incision line. Since fish scales are dermal in origin (Lee et al. 2013), this can damage the epidermis and should be accomplished with care to limit the resulting trauma to the skin and to leave the scale bed intact so that scales will regrow normally (Weber et al. 2009). Then gently flush with sterile saline or sterile water rather than typical surgical preparations (Lloyd and Lloyd 2011), as many surgical antiseptics have been reported to predispose fish to dermatitis and incisional dehiscence (Mylniczenko et al. 2007). Irrigate exposed skin and eyes with chlorine-free water throughout surgery to avoid desiccation and secondary necrosis.

For skin biopsies, use a biopsy punch or scalpel blade. Achieve hemostasis using digital pressure or hand-held electrocautery. Biopsy sites can be left open to heal by second intention. Compared to mammals, fish skin has very

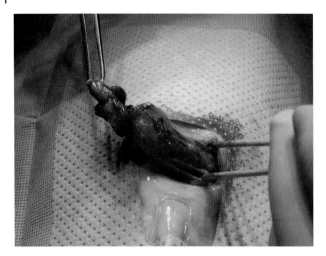

Figure 5.7 Excision of a neoplastic mass of the vent of a koi (*Cyprinus carpio*): the integrity of natural orifices and anatomy should be preserved as much as possible during mass excision. *Source:* Photo courtesy: Companion Avian and Exotic Pet Medicine Service, University of California, Davis.

low elasticity due to the dermal scales (Wildgoose 2000). External mass incisional or excisional biopsy in fish is accomplished in a manner similar to that in mammals. Surgical margins are rarely obtained for neoplasia that involves the coelomic cavity (Figure 5.7) and body wall reconstruction should be planned carefully prior to mass resection due to the low elasticity of the tissues (Boerner et al. 2000; Wildgoose 2000). Intralesional chemotherapy based on a histologic diagnosis has been reported (Figure 5.8) (Vergneau-Grosset et al. 2016; Stevens et al. 2017).

Operculoplasty is performed for esthetic purposes in fish with a laterally curled operculum, a common congenital problem in arowanas (*Osteoglossum* and *Scelopages* spp.) (Figure 5.9a). The etiology has not been determined and a genetic predisposition cannot be ruled out. Section the operculum with scissors at the level where it is still parallel to the long axis of the body (Figure 5.9b) and it will grow back straight. Some hobbyists also recommend filing the exposed opercular to the appropriate angle, but care should be taken not to damage the surrounding epithelium.

Oral surgery and incisive plate adjustments may be needed to improve food prehension due to insufficient wearing of the dental plates (Figure 5.10) or due to the presence of an oral mass. Incise the fibrous tissue with a scalpel blade in a medial to lateral direction and allow healing by second intention. Pufferfish have continuously growing incisor plates (Lécu and Lecour 2004). When fed exclusively soft food items such as pelleted diets, flakes, or soft prey instead of a natural diet that includes mollusks or crustaceans, they can develop overgrowth of their incisor plates (Figure 5.11a). Trim these plates with a dental burr or rotary tool (Dremel, Racine, WI) (Lécu

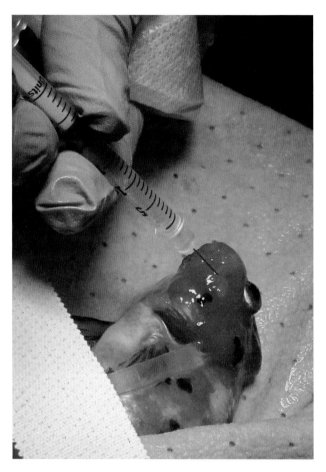

Figure 5.8 Intralesional bleomycin injection into a myxoma on the head of an oranda goldfish (*Carassius auratus*). This treatment led to a decrease of the size of the mass for the following three months and was subsequently repeated as needed. *Source:* Photo courtesy: Companion Avian and Exotic Pet Medicine Service, University of California, Davis.

and Lecour 2004) (Figure 5.11b). Take care to not overheat the incisor plates by prolonged contact with the burr. It may be necessary to fully immerse the pufferfish frequently to avoid inflation of the esophagus with air rather than water; water distention of the esophagus in these species is a normal physiologic defense, and fluid can be more easily expelled post procedure than entrapped gas (Wildgoose 2000).

Orthopedic Surgery

Successful surgical stabilization of mandibular symphyseal fractures has been reported in three arowanas (Lloyd and Sham 2014). Two 19-gauge needles were placed on each side of the mandible and a 4-metric stainless steel orthopedic wire was passed through the needle holes and tightened up to stabilize the fracture. Successful repair of a

(a) (b)

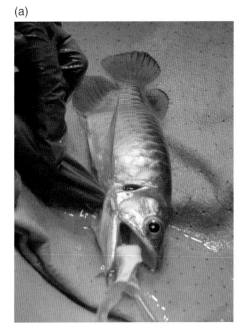 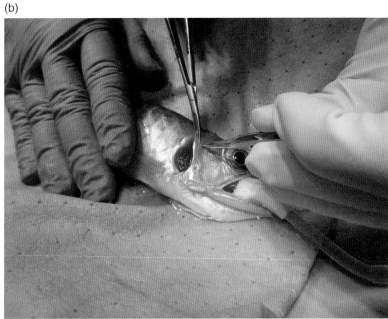

Figure 5.9 Opercular plasty in an anesthetized Asian arowana (*Scleropages formosus*): (a) the caudal part of the right operculum appears curved laterally and shortened; (b) the operculum is sectioned with scissors after butorphanol and local anesthesia have been administered. *Source:* Photo courtesy: Companion Avian and Exotic Pet Medicine Service, University of California, Davis.

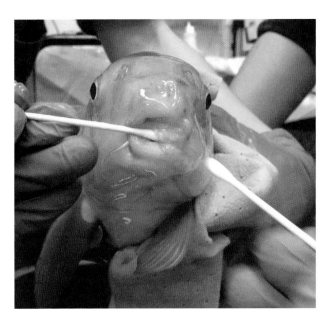

Figure 5.10 Fibrous tissue obstructing the oral cavity of a koi (*Cyprinus carpio*). *Source:* Photo courtesy: Companion Avian and Exotic Pet Medicine Service, University of California, Davis.

luxation of the dentaro-ectopterygoid joint in a fish has been performed (Dr. Freeland Dunker, Steinhart Aquarium, personal communication). The fish presented with an inability to close its dentary bone. Under general anesthesia, the mandible was closed with external manipulation, and a cerclage wire was placed on the premaxillary and

dentary bones to keep the oral cavity closed. After a few weeks, the cerclage was removed and the fish was able to open and close its mouth and to eat spontaneously. Scoliosis correction in koi has been attempted by stabilizing the vertebrate with screws, k-wire, and polymethylmethacrylate (Govett et al. 2004).

Ophthalmic Surgery

Fish eyes have marked anatomic differences compared to those of mammals (Kern 2007). Very few fish have eyelids, except some elasmobranchs. They have larger lenses comparatively to mammals of the same size, and the lens protrudes into the anterior chamber, which has implications for cataract surgery (Kern 2007). The posterior segment of the eye contains a falciform process and a choroid rete communicating with the pseudobranch in most species (Copeland and Brown 1976). An important consideration when performing an enucleation is the presence of scleral ossicles in the anterior part of the globe, as in teleosts, and scleral cartilage or scleral calcifications in the posterior part in elasmobranchs (Pilgri and Franz-Odendaal 2009).

The pupillary light reflex is usually absent, except in elasmobranchs (Duke-Elder 1958). They have a slow retinomotor reflex that takes up to two hours. During the day, retinal-pigmented epithelium granules migrate apically in the retinal epithelial cells, cones contract and rods elongate

(a)

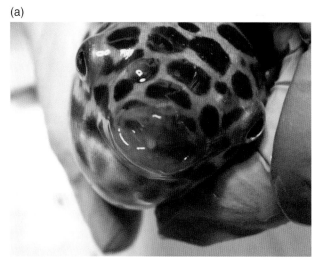

(b)

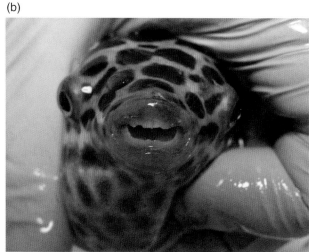

Figure 5.11 Green spotted pufferfish (*Tetraodon nigroviridis*) before (a) and after incisor plate occlusal adjustment (b). *Source:* Photo courtesy: Companion Avian and Exotic Pet Medicine Service, University of California, Davis.

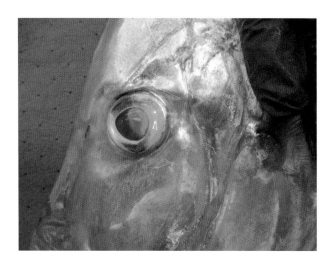

Figure 5.12 Fluorescein staining of a large corneal ulceration in a lookdown (*Selene vomer*) associated with repeated trauma on the walls of the exhibit. *Source:* Photo courtesy: Companion Avian and Exotic Pet Medicine Service, University of California, Davis.

(Burnside et al. 1983). This retinomotor reflex protects photoreceptors from bright light, but rapid exposure of anesthetized patients to a scialytic lamp may impair vision and some authors have recommended covering fish eyes with an opaque material during surgery (Wildgoose 2000).

Corneal ulcers can be highlighted by the use of fluoresceine dye (Figure 5.12). Repair corneal perforations with small diameter suture material and use periorbital tissue to cover peripheral corneal perforations, similar to a conjunctival flap.

Idiopathic gaseous exophthalmia (i.e. not due to gas oversaturation of water) has been treated with pseudobranchectomy. The pseudobranch is located dorsally in the opercular cavity in most teleosts (Harms and Wildgoose 2001).

Visually locate the pseudobranch and apply electrocautery on various points to cauterize it.

Some fancy goldfish, such as oranda and lionheads, are bred to have a fleshy outgrowth on the dorsal aspect of the skull and bilaterally in the buccal area, which is called a crown or "wen." This wen is a hyperplastic epidermal and mucous cell covering of adipose cell deposition in the hypodermis (Angelidis et al. 2006). The wen grows continuously, sometimes covering the eyes and impairing vision. Use a scalpel or electrocautery to excise the periocular tissue (Sladky and Clarke 2016).

Cataract Surgery

Cataract surgeries have been performed in fish, either with complete lens removal (Whitaker 1999; Adamovicz et al. 2015) or with phacoemulsification of the lens content in specific cases (Adamovicz et al. 2015; Bakal et al. 2005). After applying topical proparacaine and atropine, fill the anterior chamber with viscoelastic material and incise the dorsal cornea with a 2.75 mm keratome (Adamovicz et al. 2015) or a 11# scalpel blade. The authors recommend a dorsal incision of the cornea as it allows easier access to the *retractor lensis* muscle located ventral and caudal to the lens (Gustavsen et al. 2018). To prevent collapse of the anterior chamber, incise the cornea perpendicular to its surface initially, then with a more acute angle. Extract the lens, which physiologically protrudes into the anterior chamber, "en masse" with a Graefe cataract spoon through the corneal incision (Whitaker 1999). Close the cornea with simple interrupted 5-0 to 9-0 sutures. Apply a cyanoacrylate ophthalmic tissue adhesive (optional) to ensure impermeability of the cornea during healing (Whitaker 1999).

In most cases, complete phacoemulsification is not possible due to the hard texture of the lens nucleus so partial phacoemulsification is followed by enlargement of the corneal incision and extraction of the lens nucleus (Adamovicz et al. 2015). However, in the case of a sturgeon infected by intraocular digenean trematodes, complete phacoemulsification of the lens has been reported (Bakal et al. 2005). These trematodes can cause cataracts causing inflammation that can lead to softening of the lens (Adamovicz et al. 2015).

Enucleation

Enucleation is performed to alleviate pain associated with nonresolvable ocular lesions (Figure 5.13) (da Silva et al. 2010; Lair et al. 2014) or severe injury. A prosthetic eye can be placed (Nadelstein et al. 1997), but keeping the prosthesis in place long-term may be problematic (Harms and Wildgoose 2001).

After performing a local block with lidocaine, dissect and transect periorbital tissue, conjunctiva and oculomotor muscles off the globe with fine curved scissors. Branches of the trigeminal and facial nerves running along the caudolateral border of the orbit should not be transected (Wildgoose 2007b). If a hemostat is placed on the retro-orbital pedicle, minimize traction on the optic nerve to prevent damage to the optic chiasm, which will result in blindness in the contralateral eye. Transect the pedicle, remove the globe, and ligate the retro-orbital vessels. Supplement hemostasis by applying digital pressure and a hemostatic agent (Gelfoam®, Pfizer, New York, NY). Suturing the periorbital tissue, with an H-plasty if needed, enables one to close the orbit for esthetical purposes in some fish species such as cod (*Gadus morhua*) and saithe (*Pollachius virens*) (Figure 5.14). In fish where this is not possible, leave the orbit open to heal (Figure 5.15) and

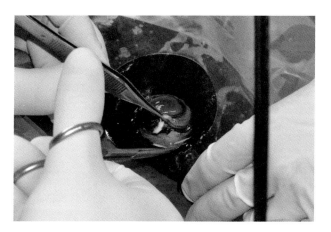

Figure 5.13 Enucleation of a rockfish (*Sebastes caurinus*) with a retinal tumor. *Source:* Photo courtesy: Aquarium du Québec.

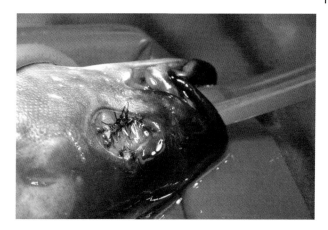

Figure 5.14 Suture of the periorbital tissue after an enucleation in a saithe (*Pollachius virens*). *Source:* Photo courtesy: Aquarium du Québec.

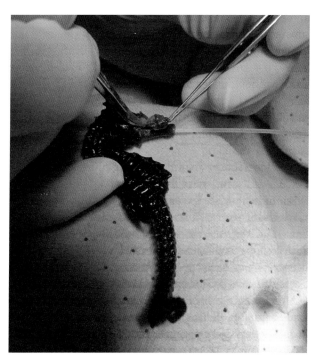

Figure 5.15 Enucleation of a sea horse (*Hippocampus erectus*) with a retro-orbital abscess. The tube on the right of the image is used for anesthesia maintenance and Harmon–Bishop's forceps were used to elevate the globe from the orbit and allow section of the optic nerve and retro-orbital pedicle. In this species, it is not possible to close the orbit after enucleation due to the dermal plates greatly reducing the elasticity of the skin. *Source:* Photo courtesy: Companion Avian and Exotic Pet Medicine Service, University of California, Davis.

expect mild hemorrhagic discharge after recovery. Some authors recommended placing a waterproof paste containing pectin, gelatin, and methylcellulose (Orabase®, ConvaTec, Bridgewater Township, NJ) into the orbit over the next 24–72 hours (Harms and Wildgoose 2001).

Coelomic Surgery

The coelomic cavity may be approached ventrally or laterally. For a ventral approach, make either an incision caudal to the pelvic fins just cranial to the vent (Figure 5.16) or an incision from the pectoral to the pelvic fins. If wider access to the coelom is needed, section the pelvic girdle on midline. The pelvic bones are joined on midline by a fibrous junction in some younger fish which becomes ossified in older specimens (Harms and Wildgoose 2001). During the approach, take care to avoid damaging the digestive tract, especially if a coelomic mass is displacing the intestine near the ventral body wall (Weisse et al. 2002; Weber 2011b). Perform a lateral approach or an L-shaped incision in the coelom to access dorsal organs such as the kidneys or the swim bladder (Harms and Wildgoose 2001). Make the craniocaudal incision just ventral to the lateral line of the fish, extending from the caudal edge of the pectoral fin to the level of the anus. Make the dorsoventral incision at the level of the anus and extend as needed for exposure; do not incise too close to the sphincter of the anus.

Coelomic adhesions are common in some species of fish including koi and are not necessarily an indication of coelomitis (Wildgoose 2000; Boone et al. 2008; Grosset et al. 2015). During the celiotomy, take care to limit traction on the coelomic wall as trauma to this delicate tissue can result in postoperative necrosis of the body wall. An assistant may gently retract the coelomic wall using a Farabeuf or Roux retractor or a self-retaining retractor such as Heiss, Lone Star, or Gelpi retractors, or a Barraquer eyelid speculum may be used depending on the size of the fish (Harms and Wildgoose 2001).

Close the coelomic wall in two layers: muscle and skin (Harms and Wildgoose 2001). During closure, take care to close the pelvic girdle in accurate apposition if it has been sectioned. A subcuticular pattern rather than cutaneous suture is recommended in goldfish, as this induces less local reaction than simple interrupted sutures or interrupted horizontal mattress sutures (Nematollahi et al. 2010). Ideally, leave no additional air in the coelom during closure to avoid buoyancy problems. Also, consider the weight of suture materials and any prosthetics or surgical devices in very small patients (Britt et al. 2002).

Do not remove sutures before four weeks (Shin et al. 2011). Sutures may be removed after four to eight weeks in temperate species (Sladky and Clarke 2016). Months may be necessary for adequate healing before suture removal in cold-water species. Carefully examine the wound margins to assess skin continuity prior to suture removal.

Swim Bladder Surgery

The swim bladder is important in maintaining neutral buoyancy. Abnormal buoyancy is a common presentation of ornamental fish (Wildgoose 2007a) with a number of etiologies that can be diagnosed using radiography or other imaging techniques. Positive buoyancy may be due to overinflating of the swim bladder (Figure 5.17), torsion (rare), or gas in the coelomic cavity or other coelomic organs. Negative buoyancy may be due the accumulation of fluid in the swim bladder, infection, neoplasia, or compression by enlarged coelomic organs, cystic kidneys or ovaries, or other coelomic masses. Swim bladder anatomy

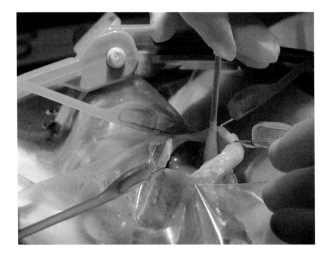

Figure 5.16 Incision of the coelom between the pelvic fins and the digestive orifice in an anesthetized goldfish (*Carassius auratus*). A Lone Star retractor is placed on the coelomic cavity to facilitate visualization. *Source:* Photo courtesy: Zoological Medicine Service, Université de Montréal.

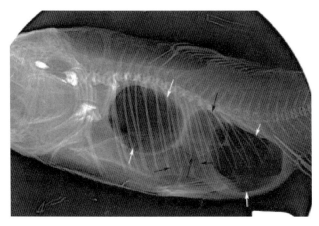

Figure 5.17 Right lateral radiograph of a positively buoyant goldfish (*Carassius auratus*) presented with multiple gas (white arrows) and fluid-filled (black arrows) structures connected to the swim bladder. *Source:* Photo courtesy: Companion Avian and Exotic Pet Medicine Service, University of California, Davis.

varies greatly among fish species and surgeons should be familiar with the anatomy of their patient (Zebedin and Ladich 2013). Some fish are physostomous (swim bladder is connected to the digestive tract), some are physoclistous (swim bladder inflation is regulated by a gas gland), and some fish do not have a swim bladder (e.g. elasmobranchs, mackerels, tunas, benthic fishes, and remoras) (McCune and Carlson 2004). Koi and goldfish have a bi-compartmentalized swim bladder with the most cranial compartment being more rigid and a pneumatic duct connecting it to the caudal compartment (Muir Evans 1925), while some catfish species have multi-compartmentalized swim bladders (Zebedin and Ladich 2013). Imaging both the patient and a normal conspecific helps identify swim bladder lesions whenever specific anatomy has not been described (Schwartz et al. 2002; Pees et al. 2010). Care should be taken to avoid trauma to and deflation of the swim bladder during a celiotomy.

In the case of swim bladder neoplasia or distension, surgical reduction of the swim bladder is indicated. This procedure has been termed pneumocystoplasty or complete pneumocystectomy depending on the volume of swim bladder reduction (Britt et al. 2002; Lewbart et al. 1995). Approach the swim bladder using a ventral coelomic midline incision (Lewbart et al. 1995; Britt et al. 2002) or a L-shaped incision through the lateral coelomic wall (Harms and Wildgoose 2001). For pneumocystoplasty, locate and preserve the pneumatic duct and/or the gas gland that is a "rete mirabile" and partially surrounds the walls of the swim bladder and furnishes a rich supply of blood often located ventrally on the most cranial aspect of the swim bladder (Harms and Wildgoose 2001). Carefully dissect the swim bladder to avoid perforation and collapse (Harms and Wildgoose 2001). The wall of the swim bladder is very thin and delicate and achieving impermeability following formation of a tear may be very challenging. This can result in free coelomic gas, abnormal buoyancy, and communication between the digestive tract and the coelom in physiostomous fish, which may cause coelomitis. Depending on the size of the fish, place an encircling ligature (Harms and Wildgoose 2001) or a vascular clip (Hemoclip, Teleflex, Morrisville, NC) prior to excising the affected part of the swim bladder (Britt et al. 2002). Alternatively, a two-layer inverting suture may be placed to close the swim bladder after excision of a section of this organ (Sladky and Clarke 2016). Negative buoyancy is a common complication immediately following pneumocystoplasty as the fish needs to adjust gas content of the swim bladder to accommodate the weight of a hemostatic clip or for decreased size of the swim bladder itself. This complication may persist for the remaining life of the fish if the resulting volume of the swim bladder is too small

(Sladky and Clarke 2016). On the Internet, several hobbyists and websites have suggested ways to create custommade flotation harnesses for goldfish using chamois material, plastic airline tubing, and cork to allow locomotion in negatively buoyant fish.

Reproductive Surgery

Determining the sex of fish through surgical incision into the coelomic cavity is performed routinely in some fish industries. Commercial sturgeon is sexed around three year of age to separate males for meat production and females for caviar production. Caviar collection itself may also be accomplished antemortem through a coelomic incision followed by closure of the body wall; this technique is employed in some commercial facilities to allow production by the same female during subsequent years. Sturgeon can be sexed using ultrasound eliminating the need for surgery (Colombo et al. 2004).

Ovariectomy has been performed in many piscine species (Stamper and Norton 2002; Lewisch et al. 2014). Indications for ovariectomy include contraception, persistent egg retention despite medical treatment, and gonadal tumors (Jafarey et al. 2015). Ovariectomy is rarely performed prophylactically in fish (Kizer and Novo 2003), with the exception of batoid species, i.e. rays and skates, kept in female-only groups (Sladky and Clarke 2016) as this group structure may predispose rays to reproductive tract lesions. Rays with an oral disc ranging from 50 to 60 cm have been reported to have a better surgical outcome (Sladky and Clarke 2016). Ovariectomy should only be attempted in mature fish for contraceptive purposes, as gonads may be extremely difficult to locate in immature fish, resulting in gonadal tissue being left behind. It should be noted that some teleost species, such as the arowana, have a single ovary located on the left side of the coelom (Yanwirsal 2013). Some elasmobranchs have a single functional ovary (left ovary in rays and the right ovary and both oviducts in sharks) (Henningsen et al. 2004).

In teleosts, use a ventral approach to the coelomic cavity and locate the ovaries. Bluntly dissect from caudal to cranial with cotton-tipped applicators or hemostats to locate the ovarian pedicle. Depending on the size of the fish, use a ligature, a hemostatic clip, or electrocautery to provide hemostasis. Transect the pedicle distal to the ligature and remove the ovaries (Figure 5.18). In some fish, the ovarian mass may be very friable and should be carefully handled with cotton-tip applicators to avoid rupture. Leaving ovarian material in the coelomic cavity may result in coelomic inflammation; use a combination of irrigation and suction

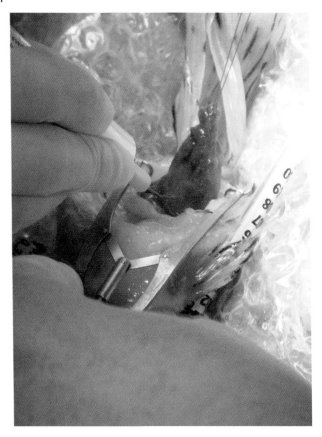

Figure 5.18 Ovariectomy in an Oranda goldfish (*Carassius auratus*): the head of the fish is toward the bottom of the picture and the caudal fin toward the top of the picture. A diseased ovary is been retracted with a stay suture. *Source:* Photo courtesy: Companion Avian and Exotic Pet Medicine Service, University of California, Davis.

to avoid this complication (Sladky and Clarke 2016). In fish with egg retention, medical management (Ovaprim®, Syndel Laboratories Ltd., Nanaimo, Canada) should be attempted before surgical ovariectomy (Hill et al. 2009).

Use a dorsal paralumbar approach in batoid species. Make a craniocaudal longitudinal incision approximately 2 cm lateral to the dorsal lumbar muscles, on the side of the functional ovary (e.g. left side for cownose rays and stingrays). Use a #10 scalpel blade in large females, as the skin and body wall are very thick. Elevate and incise the coelomic membrane. Visualize the ovary (connected to the epigonal organ), ovarian pedicle, suspensory ligament, and cranial portion of the oviduct. Ligate the ovarian vessels with suture or a hemostatic clip. Dissect the caudal pole of the ovary from the epigonal organ and excise the ovary. Inspect the coelomic cavity to assess hemostasis. Close the peritoneum with 3-0 polydioxanone or polyglyconate suture, then close the muscle and the skin in two layers (Sladky and Clarke 2016).

Ovarian and testicular tumors are frequent in koi and gonadectomy has been reported as curative in various fish species (Weisse et al. 2002; Lewisch et al. 2014). Some of these gonadal tumors become locally invasive in the coelomic cavity and surgical excision is not possible.

Cesarean section may be performed in ovoviviparous species with fry retention, or in viviparous species with dystocia. Surgery should be attempted before the dam is too debilitated. In teleosts, incise the coelomic cavity on ventral midline from the anus caudally to the pelvic symphysis cranially and locate the pouches internally on each side of the coelom. Place stay sutures in the gravid pouch and elevate it from the rest of the coelom. Make an incision with scissors where the tail of a fry is visible and exteriorize the fry through the incision. Other fry in the same pouch can be gently manually expressed through the same incision. Close each incubation pouch with a simple continuous pattern or a continuous inverting pattern using absorbable suture. If possible, remove air trapped in the incubation pouches prior to closure of the coelom, otherwise, the fish may be positively buoyant postoperatively.

In batoids species, position the fish in ventral recumbency and make a longitudinal incision 2 cm lateral to the lumbar muscles, similar to the approach used for ovariectomy. Enter the coelomic cavity after elevating the peritoneum. Locate the uterus and incise its wall, paying attention not to contaminate the coelomic cavity with uterine contents including the embryonic histotroph. After removing the young from the uterus and handing it to a team dedicated to young recovery, close the uterus in two layers with a continuous inverting suture pattern using monofilament suture. Lavage the coelomic cavity before routine closure (Sladky and Clarke 2016).

Urinary Surgery

Renal biopsies are performed in fish to obtain cultures from the posterior kidney in fish with a systemic infection or to investigate renal disease. For instance, a renal biopsy would be indicated to investigate a renal mass displacing the swim bladder ventrally on radiographs (Figure 5.19): this can be due to polycystic kidney disease in goldfish. To access the posterior kidney, make a paramedian coelomic incision midway between the lateral line and pelvic fin. Retract the gonads and the digestive tract. Gently dissect the swim bladder away from the kidney (Harms and Wildgoose 2001). Obtain a wedge biopsy of the underlying kidney. Possible complications include hemorrhage and nephrocalcinosis at the site of biopsy (Harms and Wildgoose 2001).

(a)

(b)

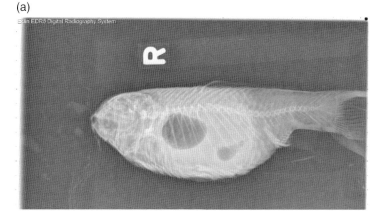

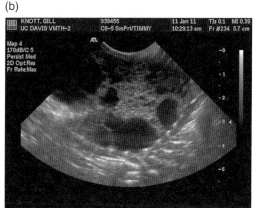

Figure 5.19 Whole body right lateral radiograph (a) and ultrasound image (b) from a goldfish (*Carassius auratus*) presenting with a cystic renal mass displacing the caudal chamber of the swim bladder ventrally. *Source:* Photo courtesy: Companion Avian and Exotic Pet Medicine Service, University of California, Davis.

Some fish species have a urinary bladder and calcium phosphate uroliths have been reported (Osborne et al. 2009). The removal of bladder stones from a bridled burrfish (*Chilomycterus antennatus*) by Howard Krum, Veterinary Medicine Doctor, aired during a Public Broadcasting Service of Scientific America in 1998.

Digestive Tract Surgery

Gastrointestinal foreign bodies have been reported in various fish species (Clark 1988; Lecu et al. 2011; Lloyd and Lloyd 2011) and are a common finding in captive and wild sharks (Lloyd and Lloyd 2011). When foreign body removal manually per *os* or via endoscopy is not possible, gastrotomy or enterotomy is performed. Depending on the fish species and location of the foreign body, use a ventral midline approach cranial to the pectoral fins or between the pectoral and anal fins (Lloyd and Lloyd 2011). Gently exteriorize the intestine (Figure 5.20) and place stay sutures. Digestive tract layers are the same as those of terrestrial vertebrates (Dos Santos et al. 2015). Make a full thickness enterotomy as close as possible to the object in a relatively healthy segment. Multiple foreign objects can often be removed through one enterotomy. If vascular integrity of the digestive segment has been compromised, a resection and anastomosis should be performed, if possible (Sladky and Clarke 2016). In large fish, close the digestive tract in two layers with a monofilament absorbable suture material (Lloyd and Lloyd 2011). Close the second layer using an inverting or simple continuous suture pattern. In smaller fish, use a single inverting suture pattern taking care to include all layers. Lavage the coelomic cavity with sterile saline and then use sterile instruments to close the coelomic wall.

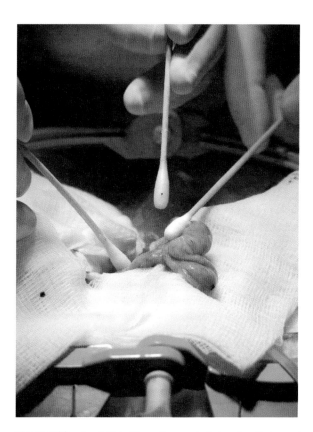

Figure 5.20 A goldfish (*Carassius auratus*) showing its impacted intestine exteriorized from the coelom and placed on wet gauze. *Source:* Photo courtesy: Zoological Medicine Service, Université de Montréal.

Minimally Invasive Surgery

Endoscopy has been described in catfish (*Ictalurus punctatus*) (Boone et al. 2008), trout (*Oncorhynchus mykiss*) (Moccia et al. 1984), wolf fish (*Hoplias aimara*)

(Weber 2011b), eel (*Anguilla Anguilla*) (Macri et al. 2014), and sturgeon (Hernandez-Divers et al. 2004; Divers et al. 2013; Falahatkar and Poursaeid 2014) among others, to determine sex, evaluate coelomic organs, remove ingested foreign bodies, and obtain biopsies (Boone et al. 2008; Stetter 2010; Divers et al. 2013). Celioscopy may be performed with the endoscope inserted directly into the coelomic cavity or within the swim bladder (Stetter 2010; Stevens et al. 2019). Deflation of the swim bladder may facilitate coelomic organ visualization depending on the species and procedure performed (Hernandez-Divers et al. 2004). Celioscopy has been used to perform minimally invasive surgical procedures in fish, such as gastrointestinal foreign body removal, organ biopsy, (Stetter 2010; Weber 2011b), and gonadectomy (Hernandez-Divers et al. 2004).

Telemetry and Microchip Implantation

Sonic or radio transmitters weighing less than 2% of the fish body weight may be implanted in free-ranging fish and because of the absence of antenna, a small celiotomy is used (Harms and Wildgoose 2001). More recently, injectable sonic transmitters that do not require surgical implantation have become available (Deng et al. 2015). Radiotelemetry transmitters are implanted with a similar technique as in other vertebrates (Wargo Rub et al. 2014). The antenna should exit through another incision rather than the incision used for insertion. It can be threaded through a cannula placed through the lateral body wall. To position the transmitter away from the surgical incision and avoid pressure on the coelomic organs, suture the transmitter to the pectoral girdle (Snelderwaard et al. 2006).

References

Adamovicz, L., Lewbart, G., and Gilger, B. (2015). Phacoemulsification and aspiration for cataract management in a dollar sunfish, *Lepomis marginatus* (Holbrook) – a case report. *Journal of Fish Diseases* 38: 1089–1092.

Andrews, M., Stormoen, M., Schmidt-Postahaus, H. et al. (2015). Rapid temperature-dependent wound closure following adipose fin clipping of Atlantic salmon *Salmo salar* L. *Journal of Fish Diseases* 38: 523–531.

Ang, J., Pierezan, F., Kim, S. et al. (2021). Use of topical treatments and effects of water temperature on wound healing in common carp (*Cyprinus carpio*). *Journal of Zoo and Wildlife Medicine* 52 (1): 103–116.

Angelidis, P., Vatsos, I., and Karagiannis, D. (2006). Surgical excision of skin folds from the head of a goldfish *Carassius auratus* (Linnaeus 1758). *Journal of the Hellenic Veterinary Medical Society* 58: 299.

Bakal, R.S., Love, N.E., Lewbart, G.A., and Berry, C.R. (1998). Imaging a spinal fracture in a Kohaku koi (*Cyprinus carpio*): techniques and case history report. *Veterinary Radiology & Ultrasound* 39: 318–321.

Bakal, R.S., Hickson, B.H., Gilger, B.C. et al. (2005). Surgical removal of cataracts due to Diplostomum species in Gulf sturgeon (*Acipenser oxyrinchus desotoi*). *Journal of Zoo and Wildlife Medicine* 36: 504–508.

Baker, T.R., Baker, B.B., Johnson, S.M., and Sladky, K.K. (2013). Comparative analgesic efficacy of morphine sulfate and butorphanol tartrate in koi (*Cyprinus carpio*) undergoing unilateral gonadectomy. *Journal of the American Veterinary Medical Association* 243: 882–890.

Baldursson, B.T., Kjartansson, H., Konradsdottir, F. et al. (2015). Healing rate and autoimmune safety of full-thickness wounds treated with fish skin acellular dermal matrix versus porcine small-intestine submucosa: a noninferiority study. *International Journal of Lower Extremity Wounds* 14: 37–43.

Benhamed, S., Guardiola, F.A., Mars, M., and Esteban, M.A. (2014). Pathogen bacteria adhesion to skin mucus of fishes. *Veterinary Microbiology* 171: 1–12.

Boerner, L., Weber, E.S., and Adams, L. (2000). Squamous cell carcinoma in a kannume (*Mormyrus kannume*). *Proceedings of the 33rd International Association of Aquatic Animal Medicine Annual Conference*, Albufeira, Portugal, p. 57.

Boerner, L., Dube, K., Peterson, K. et al. (2003). Angiogenic growth factor therapy using recombinant platelet-derived growth factor (Regranex) for lateral line disease in marine fish. *Proceedings of the International Association of Aquatic Animal Medicine*, Kohala Coast of Hawaii.

Boone, S.S., Hernandez-Divers, S.J., Radlinsky, M.G. et al. (2008). Comparison between coelioscopy and coeliotomy for liver biopsy in channel catfish. *Journal of the American Veterinary Medical Association* 233: 960–967.

Boylan, S.M., Camus, A., Waltzek, T. et al. (2015). Liquid nitrogen cryotherapy for fibromas in tarpon, Megalops atlanticus, Valenciennes 1847, and neoplasia in lined sea horse, *Hippocampus erectus*, Perry 1810. *Journal of Fish Diseases* 38: 681–685.

Britt, T., Weisse, C., Weber, E.S. et al. (2002). Use of pneumocystoplasty for overinflation of the swim bladder in a goldfish. *Journal of the American Veterinary Medical Association* 221 (690–693): 645.

Burnside, B., Adler, R., and O'Connor, P. (1983). Retinomotor pigment migration in the teleost retinal pigment epithelium. *Invest Ophthalmol Vis Sci.* 24: 1–15.

Carr, A., Weber, E.P. III, Murphy, C.J., and Zwingenberger, A. (2014). Computed tomographic and cross-sectional anatomy of the normal pacu (*Colossoma macroponum*). *Journal of Zoo and Wildlife Medicine* 45: 184–189.

Chanet, B., Fusellier, M., Baudet, J. et al. (2009). No need to open the jar: a comparative study of Magnetic Resonance Imaging results on fresh and alcohol preserved common carps (*Cyprinus carpio* (L. 1758), Cyprinidae, Teleostei). *Comptes Rendes Biologies* 332: 413–419.

Clark, P.J. (1988). Oral obstruction in a goldfish. *Veterinary Record* 122: 311.

Colombo, R.E., Wills, P.S., and Garvey, J.E. (2004). Use of ultrasound imaging to determine sex of shovelnose sturgeon. *North American Journal of Fisheries Management* 24: 322–326.

Copeland, D.E. and Brown, D.S. (1976). The anatomy and fine structure of the eye in teleosts. V. Vascular relations of choriocapillaris, lentiform body and falciform process in rainbow trout (*Salmo gairdneri*). *Experimental Eye Research* 23 (1): 15–27.

Coutant, T., Lair, S., and Vergneau-Grosset, C. (2019). Effect of a misoprostol/phenytoin gel on experimentally induced wounds in brook trout (Salvelinus frontinalis)– a preliminary study. *Journal of Aquatic Animal Health* 31: 214–221.

Da Silva, E.G., Gionfriddo, J.R., Powell, C.C. et al. (2010). Iridociliary melanoma with secondary lens luxation: distinctive findings in a long-horned cowfish (*Lactoria cornuta*). *Veterinary Ophthalmology* 13 (Suppl 1): 123–127.

Davis, M.R., Myliniczenko, N., Storms, T. et al. (2006). Evaluation of intramuscular ketoprofen and butorphanol as analgesics in chain dogfish (*Scyliorhinus retifer*). *Zoo Biology* 25: 491–500.

Deng, Z.D., Carlson, T.J., Li, H. et al. (2015). An injectable acoustic transmitter for juvenile salmon. *Scientific Reports* 5: 8111.

Divers, S.J., Boone, S.S., Berliner, A. et al. (2013). Nonlethal acquisition of large liver samples from free-ranging river sturgeon (*Scaphirhynchus*) using single-entry endoscopic biopsy forceps. *Journal of Wildlife Diseases* 49: 321–331.

Dos Santos, M., Arantes, F., Santiago, K., and Dos Santos, J. (2015). Morphological characteristics of the digestive tract of *Schizodon knerii* (Steindachner, 1875), (Characiformes: Anostomidae): an anatomical, histological and histochemical study. *Anais da Academia Brasileira de Ciencias* 87: 867–878.

Duke-Elder, S. (1958). *System of ophthalmology*. Vol., vol. I. London: The eye in evolution. Henry Kimpton.

Falahatkar, B. and Poursaeid, S. (2014). Gender identification in great sturgeon (*Huso huso*) using morphology, sex steroids, histology and endoscopy. *Anatomia Histologia and Embryologia* 43: 81–89.

Fleming, G.J., Corwin, A., McCoy, A.J., and Stamper, M.A. (2008). Treatment factors influencing the use of recombinant platelet-derived growth factor (Regranex) for head and lateral line erosion syndrome in ocean surgeonfish (*Acanthurus bahianus*). *Journal of Zoo and Wildlife Medicine* 39: 155–160.

Francis-Floyd, R., Bolon, B., Fraser, W., and Reed, P. (1993). Lip fibromas associated with retrovirus-like particles in angel fish. *Journal of the American Veterinary Medical Association* 202: 427–429.

Fredholm, D.V., Mylniczenko, N.D., and Kukanich, B. (2016). Pharmacokinetic evaluation of meloxicam after intravenous and intramuscular administration in nile tilapia (*Oreochromis niloticus*). *Journal of Zoo and Wildlife Medicine* 47: 736–742.

Govett, P.D., Olby, N.J., Marcellin-Little, D.J. et al. (2004). Stabilisation of scoliosis in two koi (*Cyprinus carpio*). *Veterinary Record* 155: 115–119.

Grant, K.R., Campbell, T.W., Silver, T.I., and Olea-Popelka, F.J. (2013). Validation of an ultrasound-guided technique to establish a liver-to-coelom ratio and a comparative analysis of the ratios among acclimated and recently wild-caught southern stingrays, *Dasyatis americana*. *Zoo Biology* 32: 104–111.

Grondel, J.L., Nouws, J.F., and Haenen, O.L. (1986). Fish and antibiotics: pharmacokinetics of sulphadimidine in carp (*Cyprinus carpio*). *Veterinary Immunology and Immunopathology* 12: 281–286.

Grosset, C., Weber, E.S. III, Gehring, R. et al. (2015). Evaluation of an extended-release formulation of ceftiofur crystalline-free acid in koi (*Cyprinus carpio*). *Journal of Veterinary Pharmacology and Therapeutics* 38: 606–616.

Gruber, S.H. (1977). The visual system of sharks: adaptations and capability. *American Zoology* 17: 453–469.

Guardiola, F.A., Cuesta, A., Abellan, E. et al. (2014). Comparative analysis of the humoral immunity of skin mucus from several marine teleost fish. *Fish & Shellfish Immunology* 40: 24–31.

Gustavsen, K.A., Paul-Murphy, J., Weber, E.S. III et al. (2018). Ocular anatomy of the black pacu (*Colossoma macropomum*): gross, histologic and diagnostic imaging. *Veterinary Ophthalmology* 21 (5): 507–515.

Hadfield, C.A., Haines, A.N., Clayton, L.A., and Whitaker, B.R. (2010). Cross matching of blood in carcharhiniform, lamniform, and orectolobiform sharks. *Journal of Zoo and Wildlife Medicine* 41: 480–486.

Harder, W. (1975). *Anatomie der Fische*. Stuttgart: Schweizerbart'sch Verlagsbuchhandlung.

Harms, C.A. and Wildgoose, W. (2001). Surgery. In: *BSAVA Manual of Ornamental Fish*, Chapter 31, 2e (ed. W. Wildgoose), 159–266. Quedgeley: British Small Animal Veterinary Association.

Harms, C.A., Lewbart, G.A., Swanson, C.R. et al. (2005). Behavioral and clinical pathology changes in koi carp (*Cyprinus carpio*) subjected to anesthesia and surgery with and without intra-operative analgesics. *Comparative Medicine* 55: 221–226.

Harms, C.A., Christian, L.S., Burrus, O. et al. (2008). Cryotherapy for removal of a premaxillary mass from a chain pickerel using an over-the-counter wart remover. *Exotic DVM* 10: 15–17.

Health Canada (2010). List of veterinary drugs that are authorized for sale by Health Canada for use in food-producing aquatic animals.

Henningsen, A., Smale, M., Garner, R., and Kinnunen, N. (2004). Reproduction, embryonic development, and reproductive physiology of Elasmobranchs. In: *Elasmobranch Husbandry Manual: Captive Care of Sharks, Rays, and their Relatives*, Chapter 16 (eds. M. Smith, D. Warmolts, D. Thoney and R. Hueter), 227–236. Columbus, OH: Ohio Biological Survey.

Hernandez-Divers, S.J., Bakal, R.S., Hickson, B.H. et al. (2004). Endoscopic sex determination and gonadal manipulation in Gulf of Mexico sturgeon (*Acipenser oxyrinchus desotoi*). *Journal of Zoo and Wildlife Medicine* 35: 459–470.

Hill, J.E., Kilgore, K.H., Pouder, D.B. et al. (2009). Survey of Ovaprim use as a spawning aid in ornamental fishes in the United States as administered through the University of Florida Tropical Aquaculture Laboratory. *North American Journal of Aquaculture* 71: 206–209.

Jafarey, Y.S., Berlinski, R.A., Hanley, C.S. et al. (2015). Presumptive dysgerminoma in an orange-spot freshwater stingray (*Potamotrygon motoro*). *Journal of Zoo and Wildlife Medicine* 46: 382–385.

Kern, T. (2007). Exotic animal ophthalmology. In: *Veterinary Ophthalmology*, Chapter 28, 4e (ed. K. Gelatt), 1370–1405. Blackwell Publishing.

Kizer, A. and Novo, R.E. (2003). Ovariectomy in rainbow trout for prevention of postovulatory stasis. *Exotic DVM* 5: 27–30.

Lair, S., Santamaria-Bouvier, A., and Marvin, J. (2014). Clusters of retinoblastoma-like neoplasms in a group of aquarium-housed striped basses (*Morone saxatilis*). *Proceedings of the 45th International Association for Aquatic Animal Medicine Annual Conference*, Gold Coast, Australia.

Larouche, C.B., Limoges, M.-J., and Lair, S. (2018). Absence of acute toxicity of a single intramuscular injection of meloxicam in goldfish (*Carassius auratus auratus*): a randomized controlled trial. *Journal of Zoo and Wildlife Medicine* 49 (3): 617–622.

Lecu, A. and Lecour, F. (2004). Teeth trimming in tetraodontidae fish. *Exotic DVM* 6: 33–36.

Lecu, A., Herbert, R., Coulier, L., and Murray, M.J. (2011). Removal of an intracoelomic hook via laparotomy in a sandbar shark (*Carcharhinus plumbeus*). *Journal of Zoo and Wildlife Medicine* 42: 256–262.

Lee, R.T., Thiery, J.P., and Carney, T.J. (2013). Dermal fin rays and scales derive from mesoderm, not neural crest. *Current Biology* 23: R336–R337.

Lewbart, G.A., Stone, E.A., and Love, N.E. (1995). Pneumocystectomy in a Midas cichlid. *Journal of the American Veterinary Medical Association* 207: 319–321.

Lewbart, G., Vaden, S., Deen, J. et al. (1997). Pharmacokinetics of enrofloxacin in the red pacu (*Colossoma brachypomum*) after intramuscular, oral and bath administration. *Journal of Veterinary Pharmacology and Therapeutics* 20: 124–128.

Lewisch, E., Reifinger, M., Schmidt, P., and El-Matbouli, M. (2014). Ovarian tumor in a koi carp (*Cyprinus carpio*): diagnosis, surgery, postoperative care and tumour classification. *Tierarztliche Praxis Ausgabe K Kleintiere Heimtiere* 42: 257–262.

Lloyd, R. and Lloyd, C. (2011). Surgical removal of a gastric foreign body in a sand tiger shark, *Carcharias taurus* Rafinesque. *Journal of Fish Diseases* 34: 951–953.

Lloyd, R. and Sham, N. (2014). Surgical repair of mandibular symphyseal fractures in three silver arowana (*Osteoglossum bicirrhosum*) using interfragmentary wire. *Journal of Zoo and Wildlife Medicine* 45: 926–930.

Love, N.E. and Lewbart, G.A. (1997). Pet fish radiography: technique and case history reports. *Veterinary Radiology & Ultrasound* 38: 24–29.

Lovy, J., Speare, D.J., and Wright, G.M. (2007). Pathological effects caused by chronic treatment of rainbow trout with indomethacin. *Journal of Aquatic Animal Health* 19: 94–98.

Macri, F., Rapisarda, G., De Stefano, C. et al. (2014). Coelioscopic investigation in European eels (*Anguilla anguilla*). *Journal of Exotic Pet Medicine* 23: 147–151.

McCune, A.R. and Carlson, R.L. (2004). Twenty ways to lose your bladder: common natural mutants in zebrafish and widespread convergence of swim bladder loss among teleost fishes. *Evolution & Development* 6: 246–259.

Mettam, J., Oulton, L., McCrohan, C., and Sneddon, L. (2011). The efficacy of three types of analgesic drugs in reducing pain in the rainbow trout, *Oncorhynchus mykiss*. *Applied Animal Behavioral Science* 133: 265–274.

Moccia, R.D., Wilkie, E.J., Munkittrick, K.R., and Thompson, W.D. (1984). The use of fine needle fibre endoscopy in fish for in vivo examination of visceral organs, with special reference to ovarian evaluation. *Aquaculture* 40: 255–259.

Muir Evans, H. (1925). A contribution to the anatomy and physiology of the air-bladder and Weberian ossicles in the cyprinidae. *Proceedings of the Royal Society B* 97: 545–576.

Mylniczenko, N.D., Harris, B., Wilborn, R.E., and Young, F.A. (2007). Blood culture results from healthy captive and free-ranging elasmobranchs. *Journal of Aquatic Animal Health* 19: 159–167.

Mylniczenko, N., Neiffer, D., and Clauss, T.M. (2014). Bony fish (lungfish, surgeon, and teleosts). In: *Zoo Animal and Wildlife Immobilization and Anesthesia*, 2e (eds. G. West, D. Heard and N. Caulkett), 209–260. Ames, IO: Wiley Blackwell.

Nadelstein, B., Bakal, R., and Lewbart, G.A. (1997). Orbital exenteration and placement of a prosthesis in fish. *Journal of the American Veterinary Medical Association* 211: 603–606.

Nematollahi, A., Bigham, A.S., Karimi, I., and Abbasi, F. (2010). Reactions of goldfish (*Carassius auratus*) to three suture patterns following full thickness skin incisions. *Research in Veterinary Science* 89: 451–454.

Nordgreen, J., Kolsrud, H. H., Ranheim B., and Horsberg, T.E. (2009). Pharmacokinetics of morphine after intramuscular injection in common goldfish Carassius auratus and Atlantic salmon Salmo salar. *Diseases of Aquatic Organisms* 88(1): 55–63.

Nouws, J.F., Grondel, J.L., Schutte, A.R., and Laurensen, J. (1988). Pharmacokinetics of ciprofloxacin in carp, African catfish and rainbow trout. *Veterinary Quarterly* 10: 211–216.

Ochandio, B., Bechara, I., and Parise-Maltempi, P. (2015). Dexamethasone action on caudal fin regeneration of carp *Cyprinus carpio* (Linnaeus, 1758). *Brazilian Journal of Biology* 75: 442–450.

Osborne, C.A., Albasan, H., Lulich, J.P. et al. (2009). Quantitative analysis of 4468 uroliths retrieved from farm animals, exotic species, and wildlife submitted to the Minnesota Urolith Center: 1981 to 2007. *Veterinary Clinics of North America: Small Animal Practice* 39: 65–78.

Pees, M., Pees, K., and Kiefer, I. (2010). The use of computed tomography for assessment of the swim bladder in koi carp (*Cyprinus carpio*). *Veterinary Radiology & Ultrasound* 51: 294–298.

Pilgrim, B.L. and Franz-Odendaal, T.A. (2009). A comparative study of the ocular skeleton of fossil and modern chondrichthyans. *Journal of Anatomy* 214 (6): 848–858.

Raidal, S.R., Shearer, P.L., Stephens, F., and Richardson, J. (2006). Surgical removal of an ovarian tumour in a koi carp (*Cyprinus carpio*). *Australian Veterinary Journal* 84: 178–181.

Rapanan, J.L., Pascual, A.S., Uppalapati, C.K. et al. (2015). Zebrafish keratocyte explants to study collective cell migration and reepithelialization in cutaneous wound healing. *Journal of Visualized Experiments* 96 https://doi.org/10.3791/52489.

Schwaiger, J., Ferling, H., Mallow, U. et al. (2004). Toxic effects of the non-steroidal anti-inflammatory drug diclofenac. Part I: histopathological alterations and bioaccumulation in rainbow trout. *Aquatic Toxicology* 68: 141–150.

Schwarz, T., Weber, E.S., Weisse, C., and Klide, A.M. (2002). Advanced imaging in selected fish patients with coelomic swelling. *Proceedings in Veterinary Radiology and Ultrasound*: 59.

Shin, S.P., Jee, H., Han, J.E. et al. (2011). Surgical removal of an anal cyst caused by a protozoan parasite (*Thelohanellus kitauei*) from a koi (*Cyprinus carpio*). *Journal of the American Veterinary Medical Association* 238: 784–786.

Sladky, K.K. and Clarke, E.O.I. (2016). Fish surgery. *Veterinary Clinics of North America: Exotic Animal Practice* 19: 55–76.

Snelderwaard, P., Van Ginneken, V., Witte, F. et al. (2006). Surgical procedure for implanting a radiotelemetry transmitter to monitor ECG, heart rate and body temperature in small *Carassius auratus* and *Carassius auratus gibelio* under laboratory conditions. *Laboratory Animals* 40: 465–468.

Stamper, M.A. and Norton, T. (2002). Ovariectomy in a brook trout (*Salvelinus fontinalis*). *Journal of Zoo and Wildlife Medicine* 33: 172–175.

Stetter, M.D. (2010). Minimally invasive surgical techniques in bony fish (osteichthyes). *Veterinary Clinics of North America: Exotic Animal Practice* 13: 291–299.

Stevens, B. N., Vergneau-Grosset, C., Rodriguez Jr., C. O., et al. (2017) Treatment of a facial myxoma in a goldfish (Carassius auratus) with intralesional bleomycin chemotherapy and radiation therapy. *Journal of Exotic Pet Medicine* 26(4): 283–289.

Stevens, B.N., Guzman, D.S., Phillips, K.L. et al. (2019). Evaluation of diagnostic coelioscopy in koi (*Cyprinus carpio*). *American journal of Veterinary Research* 80 (3): 221–229.

Stoskopf, M.K. and Posner, L.P. (2014). Anesthesia and restraint of laboratory fish. In: *Anesthesia and Analgesia in Laboratory Animals*, Chapter 21 (eds. R.E. Fish, P. Danneman, M. Brown and A. Karas), 519–534. San Diego, CA: American College of Laboratory Animal Medicine Series.

Tell, L., Oeller, M., and Craigmill, A.L. (2012). Consideration for treating minor food-producing animals with veterinary pharmaceuticals. In: *Veterinary Pharmacology and Therapeutics*, Chapter 52, 9e (eds. J.E. Riviere and M.G. Papich), 1331–1342. Ames, IO: Wiley Blackwell.

Vergneau-Grosset, C., Summa, N., Rodriguez Jr., C. O., Cenani, A., et al. (2016) Excision and subsequent treatment of a leiomyoma from the periventiduct of a koi (*Cyprinus carpio koi*), *Journal of Exotic Pet Medicine* 25(3), 194–202.

Walsh, M.T., Pipers, F.S., Brendemuehl, C.A., and Murru, F.L. (1993). Ultrasonography as a diagnostic tool in shark species. *Veterinary Radiology & Ultrasound* 34: 213–218.

Ward, J., McCartney, S., Chinnadurai, S., and Posner, L.P. (2012). Development of a minimum-anesthetic-concentration depression model to study the effects of various analgesics in goldfish (*Carassius auratus*). *Journal of Zoo and Wildlife Medicine* 43: 214–222.

Wargo Rub, A.M., Jepsen, N., Liedtke, T.L. et al. (2014). Surgical tagging and telemetry methods in fisheries research: promoting veterinary and research collaboration. *American Journal of Veterinary Research* 75: 402–416.

Weber, E.S.P. III (2011a). Fish analgesia: pain, stress, fear aversion, or nociception? *Veterinary Clinics North America: Exotic Animal Practice* 14: 21–32.

Weber, E.S.P. III (2011b). Non-lethal diagnostic and surgical procedures for fish patients. In: *Bridging America and Russia with Shared Perspectives on Aquatic Animal Health* (eds. R.C. Cipriano, A.W. Bruckner and I.S. Shchelkunov), 309–319. East Lansing, MI: Michigan State University.

Weber, E.S.P. III (2013). Itchy fish and viral dermatopathies: sampling, diagnosis, and management of common viral diseases. *Veterinary Clinics of North America: Exotic Animal Practice* 16: 687–703.

Weber, E.S.P. III, Weisse, C., Schwartz, T. et al. (2009). Anesthesia, diagnostic imaging, and surgery of fish. *Compendium Continuing Education for Veterinarians* 31: E1–E9.

Weisse, C., Weber, E.S., Matzkin, Z., and A, K. (2002). Surgical removal of a seminoma from a black sea bass. *Journal of the American Veterinary Medical Association* 22: 280–283.

Whitaker, B.R. (1999). Surgical procedures for fishes and amphibians. *Exotic DVM* 1: 63–70.

Whiteside, D. (2014). Analgesia. In: *Zoo Animal and Wildlife Immobilization and Anesthesia*, 2e (eds. G. West, D. Heard and N. Caulkett), 83–108. Ames, IO: Wiley Blackwell.

Wildgoose, W. (2000). Fish surgery: an overview. *Fish Veterinary Journal* 5: 22–36.

Wildgoose, W. (2007a). Buoyancy disorders of ornamental fish: a review of cases seen in veterinary practice. *Fish Veterinary Journal* 9: 22–37.

Wildgoose, W. (2007b). Exenteration in fish. *Exotic DVM* 9: 27–28.

Yanong, R.P.E., Curtis, E.W., Simmons, R. et al. (2011). Pharmacokinetic studies of florfenicol in koi sarp and threespot gourami *Trichogaster trichopterus* after oral and intramuscular treatment. *Journal of Aquatic Animal Health* 17: 129–137.

Yanwirsal, H. (2013). Reproductive styles of osteoglossomorpha with emphasis on *Notopterus notopterus* and *Osteoglossum bicirrhosum*. Doctor rerum agriculturarum. Humboldt University.

Zebedin, A. and Ladich, F. (2013). Does the hearing sensitivity in thorny catfishes depend on swim bladder morphology? *PLoS ONE* 8: e67049.

6

Amphibian Surgery

Claire Vergneau-Grosset and E. Scott Weber, III

Introduction

Amphibians include three orders: the Anura (frogs and toads), Urodela (newts, salamanders, and axolotls), and Gymnophiona (includes legless caecilians). There is increasing concern for amphibians because many wild populations are dwindling, making them benefactors of numerous conservation efforts globally, and the continuing evolution of the human–animal bond for pet owners is creating demands for higher quality of veterinary practice for a greater variety of animals, including amphibians. Amphibian surgery follows the same general principles as surgery in other vertebrates: surgeons should minimize blood loss, perform gentle tissue handling, and aim for aseptic techniques whenever possible. Surgeons working with amphibians should be familiar with their unique and specific anatomy. Anatomic variability is an important consideration, and there are a number of references containing information pertaining to various amphibian species (Juan Hidalgo 1989; Helmer and Whiteside 2005; James-Zorn et al. 2013).

Perioperative and Postoperative Considerations

Amphibian surgery carries specific challenges including danger of skin desiccation, water-soluble toxins, skin trauma, ocular lesions, thermal burns, and hyper- or hypothermia (Wright and Whitaker 2001a). Amphibian skin should be kept moist and should be handled gently, as it is easily damaged (Figure 6.1) and also to prevent dermatitis, xerophthalmia, and secondary osmotic imbalances (Mylniczenko 2006; Clayton and Mylniczenko 2015). Because amphibian mucus is critical for the skin's innate immunity, limit preparation of the surgical site to avoid disrupting the natural mucous layer (Green 2010; Ramsey et al. 2010; Shigeri et al. 2015). Gently flush the skin with sterile saline or 0.05% chlorhexidine solution rather than aggressive surgical scrubbing and avoid alcohol-based disinfectants (Poll 2009). Irrigate exposed skin with fresh chlorine-free and chloramine-free water throughout the surgery to avoid desiccation (Poll 2009). As a result of minimal surgical site preparation and because of the necessity for water containing appropriate electrolytes, and of the same water quality parameters as in the exhibit, achieving asepsis is challenging. Place patients over a moist nonabrasive surface such as plastic (Wright and Whitaker 2001a), a sponge covered by a plastic drape, bubble wrap, or the underside of a disposable absorbent pad. The use of towel quarter drapes is controversial in amphibians as using dry surgical drapes may disrupt the beneficial mucous coat and wet towel drapes quickly become permeable to bacteria (Green 2010). Plastic drapes are recommended and surgical procedures performed without drapes are acceptable for many Institutional Animal Care and Use Committee (IACUC) approved protocols (Green 2010). Avoid contact between the skin and the surgical drape's adhesive surface. To keep the drape in place, use sutures or very fine staples to protect the delicate skin. For short procedures, a safe surgical water-soluble lubricant can be used to hold the drape in place. Surgical lighting can be damaging because of the heat and light intensity from proximal lighting sources leading to desiccation and thermal burns causing ocular and skin lesions. Light-emitting diodes (LEDs), as commonly installed on surgical loupes, should be used to minimize these effects.

Temperature should be kept within the preferred optimal temperature zone (POTZ) of the species throughout the procedure. Like reptiles, amphibians are poikilothermic, but they rarely need supplemental heat due to their lower POTZ. It is better to keep a low room temperature and to place sealed ice packs in the water to cool it.

When handling amphibians with toxin-producing glands, the surgeon may need to wear protective eye wear as *Bufo* spp. can expel toxic parotidian secretions into the air

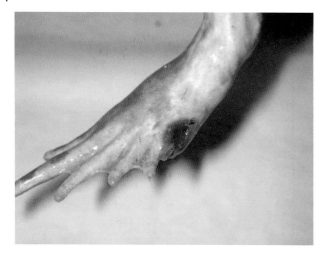

Figure 6.1 A wound on the lateral aspect of the tarsus in a laboratory African clawed frog (*Xenopus laevis*) showing granulation tissue and formation of scar tissue around the outer edge of the lesion. *Source:* Photo courtesy: Companion Avian and Exotic Pet Medicine Service, University of California, Davis.

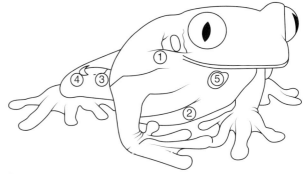

① Facial vein
② Ventral abdominal vein
③ Femoral vein
④ Plexus caudal to the stifle
⑤ Cardiocenthesis

Figure 6.2 Possible intravenous injection sites in amphibians. *Source:* Delphine Grosset, Visual Conception Communication Creator.

(Wright 2006). The choice of gloves is important as many compounds are absorbed through amphibian skin. Gloves with talcum powder should be avoided (Wright 2006). Latex is toxic to tadpoles of some amphibian species, including common frogs (*Rana temporaria*) and African clawed frogs (*Xenopus laevis*) and may result in acute mortalities (Sobotka and Rahwan 1994; Gutleb et al. 2001). Nitrile gloves have been shown to kill chytrid fungi zoospores that can infect amphibian patients, while polyethylene gloves did not (Mendez et al. 2008). Powderless vinyl gloves are preferred by many practitioners (Norton et al. 2014).

Like in other animals, perioperative antibiotics (Wright and Whitaker 2001a) and antinociception (Weber 2011) have been advocated. Antibiotics with a spectrum oriented toward Gram-negative bacteria are preferred given the predominance of Gram-negative bacteria in amphibian flora (Roth et al. 2013). Depending on the amphibian species, intravenous injections may be performed using the femoral vein, musculocutaneous vein (Sancho et al. 2012), popliteal plexus, ventral abdominal vein, or lingual venous plexus in frogs larger than 25 g (Whitaker and Wright 2001) (Figure 6.2). Alternatively, preoperative antibiotics may be administered topically (ciprofloxacin 10 mg/kg; Wright and Whitaker 2001b), subcutaneously (enrofloxacin 10 mg/kg; Wright and Whitaker 2001b) or intramuscularly (amikacin 5 mg/kg: Felt et al. 2013), or into the dorsal lymphatic sacs that are paired sacs accessible dorsally on each side of the urostyle.

Amphibian opioid receptors are similar to those of mammals (Newman et al. 2002). Amphibians appear to require higher doses of opioids to produce antinociception when compared to rodents (Koeller 2009). Opioid dosages up to hundred times the minimal dose have been reported for northern

leopard frogs (Stevens 2011). Recommended opioid dosages need to be refined in amphibians. The reader is referred to review chapters about amphibian anesthesia regarding monitoring and choice of anesthetic agents (Mitchell 2009; Braitman and Stetter 2014; O'Rourke and Jenkins 2014).

Anurans may be more resistant to the effects of hemorrhage than some mammals (Chai 2015a) due to lymph regulation and a powerful baroreceptor reflex (Hedrick et al. 2015) as long as they are maintained at their POTZ of the species (Zena et al. 2015). Hemostasis can be accomplished using techniques similar to those employed in mammals, and some authors have also recommended using cyanoacrylate tissue adhesive as an hemostatic agent for internal organs (Wright and Whitaker 2001a), but no study has investigated adverse effects associated with this technique.

Patients with skin sutures may be kept isolated in a tank with a nonabrasive substrate such as a moist plastic lining. In aquatic species, water quality should be carefully monitored during the postoperative period, especially in patients with incisional secretions that may increase nitrogenous wastes in the tank water. Skin sutures may be removed after about three weeks (Green 2010). Similar to other patients, nutritional support and postoperative antinociceptive drugs may be needed depending on the procedure performed (Gentz 2007).

Wound Healing

Epithelialization, wound contraction, and tissue remodeling takes place in amphibians similar to in mammals (Poll 2009). In immature amphibians, skin healing involves contraction and regeneration of the skin, while postmetamorphic amphibians will form scar tissue devoid of dermal mucous and granular glands (Yannas et al. 1996).

During the inflammatory phase of wound healing, wet-to-dry bandages are contraindicated in amphibians because they may result in desiccation of the tissue surrounding the wound (Poll 2009). During the proliferative phase, becaplermin (Regranex®, 0.01% gel, Ortho-McNeil Pharmaceutical Inc., Raritan, NJ, USA), recombinant human platelet-derived growth factor has been suggested to accelerate healing (Walker and Whitaker 2003; Poll 2009). Apply the gel to the wound for 60 seconds every three weeks (Fleming et al. 2008). Before applying the gel, irrigate the wound with saline to loosen external debris, necrotic skin and exudates. Gently debride the area until a small amount of hemorrhage is observed and then rinse the wound again before applying a thin layer of gel (Poll 2009). After a contact time of 60–120 seconds, rinse the gel off or leave it on the wound. The use of hydrogel has also been recommended to accelerate wound granulation (Poll 2009).

Skin Surgery

There are a number of indications for skin biopsy. Perform a local anesthesia block with lidocaine 2 mg/kg and obtain the biopsy with a sterile punch biopsy instrument or scissors. Use hand-held electrocautery to achieve hemostasis, if needed. For skin closure, use a cutaneous everting pattern (Figure 6.3), appositional sutures, and/or cyanoacrylate tissue adhesive (Tuttle et al. 2006; Gentz 2007; Van Bonn 2009; Baitchman and Herman 2015; Chai 2015a). Appositional

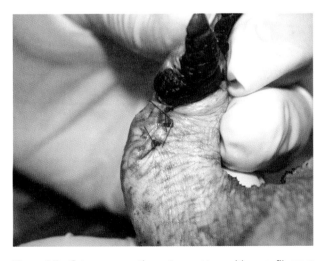

Figure 6.3 Cutaneous everting suture pattern with monofilament absorbable suture material on the right forelimb of a cane toad (*Bufo marinus*). *Source:* Photo courtesy: Zoological Medicine Service, Université de Montréal.

sutures are preferred by the authors. Take care to minimize suture tension as amphibian cutaneous tissue is less elastic than mammalian skin (Chai 2015a). This is not always possible when large margins are needed for excising neoplasms. To relieve tension, use silicone rubber tubing as stents on each side of the incision (Wright and Whitaker 2001a).

Cryosurgery and laser surgery have been used in amphibians for mass ablation (Wright and Whitaker 2001a). These modalities improve hemostasis, but do not enable histologic analysis of the mass. A protocol of three freeze-thaw cycles over 30 seconds for each phase using a thermocouple has been described. If cryosurgery is elected and histopathology is needed, first collect an incisional biopsy of the mass. Chemical cauterization, such as with formalin and metacresolsulfonic acid (Lotagen TM, Schering Plough Animal Health), has been used to remove cutaneous masses in amphibians (Chai 2015a); however, controlled studies are needed to evaluate tissue healing, adverse effects, and pain associated with this technique.

Orthopedic Surgery

Surgical stabilization is indicated for traumatic fractures as the moist environment precludes the use of bandages unless they are frequently assessed and changed. Bone healing is typically slower in amphibians than in mammals and reptiles (Pritchard and Ruzicka 1950). Cartilaginous union of the fracture fragments may appear after a month, but bony union may not occur until after 80 days, and callous remodeling may take more than seven months at the POTZ (Pritchard and Ruzicka 1950; Johnson 2003).

External fixators may be difficult to place in amphibians to achieve appropriate compression and alignment without movement due to the normal limb angulation as hind limbs are positioned in close contact with the body and other limb segments in the resting position and external fixators can cause cutaneous abrasions of the adjacent skin (Wright and Whitaker 2001a; Royal et al. 2007). Stabilization of tibiofibular fractures with type I external fixators has been reported (Johnson 2003). Insert at least two transcortical Kirschner wires on each side of the fracture. When using nonthreaded pins, vary the angle of insertion into the bone in case lateral traction is applied to the fixator. Form the connecting bar by bending the transcortical pins and joining them with epoxy putty in a ventrolateral plane compared to the tibiofibula. While bending the Kirschner wires, hold the insertion site of the pin with a wire twister applying counter pressure while bending the pin over with a second wire twister to avoid iatrogenic fracture of the bone.

Successful stabilization of a simple closed mid-diaphysis femoral fracture with an internal fixator has been reported

(Royal et al. 2007). Make a dorsolateral skin incision and dissect the underlying tissues with care to not damage the sciatic nerve. After approaching the fracture site, place at least two transcortical Kirschner wires on each side of the fracture. Place a threaded pin alongside the femur on its caudal surface and secure it to the femur with polyglyconate suture. Place cerclage wires as needed. Mold sterile polymethylmethacrylate (PMMA) over the threaded pin and the protruding transcortical pins to secure the apparatus. The PMMA device will remain internal and should not be too voluminous to close soft tissue without tension. Suture the muscular and cutaneous planes with monofilament suture. The advantage of this internal fixator is the amphibian can return in water quickly postoperatively.

A surgical technique to stabilize the stifle joint was performed in an American bullfrog (*Lithobates catesbeiana*) after a suspected cranial cruciate ligament tear (Van Bonn 2009). A tourniquet was applied at the level of the proximal femur to reduce the risk of hemorrhage. A curved incision was made over the craniomedial aspect of the stifle joint. Two extraarticular 3-0 monofilament nylon sutures were placed in a cruciate pattern along the cranial aspect of the joint capsule. The skin was closed with 5-0 monofilament nylon in a Ford interlocking pattern which was removed two weeks postoperatively. The joint remained stable with no complication.

A dorsal laminectomy was performed in a salamander to manage scoliosis (Waffa et al. 2012). Perform a 1.5 cm dorsal incision over the affected vertebrae. Use blunt and sharp dissection to expose dorsal spinous processes and laminae. Excise the dorsal laminae and facets with rongeurs. Lavage the surgical site with sterile saline. Place a hemostatic absorbable gelatin sponge (Gelfoam®, Pfizer, New York, NY) over the laminectomy site. Close the incision with subcutaneous and subcuticular suture patterns. Unfortunately, three weeks postoperatively, the patient self-mutilated caudal to the surgery site and was euthanized. Focal osteonecrosis and vertebral fractures at the laminectomy site were detected on post mortem examination. It is unknown whether the surgical technique or postoperative antinociceptive management should be modified to avoid this complication.

Mandibular fractures can be stabilized with external coaptation using bone cement, orthopedic wire, an external skeletal fixator or by gluing the mouth closed with tissue adhesive for species with limited gular respiration (Wright and Whitaker 2001a). Bilateral mandibular fractures may be stabilized more efficiently by gluing the mouth closed and placing a feeding tube to provide nutrition. Placing and maintaining a feeding tube can be challenging in small amphibian species (Wright and Whitaker 2001a), and the prognosis is guarded in most amphibians with mandibular fractures.

Larval forms and neotenic amphibians have the ability to regenerate limbs (Pearl et al. 2008; Aguilar and Gardiner 2015) and even the spinal cord after complete transection (Diaz Quiroz et al. 2014). Thus, surgery may not be indicated in cases of traumatic amputation (Baitchman and Herman 2015). Limb, toe, and tail amputations are frequently performed (Figures 6.4 and 6.5) (Pizzi and Miller 2005) especially for very comminuted, articular, infected, or pathologic fractures (Dombrowski et al. 2016). It is advisable to amputate the limb proximally by disarticulation of the humerus or at the proximal third of the femur, to avoid trauma to the stump (Wright and Whitaker 2001a). Place a tourniquet on the limb prior to amputation to reduce hemorrhage. Do not leave the tourniquet in place more than 15 minutes. Make a skin incision

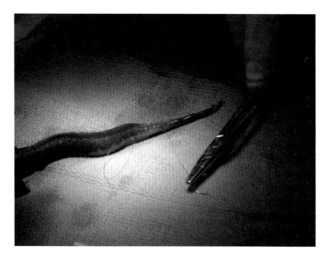

Figure 6.4 Amputation of the tip of the tail of a California newt (*Taricha torosa*). *Source:* Photo courtesy: Companion Avian and Exotic Pet Medicine Service, University of California, Davis.

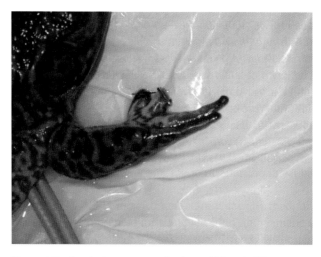

Figure 6.5 Surgical toe amputation in an African bullfrog (*Pyxicephalus adspersus*). *Source:* Photo courtesy: Companion Avian and Exotic Pet Medicine Service, University of California, Davis.

distal to the site of the planned bone transection to allow skin closure with limited tension. Prior to nerve transection, perform a local block with lidocaine and bupivacaine (Bainton and Strichartz 1994). Many newts and salamanders regenerate their limbs (Figure 6.6): the regenerated limb may contain a cartilaginous skeleton instead of bone and nerves regenerate with a resulting normal locomotion (Wright and Whitaker 2001a). Leave the stump open in these species as closure of the surgical site may prevent limb regeneration or result in abnormal regenerated tissue (Baitchman and Herman 2015).

As amphibians normally use their hind limbs during ecdysis, for nest building in females, and for amplexus in males, hind limb amputation may lead to dysecdysis and reproductive failures (Wright and Whitaker 2001a). Consequently, it is questioned whether amphibians should be released following permanent hind limb amputation.

Ophthalmic Surgery

Given the moist environment for aquatic amphibians, corneal ulcers can be difficult to treat as ophthalmic topical aqueous solutions and ointments are quickly diluted. Deep corneal ulcers may be treated with a tarsorrhaphy or with butyl cyanoacrylate tissue adhesive (Williams and Whitaker 1994). Tarsorrhaphy is performed in a similar manner as domestic animals.

Enucleation may be performed as a salvage procedure (Wright and Whitaker 2001a; Imai et al. 2009). Indications for enucleation are similar to those of other vertebrates and include nontreatable painful intraocular lesions and retro-orbital neoplasms or abscesses (Williams and Whitaker 1994).

Of note, amphibians have higher regenerative abilities than mammals and many anurans and newt are able to regenerate their retina while adult newts and African clawed frog tadpoles are able to regenerate their lenses (Filoni 2009). As a result, in patients with cataracts, removal of the lens allows the growth of a new transparent lens and retinal lesions that progress to permanent blindness in mammals may heal in amphibians. Temporary tarsorrhaphy may be performed to protect the cornea pending vision recovery.

In species that retract their globe during food swallowing, the globe is very mobile and a gauze should be placed in the mouth prior to ocular surgery (Chai 2016). After infusion of local anesthetic into the conjunctival tissue, incise the conjunctiva and dissect the extraocular muscles from the globe, which frees the globe from its attachments. Take care to not damage the tissue between the orbit and the oral cavity (Wright and Whitaker 2001a) and to not damage the facial vein (Forzan et al. 2012). Transect the optic nerve and vessels and control hemorrhage with pressure using a cotton-tipped applicator or by packing the orbit with a collagen sponge (OraPlug, Salvin, Charlotte, NC) or an absorbable gelatin hemostatic sponge. If using hemostats to clamp the retro-orbital vessels, avoid putting traction on the optic chiasm that would cause blindness in the contralateral eye. Tarsorrhaphy with nylon suture material is recommended in species with eyelids to facilitate hemostasis (Wright and Whitaker 2001a) (Figure 6.7). Second intention healing is also an option (Chai 2016).

Lens excision has been described in a milk frog (*Tachycephalus resinifictrix*) (Chai 2016). Make a two-step circumferential incision over 180° at the limbus with a

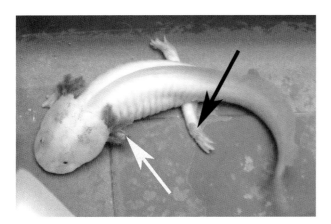

Figure 6.6 An albino axolotl (*Ambystoma mexicanum*) presented with a traumatic amputation of the left forelimb (white arrow) and multifocal bite wound on the tail and left hind limb (black arrow). The left forelimb traumatic wound is left open to allow limb regeneration. *Source:* Photo courtesy: Aquarium du Québec.

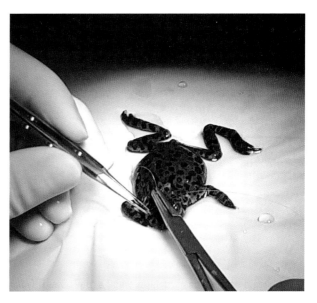

Figure 6.7 Enucleation of the right eye in an Oriental fire-bellied toad (Bombina orientalis). *Source:* Sepaq | Aquarium du Québec..

keratome with the first incision perpendicular to the globe and then a second deeper incision with a more pronounced angulation to prevent the cornea from collapsing. Inject viscoelastic medium in the anterior chamber. Retrieve the lens with a Snellen loop. Irrigate with saline. Suture the cornea in one layer with 9-0 nylon, in a simple interrupted pattern.

Coelomic Surgery

For a ventral coelomic cavity approach, position the patient in dorsal recumbency (Wright and Whitaker 2001a). A paramedian incision is recommended to avoid the ventral abdominal vein (Figure 6.8) (Wright and Whitaker 2001a). Incise the skin and coelomic muscles with a scalpel blade or iris scissors. Have an assistant, gently retract the coelomic wall or use a self-retaining retractor such as Heiss, Lone Star, or Gelpi retractors or a Barraquer eyelid speculum. After celiotomy, the coelom should be sutured with absorbable monofilament suture material (Tuttle et al. 2006) in two layers, one for the muscle and one for the skin (Wright and Whitaker 2001a; Gentz 2007; Green 2010). In small amphibians, it is possible to suture both the muscle and skin in a single layer without complication (Archibald et al. 2015). When working with aquatic amphibians, such as newts, neotenic species, and tadpoles, positive buoyancy after anesthetic recovery is an important consideration, so gas should be removed from the coelomic cavity at the end of the procedure. The weight of hemostatic clips should be considered when working with small aquatic animals due to postoperative negative buoyancy issues.

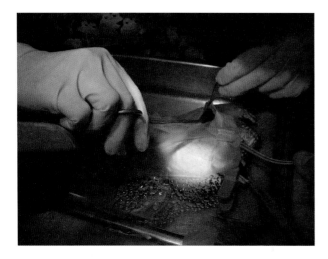

Figure 6.8 Exploratory celiotomy in an Argentine horned frog (*Ceratophrys ornata*). Intra-operative images. *Source:* Photo courtesy: Zoological Medicine Service, Université de Montréal.

A ventral coelomic hernia has been successfully repaired in a female tomato frog (Meier 1982). Distended intestines were found to prolapse subcutaneously through a right lateral coelomic hernia. To repair a coelomic hernia, make a cutaneous incision medial to the hernia and replace the prolapsed organs into the coelom. If the coelomic musculature is thin and friable, place an absorbable gelatin sponge in the coelomic cavity inside the muscular defect and suture the muscles as best as possible over the gelatin sponge. Close the skin in a simple continuous pattern with absorbable monofilament suture.

Urogenital Surgery

Cystotomy has been reported in a variety of amphibians including *Phyllomedusa* spp. (Wright and Whitaker 2001a; Archibald et al. 2015) that seem to be predisposed to ammonium urates uroliths due to their uricotelism (the production of uric acid). With the patient in dorsal recumbency, make a ventral paramedian incision using a #15 scalpel blade. Exteriorize the urinary bladder to avoid contamination of the coelom as bacteriuria is normal in amphibians (Johnson et al. 2015). Incise the bladder wall with a #15 blade. Close the bladder in a simple continuous pattern with fine poliglecaprone 25 suture after removing the calculi, and then suture the coelomic cavity with a simple continuous pattern with fine polydioxanone suture (Archibald et al. 2015).

Partial or complete cystectomy is an option in amphibians with bladder necrosis secondary to chronic bladder prolapse or with untreatable mucosal lesions because the ureters connect to the cloaca and not the urinary bladder (Archibald et al. 2015).

Surgical harvest of oocytes from laboratory amphibians is a commonly performed procedure, especially to design transgenic frogs (Green 2010). To collect ova, place the frog in dorsal recumbency and perform a paramedian ventral incision with particular care to not puncture the lungs, the urinary bladder, or the enlarged ovaries. The ovaries with mature follicles extend ventrally in the coelom and are easily visualized (Figure 6.9). Grasp the ovaries with forceps and exteriorize them onto the plastic drape, as the skin is not sterile. Excise the desired number of oocytes using scissors. No ligature is necessary to collect a small portion of the ovary (Gentz 2007). Close the coelomic incision in two layers. Place simple interrupted sutures in the muscle layer and simple interrupted, vertical, or horizontal mattress monofilament sutures in the skin (Green 2010). The procedure can be repeated every three to six months in a single female.

Ovariectomy is performed in adult females. Make a ventral paramedian incision. Use an eyelid retractor to facilitate visualization. Exteriorize the ovaries onto the plastic drape with cotton tip applicators. Use electrocautery, diode laser

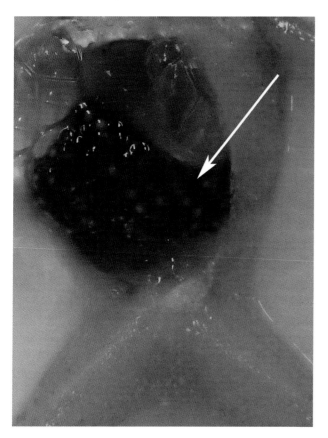

Figure 6.9 Location of the ovaries (white arrow) in a reproductively active Gray tree frog (*Hyla versicolor*). *Source:* Photo courtesy: Zoological Medicine Service, Université de Montréal.

(Chai 2016), place hemostatic clips, or ligate the ovarian pedicles with polydioxanone suture (Wright and Whitaker 2001a). Transect the pedicle and retrieve the ovary. After repeating the procedure contralaterally, lavage the coelom and suture the coelomic muscles and skin in two layers. If the muscular layer is very thin, place a collagen pad in the coelom to improve the security of the suture, especially in laying females (Meier 1982). Ovariectomy may predispose amphibians to becoming overweight (Wright and Whitaker 2001a).

Castration is performed in a similar manner to ovariectomy. Make a paramedian ventral incision and locate the intracoelomic testicles cranial to the kidneys. Testicular vessels are shorter than ovarian vessels. Gently elevate the testis to place hemostatic clips or ligating sutures. Use small overlapping hemostatic clips in large specimens rather than choosing large hemostatic clips which are more prone to slip if not closed appropriately resulting in hemorrhage. Cauterize the bilateral ductus deferens with electrocautery and transect the testicle distal to the clips. Close the coelom in two layers of monofilament suture. Testicular biopsy is used in laboratories for reproductive studies (Gentz 2007). Make a small paramedian ventral incision and locate the intracoelomic testicles located cranial to the kidneys. Obtain biopsies with a biopsy forceps: close the

forceps, wait and apply gentle pressure before pulling on the forceps to retrieve the biopsy. Apply counter-forces to the testicle with a cotton-tip applicator to avoid damage to the vasculature supplying the testicle. Close the coelomic incision in two layers with monofilament suture. Alternatively, endoscopy-assisted testicular biopsy can be performed.

Gastrointestinal Tract Surgery

For gastrotomy, after making a paramedian ventral incision into the coelomic cavity, place saline soaked gauze to isolate the area of interest and reduce the risk of contamination with gastrointestinal contents (Gentz 2007). Place stay sutures in the gastric wall (Figure 6.10) and perform the gastrostomy as in mammals. Close the stomach wall in one or two layers using monofilament absorbable suture material (Meier 1982) (Figure 6.11). If the diameter of the stomach is small, opt for a single inverting suture to decrease the risk of gastric stenosis. Postoperatively, offer the patient small meals or syringe feed a liquid diet for 4–6 weeks. Feeding live and chitinous prey items with abrasive body parts should be avoided during this period.

Cloacal prolapse is a common problem in amphibians (Wright and Whitaker 2001a; Fleming and Isaza 2000; Phillott and Young 2009). Cloacal prolapses should be differentiated from intestinal, urinary bladder, and reproductive organ prolapse, and perineal hernias.

After providing analgesia, soaking the prolapsed tissue in a hypertonic solution (e.g. 5% NaCl or 50% dextrose) for 5–10 minutes can help reduce its size (Wright and Whitaker 2001a; Hadfield and Whitaker 2005) and identify the prolapsed structures. If ureteral openings are exposed and appear necrotic, the prognosis is poor and euthanasia should be elected. If cloacal tissue is viable, cover the exposed cloaca with water-soluble lubricant and reduce the prolapse with a blunt instrument (e.g. cotton-tipped applicator or a red-rubber tube) (Wright and Whitaker 2001a). With recurrent cloacal prolapses, a purse-string suture may be placed with the cotton-tipped applicator still in the vent to assure that feces will be able to pass once the suture is secured and the applicator removed.

If the prolapsed tissue includes necrotic intestine or reproductive tract, it should be amputated (Hadfield and Whitaker 2005) if reconstruction is possible. Resection and anastomosis of an intestinal loop or the salpinx may be performed externally before replacement of the prolapsed tissue. In females, perform an ovariohysterectomy after amputation of the prolapsed salpinx. If lesions are unilateral, a unilateral ovariectomy may be elected.

Cloacotomy has been described in a waxy monkey frog (*Phyllomedusa sauvagii*) presented with recurring urolithiasis

(a)   (b)   (c)

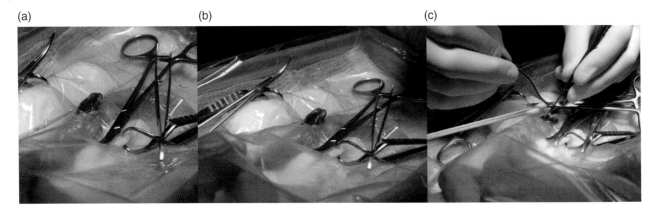

Figure 6.10 Gastrotomy in an axolotl (*Ambystoma mexicanum*) anesthetized with a continuous effusion of 5 mg/l of alfaxalone delivered through plastic tubing visible on the left of each image. (a) Stay sutures with Prolene 5-0 are placed on the coelomic cavity, (b) stay sutures are placed on the stomach on each side of the incision, and (c) rocks are exteriorized through the gastric wall incision. *Source:* Photo courtesy: Dr. Marcie Logsdon, Exotics and Wildlife Department, Washington State University.

(a)   (b)

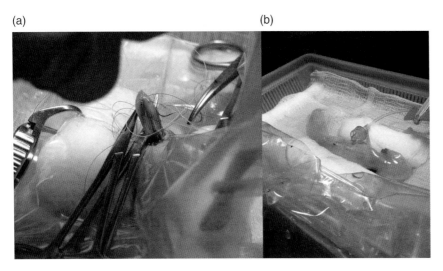

Figure 6.11 Gastrotomy in an axolotl (*Ambystoma mexicanum*): (a) suture of the stomach wall in a single layer with a continuous pattern of absorbable monofilament suture. (b) Recovery of the axolotl after suturing the skin with monofilament suture using a slightly everting continuous pattern. *Source:* Photo courtesy: Dr. Marcie Logsdon, Exotics and Wildlife Department, Washington State University.

after cystectomy (Archibald et al. 2015). Urolith formation recurred twice in the cloaca in this animal. The technique described to remove the calculus involved a paramedian coelomic incision followed by incision of the ventral cloacal wall. The cloaca was sutured with 5-0 polydioxanone suture in a simple interrupted pattern and the patient recovered from this procedure.

Minimally Invasive Surgery

Minimal invasive surgery has been described in detail for amphibians (Chai 2015b). Indications are similar to other vertebrate species and include organ biopsy, sex determination, and retrieval of gastrointestinal foreign bodies (Gentz 2007). An oral speculum may be used during gastroscopy to prevent trauma to the endoscope. To visualize the heart, liver, urinary bladder, and gastrointestinal tract via celioscopy, a paramedian incision has been recommended, whereas a lateral approach is preferred to visualize the gonads, adrenal glands, and kidneys (Gentz 2007). Celioscopy should take no more than 10 minutes to minimize anesthetic risks (Chai 2015b). Saline insufflation or carbon dioxide insufflation can be used to improve visualization during celioscopy (Chai 2015a).

Telemetry and Microchip Implantation

Passive integrated transponder devices (PIT tags) have been placed in captive and free-ranging amphibians. PIT tags are typically surgically implanted intracoelomically in urodela and caecilians, while they can be implanted subcutaneously in anurans (Wright and Whitaker 2001a). In hellbenders, subcutaneous implantation on the dorsal aspect of the tail has been described (Norton et al. 2014). Cosmetic implantation sites include the ventral thigh on either side or deep to the parotid gland in anurans (Wright and Whitaker 2001a). When inserting the microchip subcutaneously, close the insertion site with tissue glue to prevent osmotic imbalance (Norton et al. 2014). For intracoelomic implantation, make a paramedian coelotomy incision rather than inserting the microchip blindly into the coelom to avoid internal organ trauma (Wright and Whitaker 2001a). Some researchers have expressed concerns regarding microchip implantation in free-ranging amphibians of small size (Funk et al. 2005), but no reference was cited to document adverse effects of microchip implantation. A marking technique using a gun to inject pressurized fluorescent pigment was recommended (Schlaepfer 1998). Alternative marking techniques include subcutaneous visible implant elastomer tags, fluorescent pigments injected with a needle and detected with ultraviolet lights, or toe clipping, but external identification techniques can become illegible (Gibbons and Andrews 2004).

Radiotransmitters may be implanted intracoelomically (Johnson 2006) or placed externally in amphibians (Norton et al. 2014). Due to the risks associated with external radiotransmitters, many researchers opt for intracoelomic implantation. Incise the ventral skin, coelomic muscles, and coelomic lining and insert the radiotransmitter into the coelomic cavity (Norton et al. 2014). Close the muscular layer with polydioxanone suture and the skin layer with nylon. Researchers should consider removing the radiotransmitter at the completion of their study to prevent chronic coelomitis (Norton et al. 2014).

References

Aguilar, C. and Gardiner, D.M. (2015). DNA methylation dynamics regulate the formation of a regenerative wound epithelium during Axolotl limb regeneration. *PLoS ONE* 10: e0134791.

Archibald, K.E., Minter, L.J., Dombrowski, D.S. et al. (2015). Cystic urolithiasis in captive waxy monkey frogs (*Phyllomedusa sauvagii*). *Journal of Zoo and Wildlife Medicine* 46: 105–112.

Bainton, C. and Strichartz, G. (1994). Concentration dependence of lidocaine-induced irreversible conduction loss in frog nerve. *Anesthesiology* 81: 657–667.

Baitchman, E.J. and Herman, T.A. (2015). Caudata (Urodela). In: *Fowler's Zoo and Wild Animal Medicine*, 8e (eds. R.E. Miller and M.E. Fowler), 13–19. St. Louis, MO: Elsevier.

Braitman, E. and Stetter, M. (2014). Amphibians. In: *Zoo Animal and Wildlife Immobilization and Anesthesia*, 2e (eds. G. West, D. Heard and N. Caulkett), 303–312. Ames, IO: Wiley Blackwell.

Chai, N. (2015a). Anurans. In: *Fowler's Zoo and Wild Animal Medicine*, 8e (eds. R.E. Miller and M.E. Fowler), 1–12. St. Louis, MO: Elsevier.

Chai, N. (2015b). Endoscopy in amphibians. *Veterinary Clinics of North America: Exotic Animal Practice* 18: 479–491.

Chai, N. (2016). Surgery in amphibians. *Veterinary Clinics of North America: Exotic Animal Practice* 19: 77–95.

Clayton, L.A. and Mylniczenko, N.D. (2015). Caecilians. In: *Fowler's Zoo and Wild Animal Medicine*, 8e (eds. R.E. Miller and M.E. Fowler), 20–26. St. Louis, MO: Elsevier.

Diaz Quiroz, J.F., Tsai, E., Coyle, M. et al. (2014). Precise control of miR-125b levels is required to create a regeneration-permissive environment after spinal cord injury: a cross-species comparison between salamander and rat. *Disease Models & Mechanisms* 7: 601–611.

Dombrowski, D.S., Vanderklol, C., and Van Wettere, A.J. (2016). Curative surgical excision of a squamous cell carcinoma associated with the digit of an Amercian bullfrog (*Lithobates catesbeianus*). *Journal of Herpetological Medicine and Surgery* 26: 42–45.

Felt, S., Papich, M., Howard, A. et al. (2013). Tissue distribution of enrofloxacin in African clawed frogs (*Xenopus laevis*) after intramuscular and subcutaneous administration. *Journal of the American Association for Laboratory Animal Science* 52: 186–188.

Filoni, S. (2009). Retina and lens regeneration in anuran amphibians. *Seminars in Cell & Developmental Biology* 20: 528–534.

Fleming, G.J. and Isaza, R. (2000). What is your diagnosis? A 4-cm mass protruding from the dorsal area of the cloaca. *Journal of the American Veterinary Medical Association* 217: 325–326.

Fleming, G.J., Corwin, A., Mccoy, A.J. et al. (2008). Treatment factors influencing the use of recombinant platelet-derived growth factor (Regranex) for head and lateral line erosion syndrome in ocean surgeonfish (*Acanthurus bahianus*). *Journal of Zoo and Wildlife Medicine* 39: 155–160.

Forzan, M.J., Vanderstichel, R.V., Ogbuah, C.T. et al. (2012). Blood collection from the facial (maxillary)/musculo-cutaneous vein in true frogs (family Ranidae). *Journal of Wildlife Diseases* 48: 176–180.

Funk, W.C., Donnelly, M.A., and Lips, K.R. (2005). Alternative views of amphibian toe-clipping. *Nature* 433: 193.

Gentz, E.J. (2007). Medicine and surgery of amphibians. *ILAR Journal* 48: 255–259.

Gibbons, J.W. and Andrews, K. (2004). PIT taggining: simple technology at its best. *BioScience* 54: 447–454.

Green, S.L. (2010). *The Laboratory Xenopus sp.* Boca Raton, FL: CRC Press.

Gutleb, A.C., Bronkhorst, M., Van Den Berg, J.H. et al. (2001). Latex laboratory-gloves: an unexpected pitfall in amphibian toxicity assays with tadpoles. *Environmental Toxicology and Pharmacology* 10: 119–121.

Hadfield, C.A. and Whitaker, B.R. (2005). Amphibian emergency medicine and care. *Seminars in Avian and Exotic Pet Medicine* 14: 79–89.

Hedrick, M.S., McNew, K.A., and Crossley, D.A. (2015). Baroreflex function in anurans from different environments. *Comparative Biochemistry and Physiology - Part A: Molecular & Integrative Physiology* 179: 144–148.

Helmer, P. and Whiteside, D. (2005). Amphibian anatomy and physiology. In: *Clinical Anatomy and Physiology of Exotic Species: Structure and Function of Mammals, Birds, Reptiles and Amphibians* (ed. B. O'Malley), 5–16. Edinburgh, Ireland: Elsevier.

Imai, D.M., Nadler, S.A., Brenner, D. et al. (2009). Rhabditid nematode-associated ophthalmitis and meningoencephalomyelitis in captive Asian horned frogs (*Megophrys montana*). *Journal of Veterinary Diagnostic Investigation* 21: 568–573.

James-Zorn, C., Ponferrada, V.G., Jarabek, C.J. et al. (2013). Xenbase: expansion and updates of the *Xenopus* model organism database. *Nucleic Acids Research* 41: D865–D870.

Johnson, D. (2003). External fixation of bilateral tibial fractures in an American bullfrog. *Exotic DVM* 5: 27–29.

Johnson, J.R. (2006). Success of intracoelomic radiotransmitter implantation in the treefrog (*Hyla versicolor*). *Lab Animal (NY)* 35: 29–33.

Johnson, J.G., Brandao, J., Perry, S.M. et al. (2015). Urinary system. In: *Current Therapy in Exotic Pet Practice* (eds. M.A. Mitchell and T.N. Tully), 494–548. St. Louis, MO: Elsevier.

Juan Hidalgo, F.S. (1989). *Human and Frog Anatomy Atlas: A Comparative Study*, 161. Manila, PH: Rex Book Store.

Koeller, C.A. (2009). Comparison of buprenorphine and butorphanol analgesia in the eastern red-spotted newt (*Notophthalmus viridescens*). *Journal of the American Association for Laboratory Animal Science* 48: 171–175.

Meier, J. (1982). Surgical repair of a ventral abdominal hernia in Madagascan tomato frog *Dyscophus antongilii*. *Journal of Zoo and Wildlife Medicine* 13: 123–124.

Mendez, D., Webb, R., Berger, L. et al. (2008). Survival of the amphibian chytrid fungus *Batrachochytrium dendrobatidis* on bare hands and gloves: hygiene implications for amphibian handling. *Diseases of Aquatic Organisms* 82: 97–104.

Mitchell, M.A. (2009). Anesthetic considerations for amphibians. *Journal of Exotic Pet Medicine* 18: 40–49.

Mylniczenko, N.D. (2006). A medical health survey of diseases in captive caecilian amphibians. *Journal of Herpetological Medicine and Surgery* 16: 120–128.

Newman, L.C., Sands, S.S., Wallace, D.R. et al. (2002). Characterization of mu, kappa, and delta opioid binding in amphibian whole brain tissue homogenates. *Journal of Pharmacology and Experimental Therapeutics* 301: 364–370.

Norton, T.M., Andrews, K., and Li, S. (2014). Techniques for working with wild reptiles. In: *Current Therapy in Reptile Medicine and Surgery* (eds. D. Mader and S. Divers), 310–340. St. Louis, MO: Elsevier.

O'Rourke, D.P. and Jenkins, A.L. (2014). Anesthesia and analgesia in amphibians. In: *Anesthesia and Analgesia in Laboratory Animals* (eds. R.E. Fish, M.J. Brown, P.J. Danneman and A.Z. Karas), 511–518. San Diego, CA: American College of Laboratory Animal Medicine Series.

Pearl, E.J., Barker, D., Day, R.C. et al. (2008). Identification of genes associated with regenerative success of *Xenopus laevis* hindlimbs. *BMC Developmental Biology* 8: 66.

Phillott, A.D. and Young, S. (2009). Occurrence of cloacal prolapse in wild hylids in the Wet Tropics, Australia. *Diseases of Aquatic Organisms* 86: 77–80.

Pizzi, R. and Miller, J. (2005). Amputation of a *Mycobacterium marinum*-infected hindlimb in an African bullfrog (*Pyxicephalus adspersus*). *Veterinary Record* 156: 747–748.

Poll, C.P. (2009). Wound management in amphibians: etiology and treatment of cutaneous lesions. *Journal of Exotic Pet Medicine* 18: 20–35.

Pritchard, J.J. and Ruzicka, A.J. (1950). Comparison of fracture repair in the frog, lizard and rat. *Journal of Anatomy* 84: 236–261.

Ramsey, J.P., Reinert, L.K., Harper, L.K. et al. (2010). Immune defenses against *Batrachochytrium dendrobatidis,* a fungus linked to global amphibian declines, in the South African clawed frog, *Xenopus laevis. Infection and Immunity* 78: 3981–3992.

Roth, T., Foley, J., Worth, J. et al. (2013). Bacterial flora on Cascades frogs in the Klamath mountains of California. *Comparative Immunology, Microbiology and Infectious Diseases* 36: 591–598.

Royal, L.W., Grafinger, M.S., Lascelles, B.D.X. et al. (2007). Internal fixation of a femur fracture in an American bullfrog. *Journal of the American Veterinary Medical Association* 230: 1201–1204.

Sancho, J.M., Morgades, M., Grifols, J.R. et al. (2012). Predictive factors for poor peripheral blood stem cell mobilization and peak CD34[+] cell count to guide pre-emptive or immediate rescue mobilization. *Cytotherapy* 14: 823–829.

Schlaepfer, M.A. (1998). Use of fluorescent marking technique on small terrestrial anurans. *Herpetological Review* 29: 25–26.

Shigeri, Y., Yasuda, A., Hagihara, Y. et al. (2015). Identification of novel peptides from amphibian (*Xenopus tropicalis*) skin by direct tissue MALDI-MS analysis. *FEBS Journal* 282: 102–113.

Sobotka, J.M. and Rahwan, R.G. (1994). Lethal effect of latex gloves on *Xenopus laevis* tadpoles. *Journal of Pharmacological and Toxicological Methods* 32: 59.

Stevens, C.W. (2011). Analgesia in amphibians: preclinical studies and clinical applications. *Veterinary Clinics of North America: Exotic Animal Practice* 14: 33–44.

Tuttle, A.D., Law, J.M., Harms, C.A. et al. (2006). Evaluation of the gross and histologic reactions to five commonly used suture materials in the skin of the African clawed frog (*Xenopus laevis*). *Journal of the American Association for Laboratory Animal Science* 45: 22–26.

Van Bonn, W. (2009). Clinical techniques: extra-articular surgical stifle stabilization of an American bullfrog (*Rana catesbeiana*). *Journal of Exotic Pet Medicine* 18: 36–39.

Waffa, B.J., Montgerard, A.C., Grafinger, M.S. et al. (2012). Dorsal laminectomy in a two-toed amphiuma (*Amphiuma means*). *Journal of Zoo and Wildlife Medicine* 43: 927–930.

Walker, I. and Whitaker, B. (2003). Published. Topical administration of recombinant human pletelet-derived growth factor to aid healing of chronic, dermal ulcerations in a giant leaf tree frog (*Phyllomedusa bicolor*). *Proceedings of the International Association of Aquatic Animal Medicine*, Waikoloa, HI, p. 178.

Weber, E.S. III (2011). Fish analgesia: pain, stress, fear aversion, or nociception? *Veterinary Clinics of North America: Exotic Animal Practice* 14: 21–32.

Whitaker, B. and Wright, K. (2001). Clinical techniques. In: *Amphibian Medicine and Captive Husbandry* (ed. K. Wright), 89–122. Malabar, FL: Krieger Publishing Company.

Williams, D.L. and Whitaker, B.R. (1994). The amphibian eye—a clinical review. *Journal of Zoo and Wildlife Medicine* 25: 18–28.

Wright, K. (2006). Overview of amphibian medicine. In: *Reptile Medicine and Surgery* (ed. D. Mader), 941–971. Philadelphia, PA: Saunders Elsevier.

Wright, K. and Whitaker, B. (2001a). Surgical techniques. In: *Amphibian Medicine and Captive Husbandry* (ed. K. Wright), 273–283. Malabar, FL: Krieger Publishing Company.

Wright, K. and Whitaker, B. (2001b). Pharmacotherapeutics. In: *Amphibian Medicine and Captive Husbandry* (ed. K. Wright), 309–330. Malabar, FL: Krieger Publishing Company.

Yannas, I.V., Colt, J., and Wai, Y.C. (1996). Wound contraction and scar synthesis during development of the amphibian *Rana catesbeiana*. *Wound Repair and Regeneration* 4: 29–39.

Zena, L.A., Gargaglioni, L.H., and Bicego, K.C. (2015). Temperature effects on baroreflex control of heart rate in the toad, *Rhinella schneideri*. *Comparative Biochemistry and Physiology - Part A: Molecular & Integrative Physiology* 179: 81–88.

7

Reptile Orthopedic Surgery
Michael S. McFadden

Introduction

Reptiles are commonly presented for a variety of disorders of the musculoskeletal system. There is a wide variety of species that are included in this group, but many principles can be applied across taxa. Many veterinarians are familiar with common orthopedic diseases in domestic species. In many cases, the same diagnostic approach and treatments can be applied to reptiles, while in other cases, the pathophysiology and treatment are more specific. Once a knowledge base in the diagnosis and treatment of musculoskeletal diseases has been established, the diseases and diagnostics that are unique to reptiles can be added.

Anatomy and Physiology

Reptiles are a diverse group of animals that may be kept as pets including crocodilians, snakes, lizards, and chelonians (turtles and tortoises), and a basic understanding of anatomy and physiology of reptiles is crucial for successful orthopedic surgery. There are many anatomic differences among different reptile species specifically related to the musculoskeletal system. This can affect diagnosis and treatment of different diseases. Differences in body organization (limb number, limb function) and histologic differences in bone structure may affect bone healing. Due to the diversity among different reptile species only a brief review of the anatomy relevant to the musculoskeletal system is presented here.

Snakes have a musculoskeletal system that is similar across species (Mitchell 2009). The skull of snakes is adapted to ingest large prey items and it lacks a mandibular symphysis. The vertebral column consists of several hundred vertebrae with very little variation in configuration along the length of the animal. Large groups of epaxial muscles are present along the length of the animal with multiple attachments to aid in locomotion. There is no sternum and ribs connect to the ventral scales to allow locomotion. Some groups have vestigial pelvic and hind limb remnants including external spurs that are used in courtship and mating (Funk 2006).

The musculoskeletal system is similar in most lizard species. They have well-developed extremities and tails that are adapted for different locomotion strategies (running, climbing, and swimming). Most lizards have a rib attached to every vertebral body except the sacral vertebrae (Barten 2006a).

Chelonians (turtles, tortoises, and terrapins) are one of the most recognizable groups of animals due to their shells. There are over 285 species of chelonians in the world, and these are the only tetrapod that has both the pelvic and pectoral girdle within the rib cage and encased in bone (Boyer and Boyer 2006; Kirchgessner and Mitchell 2009). The shell consists of an upper carapace and lower plastron connected by bony bridges. Some species, particularly aquatic species, have large portions of the bony carapace and plastron replaced with thick leathery skin (Boyer and Boyer 2006). Chelonians have thoracic and lumbar ribs that are incorporated into the shell and no sternum is present. The trunk vertebrae are fused together, but the cervical and coccygeal vertebrae are able to move independently allowing for retraction of the head and tail to within the shell. Modified pectoral and pelvic girdles are present and are fused to the carapace. The pectoral girdle consists of the epiplastron (clavicle), entoplastron (interclavicle), the scapula, acromion process, and coracoid bone. The pelvic girdle consists of paired ilium, ischium, and pubic bones. The humerus and femur are reduced in length and the limbs extend more laterally than mammalian limbs.

Surgery of Exotic Animals, First Edition. Edited by R. Avery Bennett and Geoffrey W. Pye.
© 2022 John Wiley & Sons, Inc. Published 2022 by John Wiley & Sons, Inc.

Diagnostics

Radiographs can be used to assess bone density in metabolic bone disease as well as evaluate the skeletal system for any fractures, luxations, or other joint problems (Figure 7.1). Standard radiographic equipment can be used, although in smaller species dental film and dental radiography units are preferred due to patient size or if detailed focal areas of interest are needed (Stetter 2001). The availability of digital radiography in most practices can be adapted to use in reptiles, including digital dental radiography units.

Sedation or immobilization with proper restraint will help obtain the correct lateral and dorsoventrally projections. Radiographic standards for other species apply to reptiles and collimated views over the area of interest are preferred as opposed to full body radiographs. For spinal radiographs in snakes, obtaining multiple images taken of segments of the snake is preferred over a single image of the snake coiled up.

Computed tomography (CT) and magnetic resonance imaging (MRI) studies have been performed in reptiles; however, availability, cost, and the need for sedation or anesthesia may be limiting factors. Newer CT scans allow rapid acquisition of images making anesthesia or sedation unnecessary in some cases. The main benefit of CT over

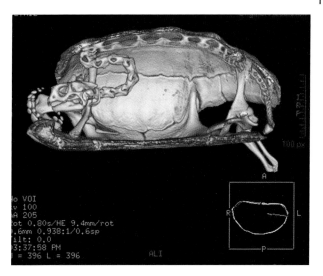

Figure 7.2 A CT reconstruction of a juvenile African spurred tortoise (*Centrochelys sulcata*) showing the skeleton with soft tissues digitally removed. The patient was having a CT for disease unrelated to the musculoskeletal system, and reconstruction was performed as an example of the detail that can be seen with CT scans.

conventional radiography is the increased sensitivity and ability to create 3-D reconstructions (Figure 7.2). An added benefit in chelonians is the ability to obtain cross-sectional images of various structures without superimposition of the bones of the carapace and plastron. A case series demonstrating lesions that were missed on plain radiographs but detected on CT scans has been published (Abou-Madi et al. 2004). A radiated tortoise was diagnosed with a shoulder luxation using CT and two snapping turtles were diagnosed with fractures that were not seen on plain radiographs.

In addition to standard imaging techniques, other diagnostic modalities utilized for musculoskeletal abnormalities in reptiles include joint aspirates and muscle and bone biopsies (Hernandez-Divers 2006). Joint aspirates and cytologic evaluation of joint fluid should be evaluated for any swollen or painful joint (Figure 7.3). Aseptic preparation of the skin over the joint is critical to prevent iatrogenic introduction of skin flora. Assessment of joint fluid, depending upon the volume obtained, can include color, volume, viscosity, protein concentration, and total and differential cell counts (Alleman and Kupprion 2007). This can help differentiate between degenerative joint disease and septic arthritis. Many reptiles have very small volumes of joint fluid, even in an infected joint. If there is only a small volume of fluid available, a small amount of sterile saline can be aspirated into the syringe after slides are prepared. The saline and any remaining joint fluid in the needle and hub can be submitted for culture and sensitivity testing. Reptiles often produce inspissated pus and joint

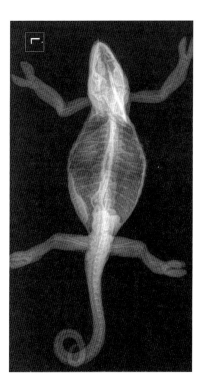

Figure 7.1 A dorso-ventral (DV) projection of the entire skeleton of a chameleon (exact species unknown) showing significant decrease in bone density and multiple pathologic fractures.

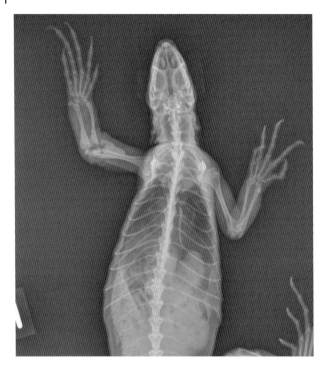

Figure 7.3 A DV projection of a green iguana (*Iguana iguana*) showing chronic changes to the left elbow joint. There is destruction of the joint surface and periosteal reaction in the distal humerus, proximal radius, and proximal ulna. The patient was being evaluated for chronic lameness after a fight with a cage mate.

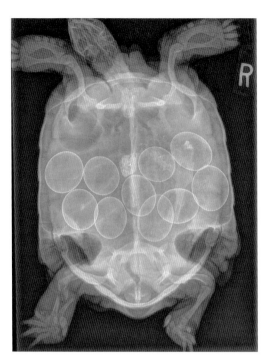

Figure 7.4 Full body DV projection of a female African spurred thighed tortoise (*Centrochelys sulcata*) showing a displaced fracture of the left tibia and fibula.

aspirates may not always produce fluid that is able to be analyzed. Surgical debridement is often required and samples can be obtained for analysis at that time.

Bone biopsies can be obtained using bone biopsy instruments of the appropriate size for the patient. The bone can be submitted for histopathology and/or for culture and sensitivity testing. In smaller species, hypodermic needles can be used to obtain samples for cytologic evaluation and culture. Many fractures seen in reptiles are secondary to nutritional secondary hyperparathyroidism (NSHP), and any individual presenting with a fracture should be closely evaluated for evidence of NSHP. The diagnosis and management of NSHP are beyond the scope of this chapter but must be considered in most cases of reptile fractures. Assessment of blood work and bone density should be included in the diagnostic work up if NSHP is suspected. Pathologic fractures vary but are commonly greenstick or folding fractures. Successful treatment of these fractures relies heavily on restoring normal calcium metabolism. Fractures secondary to NSHP heal rapidly once calcium metabolism is corrected.

Trauma

Traumatic fractures in companion reptiles are usually caused by low-impact trauma resulting in simple

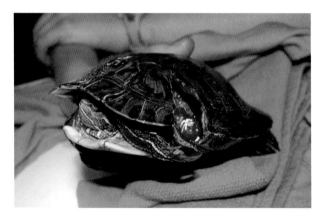

Figure 7.5 Typical motor vehicle trauma to the plastron of a red-eared slider (*Trachemys scripta*) with significant bone loss and communication with the coelomic cavity.

fractures (Figure 7.4). Wild reptiles can be presented after high-impact trauma such as being hit by a car or run over by a lawnmower. Fractures from high-impact trauma are often open and comminuted with significant soft tissue trauma (Figure 7.5). Skeletal injuries may be obvious on initial examination, as in the case of a chelonian after being hit by a car, or they can be very subtle. Postural abnormalities, lameness, swelling, or changes in limb alignment can be signs of a fracture or luxation. As in any other species, reptiles presenting with fractures may have significant injuries and a complete assessment should be performed. The fracture should only be addressed when any life-threatening abnormalities have been managed.

Bone Composition, Bone Healing, and Fracture Repair

Understanding bone biology and fracture healing is important when addressing fractures. Bone composition, bone structure, and mechanisms of bone healing are all important in fracture fixation and differences in these principles exist among species. These differences can affect fracture configurations and may affect bone healing.

Bones are a mixture of organic and inorganic material. The inorganic material consists of calcium hydroxyapatite ($Ca_{10}[PO_4]_6[OH]_2$) which gives bone its strength and rigidity (Dunning 2002). The amount of calcium can vary among species and this ultimately affects bone strength, stiffness, and density. The organic component of bone consists of cells (osteocytes, osteoblasts, and osteoclasts) and the extracellular matrix (glycoproteins, proteoglycans, and collagen).

The bone cortex of snakes and lizards contains bone of periosteal and endosteal origin. Seasons or periodic growth leads to layering or laminar arrangement. Cortical bones of snakes and lizards are composed of a mixture of lamellar and nonlamellar bone with no Haversian systems. Major differences between cortical bone in snakes and lizards compared to other reptiles are the presence of compact bone that is virtually nonvascular with a marked reduction of vascular channels and limited extent of cancellous trabeculae (Enlow 1969). The cortex in chelonian and crocodilian bones is arranged in circumferential broad laminae each containing rows of vascular canals. Each lamination is a result of periods of growth, and in young individuals, the cortex may be composed of a single lamina with the number increasing as the animal ages (Enlow 1969). Chelonians and crocodilian bones also contain incomplete Haversian systems that are limited to localized areas of the cortex (Foote 1911; Enlow 1969). The metaphysis of long bones is composed of cancellous bone that is structurally different from mammalian cancellous bone. Chelonians also lack a medullary cavity in long bones. This affects the ability to use intraosseous catheters and affects selection of implants used in orthopedics such as intramedullary (IM) pins.

Bone Healing

Bone healing occurs by different mechanisms depending on contact between fracture fragments and stability. There are also potential inter- and intraspecies differences in bone healing. The classic description of bone healing is through formation of a callus (secondary or indirect bone healing). When the fracture occurs, a hematoma develops at the fracture site. The cells within the hematoma initiate an inflammatory response and release cytokines. Once the inflammatory phase subsides, pluripotent mesenchymal cells arising from the periosteum, endosteum, and surrounding soft tissues are induced and differentiate into fibroblasts, chondroblasts, and osteoblasts. These cells produce fibrous tissue, cartilage, and woven bone, respectively, resulting in the formation of a callus that bridges the fracture and continuously reorganizes into progressively stiffer tissue until a bony callus bridges the fracture gap. The later stages can be evaluated radiographically and clinical healing is complete when the bony callus bridges the fracture gap.

The considerable variation in bone structure may affect how fractures heal. Many species lack Haversian systems, while in others, they are incomplete. Due to the arrangement of cutting cones with the osteon during primary or direct bone healing, this type of healing may not occur in species that do not have well-developed Haversian systems. Primary or direct bone healing has not been studied in reptiles and may not occur in the same manner that is seen in mammals.

The mechanism of indirect or callus bone healing is similar among species, although some differences exist. The main differences noted among species are the rate of repair and the relative contribution of the periosteum, endosteum, and surrounding soft tissues to the healing process.

It takes longer for fractures of reptile bones to heal than most other animals, and in some cases, it can be as long as 6–30 months (Mitchell 2002). In one study, full union of tibial fractures took 50% longer in lizards compared to rats (Pritchard and Ruzicka 1950). Also fracture healing in lizards maintained at lower environmental temperatures (26 °C) takes longer than in lizards kept within their preferred temperature range (32–37 °C) (Pritchard and Ruzicka 1950; Raftery 2011).

In reptile fractures, a majority of the hematoma and subsequent callus are derived from the periosteum compared to mammalian fractures that derive much of the blood supply from the surrounding soft tissue (Pritchard and Ruzicka 1950). These differences can be important in fracture repair and may affect the implants that are selected in order to minimize any detrimental effects on the endosteum or periosteum, and it is important to take these differences into consideration to ensure careful dissection with proper surgical technique to minimize disruption of the soft tissues surrounding the fracture.

Principles of Fracture Stabilization

The principles of fracture fixation are similar regardless of species. The goal is reduction of the fracture with correct alignment, rigid immobilization, and preservation of the soft tissues. All fractures have forces acting on them such as bending, rotation, axial load (compression and tension), and shear. The method chosen to immobilize fractures must be able to counteract all forces acting on the fracture. The methods for fixation can vary, and in some cases, the options available are limited by the size of the patient, anatomy, skill of the veterinarian in orthopedic surgery, and costs (for the owner as well as to the veterinarian).

External coaptation refers to the use of a sling, splint, bandage, or cast to immobilize the fracture. Internal fixation refers to the use of orthopedic implants such as IM pin, orthopedic wire, bone plates and screws, and interlocking nails. External skeletal fixation (ESF) refers to the use of fixation pins that are inserted percutaneously through the cortices of the bone and are connected externally to a bar or acrylic frame. In all cases of fracture stabilization, it is important to restrict the animals' activity until the fracture has healed. Any additional movement can cause bandage complications or stress implants leading to implant failure. Other complications associated with fracture fixation include osteomyelitis, malunion, delayed union, nonunion, and diseases in other limbs due to changes in weight bearing. External coaptation, internal fixation, and ESF have all been applied in reptiles.

External Coaptation

Ideally, external coaptation is limited to simple, closed, minimally displaced fractures. These are generally characteristics of pathologic fractures secondary to NSHP making external coaptation the treatment of choice for these fractures. It is a simple, inexpensive technique that can be used to stabilize certain fractures. In many cases, external coaptation is chosen when surgery is not possible due to patient size or because of financial constraints; however, it must be noted that the cost of treatments may be similar when factoring in bandage changes and problems associated with bandaging. In other cases, external coaptation is applied for temporary immobilization until surgical stabilization can be performed.

To be effective, the splint or cast must immobilize the joints proximal and distal to the fracture. A properly applied splint or cast will counteract bending and rotational forces, but will not counteract axial forces applied to the fracture. In reptiles, external coaptation can be used for fractures of the humerus and femur more successfully than domestic species because their extremities are usually more perpendicular to the long axis of the body.

General principles for external coaptation in mammals can be applied to reptiles. Due to environment and husbandry practices, be careful when choosing bandaging materials since some can swell or shrink when moistened. The bandage should be changed regularly to assess for any skin irritation, and radiographs can be obtained to assess the presence of a callus and bone healing. Keep in mind that every time a bandage is changed, the fracture fragments are likely to move, which can delay fracture healing.

In some lizards and crocodilians, forelimb fractures can be managed by retracting the limb caudally and securing it to the lateral body as described for applying a splint (cast padding, roll gauze, and a self-adhering wrap). If these types of bandages are used, care must be taken to prevent interruption of respiration. Hind limb fractures can be immobilized by pulling the limb caudally and securing it to the tail. Careful application is needed to prevent tail autonomy and/or incorporation of the vent into the bandage. Some chelonians present a unique obstacle due to the difficulty in applying a splint or bandage due to the shell. In most cases, the fractured limb can be folded into the fossa, and then tape applied from the carapace to the plastron to hold the limb in place. When the limb is folded in the same position as the animal would keep it within the fossa, the fracture fragments are often reduced in close approximation.

Although there are some variations, the bandages used for external coaptation have many similar components regardless of the species. Cast padding, conforming cotton roll gauze, and an outer protective layer. Cast padding is the primary layer and is used to protect soft tissues. Any wounds that are present from the initial injury should be treated appropriately with a debriding or nonadherent dressing based on the type of wound. When placing cast padding, it should be snug to prevent the bandage from slipping. In most cases, it is impossible to place the cast padding too tight since most brands will tear before they reach sufficient tension to cause vascular compromise to the distal limb. After the cast padding is applied, the conforming roll gauze is used to gently compress the cast padding to help provide immobilization. Unlike the cast padding, the roll gauze can be placed too tight causing vascular compromise.

Splints are used to reinforce the bandage and can be made from a variety of materials. Prefabricated plastic or metal splints are available but of very limited value in reptiles because they are made for dog and cat legs. A splint can be made from acrylic casting material, thermoplastic polymers, syringe cases, tongue depressors, aluminum rods, or other stiff material. Most prefabricated splints require the limb to be placed in extension and long-term immobilization in extension can lead to decreased range of motion in the joints. This can ultimately affect the ability to ambulate normally. Apply the splint with the joints in a normal resting position so any long-term effects of immobilization are minimized (Mader et al. 2006). This is most easily accomplished with thermoplastic or acrylic cast material. Apply the splint on top of the roll gauze, secure it with additional roll gauze or tape, and then apply a protective layer of self-adhering wrap or elastic tape over the top.

Bandages must be monitored carefully after they are applied to ensure that they do not cause any vascular constriction to the distal extremity. They must also be monitored for the duration of treatment to ensure they do not slip, fall off, or become wet or soiled. If any of these occur, the bandage and splint must be evaluated immediately and replaced. Again, each time external coaptation must be changed, you risk moving fracture fragments and delaying fracture healing. The fewer the number of bandage changes the more likely the fracture will heal in a timely manner.

Complications associated with external coaptation involve the development of skin irritation, pressure sores, or full thickness wounds. Any animal that has a bandage, splint, or cast should have the area checked regularly to catch any areas of irritation early before significant wounds are present. In some cases, the soft tissue wounds caused by the bandages can be worse than the original injury, requiring amputation in severe cases. Another complication of external coaptation is atrophy and contracture of the musculature and decreased range of motion in the joints due to long-term immobilization. Since closed reduction is often used when external coaptation is selected, anatomic apposition is not always achieved and malunion can develop. The severity of the malunion and magnitude of any alterations in limb alignment can determine if the malunion causes any functional deficits. To minimize the complications associated with immobilization, external coaptation should be removed as soon as possible and rehabilitation should be initiated to regain range of motion and muscle mass.

Internal Fixation

Open reduction and internal fixation are indicated for more complicated fractures or those in which external coaptation is not tolerated or not possible (as in aquatic and semiaquatic reptiles) (Bennett 1996). Internal fixation involves placement of orthopedic implants to provide rigid immobilization. Orthopedic wire, Kirschner wires, IM pins, interlocking nails, and plates and screws are common orthopedic implants that can be applied to reptiles.

Orthopedic implants are made of 316L stainless steel or titanium alloys. The composition of 316L stainless steel and the method in which the metal is manufactured will determine the mechanical properties of the implant, specifically stiffness, strength, and ductility. Cold working and annealing can be used to attain the desired properties for each type of implant and allow variations among implant types. For example, orthopedic wire is more ductile than bone plates, which are in turn more ductile than IM pins. Orthopedic implants can also be made of titanium alloys. Titanium implants have a higher strength to weight ratio than stainless steel, have improved corrosion resistance, and produce less tissue reaction. Other advantages include increased flexibility compared to steel which reduces stress protection when applied to bone, and titanium implants may offer increased resistance to infection. The main disadvantage of titanium implant is the increased cost.

IM pins can be used for diaphyseal fractures in long bones. Benefits of IM pins include the relatively low cost of the implants and placing pins does not require a significant investment of specialized equipment. IM pins have a biomechanical advantage as placement in the center of the bone provides resistance to bending in all directions. This is particularly advantageous biomechanically in comminuted fractures were a fracture gap is present. Disadvantages of IM pins include poor resistance to axial loads and rotational forces. IM pins should always be combined with another form of fixation to counteract these forces such as plates, orthopedic wire, or external skeletal fixators. The most commonly used pins are Kirchner wires and Steinmann pins. Kirchner wires are available in sizes from 0.028″ to 0.062″ (0.7–1.6 mm) and Steinmann pins are available from 1/16″ to 1/4″ (1.6–6.3 mm) making them versatile for patients of many different sizes. In very small patients, spinal needles can be used as IM pins, and they are available in multiple sizes as small as 25 gauge × 3.5 in. (Bennett 1996).

Orthopedic wire has many applications in fracture stabilization. The most common uses are for cerclage or hemicerclage wire and interfragmentary wire. Cerclage wire can be applied to long oblique or spiral fractures where the length of the fracture line is at least twice the diameter of the bone and the entire bony column can be reconstructed. Cerclage wire should never be used as a sole method of fixation, but properly placed cerclage wire can provide interfragmentary compression and counteract rotational and axial forces when combined with an IM pin. Rules for the use of cerclage wires include placing a minimum of two wires and spacing them the appropriate distance from each other and from the fracture ends. As a general rule wires are spaced approximately one bone diameter away from each other and away from the fracture ends. This rule allows some adaptation for changes in patient size. Cerclage wires are often applied improperly, which can have negative effects on fracture reduction and bone healing. If the bony column is not reconstructed or if soft tissue is trapped between the wire and the bone, the wires will loosen decreasing fracture stability and disrupting periosteal blood supply. Hemicerclage wire and interfragmentary wire are utilized in certain short oblique and transverse fractures to prevent rotation, secure bone fragments, and stabilize fissures.

Interlocking nails are pins placed in the medullary canal and locked in place with screws or bolts placed through the proximal and distal fracture fragments. These screws or bolts also pass through special holes within the nail counteracting all forces acting on the fracture. The pin resists bending and the screws or bolts counteract rotation and axial forces. The largest nail that fits in the medullary canal should be used, and many sizes are available ranging from 4.0 to 10 mm. Their use in reptiles has not been documented but may be an option in some large lizards and crocodilians.

Stabilization of fractures with bone plates and screws is one of the most common methods of internal fixation for diaphyseal fractures in domestic mammals. The goal of fixation with bone plates and screws is to achieve early return to function and decreased morbidity that can be seen with other fixation systems. Implant design and application methods are adapting to decrease surgical trauma and maintain optimal bone biology to augment fracture healing.

Plates can be load-sharing or load-bearing devices. Neutralization plates neutralize the physiologic forces acting on a section of bone that has been anatomically reconstructed and stabilized. Indications for neutralization include reducible comminuted fractures and long oblique fractures. Compression can be achieved through proper use of a compression plate. Compressing the fragments together will minimize any gap at the fracture and will lead to direct bone healing with minimal to no callus production. Compression is limited to transverse and short oblique fractures since compressing long oblique fractures will lead to shear and displacement of the fracture ends. Buttress or bridging plates span a nonreducible comminuted fracture. The function of the plate is to maintain length and alignment, and prevent axial deformity by resisting bending, shear, and torsional forces.

There are a wide variety of plates available in veterinary orthopedic surgery. Semitubular plates, veterinary cuttable plates (VCPs), dynamic compression plates (DCPs), limited contact dynamic compression plates (LC-DCPs), and locking compression plates (LCPs) have all been used in reptiles. In general, plates area available in sizes from 1.5 mm round hole plates to 5.5 mm LCPs. VCP are versatile plates that have many properties that make them well suited for use in reptiles. These plates are available in two sizes

(1.5/2.0 and 2.0/2.7) based on the screws that can be used with the plates. They are available in one length of 50 holes and can be cut to the length of the bone that needs to be plated. The holes are spaced close together to allow a sufficient number of cortices to be captured with screws when small fracture fragments are present, and they can be stacked in situations where increased strength is needed. The use of plates in reptiles is often limited by the patient size. A general rule in plate fixation is to limit the size of the screw core diameter to 40% of the width of the bone (Koch 2005). Using this guideline 1.5 mm (screw core diameter 1.1 mm) round hole plates, 1.5–2.0 mm (1.5 mm screw core diameter) VCP, and 2.0 compression plates can be used in many small reptiles with a minimum bone diameter of 3 mm (Figure 7.6). A new system has recently been released with 1.0, 1.4, and 1.6 mm plate sizes (IMEX Veterinary, Longview, TX). These have not been used specifically in reptiles but could be an option for small patients.

A disadvantage of plate fixation is the cost associated with their applications. Plating systems also require an extensive approach to the bone, which disrupts the soft tissues around the bone. Minimally invasive plating techniques can minimize the amount of soft tissue disruption and could be applied to certain fractures in reptiles.

Fractures of the humerus and femur are seen in chelonians. Humeral fractures can occur in very large chelonians when they slip off during breeding and humeral and femoral fractures can occur when the leg is pinched between the carapace and plastron during hit by car incidents. Consider performing a carapacial osteotomy to gain access for fixation of proximal fractures of these bones with a bone plate.

Traumatic injuries can be seen in wild, farmed, and captive crocodilians. Many of these injuries are the result of fighting with other individuals (Nevarez 2009). Fracture fixation in crocodilians can be a challenge due to the large size, demeanor, and aquatic environment. Internal fixation with plates and screws is often preferred.

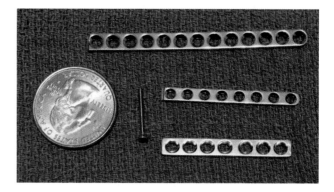

Figure 7.6 Examples of commonly available small bone plates. (a) A 2.0/2.7 mm veterinary cuttable plate (VCP), (b) a 1.5/2.0 mm veterinary cuttable plate (VCP), and (c) a 7 hole 2.0 mm dynamic compression plate. A United States quarter is shown for size comparison.

External Skeletal Fixation

ESFs involve placement of two to four transcutaneous pins into each major fracture fragment and connecting those pins to a connecting system outside the body. There are a variety of systems available for use in veterinary surgery with variations on clamp design. The stainless steel fixation pins are inserted through small skin incisions and penetrate both cortices of the proximal and distal major fragments. If the pin only exits the skin on one side of the limb, it is a half pin and if it exits the skin on both sides of the fracture, it is a full pin. A minimum of two pins should be placed in each fragment up to a maximum of four pins per fragment. Any additional pins after the fourth pin will not add any biomechanical advantage and only add to patient morbidity. Positive-profile threaded pins are recommended to prevent premature loosening. Important principles must be followed when placing fixation pins to maximize results. The pins should be inserted at a low rpm (150–300 rpm) to minimize any chance for thermal necrosis at the bone-implant interface. If the pins are placed at a high speed and there is thermal necrosis, the pins will prematurely loosen as the bone at the implant interface is resorbed. Hand chucks can be used; however, wobble can also lead to premature loosening. Connecting systems are made of a variety of materials including carbon fiber, aluminum, titanium, acrylic, polymethylmethacrylate (PMMA), or epoxy resins. Acrylic, epoxy, and PMMA connecting bars are particularly useful in reptiles due to their ease of application, low cost, and light weight. Once the fixation pins are in place, various types of tubing (Penrose drains or anesthesia tubing) are filled with acrylic or PMMA while the fracture is held in reduction. Similarly, the epoxy resin can be molded around the fixation pins while the fracture is reduced. The number and configuration of connecting bars can vary depending on the fracture and arrangement of the fixation pins.

The benefits of ESF systems include their versatility as they can be used in most long bone, mandibular, and even some spinal fractures. The components are less expensive than plating systems, and there is a significant reduction in the equipment required to apply an external fixator. There is also considerable versatility allowing them to be applied to different sized patients. In general, the diameter of the fixation pins should not exceed 25–30% of the bone diameter. IMEX ESF systems (IMEX Veterinary, Longview, TX) produces a miniature ESF system with positive profile pins ranging from 0.9 to 2.5 mm pins that can be used in a variety of small patients with bones as narrow as 3.6 mm diameter. These pins can be used with connecting bars and clamps or connected with acrylic or epoxy. In smaller reptiles, hypodermic needles or spinal needles have been used as fixation pins and connected with epoxy or acrylic

(Bennett 1996; Wellehan et al. 2001). The ability to adapt ESF to very small patients, and the affordability have made external skeletal fixators a favorite method of fixation among reptile veterinarians.

Disadvantages of ESF systems include patient morbidity associated with transcutaneous fixation pins. Patient morbidity will vary depending on the fracture. When fixation pins are passed through a large muscle mass, they cause more patient morbidity and pin loosening due to muscle contraction causing pin movement. Some use bandages for external fixators to protect the pins, clamps, and connecting bars and to keep the pin tracts clean, but they are not considered essential. If used, these bandages must be changed and the pin tracts inspected regularly which can add to costs associated with the treatment.

Virtually, all methods of fracture fixation have been applied to reptiles, and the surgical approach and principles of application are similar to mammalian species; however, some differences do exist (Bennett 1996). When placing ESF constructs in many reptiles, the orientation of the pins should be in a cranial to caudal direction that is parallel to the substrate instead of a medial to lateral orientation used in mammals because they rest their limbs perpendicular to the long axis of the body parallel to the substrate. Bone plating has been performed in larger reptiles. In some species, the long bones are curved which makes precise plate contouring challenging. In these cases, reconstruction and string-of-pearl plates that allow contouring in multiple planes may be preferred. An alternative would be to use locking plates since these do not require the plate to be contoured precisely to the surface of the bone.

In some cases, the severity of the trauma, patient size, or other confounding factors makes surgical or nonsurgical management of the fracture impossible. In very select cases, amputation may be the best option for fracture management. Complications associated with fracture repair occur due to inappropriate choice of implants, improper placement of the implants, poor owner compliance with postoperative instructions, or, in some cases, bad luck. Delayed unions, nonunions, and malunions can all occur. Depending on the severity, treatment may not be required, the fracture may need revision, or, in the worst cases, amputation may be indicated.

Shell Fractures

The chelonian shell is a dynamic, metabolically active structure composed of 60 dermal bones covered with keratinized epidermal scutes (Adkesson et al. 2007). Traumatic injuries to chelonian shells are common after patients are hit by cars, run over by lawnmowers, or attacked by carnivores (Mitchell 2002). A detailed understanding of anatomy is important because shell fractures can affect other body systems. The pelvic and pectoral girdles, and the spine are incorporated into the shell and fractures can affect all of these (Mitchell 2002). Animals with shell fractures crossing the dorsal midline should be examined carefully for evidence of paraparesis or paralysis, which carry a guarded to poor prognosis (Figure 7.7). If neurologic signs are present, a CT or MRI can further evaluate any compromise to the spinal cord. Culture of the fracture sites and empirical antibiotic therapy is crucial since shell fractures are considered open fractures and osteomyelitis can occur. Many shell fractures communicate with the coelomic cavity and infection can affect soft tissues and organs within. Chelonians do not have a diaphragm and respiration will not be affected by fractures that penetrate the coelomic cavity; however, any damage to or contamination of the lung can lead to complications and affect the prognosis. Broad spectrum antibiotic therapy should be started until culture results are available and aggressive wound therapy should be initiated once the patient is stable to decrease gross contamination and devitalized tissue.

Many traumatic shell injuries are associated with serious wounds. Proper wound care with copious lavage and debridement are needed before shell fracture repair can be planned. Wound management techniques used in other species can be applied to chelonians such as wet to dry bandages, sugar bandages, honey bandages, or negative pressure wound therapy can all be used depending on the nature of the wounds.

Epoxy resin and fiberglass patches were once the standard treatment for shell fractures; however, these were associated with abscesses and osteomyelitis that developed underneath the fiberglass patch, and this technique is no longer recommended (Barten 2006b). Other techniques have been used including orthopedic screws, orthopedic wire, bone plates, and cable ties (Figure 7.8). Screws with orthopedic wire is a simple, inexpensive technique for fracture fixation and compression and allows for continued

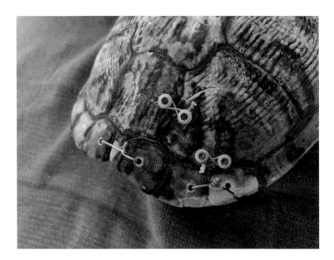

Figure 7.8 Fractured carapace in a red-eared slider (*Trachemys scripta*) showing interfragmentary wire and screws to compress the fractures.

wound care (Fleming 2008). A similar technique uses epoxy and cable ties and avoids penetration of healthy bone (Forrester and Satta 2005). With either technique, wounds can be treated as the fractures heal and the implants can be easily removed after healing.

Joint Disease

Joint disease can be caused by a variety of mechanisms and diseases. Arthritis (osteoarthritis and septic arthritis), joint instability or luxations, and gout can cause pain, joint swelling, and lameness (Figure 7.9).

Iguanas and other lizards are commonly found to have bacterial septic arthritis (Maxwell 2003). Clinical signs include lameness and painful swollen joints. Radiographs show lysis of the epiphyses and widening of the joint space. In some cases, subluxation or luxation of the joint may occur. Joint aspirates can be used to obtain a definitive diagnosis, and culture of the joint contents or synovium can be used to guide antibiotic treatment. If the infection does not respond to conservative treatment, arthrotomy with lavage and debridement is required. In some cases, antibiotic impregnated beads are helpful for the treatment of septic arthritis (Bennett 1999). Beads that are not absorbable should be removed from the joint after the infection has resolved.

Stifle instability was documented in a spur-thighed tortoise that was presented for acute left hind limb lameness (Hernandez-Divers 2002). Stifle instability was diagnosed based on clinical findings and diagnostic imaging. A modification of the over-the-top method for cranial cruciate reconstruction using a vastus muscle autograft was performed with lateral imbrication of the joint capsule.

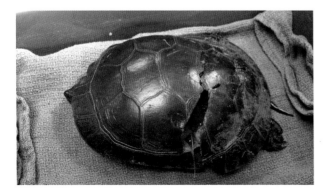

Figure 7.7 Severe fracture of the carapace in a painted turtle (*Chrysemys picta*). Note the fracture line extends past the midline (red arrow). This patient showed neurologic deficits to the hind limbs with loss of motor activity.

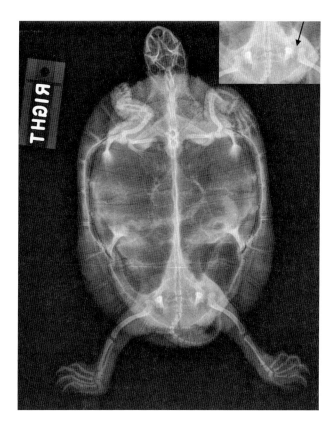

Figure 7.9 A full body DV view of a chelonian (species unknown) showing luxation of the left coxofemoral joint.

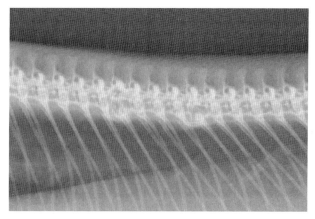

Figure 7.10 A lateral radiograph of a red-tailed Boa (*Boa constrictor*) showing proliferative spinal osteopathy.

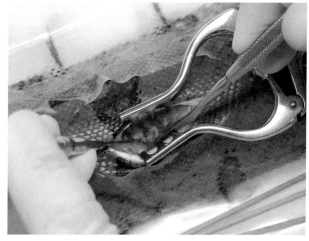

Figure 7.11 Intraoperative photograph showing approach to the spine to obtain samples for histopathology and/or culture, or to place antibiotic impregnated beads.

Proliferative Spinal Osteopathy

Proliferative spinal osteopathy affects the joints of the spinal column and has been described in turtles, lizards, and most commonly snakes (Isaza et al. 2000; Fitzgerald and Vera 2006). The exact cause remains unclear and many etiologies have been proposed such as trauma, nutritional deficiencies, viral infections, neoplasia and bacterial infections. Clinical signs vary depending on location and extent of the lesions and can include stiffness, scoliosis, and kyphosis. Spinal lesions can lead to weakness and affect spinal reflexes. In severe cases, it can affect an animal's ability to move, strike, constrict, or swallow prey. Radiographs show segmental vertebral bone proliferation with exostosis predominantly on the ventrolateral aspects of the vertebrae (Figure 7.10). Biopsies of affected bone for culture and histopathology is recommended as well as blood cultures since there can be a strong correlation between blood cultures and bone culture results (Figure 7.11) (Isaza et al. 2000; Fitzgerald and Vera 2006). Many of the lesions can cause spinal cord compression or nerve root compression and animals may present for neurologic abnormalities.

Treatment of spinal osteopathy involves long-term antibiotic therapy and early recognition is essential for a favorable long-term prognosis. Antibiotics with good bone penetration should be selected and administered. Antibiotic-impregnated beads can also be used in selected cases with focal lesions, and the antibiotics impregnated within the beads should be based on culture and sensitivity results. Aggressive analgesia should also be implemented. Overall, the prognosis is poor since animals are often presented with advanced clinical disease (Fitzgerald and Vera 2006).

References

Abou-Madi, N., Scrivani, P.V., Kollias, G.V., and Hernandez-Divers, S.M. (2004). Diagnosis of skeletal injuries in chelonians using computed tomography. *Journal of Zoo and Wildlife Medicine* 35: 226–231.

Adkesson, M., Travis, E.K., Weber, M.A. et al. (2007). Vacuum assisted closure for treatment of a deep shell abscess and osteomyelitis in a tortoise. *Journal of the American Veterinary Medican Association* 231: 1249–1254.

Alleman, A. and Kupprion, E. (2007). Cytologic diagnosis of disease in reptiles. *Veterinary Clinics of North America: Exotic Animal Practice* 10 (1): 155–186.

Barten, S.L. (2006a). Lizards. In: Reptile Medicine and Surgery (ed. D. Mader), 59–77. St. Louis, MO: Saunders.

Barten, S.L. (2006b). Shell damage. In: Reptile Medicine and Surgery (ed. D. Mader), 893–899. St. Louis, MO: Saunders.

Bennett, R. (1996). Fracture management. In: Reptile Medicine and Surgery (ed. D. Mader), 281–286. Philadelphia, PA: Saunders.

Bennett, R. (1999). Antibiotic PMMA beads for septic arthritis in a green iguana. *Exotic DVM* 1 (3): 27–28.

Boyer, T. and Boyer, D. (2006). Turtles, tortoises, and terrapins. In: Reptile Medicine and Surgery (ed. D. Mader), 78–99. St. Louis, MO: Saunders.

Dunning, D. (2002). Basic mammalian bone anatomy and healing. *Veterinary Clinics of North America: Exotic Animal Practice* 5 (1): 115–128.

Enlow, D. (1969). The bone of reptiles. In: Biology of the Reptilia (ed. C. Gans), 45–80. London: Academic Press.

Fitzgerald, K. and Vera, R. (2006). Spinal osteopathy. In: Reptile Medicine and Surgery (ed. D. Mader), 906–912. St. Louis, MO: Saunders.

Fleming, G. (2008). Clinical technique: chelonian shell repair. *Journal of Exotic Pet Medicine* 17 (4): 246–258.

Foote, J. (1911). The comparative histology of femoral bones. *Transactions of the American Microscopical Society* 30 (2): 87–140.

Forrester, H. and Satta, J. (2005). Easy shell repair. *Exotic DVM* 6 (6): 13.

Funk, R. (2006). Snakes. In: Reptile Medicine and Surgery (ed. D. Mader), 42–58. St. Louis, MO: Saunders.

Hernandez-Divers, S. (2002). Diagnosis and surgical repair of stifle luxation in a spur-thighed tortoise (*Testtudo graeca*). *Journal of Zoo and Wildlife Medicine* 33 (2): 125–130.

Hernandez-Divers, S. (2006). Diagnostic techniques. In: Reptile Medicine and Surgery (ed. D. Mader), 490–532. St. Louis, MO: Saunders.

Isaza, R., Garner, M., and Jacobson, E. (2000). Proliferative osteoarthritis and osteoarthrosis in 15 snakes. *Journal of Zoo and Wildlife Medicine* 31 (1): 20–27.

Kirchgessner, M. and Mitchell, M. (2009). Chelonians. In: Manual of Exotic Pet Practice (eds. M. Mitchell and T. Tully), 207–249. St. Louis, MO: Saunders.

Koch, D. (2005). Screws and plates. In: AO Principles of Fracture Management in the Dog and Cat (eds. A. Johnson, J. Houlton and R. Vannini), 27–52. Switzerland: AO Publishing.

Mader, D. et al. (2006). Surgery. In: Reptile Medicine and Surgery (ed. D. Mader), 581–630. St. Louis, MO: Saunders.

Maxwell, L. (2003). Infectious and non infectious diseases. In: Biology, Husbandrym and Medicine of the Green Iguana (ed. E. Jacobson), 108–132. Malabar: Krieger.

Mitchell, M. (2002). Diagnosis and management of reptile orthopedic injuries. *The Veterinary Clinics of North America: Exotic Animal Practice* 5 (1): 97–114.

Mitchell, M. (2009). Snakes. In: Manual of Exotic Pet Practice (eds. M. Mitchell and T. Tully), 136–163. St. Louis, MO: Saunders.

Nevarez, J. (2009). Crocodilians. In: Manual of Exotic Pet Practice (eds. M. Mitchell and T. Tully), 113–135. St. Loius, MO: Saunders.

Pritchard, J. and Ruzicka, A. (1950). Comparison of fracture repair in the frog, lizard, and rat. *Journal of Anatomy* 84: 236–261.

Raftery, A. (2011). Reptile orthopedic medicine and surgery. *Journal of Exotic Pet Medicine* 20 (2): 107–116.

Stetter, M. (2001). Diagnostic imaging of Amphibians. In: Amphibian Medicine and Captive Husbandry (eds. B. Whitaker and K. Wright), 253–272. Malabar: Kreiger.

Wellehan, J. et al. (2001). Type I skeletal fixation of radial fractures in microchiropternas. *Journal of Zoo and Wildlife Medicine* 32 (4): 487–493.

8

Surgical Approaches to the Reptile Coelom

Geoffrey W. Pye and R. Avery Bennett

The surgical approach to the coelomic cavity of reptiles varies with taxonomic group. The approach is basically the same in lizards and crocodilians and is a function of their body conformation. Chelonians have the shell that protects them from predators and trauma but makes it difficult to get into the coelom. The internal anatomic location of organs and their mode of locomotion affect the approach used in snakes.

Chelonian Coelom

Prefemoral Approach

A prefemoral approach can be used to access the bladder, kidney, caudal intestine, and reproductive tract. The benefits of this approach over a plastron osteotomy are incising through soft tissues only and a faster healing time resulting in a quicker return to normal function, especially in aquatic chelonians. It is recommended as the approach of choice in species with a small plastron (e.g. marine and snapping turtles) if it will provide access to the structure of interest. The disadvantages are that it only allows access to the caudal coelom, provides a small working space, is difficult to exteriorize organs, and limitations of the shell may prevent the removal of large bladder stones.

The chelonian is placed in either dorsal or ventral recumbency. The former makes the surgery easier, while the latter allows for better ventilation; however, assisting ventilation is recommended with either position. Elevate the cranial aspect of the body to allow viscera to fall caudally. With the hind limb pulled caudally to open up the prefemoral fossa, make a cranial to caudal incision through the skin and subcutaneous tissues starting at the bridge midway between the carapace and plastron extending it toward the leg (Figure 8.1a). Identify the muscle layer, and separate the abdominal oblique and transverse abdominal muscle fibers using a grid technique or tent the muscles and make a stab incision and extend it cranially and caudally with Metzenbaum scissors (Figure 8.1b). Identify the coelomic membrane and carefully incise it by tenting and cutting it with Metzenbaum scissors (Figure 8.1c). Avoid accidentally incising the bladder wall which can look very similar to the coelomic wall.

Close in three layers. Close the coelomic membrane with a simple continuous pattern using absorbable monofilament material (Figure 8.1d), the muscle and subcutaneous tissues with a simple continuous pattern and the skin with a simple interrupted or everting pattern (Figure 8.1e). In aquatic species, test the seal of the wound closure by applying positive pressure ventilation. Put water over the incision, and if there is a leak, it will bubble when the lungs expand. Application of tissue glue on the wound can help protect it from the aquatic environment. Keep aquatic chelonians out of water (dry dock) overnight and then monitor for wound leakage indicated by sudden weight gain or changes on survey radiographs (e.g. fluid-filled coelom). This can be confirmed with ultrasound.

Scope-assisted Celiotomy in Large Chelonians

In large chelonians such as Galapagos tortoises, make a prefemoral approach as described above large enough to insert a gloved arm. Use sterile obstetric gloves to maintain aseptic technique. In the other prefemoral fossa, make a smaller approach large enough to insert a rigid endoscope and endosurgical instruments. The approaches will create pneumocoelom providing a working space within which a procedure can be performed. Use the scope to view what the arm is doing inside the coelom. Endosurgical instruments and tissue sealing devices can be inserted into either celiotomy incision depending on the procedure to be performed. Many complicated procedures can be accomplished with the aid of an arm and endosurgical instruments while visualizing the procedure with the endoscope.

Surgery of Exotic Animals, First Edition. Edited by R. Avery Bennett and Geoffrey W. Pye.
© 2022 John Wiley & Sons, Inc. Published 2022 by John Wiley & Sons, Inc.

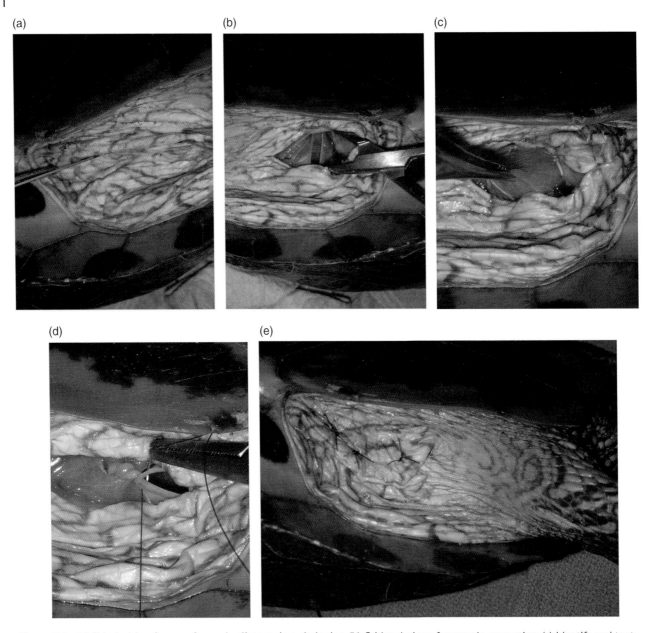

Figure 8.1 (a) Skin incision for a prefemoral celiotomy in a chelonian. (b) Grid technique for muscle separation. (c) Identify and tent the coelomic membrane prior to making a stab incision. (d) Close the coelomic membrane with a simple continuous suture pattern. (e) Close the skin with a slightly everting suture pattern.

Plastron Osteotomy

For greater access to the chelonian coelom, a plastron osteotomy is indicated. Computed tomography (CT) is a useful aid in determining the size, position, and depth of the osteotomy (Figure 8.2a–d). Use imaging to determine the location of the pelvic bones, which insert on the plastron, to avoid damaging them when making the osteotomies. In most cases, the osteotomy will involve the femoral and abdominal shields. With the chelonian in dorsal recumbency, mark the corners of the planned osteotomy site

using a low-speed drill or burr. This allows for easy identification of the margins of the osteotomy following aseptic preparation of the surgical site. Using an oscillating saw or diamond edge-cutting wheel (Figure 8.3), cut the plastron along the straight lines between the marked corners. Use the thinnest blade possible to reduce the size of the gap created. Bevel each cut toward the center of the plastron to be elevated (Figure 8.4a). During closure, when the bone flap is replaced, it will drop slightly (the amount will depend on the thickness of the saw), but there will be bone-on-bone contact to facilitate bone healing. If a thick blade or bur is

(a)

(b)

(c)

(d)

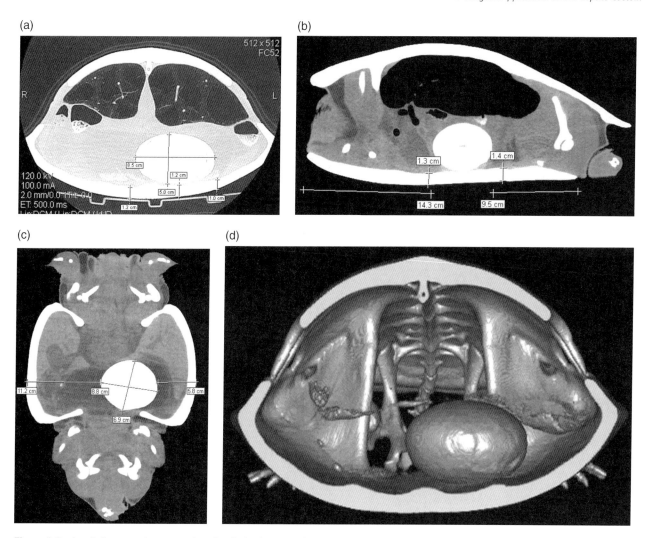

Figure 8.2 (a–d) Computed tomography of a chelonian used for surgical planning for the removal of a bladder stone. This stone was too large for a prefemoral approach so a central plastron osteotomy was used. Measurements were made on the CT to help plan the osteotomy site.

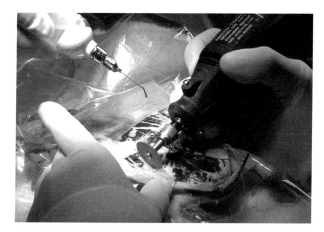

Figure 8.3 A diamond-edged cutting wheel is used to create the plastron osteotomy in a chelonian.

used, the gap might be too large to achieve bone-to-bone contact. The corners will usually need to be cut using an osteotome because the round blade will not cut through at the corners unless the cut is made beyond them. When all four cuts have been made, lever the osteotomized piece (Figure 8.4b) from the caudal and lateral edges and flip it cranially or the cranial and lateral edges and flip it caudally depending on which direction will provide the best exposure for the procedure to be performed. Keep the muscle attachments intact because they provide blood supply to the section of plastron (Figure 8.4c). Cover the bone flap and the edges of the cut plastron with saline-soaked sponges to keep the bone moist and to protect any exteriorized coelomic contents from the sharp edges. If the bone flap becomes detached creating a free section of plastron, preserve it in saline moistened sponges, and incorporate it

(a)

(b)

(c)

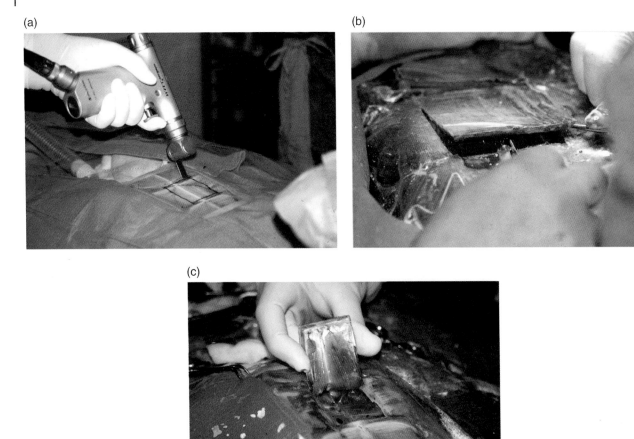

Figure 8.4 (a) An oscillating saw is used to create the plastron osteotomy in a chelonian. Note that the blade is cutting at an angle toward the center of the osteotomy site. (b) After cutting is completed, the plastron osteotomy piece is elevated on the caudal and lateral sides and flapped cranially. In this case, the plastron section is being elevated caudally. Use a periosteal elevator to elevate the pectoral muscles from the inner surface of the plastron to allow the section to be reflected caudally. (c) Attempt to keep muscle attachments to the section of plastron. This should improve bone healing by preserving some of the blood supply to the section.

into the closure. While there are no studies evaluating the healing of the plastron after plastron osteotomy, it is a well establish principle of orthopedic surgery that preserving muscle attachments to bone helps maintain the periosteal blood supply to the bone and improves bone healing. Early reports of plastron osteotomy describe removing the segment of bone and do not report necrosis of the segment of bone (Frye 1991). The authors have had similar experience.

Elevate the muscle off the internal aspect of the plastron section using a periosteal elevator. If the flap is reflected caudally, elevate the pectoral muscles off the internal aspect of the plastron, and if the flap is reflected cranially, elevate the pelvic muscles off the plastron section. Again, preserve the pelvic muscle attachments if the section is reflected caudally or preserve the pectoral muscles if the section is to be reflected cranially. It is essential to maintain as many soft tissue attachments to the plastron as possible

for proper healing of the osteotomy. The coelomic membrane is thin and translucent with no muscles detectable (Figure 8.4c). There is a large venous sinus on each side about halfway between midline and the bridge. This sinus quickly spasms and becomes difficult to identify. Be careful to avoid damaging these; however, it appears they can be sacrificed if necessary. It would seem that if the sinus is damaged during the procedure, once the patient's blood pressure increases a defect in the sinus could cause severe hemorrhage although this has not specifically been observed. Tent the coelomic membrane and incise it with Metzenbaum scissors along midline to avoid any major vasculature. Use a ring retractor or other self-retaining retractor on the coelomic membrane if greater visualization is needed (Figure 8.5).

In species with a hinge, the flap can be based on the hinge. Make three cuts, usually in the abdominal and femoral shields, and elevate the flap cranially preserving the pectoral muscle attachments. There is no need to cut the fourth side because the hinge will allow the flap to be reflected cranially providing exposure to the caudal coelomic contents.

Close the coelomic membrane using an absorbable suture in a simple continuous pattern. Place the plastron flap back in place. The coelomic membrane prevents it from dropping too far, but if the osteotomy is well planned the section will make contact with the perimeter plastron as well (Figure 8.6). The plastron flap can be secured in place with fiberglass and resin, acrylic glues, orthopedic

wire, and/or orthopedic screws and wire (Figure 8.7a,b). Foreign material between the cut surfaces of bone can inhibit healing. Prevent resin or glue from getting into the defect by carefully avoiding the edges, placing an antibiotic ointment along the defect, or packing or taping the osteotomy lines (Figure 8.8). Dry dock aquatic chelonians overnight and then monitor for wound leakage indicated by sudden weight gain or changes on survey radiographs or ultrasound (fluid-filled coelom).

The authors have been unable to find any scientific studies on plastron healing after this procedure. It seems to take 2–12 months for the osteotomy to heal (Tamukai 2010; Boyer 2015). These patches can remain in place for many

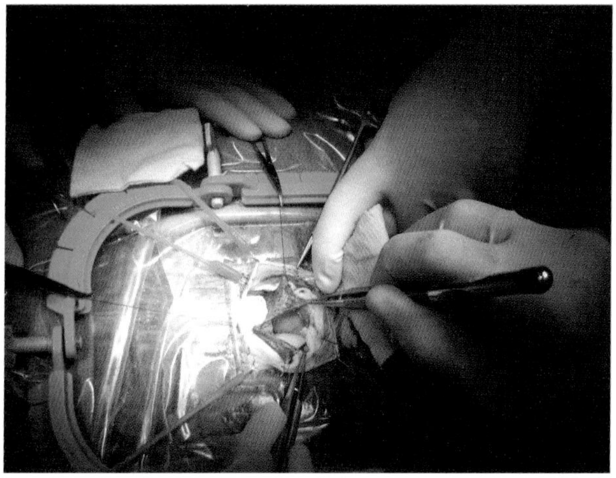

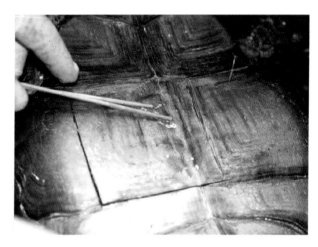

Figure 8.5 A ring retractor can be used to improve exposure of the coelomic contents. The hooks are placed in the coelomic membrane, and a cystotomy has been performed to remove eggs from the urinary bladder.

Figure 8.6 If the plastron osteotomy flap is cut with an inward beveled edge, it will provide bone-on-bone contact for improved healing of the osteotomy.

(a)   (b)

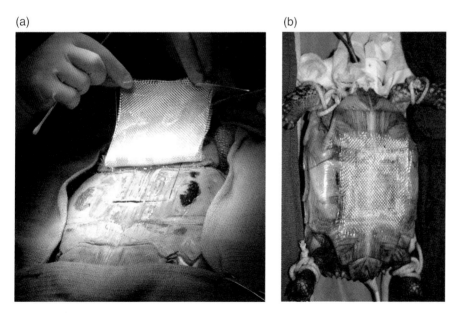

Figure 8.7 (a, b) Fiberglass and epoxy resin can be used to stabilize the plastron section as well as provide waterproofing in aquatic chelonians.

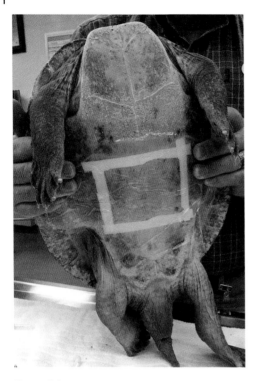

Figure 8.8 Placing tape directly over the edges of the plastron osteotomy site will prevent seepage of epoxy into the gap that might inhibit healing.

years before falling off on their own (>10 years). Anecdotally reported complications include failure of the osteotomy to heal resulting in a dead segment of plastron under the patch and possibly infection. In one report, 8 of 18 plastron segments had not healed after the patch was removed 12 months postoperatively (Tamukai 2010). This is likely the result of completely detaching the segment resulting in flap necrosis, emphasizing the need to maintain muscle and other soft tissue attachments. Remove the patch after 6–12 months as it should be healed by then. If it is not, initiate open-wound management.

In chelonians that are still growing, a patch will potentially alter normal shell growth. Either remove the patch in about eight weeks or remove it from the junction of the shields to allow free growth or use an alternate method for maintaining the segment of plastron immobilized.

In young animals where the plastron is not well mineralized, it is possible to incise the plastron with a scalpel. Be very careful not to cut deeper structures. Follow the lines between epidermal shields. Remember that the epidermal shields and bone plates only match up at the hinge and midline. Use heavy suture material to suture the plastron back together. Cover the incision site with a bandage for at least two weeks to allow healing to commence.

Other methods reported for stabilizing the segment including interfragmentary orthopedic wires, bone plates, bone screws and figure of eight orthopedic wires, zip ties, and epoxy putty (Tamukai 2010). When these methods are employed, the osteotomy should be protected from the substrate and environmental contaminants keeping the osteotomy covered with a bandage for a couple of weeks or more (Tamukai 2010).

Partial Plastron Ostectomy

An alternative method for celiotomy in chelonians is a partial plastron ostectomy (Rodriguez de la Rosa and Martorell Monserrat 2009). The approach is as described above; however, the segment of plastron is completely removed and discarded (Figure 8.9). Close the coelomic membrane with a simple continuous or interrupted monofilament absorbable material. Place a hydrocolloidal dressing cut to fit the defect over the coelomic membrane and cover the dressing with a gas permeable film. Change the bandage weekly. In their patient, at two months, the coelomic membrane had healed and became firm. Mineralization was noted to be occurring peripherally migrating centrally. At this point, there is no need to continue to bandage. At six months epithelization and pigmentation had occurred. At 10 months, mineralization and epithelialization were nearly complete. After six years, it was difficult to distinguish where the piece of plastron had been removed.

One author (RAB) has had similar experience in a green turtle where part of the segment of plastron necrosed. The defect was managed as an open wound, and eventually, the defect filled in and the turtle was released.

Lateral Plastron Osteotomy Combined with Prefemoral Approach

A celiotomy that combines a lateral plastron osteotomy with the prefemoral approach can be used to increase exposure of the coelomic contents (Figure 8.10). Improved postsurgical waterproofing, faster healing, and fewer complications have been reported with this method (McArthur and Hernandez-Divers 2004). With the chelonian in dorsal recumbency, cut a section of the plastron immediately adjacent to prefemoral fossa and reflect it toward the middle of the plastron. Extend the prefemoral incision into the tissues underlying the plastron. Following closure of the soft tissues, stabilize the plastron flap with one of the methods as described for a central plastron osteotomy (Figure 8.11) or with crossed K wires that can be removed in four weeks (McArthur and Hernandez-Divers 2004).

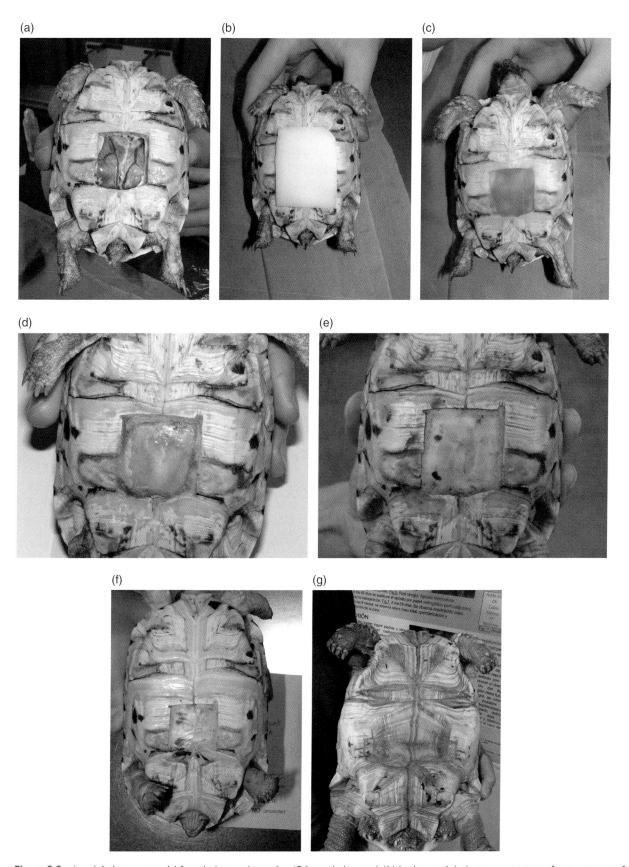

Figure 8.9 (a–g) A three-year-old female leopard tortoise (*Stigmochelys pardalis*) had a partial plastron ostectomy for treatment of a gastric foreign body. (a) The coelomic membrane was closed with a simple continuous pattern. (b) A hydrocolloid was cut to fit the defect before placing it onto the defect for moist wound management then (c) a gas-permeable thin film was placed over the hydrocolloid to protect the wound. (d) After 68 days, the membrane became firm with evidence of mineralization occurring at the periphery migrating centrally. (e) At six months, mineralization had progressed and epithelization was nearly complete. Note there is pigmentation which is interesting because scar tissue is not usually pigmented. (f) In 10 months, keratinization was complete and was thicker. Notice how much growth had occurred at the seams (g) The appearance following partial plastron ostectomy six years later. At this point, it is difficult to determine where the segment of plastron had been removed.

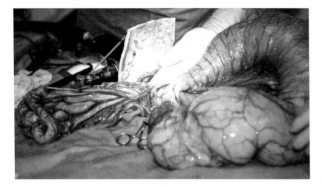

Figure 8.10 A combination of a prefemoral approach with an adjacent plastron osteotomy will facilitate additional exposure of the coelomic contents in this case of a mesenteric volvulus in a green sea turtle (*Chelonia mydas*).

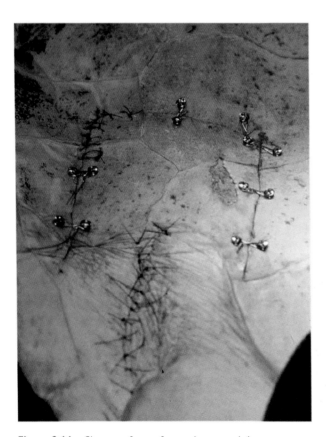

Figure 8.11 Closure of a prefemoral approach in combination with adjacent plastron osteotomy using both suture and orthopedic screws with wire for stabilization of the osteotomy site.

Snake Coelom

Lateral Approach

Due to the elongated body, it is important to know the region that is needed to be accessed. Palpation, radiographs, ultrasound, CT, or MRI can help determine the site of the celiotomy. In some circumstances (e.g. dystocia), multiple celiotomies may be needed to be able to get all of the eggs or feti out.

Historically, a ventral midline celiotomy has been used. In one report, the authors indicated they did not observe any problems in healing using a ventral midline compared to a lateral celiotomy (Millichamp et al. 1983). Making a lateral incision is preferred by the authors because it is less subject to contamination by the substrate and is less likely to be traumatized during locomotion. Additionally, snakes have a ventral abdominal vein along the ventral midline that is best to avoid.

Make the incision between the first two rows of scales dorsal to the wide ventral scutes. By making the incision in this location, when the incision is closed, the two rows of scales will be everted slightly, rather than everting the lateral edge of the scutes against the first row of scales and the incision will not be in contact with the substrate. Elevate a scale and identify the underlying skin between the two most ventral rows of scales lateral to the large ventral scutes (Figure 8.12a,b). Make a longitudinal zigzag skin incision between the scales using a #11 scalpel or radiofrequency electrosurgical unit (Figure 8.12c). Avoid cutting the ventral rib ends. Lift a scale and insert the sharp tip of the #11 blade, sharp edge directed outward, and stab a couple of millimeters deep between two scales. Lift the blade outward cutting the skin, not the scales. Repeat this process in a zigzag fashion a couple of times always cutting between scales and away from the body wall and internal organs. Once the incision is about 1 cm long, it becomes easier to identify the skin and make the zigzag cut always lifting the tip of the blade away from the body. Stab and lift between two scales, change the direction to go between the next two scales, and repeat the process until the incision is long enough. If the blade is used in a traditional manner, because the skin is so thick and tough, there is a risk the incision will also cut through the body wall and into viscera. After completing the skin incision, lift the body wall with forceps and incise a few millimeters ventral to the end of the ribs. Make the incision in the body wall with closure in mind allowing sufficient body wall on both sides of the incision to hold suture.

Close the body wall with an absorbable monofilament suture swaged on an atraumatic needle in a simple continuous pattern. The body wall muscle is thin with no fascial covering and does not hold suture well, so roll the skin outwards to place the needle between the skin and muscle, follow the curve of the needle through the muscle, and do not pull too tightly on the suture or it will tear through. For skin closure, use an interrupted everting suture pattern (e.g. vertical or horizontal mattress) as the skin's tendency is to invert. Tighten the sutures to produce slight eversion

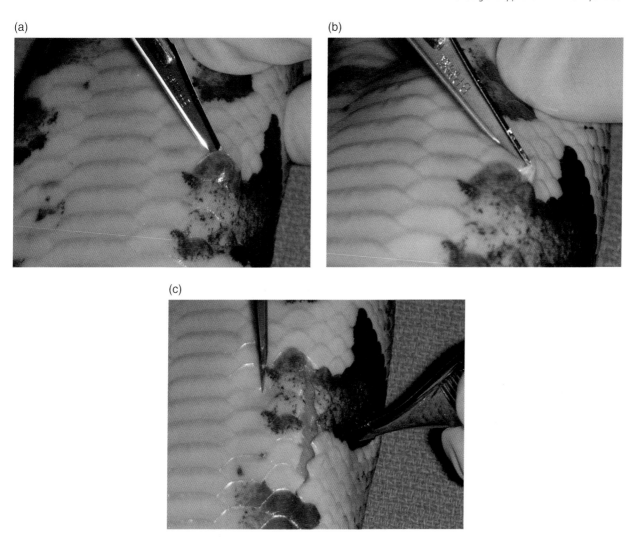

Figure 8.12 (a–c) For a snake celiotomy, (a) elevate the second scale from the ventral scute, (b) identify the skin, and (c) make a longitudinal zigzag skin incision between the first and second row of scales.

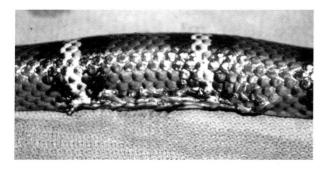

Figure 8.13 Closure of snake skin following a celiotomy using a horizontal mattress pattern. Tighten the sutures to produce slight eversion to ensure the cut surfaces are in contact.

with the cut surfaces in contact rather than the surfaces of the scales being in contact (Figure 8.13). Overtightening will result in a ridge with exposure of the cut skin edges to the environment and can compromise blood supply to the incision causing necrosis and sloughing.

Lizard and Crocodilian Coelom

Ventral Paramedian Approach

The skin is thick and tough, and the body wall is thin in lizards with the absence of subcutaneous tissues. The ventral abdominal vein runs along the midline from the umbilical scar to the liver, immediately dorsal to the body wall (Figure 8.14). Clinical evidence suggests that if it is incised, it can be ligated without consequence, but the authors prefer to avoid it. The muscle of the body wall has no fascial covering and is very thin. There is no linea alba. Make a paramedian skin incision several millimeters lateral to midline caudal to the umbilical scar and extend it cranially (Figure 8.15). Use a #11 blade to stab and lift outward as described above to avoid damaging the underlying body wall and coelomic organs. Once the skin has been incised, lift the body wall with forceps and make a small stab incision. Insert hemostats or atraumatic forceps to lift the body wall and protect the coelomic organs including the ventral abdominal vein from iatrogenic damage. Extend the incision in small increments repositioning the hemostats or forceps each time.

Closure is similar to that in snakes. Use a monofilament absorbable suture with a swaged-on, atraumatic needle in a simple continuous pattern. Roll the skin outward to insert the needle between the skin and body wall (Figure 8.16a), follow the curve of the needle to engage body wall, and avoid pulling the suture too tight. Close the skin using an everting suture pattern (Figure 8.16b). Take care to not overtighten. The cut skin edges should just meet.

The ventral paramedian approach in crocodilians is similar to that in lizards, though the scales are thicker, and body wall is more robust.

Paracostal Approach

For laterally compressed lizards, a lateral approach is preferred. With the lizard in lateral recumbency, make a skin incision 2–3 mm caudal and lateral to the last rib. In some species where the ribs protect the majority of the coelom (e.g. chameleons), an intercostal approach may

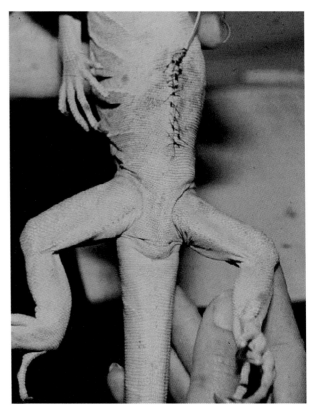

Figure 8.15 A paramedian celiotomy incision closure following castration in this green iguana (*Iguana iguana*).

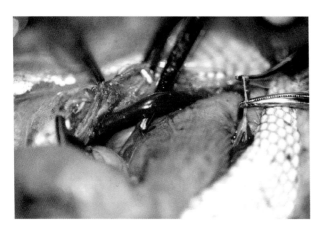

Figure 8.14 The ventral abdominal vein in a lizard runs directly dorsal to the body wall. Making a paramedian approach avoids this vein during approach and closure.

(a)

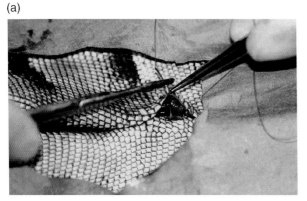

(b)

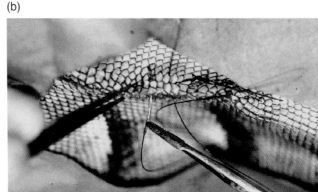

Figure 8.16 (a, b) For closure of a celiotomy in a snake or lizard, (a) roll the skin outwards to engage the needle in the body wall, follow the curve of the needle, and avoid pulling the suture too tight. (b) Close the skin using an everting suture pattern taking care to not overtighten; the skin edges should just meet.

be required. To gain greater exposure to the coelom, ventrally extend the incision paramedianly to avoid the ventral abdominal vein by creating an L-shaped incision. Make a similar incision in the body wall, taking care to avoid iatrogenic damage to the underlying coelomic contents. Flap the skin and body wall caudodorsally to maximize exposure of the coelom. Closure is as described above.

Postfemoral Approach for Renal Biopsy in Iguanids

The kidneys lie in the caudal abdomen with the caudal pole deep in the femoral region. With the iguanid in ventral recumbency, flex the hind limb as far cranially as possible. Make a horizontal skin incision at the juncture of the hind limb and the lateral tail (Figure 8.17). Separate the muscle in a grid manner to expose the caudal pole of

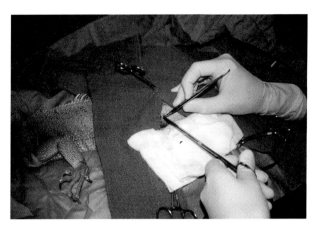

Figure 8.17 To approach the kidney for biopsy in a lizard, make an incision at the junction of the tail with the hind limb.

the kidney. Collect a sample using biopsy forceps. Close the muscle with a single cruciate suture and the skin with a one or two everting mattress sutures.

References

Boyer T.H. (2015). Chelonian surgery. *Proceedings, Pacific Veterinary Conference*, PacVet 2015, Long Beach, CA.

Frye, F.L. (1991). Surgery. In: *Biomedical and Surgical Aspects of Captive Reptile Husbandry*, vol. II (ed. F.L. Frye), 441–471. Malabar, FL: Krieger Publishing Company.

McArthur, S. and Hernandez-Divers, S. (2004). Surgery. In: *Medicine and Surgery of Tortoises and Turtles* (eds. S. McArthur, R. Wilkinson, J. Meyer, et al.), 403–464. Oxford: Blackwell Publishing Ltd.

Millichamp, N.J., Lawrence, K., Jacobson, E.R. et al. (1983). Egg retention in snakes. *Journal of the American Veterinary Medical Association* 183: 1213–1218.

Rodriguez de la Rosa, L. and Martorell Monserrat, J. (2009). Intestinal obstruction and secondary mild coelomitis after barium administration in a leopard tortoise (*Stigmochelys pardalis*). Poster. *Southern European Veterinary Conference*, Barcelona, Spain.

Tamukai, K. (2010). Flap closure method using epoxy putty in plastron osteotomy in chelonians. *Exotic DVM* 12: 5–11.

9

Reptiles: Soft Tissue Surgery

Stephen J. Mehler and R. Avery Bennett

Anatomy

Prior to undertaking a surgical procedure in a reptile patient, the surgeon must become familiar with the unique anatomy that varies among and within families of reptiles. For example, in green iguanas, the kidneys are normally located within the pelvic canal, while in monitor lizards, they are within the coelomic cavity (Bennett 1989a,b; Mehler and Bennett 2006).

Some features are relatively consistent across species of reptiles. In general, reptiles do not have a muscular diaphragm and, as such, have a coelomic cavity rather than thoracic and abdominal cavities. Crocodilians do have a relatively well-developed septum or fibrous diaphragm between the thoracic viscera and the abdominal viscera. Reptiles do not have lymph nodes. They do not store fat in the subcutaneous tissue but have discrete fat bodies within the coelom that can become quite large and well vascularized.

The urinary system of reptiles is substantially different from that of mammals. Reptiles have a renal portal system. When the renal portal vein is open, blood from the caudal half of the body passes through the kidneys prior to reaching the systemic circulation. Drugs that are eliminated by or toxic to the kidneys may be less effective if eliminated by the kidneys or more toxic to them if given in the caudal body. Urine leaves the kidneys through the ureters which empty into the cloaca, not the urinary bladder. Urine then travels from the cloaca into the bladder of those species with a urinary bladder (chelonians and some lizards) or into the colon in those species without a bladder (snakes, crocodilians, and some lizards), where water absorption and ion exchange occur. Urine does not flow through the reproductive system and the short urethra only connects the bladder to the cloaca.

The cloaca receives excretions from the reproductive tract, ureters, colon, and urinary bladder in those species with a bladder (Figure 9.1). It consists of three compartments: the coprodeum, the urodeum, and the proctodeum. The coprodeum is the most cranial compartment of the cloaca and is where the rectum enters. This compartment receives urinary and fecal wastes from the terminal colon. Urinary wastes of reptiles pass into the urodeum and then into the urinary bladder (chelonians and most lizards) or into the terminal colon (snakes and some lizards) where water absorption occurs. The urodeum is the middle section of the cloaca in which the ureters and the reproductive systems terminate. The female reproductive tract is bilateral in reptiles with each oviduct having a separate opening into the cloaca. The proctodeum is the caudal compartment of the cloaca and is a reservoir for fecal and urinary wastes prior to excretion.

Surgery of the Female Reproductive Tract

Female reptiles have a bilaterally symmetrical reproductive tract, but there is no structure equivalent to the uterus of mammals. The reproductive physiology of reptiles varies considerably. Some reptiles lay eggs (crocodilians, chelonians, and some squamates), while others deliver live babies (some squamates) (Figure 9.2). Dystocia and prevention of reproduction are the major indications for surgery of the female reproductive tract (Bennett 1989b; Lock 2000; Mehler and Bennett 2006). Surgical management of dystocia is indicated when husbandry changes and medical management have failed to relieve the dystocia. Salpingotomy is performed to treat dystocia. Ovariosalpingectomy is performed to treat or prevent future problems related to the reproductive tract such as yolk coelomitis, dystocia, and salpingitis. For reproductively valuable animals, an oviduct resection and anastomosis can be performed to remove a diseased section of oviduct (Figure 9.3). To control reproduction, perform an ovariectomy. If the oviducts are removed but the ovaries are not (or a piece of ovary remains), they will release yolks into the coelom and likely cause yolk coelomitis; however, if the ovaries are removed but the oviducts left, they will atrophy.

Surgery of Exotic Animals, First Edition. Edited by R. Avery Bennett and Geoffrey W. Pye.

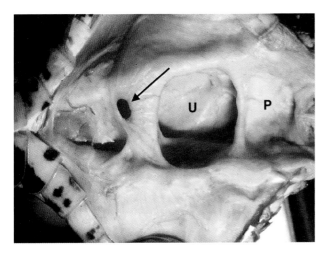

Figure 9.1 A postmortem image of a boa constrictor demonstrating the three chambers of the cloaca. The cloaca was opened along the ventral midline. The coprodeum is the most cranial compartment of the cloaca and is where the rectum enters (arrow). Urinary wastes of reptiles pass into the urodeum (U) and then into the urinary bladder (chelonians and most lizards) or into the terminal colon (snakes and some lizards) where water absorption occurs. The urodeum is the middle section of the cloaca in which the ureters, the urethra, and the reproductive system terminate. The proctodeum (P) is the caudal compartment of the cloaca and is a reservoir for fecal and urinary wastes prior to excretion.

In regard to reproductive disorders, it is often difficult to determine whether a female reptile is undergoing a normal physiologic or a pathologic process. Gestational duration, clutch size, egg size, and egg type vary among species. Therefore, an in-depth understanding of each species' reproductive cycle is required.

Preovulatory egg stasis is characterized by the development of yolks on the ovary that are not released (Lock 2000; Millichamp et al. 1983). Postovulatory stasis occurs when the eggs or feti are within the oviduct but do not pass causing systemic signs of illness such as anorexia, weight loss, dehydration, or failure to pass feces and urates for an extended period of time. In either case, it is recommended that the ovaries be removed; however, in cases of postovulatory stasis, remove the ovaries as well as the oviducts. If the oviduct is removed without removing the ovary, yolks will be released into the coelom potentially inducing yolk coelomitis. If the ovaries are removed and the oviducts left, they simply atrophy and should not cause problems in the future. Removal of one side of the reproductive tract (unilateral ovariosalpingectomy) for treatment of reproductive disease allows the patient to remain reproductively viable if the contralateral side is unaffected. In lizards and chelonians, the ovaries and oviducts are readily accessible through a standard celiotomy (see Chapter 8). In snakes, the tract is elongated and if the entire oviduct contains eggs

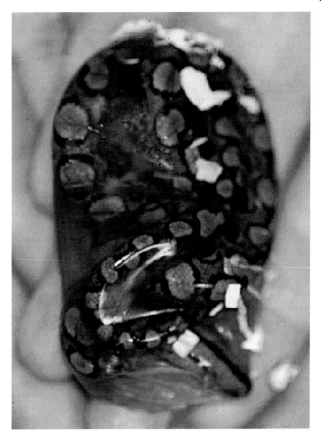

Figure 9.2 Dystocia in this Brazilian rainbow boa (*Epicrates cenchria*) was treated with oxytocin and it delivered its live offspring naturally.

or feti that must be removed, it is often necessary to make several celiotomies to access the entire oviduct (Figure 9.4).

When reproductively active, the blood vessels supplying the ovary and oviduct become engorged and hypertrophied making surgical removal more challenging. For this reason, in pet reptile species with a high incidence of dystocia, prepubertal elective ovariectomy should be discussed with the owner. The procedure is much easier to perform when the vessels and ovaries are small, and the patient is in good health.

Ovariectomy

Ovariectomy is recommended for juveniles to prevent dystocia and for preovulatory ovostasis where the patient is not stable enough to remove the oviducts simultaneously. The right ovary is near the right external iliac vein, while the left is more loosely attached with the left adrenal gland interposed between the left external iliac vein and the ovary (Figure 9.5). When the ovaries are active as with preovulatory egg stasis, the ligaments are stretched, and it is easy to apply hemostatic clips to the vessels supplying the ovaries.

(a)

(b)

(c)

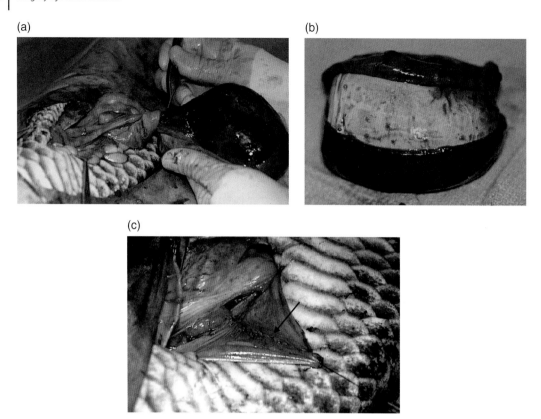

Figure 9.3 This python suffered dystocia and an oviduct volvulus around a single egg (a). The segment was resected without derotating the volvulus (b). An anastomosis of the oviduct was performed (c) and the snake delivered eggs normally the following year.

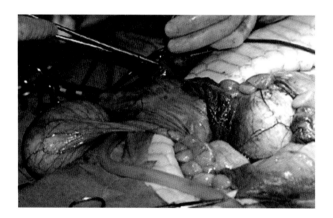

Figure 9.4 This albino Burmese python developed dystocia requiring multiple celiotomies and salpingotomies. One salpingotomy is being closed with a simple continuous pattern and other salpingotomies have already been closed. In general, three to five eggs can be removed from each salpingotomy and three to four salpingotomies can be performed through each celiotomy.

Apply two clips to each vessel and transect the vessel between the clips. Continue the process until all vessels are sealed and transected and the ovary with its yolk follicles is removed (Figure 9.6). This can also be accomplished using vessel sealing devices without the need for hemostatic clips.

The LigaSure™ (Medtronics, Minneapolis, MN) and the Harmonic® (Ethicon, Cincinnati, OH) scalpel are examples of such devices available for use in exotic animals. The LigaSure is approved to seal vessels up to 7 mm in diameter LigaSure™. Place the tips of the vessel sealing device on the blood vessels supplying the ovary, activate the bipolar energy source, and transect the vessel (Figure 9.6).

When the ovaries are not active, ovariectomy can be more challenging (Bennett 1989b; Lock 2000; Mehler and Bennett 2006). Gently elevate the right ovary, apply one or two clips between the right ovary and the right external iliac vein, and then transect the tissue distal to the clip to allow removal of the ovary. Remove the left ovary in a similar manner, applying the clips between the ovary and the left adrenal gland. Transect the tissue distal to the clips allowing removal of the left ovary without damaging the adjacent adrenal gland. A bipolar vessel sealing device can also be used instead of clips.

Salpingotomy

Salpingotomy is indicated in female reptiles with dystocia in which the owner elects to preserve reproductive function or in snakes to minimize the invasive nature of removing the entire oviduct. The oviduct wall is thin and transparent.

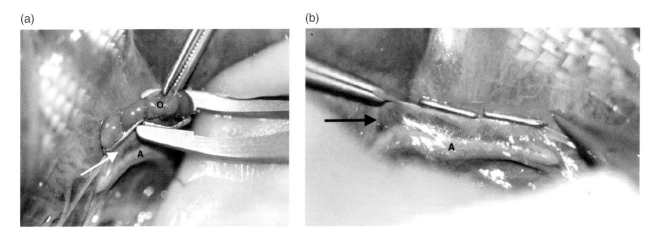

Figure 9.5 Cadaveric image of a sexually immature green iguana undergoing bilateral ovariectomy. The right ovary (O) is near the right external iliac vein (arrow) and the adrenal gland (A) is on the other side of the right external iliac vein. The left ovary is more loosely attached with the left adrenal gland interposed between the left external iliac vein and the left ovary. Apply clips between the external iliac vein (arrow) and ovary (O) on the right and between the external iliac and adrenal gland on the left. Incise along and distal to the clips to remove the ovary.

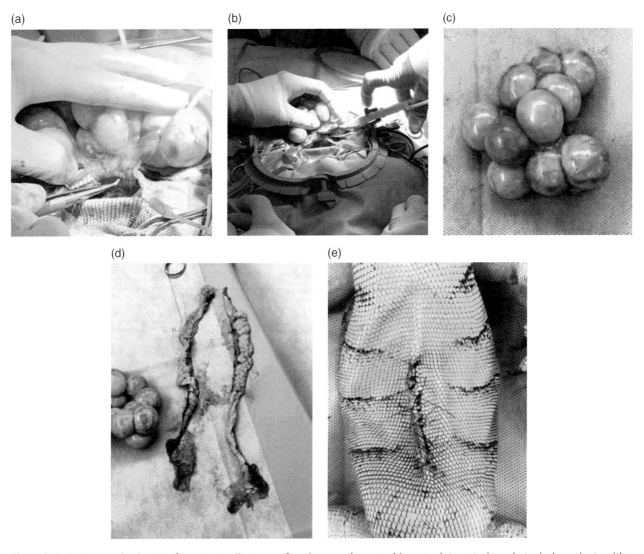

Figure 9.6 Intraoperative images from a sexually mature female green iguana with preovulatory stasis or dystocia. In patients with large ovarian follicles, the ovarian ligament is stretched out making it easier to identify and ligate vessels (a). A vessel sealing device (LigaSure™) was used to seal the arteries and veins in the mesovarium and transect them to complete the bilateral ovariectomy (b). Once the ovaries were removed (c), a salpingectomy was also performed (d) using the vessel sealing device. The patient after surgery with 3-0 nylon vertical mattress sutures in the skin (e).

When inflamed the wall becomes thicker, but more friable making it a challenge to suture it closed. Identify the oviduct and incise it in a healthy appearing section, often immediately adjacent to an egg or fetus. The stretched, friable, and often compromised tissue directly over the egg will have decreased healing potential and should be spared from surgical trauma. Gently palpate and maneuver the egg or fetus into the incision and remove it from the oviduct. If the salpingotomy incision is too small, the oviduct will tear while the eggs/feti are manipulated through the incision. The first egg/fetus is generally removed without much effort. Eggs/feti that have been in place a long period of time adhere to the oviduct wall. Insert an appropriately sized catheter between the egg/fetus and oviduct wall, connect it to a saline filled syringe and inject the saline to separate the wall from the egg/fetus. This will not only free the egg/fetus from its adhesions to the oviduct but also provide some lubrication to allow more eggs/feti to be removed from that salpingotomy site. If the egg/fetus had been in place a long time, the oviduct may not free from the egg/fetus with saline alone. In these cases, add a sterile water soluble lubricant to the saline and try again. Mix 1 : 10 lubricant to water or it will be too thick to go through the syringe. After the first egg/fetus is removed, massage and manipulate adjacent eggs/feti toward the salpingotomy using saline, finger dilation in larger reptiles or lubricated cotton-tipped applicators in smaller reptiles, and digital manipulations to separate adhesions between the egg/fetus and oviduct (Bennett 1989b; Lock 2000; Mehler and Bennett 2006).

In snakes, if the entire oviduct contains eggs or feti that must be removed, it is often necessary to make several celiotomies to access all of the oviduct (Figure 9.4). Generally, about three to five eggs can be manipulated through a single salpingotomy incision in snakes. Once the eggs/feti have been removed close the salpingotomy with a fine (5-0 to 8-0) monofilament synthetic absorbable material on a fine atraumatic needle in a two layer inverting pattern or a simple continuous oversewn with an inverting pattern. Following a properly performed salpingotomy, the prognosis for reproductive viability is good. In general, reptiles will not become gravid for months to as long as a year allowing plenty of time for incisional healing.

Ovariosalpingectomy

Where there is irreparable damage to the reproductive tract or when the owner desires to prevent future episodes of dystocia, perform an ovariectomy or ovariosalpingectomy. When the ovaries are active as with preovulatory egg stasis, the ligaments are stretched, and it is easy to apply hemostatic clips or a vessel sealing device to the vessels supplying the ovaries prior to transecting them as described above. When the ovaries are not active, ovariectomy can be more challenging as described above.

Following removal of the ovaries, remove the oviducts. Begin the dissection at the infundibulum and continue toward the cloaca. With preovulatory egg binding, the oviduct will be empty, and vessels are easily controlled either with hemostatic clips, bipolar electrosurgery, or a vessel sealing device. Once the oviduct has been isolated from its blood supply to the level of the cloaca, apply one or two hemostatic clips to the base of each oviduct at the cloaca, and then transect and remove the oviducts.

In animals with postovulatory egg binding, the oviducts will be full of eggs, but the ovaries are usually relatively small and inactive as they have already released their yolks. The oviducts full of eggs will obscure visualization of the ovaries so perform the salpingectomies prior to ovariectomy. There will be numerous large vessels supplying the oviducts. Starting as close to the ovary as possible, identify each vessel, apply two hemostatic clips, and transect the vessel between them (Figure 9.7). Continue caudad until the oviducts can be ligated or clipped at the cloaca prior to being transected. Vessels can be managed with a vessel sealing device as well. In many cases, the oviduct will be large enough to require a ligature or sealing device. After the oviducts have been removed, visualize the ovaries and remove them as described above.

In snakes with their longitudinal configuration, the ovaries are cranial to the oviduct and must be approached through separate incisions or by extending the celiotomy craniad until the ovaries are identified.

Orchidectomy

Orchidectomy is primarily performed in male green iguanas that have become aggressive or to prevent aggression from developing. Orchidectomy has been shown to decrease

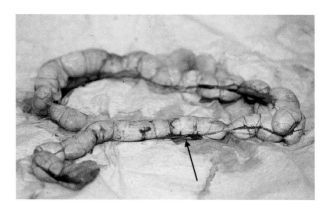

Figure 9.7 Removed oviducts full of eggs following salpingectomy in a green iguana (*Iguana iguana*) with postovulatory egg stasis. Hemostatic clips were used to control hemorrhage. Two clips were placed on each vessel, and vessels were transected between clips. Arrow points to a clip on the oviduct side of the transected vessels.

testosterone levels and sexual aggressive behaviors (Mason and Adkins 1976; Moore 1987; Lock and Bennett 2015). Most commonly, orchidectomy is performed in iguanas after the aggressive behavior has developed; however, it is likely to have more influence on behavior when performed in prepubertal iguanas before the inappropriate behaviors have developed. When performed in an aggressive animal, it appears that the aggression is not ameliorated until the following breeding season (Lock and Bennett 2015). The prognosis for ameliorating the behavior has anecdotally been reported to be around 50% following orchidectomy.

Perform orchidectomy through a standard ventral celiotomy. As with the ovaries, the right testicle is more closely attached to the right external iliac vein by its short, vascular mesorchium. The right adrenal gland is located on the other side of the external iliac vein. The left testicle is more loosely attached to the left external iliac vein, and the left adrenal gland is located between the left testicle and the external iliac vein. The adrenals are elongated and pale pink, readily distinguished from the smooth, white testicles. The testicles are covered by a capsule that is easily ruptured during aggressive manipulations. Rupture of the capsule does not result in hemorrhage, but the contents will protrude from the capsule making it difficult to continue with the dissection and definitive removal. If contents contaminate the coelom, use small gauze squares and cotton-tipped applicators combined with local lavage to remove all of the material.

Remove the testicles in a manner similar to that described for removal of inactive ovaries (Figure 9.8). Gently elevate the right testicle and apply hemostatic clips between the testicle and the external iliac vein. Transect the tissue distal to the clips allowing removal of the testicle. If the testicles are large, they may require several clips to engage all of the vessels in the mesorchium. In these animals, lift the caudal pole of the testicle and apply a clip from caudal to cranial, and then incise along the clip, which will allow the testicle to be elevated farther. With the testicle elevated, insert another clip cranial to the first clip along the mesorchium. Continue the process until the entire mesorchium has been incised and the testicle removed. Remove the left testicle in a similar manner following application of hemostatic clips between the left adrenal gland and the testicle (Figure 9.9). Vessel sealing devices can be used in place of clips for hemostasis if the patient is large enough. If there is hemorrhage from the external iliac vein apply one or two hemostatic clips tangentially along the damaged side of the vessel to control hemorrhage. Partial occlusion of the external iliac vein has not been associated with clinical problems; however, if over half of the diameter of the external iliac vein is attenuated, signs of vascular obstruction might be anticipated.

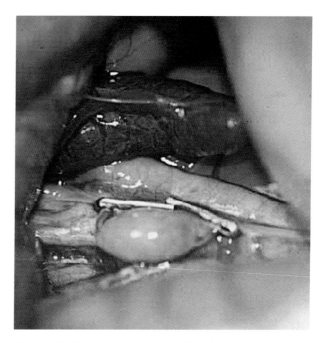

Figure 9.8 In a young green iguana, it only requires one or two hemostatic clips to control hemorrhage during orchidectomy. After applying the clips, incise distal to the clips to allow removal of the testicle.

Reproductive Organ Prolapse

The cloaca of reptiles consists of three compartments: the coprodeum, the urodeum, and the proctodeum (Figure 9.1). Each of these compartments and their associated structures can prolapse. The coprodeum is the most cranial compartment of the cloaca and is where the rectum enters. This compartment receives urinary and fecal wastes from the terminal colon. Urinary wastes of reptiles pass into the cloaca and then into the urinary bladder (chelonians and most lizards) or into the terminal cloaca (snakes and some lizards), where water absorption occurs. The urodeum is the middle section of the cloaca in which the ureters, the urethra, and the reproductive system terminate. The proctodeum is the caudal compartment of the cloaca and is a reservoir for fecal and urinary wastes prior to excretion (Bennett and Mader 2006; Mehler and Bennett 2006).

The anatomy and location of the male copulatory organ varies among reptile orders. Squamate reptiles (lizards and snakes) primarily have hemipenes (paired copulatory organs, singular is hemipenis). Hemipenes in these reptiles are hollow organs that are inverted within the tail and evert during copulation. Some lizards, crocodilians, and chelonians have a single penis or phallus that is within the cloaca or coelomic cavity. It is a solid organ with a groove for the transport of semen that everts during copulation. Neither the reptile penis nor hemipenis

(a)

(b)

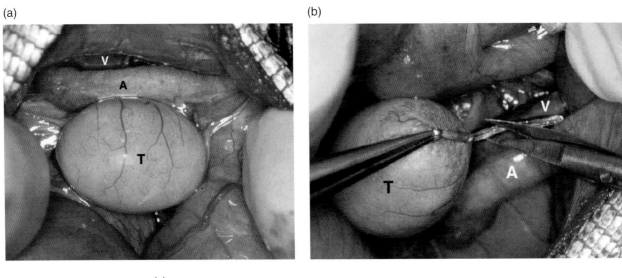

(c)

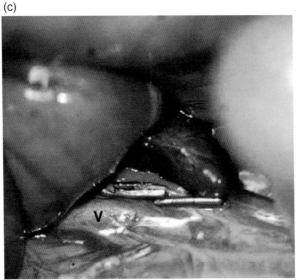

Figure 9.9 Intraoperative picture of a sexually active male green iguana undergoing orchidectomy. (a) Gently elevate the left testicle (T) and apply one or two hemostatic clips between the testicle and the adrenal gland (A). The left external iliac vein (V) is on the other side of the left adrenal gland. Transect the tissue distal to the clips allowing removal of the testicle. The right testicle is removed (b and c) following application of hemostatic clips between the left adrenal gland (A) and the left iliac vein (V). Vessel sealing devices can be used in place of clips for hemostasis if the patient is large enough.

contains a urethra. These organs are not for urination, but strictly for the transport of semen.

Paraphimosis occurs more commonly in chelonians than in squamates reptiles. Causes include excitement, stress, and trauma to the exposed organ from cage mates or the substrate, forced separation during copulation, iatrogenic trauma secondary to probing for sex determination, infection or inflammation, neurologic deficits, and cloacal impaction (Bennett and Mader 2006).

The prolapsed organ is often edematous from venous engorgement and lacerated from cage mates or the substrate and may be infected, necrotic, and covered with an inflammatory exudate. If the tissue is very edematous and

necrotic, it may be difficult to determine if the prolapsed tissue is penis/hemipenes or another cloacal structure. It is simple to ascertain the nature of the tissue in most squamates. If the base of the prolapsed tissue is coming from the caudal aspect of the vent (coming from the tail), it is most likely to be a hemipenis, and if there are two, they are the hemipenes. If the prolapsed tissue is coming from the cloaca in a squamate, it is unlikely to be hemipenes. Prolapse of the oviduct in females and the urinary bladder have been reported (Hedley and Eatwell 2014). These structures should have a lumen while an everted hemipenis does not. As in squamates, the urinary bladder of chelonians and the oviducts of crocodilians and chelonians have a lumen, but if there is severe tissue damage or necrosis, it can be difficult to determine the origin of the tissue without entering the coelomic cavity.

Sedate or anesthetize the patient, then clean and lubricate the prolapsed organ. If lacerations are noted, attempt to suture them, but typically edematous tissues will not hold sutures well. Replace the penis/hemipenis into the tail in squamate reptiles or into the cloaca in chelonians and crocodilians. Reduce the prolapsed tissue with moistened cotton-tipped applicators (Figure 9.10). Place stay sutures in the center of the vent, both cranial and caudal and apply traction to open the vent to make it easier to replace the tissue. Alternatively, incise the vent laterally on one or both sides. Once the prolapse is reduced, keep it in place with a purse string suture or transverse sutures in the vent. Transverse vent sutures have the benefit of allowing fecal and urinary wastes to be passed. In squamate reptiles, place a purse string in the caudal aspect of the vent at the

base of the tail. This technique allows for normal cloacal function but prevents the hemipenis from coming out again. Regardless of the technique used, remove the sutures in two to three weeks.

If the tissue is necrotic or infected, it should be amputated. Amputation of the penis, hemipenis, or hemipenes will not compromise urination. In snakes and lizards, amputation of a single hemipenis still allows reproductive viability (Bennett and Mader 2006; Lock 2000). Place mattress sutures or encircling sutures at the base of the prolapsed tissue and amputate the organ distal to the suture. Suture the mucosa of the stump with a simple continuous pattern and replace the stump into its normal anatomic location.

Prolapse of the oviducts occurs in female reptiles (Figure 9.11). In some cases, it is possible to reduce the prolapsed tissue; however, the viability of the tissue and assessment of damage to the suspensory ligament of the

(a) (b)

(c) (d)

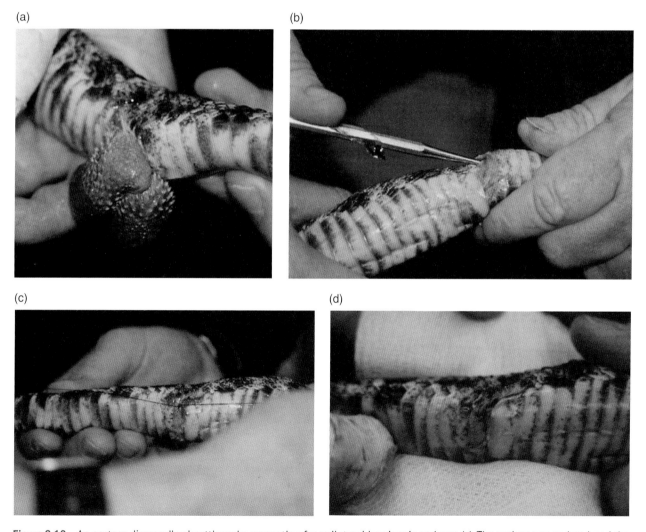

Figure 9.10 An eastern diamondback rattlesnake presenting for unilateral hemipenis prolapse (a). The patient was sedated, and the hemipenis was replaced into the vent and directed caudally toward the tip of the tail using a sterile sexing probe and sterile water soluble gel (b). Once reduced, keep the prolapse in place with a purse string suture or transverse vent sutures (c and d).

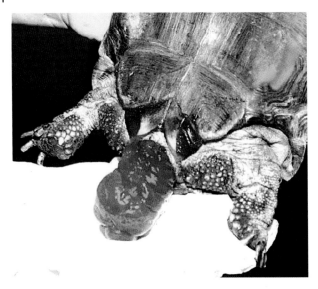

Figure 9.11 Prolapsed oviduct in a California desert tortoise (*Gopherus agassizii*) secondary to straining related to a cystic calculus. The prolapse was reduced and a celiotomy was performed to remove the cystic calculus.

oviduct is limited. If it is able to be reduced, it is important to push it back into the coelomic cavity and not leave it balled up within the cloaca because if it is not repositioned correctly it will prolapse again when the retention sutures are removed. Amputation of the tissue has been performed, but celiotomy for complete assessment of the prolapsed tissue and repair or removal of the reproductive tract is recommended. If only one side of the reproductive tract is removed, the contralateral side allows for reproductive viability.

Non Reproductive Cloacal Organ Prolapses

Other organs may prolapse from the cloaca of reptiles, including cloacal tissue, the urinary bladder, and intestine. Prior to definitive therapy, identification of the prolapsed tissue is paramount. If the tissue appears viable, reposition the prolapse under sedation or general anesthesia. Apply a hyperosmotic solution and gently apply pressure with cotton-tipped applicators to reposition the tissue. Then place two sutures at the side of the vent to reduce the chances of further prolapse. There is some controversy over the use of a purse string suture vs. transvent sutures (Girolamo and Mans 2016), because of the potential damage to the cloacal sphincter a purse string suture might cause. If these techniques fail to prevent recurrence of cloacal tissue prolapse, then cloacopexy and/or colopexy should be considered.

Extracorporeal colonic resection and anastomosis are performed if the colon is prolapsed and the tissue has sustained significant trauma or is devitalized. Anesthetize the

patient and place it in dorsal recumbency. Clean the prolapsed tissue. Place a syringe case in the lumen of the prolapsed colon and transfix the tissue with hypodermic needles placed perpendicular into the syringe case. Excise the nonviable tissue and apply mattress sutures through both layers of the colon to achieve the anastomosis. When the syringe case is removed, the anastomosis will invert and the sutures will be within the lumen.

Cystotomy

Urinary calculi can develop in any species of reptile that has a urinary bladder but seem to occur most frequently in green iguanas and certain tortoises. Improper nutrition and inadequate access to water or chronic dehydration have been suggested as an initiating cause (Reavill and Schmidt 2010). Clinical signs of cystic calculi include anorexia, depression, constipation from occlusion of the colon, dystocia from occlusion of the oviduct, cloacal prolapse from tenesmus, and paraparesis secondary to compressive injury to the pelvic nerves (Figure 9.12). A definitive diagnosis is made based on radiographs or other imaging (Figure 9.13). Calcium urate calculi are most common and are radiopaque while ammonium urate calculi are radiolucent and best visualized using ultrasound.

In chelonians, large cystic calculi can often be palpated in the left inguinal fossa (Mader 2006). The urinary bladder of chelonians is bilobed and the right liver lobe extends farther caudal than the left laying over the right lobe of the

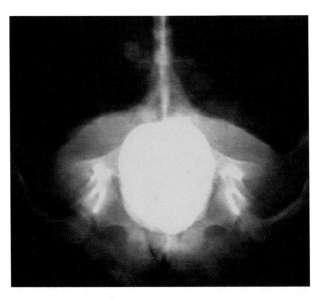

Figure 9.12 This tortoise presented for paraparesis. This radiograph showed the cause was related to a cystic calculus lodged in the pelvic canal. The stone had to be broken to free it, and once it was removed, neurologic function quickly recovered.

(a)

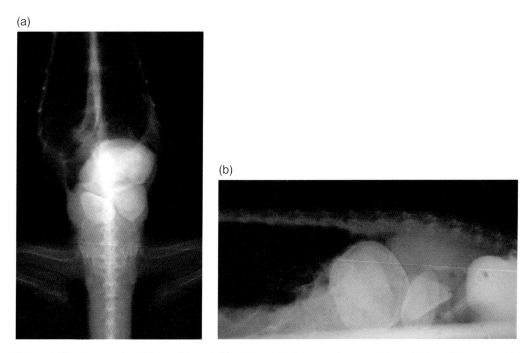

Figure 9.13 A ventrodorsal (a) and lateral (b) radiograph of a green iguana with multiple radiopaque cystic calculi.

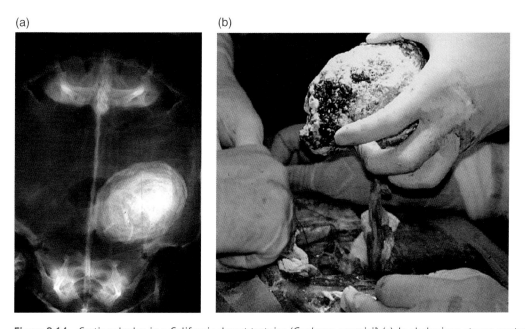

Figure 9.14 Cystic calculus in a California desert tortoise (*Gopherus agassizii*) (a). In chelonians, stones are typically located on the left side because of the bilobed anatomy of the urinary bladder. It was removed by cystotomy via plastron osteotomy. Radiograph of a cystic calculus in a California desert tortoise (a) and intraoperative cystotomy for removal of the stone (b).

urinary bladder. Because the right portion of the bladder is compressed by the right liver lobe, most cystic calculi are present in the left lobe of the bladder (Figure 9.14). Insert a finger into the fossa with the chelonian in a sternal recumbency. With the finger left in place, tip the tortoise vertically (head up) and feel the stone hitting the finger as it falls to the gravity-dependent portion of the bladder. In lizards, cystic calculi are easily identified by abdominal palpation. Imaging provides the advantages of identifying the number and size of stones, as well as their location potentially not palpable within the pelvic canal.

Cystotomy is performed through a standard celiotomy approach (Bennett and Lock 2000; Mader 2006; Mader et al. 2006; Mehler and Bennett 2006) (see Chapter 8).

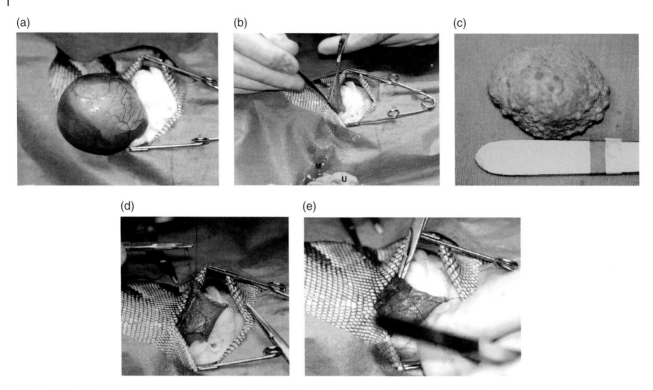

(a) (b) (c)

(d) (e)

Figure 9.15 Intraoperative images of a ventral cystotomy in a green iguana with cystic calculi. Isolate the bladder with moist gauze sponges (a) or laparotomy pads prior to making the cystotomy to minimize coelomic contamination. The urine of reptiles contains mucus (M) and urates (U) giving it a thick, cloudy appearance that is not easily aspirated through suction tips (b). Following removal of the calculus (c), the bladder was irrigated to remove residual debris. Close using a fine monofilament, absorbable material on a small, swaged-on, atraumatic needle in a simple continuous appositional pattern (d) oversewn with a Connell pattern (e).

The bladder is large and easily identified when calculi are present (Figure 9.15). The bladder wall is normally very thin and transparent but becomes somewhat thicker because of the cystitis usually associated with calculi. Isolate the bladder with moist gauze sponges or laparotomy pads prior to making the cystotomy to minimize coelomic contamination. The urine of reptiles contains mucus and urates giving it a thick, cloudy appearance that is not easily aspirated through suction tips. Following removal of the calculus, irrigate the bladder to remove residual debris. Close using a fine monofilament, absorbable material on a small, swaged-on, atraumatic needle in a simple continuous appositional pattern oversewn with an inverting pattern. If the bladder wall is too thick to accommodate an inverting pattern, a single layer closure is acceptable.

An interesting phenomenon observed in chelonians is passage of egg(s) into the urinary bladder. This seems to occur more commonly in chelonians following trauma. An egg(s) enters the urodeum and then travels into the urinary bladder via the short urethra that also opens into the urodeum when external force is applied. Eggs in the bladder are often discovered in wild chelonians following radiographic assessment for traumatic injury. It is unknown if they cause serious pathology since some have evidence of being in the bladder for a prolonged period of time having multiple layers of urates deposited on the egg(s) (Figure 9.16). This has not been reported in other species. It is important to recognize that the urinary bladder extends very cranially when distended (Figure 9.17).

Gastrointestinal Procedures

Gastrotomy, partial gastrectomy, enterotomy, and intestinal resection and anastomosis are similar to those in mammals, although tissues are often thin and friable in reptiles and call for the use of smaller diameter, swaged-on, suture, atraumatic forceps, and atraumatic taper needles (Figure 9.18). In general, standard intestinal closure techniques are used, allowing for one or two layer closure of gastric incisions and single-layer appositional closure of the small intestine. If possible, the large intestine should be closed in two layers to reduce the risk of incisional leakage. The mesentery that suspends the gastrointestinal tract is variable and may

(a)　　　　　　　　(b)　　　　　　　　(c)

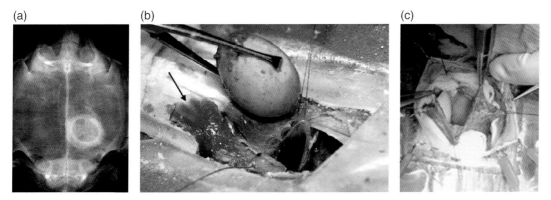

Figure 9.16 Image of an egg in the urinary bladder of a tortoise (a). Note there are multiple layers of urates on the egg, indicating it has been in the bladder for a period of time. The egg was removed through a cystotomy via plastron osteotomy (b). Note the muscle attachments preserved on the segment of plastron (arrow) and the yellow discoloration indicating chronicity. Intraoperative image of a different chelonian with two eggs visible in the urinary bladder (c).

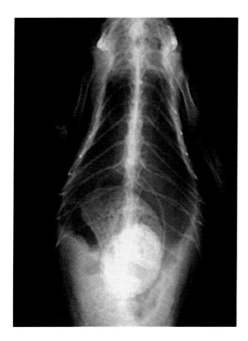

Figure 9.17 A cystic calculus in a green iguana (*Iguana iguana*) that was misdiagnosed as an egg in the urinary bladder.

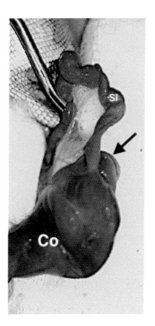

Figure 9.18 The ileocecocolic junction in a green iguana (*Iguana iguana*) demonstrating the thin wall of the intestine. The green color is from ingesta, indicating the wall is so thin that it is transparent (SI = small intestine, Co = colon, arrow points at the cecum).

prevent exteriorization through the celiotomy incision. Isolating the exteriorized gastrointestinal tract with multiple layers of gauze or laparotomy sponges is necessary to prevent coelomic contamination. In addition, copious irrigation prior to closure is recommended. Gastrointestinal foreign body removal and intestinal resection and anastomosis are commonly performed. Anastomosis for colorectal atresia, a congenital condition in which the colon and/or rectum have not formed completely causing partial or complete obstruction of the terminal large bowel, has been performed successfully in reptiles (Frye 1994).

Gastrotomy

Perform a standard celiotomy as previously described (see Chapter 8). Identify the stomach and place full thickness stay sutures to maintain the stomach at the level of the surgical site and prevent spillage of contents into the coelom. Make a stab incision along the ventral surface between greater and lesser curvatures in a relatively avascular area. Enlarge the incision with fine scissors. Remove the stomach contents and foreign bodies (Mehler and Bennett 2006; Girolamo and

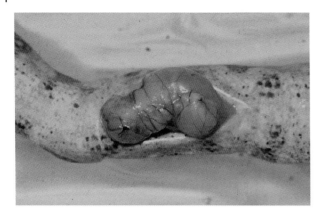

Figure 9.19 Intraoperative image of a boa constrictor undergoing gastrotomy for removal of a foreign body. A simple continuous closure was performed using monofilament rapidly absorbable material.

Mans 2016). Perform a one or two layer closure using monofilament rapidly absorbable suture (Figure 9.19).

Enterotomy

Perform a standard celiotomy. In large chelonians, the prefemoral fossa approach may be used. In snakes, celiotomy is performed in close proximity to the intestinal section of interest. Inspect and palpate the intestinal wall to identify the area of interest. Depending on the species, the mesentery may have a variable length and may prevent exteriorization through the celiotomy incision. Place full thickness stay sutures aboral to the location of the foreign body in an area

of normal appearing intestine (Figure 9.20). Make a stab incision between the sutures. Extend the incision with a scalpel blade or fine scissors. Manipulate the foreign material into the enterotomy incision. In snakes with multiple foreign body obstructions, multiple celiotomies and intestinal incisions may be required (Bennett and Lock 2000; Mehler and Bennett 2006; Girolamo and Mans 2016). Locally lavage the intestine with warm saline. Close the enterotomy with monofilament absorbable suture in a single-layer simple interrupted or continuous pattern (Figure 9.21).

Many reptiles ingest stones, sticks, and other materials from the substrate. In captivity, it is recommended not to use ingestible substrates. Most often, once the material is removed from the enclosure, they will pass the material over time (Figure 9.22). It is best to avoid colotomy if impaction is considered. Medical management is recommended giving plenty of time to allow the material to pass. In general, if material makes it to the colon, it should be able to be passed. If it is not possible to break up an impaction, surgery may be considered (Figure 9.23). Be sure to use pre- and postoperative broad spectrum antibiotics, minimize coelomic contamination, and close in two layers with the second layer being an inverting pattern to achieve serosa to serosa contact. Consider placing a closed suction drain to be able to monitor for dehiscence.

Intestinal Resection and Anastomosis

Perform an end-to-end anastomosis of the small or large bowel when resecting intestine secondary to damage or perforation from a foreign body, neoplasia, or any

(a)   (b)   (c)

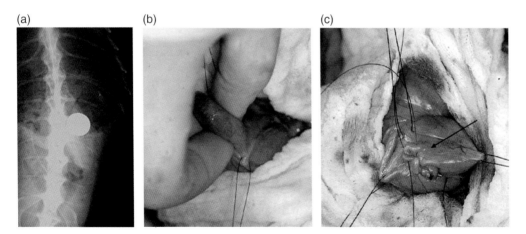

Figure 9.20 Ventrodorsal radiograph of a green iguana (*Iguana iguana*) with clinical signs suggestive of heavy metal intoxication (a). The foreign material was thought to be coins in the stomach. A celiotomy was performed, and the coins were determined to be within the cecum (b). They were removed by typhlotomy which was closed with an inverting suture pattern (c) (arrow is pointing at the typhlotomy site).

(a)

(b)

(c)

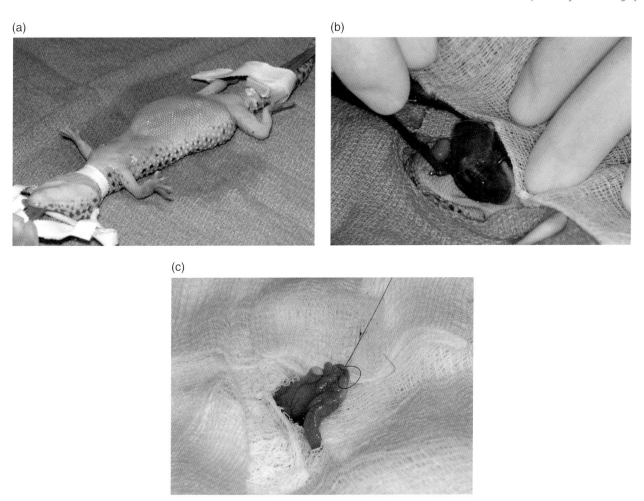

Figure 9.21 Intraoperative image of leopard gecko diagnosed with a small intestinal foreign body obstruction (a). A standard ventral midline incision was performed and the object isolated (b). Place full thickness stay sutures aborad to the location of the foreign body in an area of normal appearing intestine. Make a stab incision between the sutures. Extend the incision with a scalpel blade or fine scissors. Manipulate the foreign material out the enterotomy. Locally lavage the intestine with warm fluid. Close the enterotomy with monofilament absorbable suture in a single-layer simple interrupted or continuous pattern (c).

cause of ischemia. Use hemostatic clips, suture ligation, or a vessel sealing device to ligate the vessels supplying the segment of bowel to be removed. Apply crushing clamps to the region of bowel being removed to prevent spillage during excision. Use noncrushing forceps or an assistant's fingers on the healthy bowel that will remain in the patient to prevent spillage. Transect the bowel between the crushing and noncrushing clamps leaving enough tissue away from the noncrushing forceps in which to place the sutures. Use simple interrupted or continuous sutures with a fine, monofilament suture on a taper needle to complete the anastomosis. Start the first continuous line at the mesenteric border and finished at

the antimesenteric border. Initiate the second continuous line at the antimesenteric border and continue it on the other side to the mesenteric border. Complete the anastomosis by tying the two strands together at the mesenteric border (Bennett and Lock 2000; Mehler and Bennett 2006; Girolamo and Mans 2016; Romeijer et al. 2016). Disparities in luminal diameter can often be resolved by suture spacing techniques. Place suture bites closer together on the narrower luminal segment of bowel and farther apart on the larger luminal diameter segment. Alternatively, spatulate the smaller diameter segment and/or close the antimesenteric portion of the larger segment (Figure 9.24).

(a)

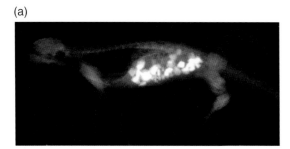

(b)

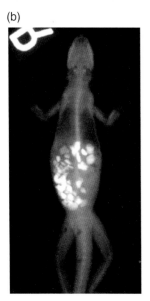

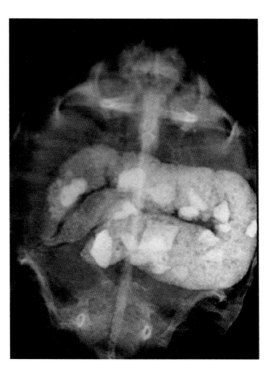

Figure 9.22 Radiographs of a green iguana (*Iguana iguana*) that was housed on a gravel substrate. The owner observed the animal eating stones and presented it for radiographs. The substrate was changed to artificial grass and a month later no stones remained. Lateral (a) and dorsoventral (b) radiographs of a green iguana.

Figure 9.23 This tortoise was diagnosed with colonic impaction. Medical management is recommended. It may take several weeks for the material to pass. Colotomy should be performed only if medical management fails.

(a)   (b)

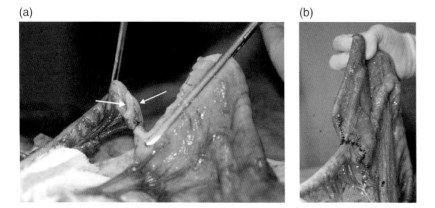

Figure 9.24 Intraoperative image of a green sea turtle with a small intestinal leiomyoma causing a partial mesenteric torsion. A distal small intestinal resection and anastomosis was performed. Significant luminal disparity was present (a). The smaller aborad segment was spatulated (arrows), but there was still a large disparity. The dilated orad segment of intestine was sutured to aborad narrow segment with 4-0 polydioxanone (PDS) in a simple interrupted pattern beginning at the mesenteric aspect. The antimesenteric portion of the dilated intestine was closed with 4-0 PDS in a simple interrupted pattern to further address the luminal disparity (b). This turtle did well postoperatively and was eventually released back into the Atlantic Ocean.

References

Bennett, R.A. (1989a). Reptilian surgery. Part I. Basic principles. *Compendium on Continuing Education for the Practicing Veterinarian* 11: 10–20.

Bennett, R.A. (1989b). Reptilian Surgery. Part II. Management of surgical diseases. *Compendium on Continuing Education for the Practicing Veterinarian* 11: 122–133.

Bennett, R.A. and Lock, B.A. (2000). Nonreproductive surgery in reptiles. *Veterinary Clinics of North America: Exotic Animal Practice* 3: 715–732.

Bennett, R.A. and Mader, D.R. (2006). Cloacal prolapse. In: *Reptile Medicine and Surgery*, 2e (ed. D.R. Mader), 751–755. Philadelphia, PA: W.B. Saunders.

Frye, F.L. (1994). Colorectal atresia and its surgical repair in a juvenile amelanistic Burmese python (*Python moluurs bivittatus*). *Journal of Small Exotic Animal Medicine* 2: 149–150.

Girolamo, N. and Mans, C. (2016). Reptile soft tissue surgery. *Veterinary Clinics of North America: Exotic Animal Practice* 19: 97–131.

Hedley, J. and Eatwell, K. (2014). Cloacal prolapse in reptiles: a retrospective study of 56 cases. *Journal of Small Animal Practice* 55: 265–268.

Lock, B.A. (2000). Reproductive surgery in reptiles. In: Soft Tissue Surgery. *Veterinary Clinics of North America: Exotic Animal Practice* 3: 733–752.

Lock, B.A. and Bennett, R.A. (2015). Changes in plasma testosterone and aggressive behavior in male green iguanas (*Iguana iguana*) following orchidectomy. *Journal of Herpetological Medicine and Surgery* 25: 107–115.

Mader, D.R. (2006). Calculi: urinary. In: *Reptile Medicine and Surgery*, 2e (ed. D.R. Mader), 763–771. Philadelphia, PA: W.B. Saunders.

Mader, D.R., Bennett, R.A., Funk, R.S. et al. (2006). Surgery. In: *Reptile Medicine and Surgery*, 2e (ed. D.R. Mader), 581–630. Philadelphia, PA: W.B. Saunders.

Mason, P. and Adkins, E.K. (1976). Hormones and social behavior in the lizard, *Anolis carolinesis*. *Hormones and Behavior* 7: 75–86.

Mehler, S.J. and Bennett, R.A. (2006). Soft tissue surgery in reptiles. In: *Current Techniques in Small Animal Surgery*, 5e (ed. M.J. Bojrab), 692–699. Jackson, WY: Teton New Media.

Millichamp, N.J., Lawrence, K., Jacobson, E.R. et al. (1983). Egg retention in snakes. *Journal of the American Veterinary Medical Association* 183: 1213–1218.

Moore, M.C. (1987). Castration affects territorial and sexual behavior of free-living male lizards, *Sceloporus jarrovi*. *Animal Behavior* 35: 1193–1199.

Reavill, D.R. and Schmidt, R.E. (2010). Urinary tract disease of reptiles. *Journal of Exotic Pet Medicine* 19: 280–289.

Romeijer, C., Beaufrère, H., Laniesse, D. et al. (2016). Vomiting and gastrointestinal obstruction in a red-footed tortoise (*Chelonoidis carbonaria*). *Journal of Herpetological Medicine and Surgery* 26: 32–35.

10

Avian Orthopedics

Brett Darrow and R. Avery Bennett

Biology of Bone Healing

The goals of orthopedic stabilization in birds are to maximize comfort, neutralize forces, maintain function, preserve soft tissues, promote load sharing, accelerate healing, minimize secondary complications, predict outcome, and balance caregiver expectations and finances. Make every attempt to lay out expectations early. In wild animals, expect the bird to recover adequate flight and foot function to carry out daily tasks. Companion species may compensate with a physical deficiency if the animal receives care; however, it should still be the goal to achieve an optimal outcome unless limited by owner circumstances.

Avian bones are unique in several ways. Compared to mammals, birds have thinner cortices relative to the diameter of the bone, some bones have pneumatic medullary canals that help reduce weight and increase respiration during movement, and they are more brittle as a result of increased ratios of mineral to organic components. The primary forces acting on the avian wing are bending and torsion, while primary forces in four-legged mammals are axial compression and bending, with only mild torsion. Considerable force is placed on the humerus when initiating and sustaining flight as the result of strong pectoral musculature. Safety factors, defined as the maximum strain of bone at failure divided by expected maximum physiologic strain of normal activity, have been reported for the tibiotarsus and humerus (Biewener and Dial 1995; Dumont 2010). In the humerus, the safety factor is approximately 1.9 in torsion and 3.5 in bending (Biewener and Dial 1995), indicating that torsion is an inherent weakness in avian bone evolution and should be a top consideration in fracture stabilization. Brittle cortices and high-stored energies mean comminuted fractures that are more common, while high amounts of torsional stress predispose

them to spiral fractures. Small amounts of soft tissue coverage, particularly over the distal extremities and distal humerus, predispose birds to having opened fractures with compromised blood supply.

The exact stiffness required for healing of avian fractures is unknown, though it is known that in small mammals <2% strain results in direct bone healing and <10% strain results in indirect bone healing (Griffon 2005). Studies observing avian fracture stabilization are limited and dated. Newton and Zeitlin showed that differences in fixation methods lead to different rates of healing – healing was accelerated with internal fixation vs. external skeletal fixation (ESF) as evidenced by increased mineralized callus formation at five and eight weeks, respectively (Newton and Zeitlin 1977). Although healing appeared to occur sooner with internal fixation, the functional outcome of the wing was better with ESF demonstrating that soft tissue structures must be preserved as best as possible. This study also found that segmental fractures healed best when soft tissue attachments were preserved. While soft tissue coverage is often minimal in birds, it plays an important role in providing fracture nutrition. West looked at mid-diaphyseal humeral fractures in pigeons stabilized with a figure-of-eight bandage for 42 days (West et al. 1996). Periosteal blood supply was by an extensive network of vessels from surrounding soft tissues. The endosteal blood supply was increased by four days suggesting it also has an important role in fracture healing that is not well described in mammalian species (West et al. 1996). This would suggest preserving the medullary canal should be of benefit. Indeed, healing has been described as both endosteal and periosteal (Bennett and Kuzma 1992). While fracture healing appears to be accelerated in avian species, extrapolation of the avian musculoskeletal system from the mammalian system is generally appropriate (Tully 2002).

Patient Evaluation

Perform a full physical exam once the patient is stable. Minimally handle a patient that is in distress. Supplement oxygen and warmth until the patient appears calm and may be handled. Take a detailed history. Concurrent diseases or comorbidities should be investigated including breeding habits. Nutritional imbalances of vitamin K, vitamin D, and calcium will affect bone quality and healing. In chickens, producing a single eggshell requires up to 10–15% of the total body calcium (Newberry et al. 1999) with 25–40% of the calcium in each egg originating from bone and other calcium stores (Comar and Driggers 1949; Mueller et al. 1964). Using densitometry, radiographs may aid in an osteopenia diagnosis.

Postural changes indicative of orthopedic disease may include wing droop, swelling, or inappropriate balance or gait. These signs and the inability to demonstrate full flight may be the only signs, such as with fractures of the thoracic girdle. Consider anesthesia to facilitate a full examination. Obtain a minimum database consisting of a hematologic panel, serum biochemistry panel, and radiographs. Open fractures of pneumatic bones should not cause respiratory compromise.

Methodically assess the injury. Evaluate the skin closely to determine the status of soft tissues. Emphysema can occur from a fracture of a pneumatic bone without it being an open fracture. This will usually resolve spontaneously. Address wounds regularly (initially daily) until viability is assured. Initiate antibiotic therapy and continue until the wounds are closed or a bed of granulation tissue is present. Infection impedes both bone and soft tissue healing, but healing can still occur if appropriate antibiotics are initiated.

Evaluate radiographs to determine the nature of the injury. Comminuted fractures are the result of high-energy release, which also creates loss of soft tissue integrity. These fractures often do not allow reconstruction of the bony column and, thus, require robust fixation. Give priority to ESF and biologic osteosynthesis over open reduction and internal fixation (ORIF) in open fractures to reduce the risk of infection. Remove any large bone fragments that lack adequate soft tissue attachment and cannot be rigidly immobilized to prevent sequestration. Use a bone graft if osteoconductivity is in question. Cancellous bone graft is preferred in contaminated areas; however, if the wound is minimally contaminated, the fracture may heal with large defects as long as the wound biology is maintained.

Examine the radiographs to evaluate the quality of bone. Inadequate bone mineral is more often a problem of improper nutrition or high-intensity breeding practices in domestic birds. A fracture located near a joint will be more difficult to stabilize – they have less bone to establish fixation and increased risk of delayed healing, arthritis, and/or ankylosis. Finally, attempt to establish chronicity by evaluating radiographs and any soft tissue injuries. If a lesion appears chronic, establish rigid fixation, preferably with compression. Consider using an osteoinductive material such as a bone graft or exogenous bone morphogenetic protein (BMP) to reinitiate the inflammatory phase and stimulate healing.

Initial fracture management should accomplish three goals – relieve pain, prevent further wound contamination, and prevent further trauma. Remove devitalized tissue and necrotic debris by flushing the wound copiously with saline. Take care with pneumatic bones as it is reported that fluids flushed into these wounds can enter the air sac system resulting in asphyxiation or infection (Martin and Ritchie 1994). Place a hydrophilic dressing over any skin wounds beyond the superficial epidermis. A topical medication may be applied to retain moisture and prevent or treat infection. The authors prefer Manuka medical honey or silver sulfadiazine. Place a motion-limiting bandage to temporarily stabilize the fractured limb.

Fracture Management Options

Cage Confinement

Reserve cage confinement to fractures not amenable to surgical stabilization such as pelvic fractures and those of very small birds. The cage should consist of smooth sides with a perch that allows the bird to be high enough to avoid contacting the ground with their tail. Ensure that there is deep, soft, and clean bedding, particularly if the injury neurologically or orthopedically impairs the bird's ability to stand. Keep lights, visibility, noxious or stressful odors, and noise to a minimum while providing a heat source as necessary.

Coaptation

Consider coaptation for initial or temporary stabilization. Coaptation may also be used as definitive treatment for very small birds, patients unfit for surgery, and those that do not require full function. It is the treatment of choice for a few specific fractures: shoulder girdle fractures and carpometacarpal fractures. Due to insufficient stability afforded by coaptation and the potential for muscle contraction, do not use as a definitive fixation for humeral, femoral, and proximal tibiotarsal fractures. Malalignment, joint ankylosis, limb-shortening, and tendon contractures or entrapment within excessive callus frequently occur with coaptation and result in poor limb function (Bennett and Kuzma 1992). External coaptation typically requires longer convalescence, which can lead to secondary complications such as pododermatitis. With slings and splints, avoid obstructing the vent and compressing the sternum. If tape is directly applied to the feathers, clean the feathers of all adhesive before release.

Bandages and Splints

Body Wrap

A body wrap is indicated for coracoid and other shoulder girdle fractures with Scheelings reporting 89% of birds returning to the wild (Scheelings 2014; Ponder and Redig 2016). To apply, first position the affected wing in a normal resting position. Keep the hips extended to avoid structures associated with the pelvic limbs. Starting at mid-keel, apply a layer of cast padding wrapping in a dorsal to ventral direction on the side of the affected limb. Next, apply self-adherent tape or masking tape in the same man-

ner. Wrap only the torso on the first pass. Incorporate the affected wing in a folded position on the second pass, and then pass cranial and caudal to, but not over the unaffected wing. Wrap until the final tape crosses the affected wing at the midpoint between the shoulder and elbow, centered mid-keel. The tape should be snug, but not impair respiration. Keep the body wrap applied until the bird is able to hold the wing up, which is often about a week.

Figure-of-Eight Bandage

A figure-of-eight bandage is indicated for elbow luxations and fractures distal to the elbow including radius, ulna, and carpometacarpus but is contraindicated as stand-alone coaptation for humeral fractures because it will create a fulcrum. Apply a loose layer of conforming gauze two times around the wing encircling the carpus cranially first and then cross the wrap on the lateral surface of the wing caudally to encircle the elbow and flight feathers in a figure-of-eight pattern (Figure 10.1). Attempt to wrap as

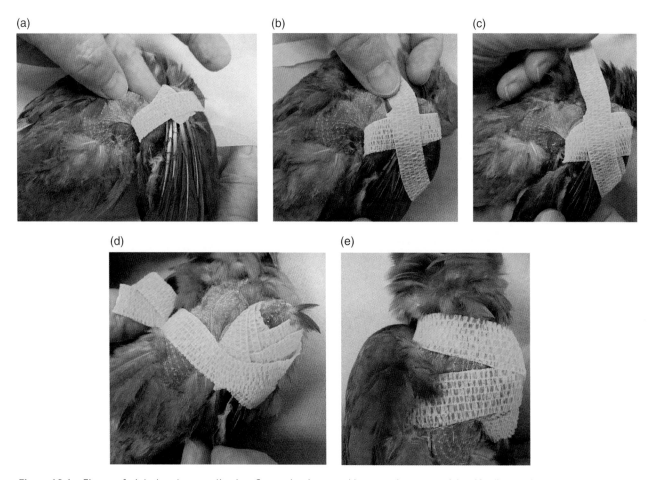

Figure 10.1 Figure-of-eight bandage application. Coaptation is started by wrapping a nonstick self-adherent bandage material around the flexed carpus and flexed elbow (a), crossing dorsally (b). It is important to wrap the humerus and not just feathers. Feathers have been plucked in this cadaver for illustrative purposes. Repeat this pattern several times (c) and the figure-of-eight may be incorporated into a body wrap (d). Wrap around the body both cranial and caudal to the contralateral wing (e). *Note:* Apply an additional gauze layer first in birds >200 g.

proximally on the humerus and carpometacarpus and primary flight feathers as possible. With proximal radius and ulna fractures, the resulting cranial overriding of the distal segment may traumatize the basilic artery and vein and the radial nerve, resulting in vascular and neurologic compromise (Martin and Ritchie 1994). Follow this procedure with two to three layers of self-adherent bandage material. Use only the self-adherent bandage in small birds <200 g. Take care to incorporate the distal humerus, not just feathers, to immobilize the elbow. With fractures of either the radius or ulna, but not both, external coaptation generally results in good fracture healing with a functional outcome unless synostosis develops. Do not use a figure-of-eight bandage as a sole means of stabilization for concurrent radius/ulna fractures, where precision flight is necessary

due to the possibility of synostosis. Radius-ulna synostosis prevents pronation and supination which are essential for birds that hover to hunt. While synostosis will be unacceptable for many wild-flighted birds, companion birds will tolerate a synostosis with acceptable function (Figure 10.2).

Do not apply coaptation excessively tight as this may lead to excessive compression and contraction of soft tissues, including the patagium. Change the bandage every two to three days, being cautious to support the wing and prevent movement at the fracture site. Keep the bandage on as long as needed to verify palpable stability and radiographic healing. Be aware that application beyond 7–10 days has a higher risk of complications. Perform physical therapy under heavy sedation or general anesthesia to reduce the risk of motion at the fracture including gentle passive

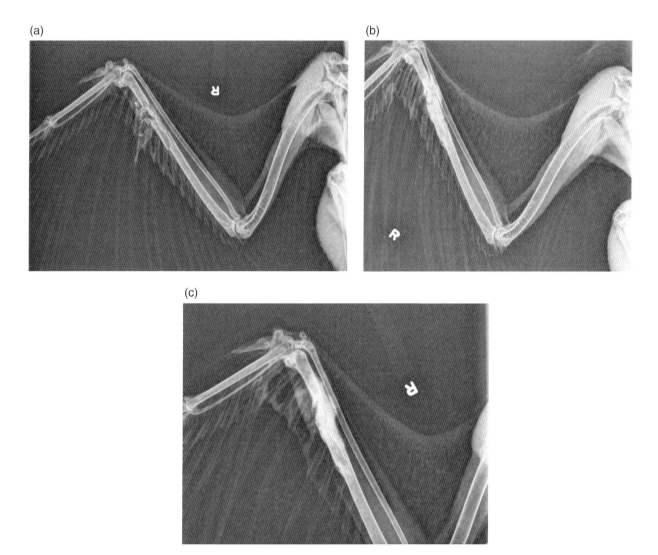

(a)

(b)

(c)

Figure 10.2 Radiographs of an adult bald eagle (*Haliaeetus leucocephalus*), treated with a figure-of-eight bandage for a highly comminuted fracture of the right ulna with surrounding metallic fragments consistent with ballistic injury. Radiographs at presentation (a), four weeks after presentation (b), and eight weeks following presentation (c). Note the radius is intact providing support to maintain reduction and alignment of the ulna.

range of motion, massaging the propatagial tendon, and addressing any soft tissue injury at each bandage change.

Humerus fractures may be stabilized using a figure-of-eight wrap combined with a body wrap to immobilize the shoulder. This can be accomplished by first applying a figure-of-eight wing wrap and then adding a body wrap as described above, or by continuing the figure-of-eight wing wrap dorsally around the body to bind the wing.

Modified Robert Jones

Apply a modified Robert Jones bandage to provide temporary support to tibiotarsal or tarsometatarsal fractures in medium-to-large birds, extending beyond the joints proximal and distal to the fracture. Do not use for femoral fractures (it does not immobilize the coxofemoral joint). First, treat and cover any wound with a nonadherent dressing. Place the limb in a normal perching angle. Apply tape stirrups on opposite sides extending from the mid-tibiotarsus to beyond the toes by approximately the same distance. Apply four to six layers of cast padding starting just proximal to the toes and wrapping proximally as far as possible into the inguinal region, overlapping each previous wrap by approximately 50%. Alternate the direction of each layer of cast padding to prevent torsional malalignment. Pad around not over bone protuberances, such as the tarsus, by adding two to three extra layers of cast padding immediately proximal and distal to the joint, or a "donut" over the protuberance. Apply two layers of roll gauze in the same manner, also alternating direction. At this point, reverse the distal portion of the stirrups folding them 180° up the leg with the adhesive side toward the limb over the gauze. Finally, add one to two layers of a water-resistant material (VetRap, 3M St. Paul, MN). Do not allow the bandage to become wet. Remove a modified Robert Jones every 1-3 days and perform passive range of motion exercises to prevent ankylosis minimizing any motion at the fracture site. Monitor the distal extremity for swelling and remove the bandage if it occurs.

Lateral Splint

The indications for a lateral splint are the same as for a modified Robert Jones bandage, but when more support is indicated and they can be used for more than temporary stabilization. The tibiotarsus is particularly suited for a lateral splint, but internal or ESF is more likely to achieve a desirable outcome and repeated bandaging may cost more than what many owners expect. A splint may be composed of any material suitable to provide stiffness to a bandage. Examples include wood (tongue depressors), plastics (syringe cases), metals (aluminum rods), cast materials, and thermoplastics. Orthoplast (Johnson & Johnson Products Inc., New Brunswick, NJ) and Hexcelite (Hexcel Medical, Dublin, CA) are especially useful thermoplastics that become malleable when hot and conform to the leg but become firm once cool. Apply a bandage with two to four layers of cast padding. Prior to applying the final layer, apply the splint material, adhere it to the underlying bandage with either tape or roll gauze, and cover with the outer layer. Apply the splint so it extends beyond the joints proximal and distal to the fracture with the leg in a standing position. If a fracture is of proximal or distal metaphyseal bone, the splint may not provide sufficient stability for healing and may act as a lever arm, doing more harm than good.

Spica Splint (Femoral Fractures)

Place a spica splint to provide temporary stability to the femur by immobilizing the hip. While it may be used in conjunction with an intramedullary (IM) pin as a means of definitive stabilization, do not use it as the sole means for fixation. Apply in a similar manner as a lateral splint. After applying the first layer of cast padding, continue the wrap dorsally over the bird's lumbosacral spine and around the other side, wrapping around the body two to three times. When applying a spica splint, do not cover the cloaca or entrap the wings. Avoiding the cloaca can be difficult, and if the bandage migrates, it will become soiled and must be changed. After applying two to three layers of cast padding, apply two to three layers of roll gauze. After applying roll gauze, conform a splint to the lateral aspect of the leg, extending from the distal tarsometatarsus over the dorsal midline of the lumbar spine with joints in normal standing angles. Apply two to three more layers of roll gauze followed by one to two layers of a water-resistant, self-adherent elastic material. As with other bandages, remove every 1–3 days for rehabilitation.

Curved Edge/Metacarpal Splint

Metacarpal fractures may be treated with either a figure-of-eight bandage (authors' preference) or with a metacarpal splint and body wrap. For a metacarpal splint, mold a strip of thermoplastic extending from the carpus to the distal phalanx to the ventral aspect of the metacarpus with the wing in a folded position, with a small cranial and lateral lip folding 90° over the leading edge of the carpus (Figure 10.3). Do not allow the edge to protrude much above the plane of the dorsal aspect of the carpus so the splint remains snug. Apply tape to the dorsal and ventral aspects of the wing, effectively sandwiching the distal wing in the splint. Apply a body wrap as previously described to provide additional stability. Treat this splint as others – keep dry and remove every 1–3 days to perform rehabilitation. Apply a figure-of-eight wing wrap following removal of the metacarpal splint if still unstable.

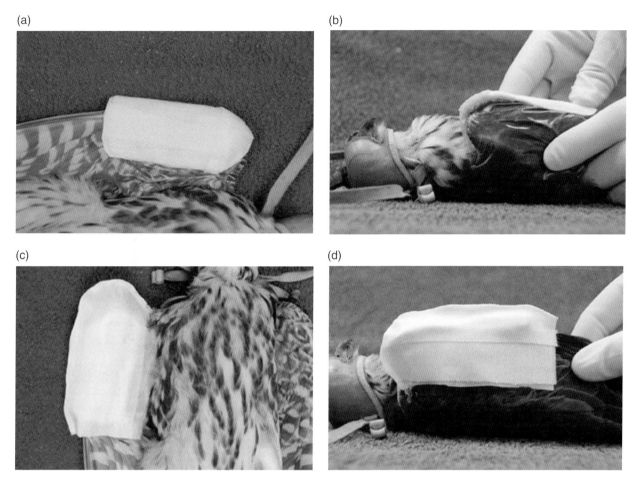

Figure 10.3 Curved edge splint application (Ponder and Redig 2016). Select and cut a moldable piece of thermoplastic to fit the ventral aspect of the radius, carpus, and metacarpus (a). Mold the plastic such that there is a 90° lip on the leading edge (b). Sandwich the splint and wing using multiple layers of tape applied to the ventral (c) and dorsal wing (d).

Tape Leg Splint

The tape splint is indicated for tibiotarsal and metatarsal fractures in small birds (<300 g). Extend the tape to encompass the mid-to-distal femur proximally down to the pes, distal to the tarsometatarsus (Figure 10.4). Following fracture reduction, place the leg into a normal perching position. Stack two pieces of porous adhesive tape together and apply to the medial and lateral aspects of the limb, sandwiching it between the stacks of tape. Pinch the tape together as close to the limb as possible. Crimp with hemostats to create optimal tape apposition as close to the skin as possible to minimize bone movement. Trim the excess tape and coat the apparatus with cyanoacrylate glue for additional support.

Schroeder–Thomas Splint

Schroeder–Thomas (ST) splints are currently not used frequently but are inexpensive and can be used as a primary means to stabilize distal femoral, tibiotarsal, and tarsometatarsal fractures (Figure 10.5). ST splints can also be used as an adjunct to an IM pin in the tibiotarsus preventing rotation and allowing weight bearing. ST splints provide traction at the fracture using a combination of tape slings attached to a rigid frame. These slings can counter muscle forces to align and immobilize a fractured bone. They are not intended to maintain all joints in hyperextension and traction. Place the limb in a functional position with tension applied to separate the joints at each end of the fractured bone to allow distraction and alignment (Bennett and Kuzma 1992).

Surgical Stabilization

In most circumstances, surgery offers the highest chance of a successful outcome when full function is desired. The anatomy of the avian thoracic and pelvic limbs has been accurately described in detail (MacCoy 1987; MacCoy and Redig 1987; Redig and Roush 1987; Orosz et al. 1992; Lumeij 1994). An ideal fixation is rigid,

(a)

(b)

(c)

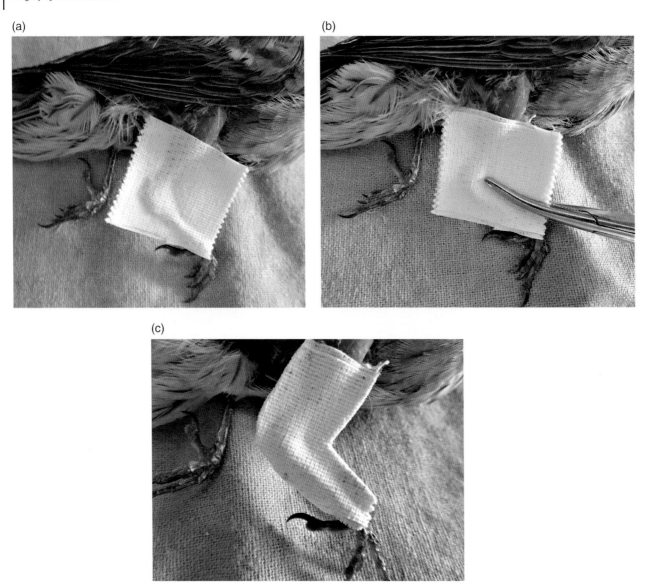

Figure 10.4 Tape splint application. Apply two layers of tape on the medial and lateral aspects of the tibiotarsus, tarsus, and tarsometatarsus, ensuring the instability is encompassed well within the tape margins (a). Use hemostats to achieve strong adhesion near the limb (b). Trim the tape a small distance from the leg and apply cyanoacrylate glue to the outside of the tape to increase stiffness (c).

lightweight, versatile, and preserves soft tissues. Given the requirements for avian performance, some would argue that the fixation should also be removable, though this has not been documented. With different fracture configurations and requirements for fixation, it is best to have a repertoire of surgical fixation options.

Internal Fixation

The best chance for anatomic fracture healing occurs with internal fixation; however, internal fixation requires an open approach, which results in increased risk of osteomyelitis related to compromise of soft tissues and blood supply during dissection, greater volume of foreign implants, prolonged general anesthesia, and surgical inexperience associated with these procedures. Surgical expertise required depends on the method of fixation proposed. Internal fixation requires implants and equipment that may be sophisticated and expensive. As our understanding of avian wound healing and fracture stabilization advances, and with technological advancements in surgical instruments and fixation devices, internal fixation may become even more common. In avian orthopedics, because of the small patient size, internal fixation is often combined with external coaptation, which is less than ideal as the disadvantage of both come into play.

(a)   (b)

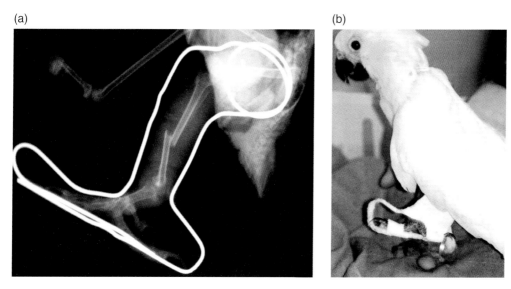

Figure 10.5 Lateral radiograph showing a short oblique mid-tibiotarsal fracture stabilized with a Schroeder–Thomas splint in a yellow-crested cockatoo (*Cacatua galerita*). Note that ideally the fracture would be reduced to involve 50% overlap of fracture ends (a). The bird is afforded early weight bearing with this splint (b).

Intramedullary (IM) Pin

IM pins are versatile especially in combination with ESF. An IM pin provides excellent resistance to bending and some resistance to axial compression but fails to counteract torsional forces. Thus, except for a fractured radius and stable ulna or vice versa, use an IM pin only in conjunction with additional torsional fixation.

Insert an IM pin either in a retrograde (into the fracture and directed proximally or distally) or normograde fashion (inserted at the proximal or distal end of the bone and directed past the fracture into the other segment) (see Table 10.1). Normograde application is less likely to result in soft tissue/joint impairment because the point of insertion is controlled, though retrograde application can avoid this in the humerus and femur where careful aim can result in pin placement outside the joint. While an IM pin intuitively will cause some level of trauma when placed within the stifle joint, long-term sequelae are uncommon. In a series of 37 tibiotarsal fractures where IM pins were placed both normo- and retrograde for a tie-in fixation, severe

Table 10.1 Preferred and alternative methods of IM pin fixation.

Bone	Preferred IM insertion method	Alternative methods	ESF-IM
Coracoid	Retrograde (cranial and seat caudal)	Normograde (cranial to caudal)	NA
Humerus	Retrograde (proximal and seat distal)	Normograde (proximal to distal[a] or distal to proximal)	Tie-in proximal[a] or distal
Ulna	Normograde (proximal to distal)	Retrograde (proximal and seat distal)	Tie-in proximally[b]
Radius	Retrograde (distal and seat proximal)	NA	NA
Carpometacarpal	Normograde (proximal to distal)	Retrograde (proximal and seat distal)	NA
Femur	Normograde (proximal to distal)	Retrograde (proximal and seat distal). Extend hip and adduct leg to avoid sciatic	Tie-in proximal
Tibiotarsus	Normograde (proximal to distal)	Retrograde (proximal and seat distal)	Tie-in proximal
Tarsometatarsus	NA	NA	NA

[a] Preferred method (if more than one option is listed in that category).
[b] Insert the pin away from the elbow into the caudal curvature of the ulna to avoid the elbow joint.

osteoarthritis resulting in euthanasia occurred in one raptor secondary to stifle IM pin placement (Bueno et al. 2015).

When placing an IM pin normograde, make a stab incision at the location of the planned placement. For a femoral fracture, advance the pin into the trochanteric fossa and insert it into the medullary canal of the proximal segment. Normograde placement helps and avoids injuring the sciatic nerve. Make a stab incision at the medial aspect of the proximal tibiotarsus for normograde placement of a pin. Insert the pin to engage the proximomedial aspect and, while holding the tibiotarsus in the nondominant hand for orientation, advance the pin into the medullary canal. An IM pin can be placed normograde in the humerus at the deltoid crest. Palpate the humerus with the nondominant hand for alignment and insert the pin into the medullary canal. The proximal ulna has a curve and a pin can be inserted normograde usually between the second and third flight feathers distal to the elbow (Figure 10.6). Insert the pin between the feathers perpendicular to the long axis. Once the trocar engages the

bone, gradually increase the angle to be parallel to the bone and into the medullary canal.

Once a hole has been made during normograde insertion, if the pin is not within the medullary canal, it is difficult to change the direction of the pin to create a new hole. Attempts typically fail and the pin ends up exiting the bone in the same location. Therefore, if the pin exits the bone rather than advancing into the medullary canal, it is often best to convert and place the pin retrograde if that is an option.

Because the proximal humerus curves at the head, retrograde an IM pin at the caudal edge of the fracture and direct it cranially to exit as far from the shoulder joint as possible out the deltoid crest (Figure 10.7). Similarly, to retrograde a pin out the proximal ulna, insert the pin at the cranial edge of the fracture and direct it caudally to exit the ulna caudal to the elbow joint. Do not insert a pin retrograde such that it exits the proximal ulna or distal humerus near the elbow joint in uncontrolled orientation. Retrograde an

(a)　　　　　　　　　　　　　　　　　　(b)

(c)

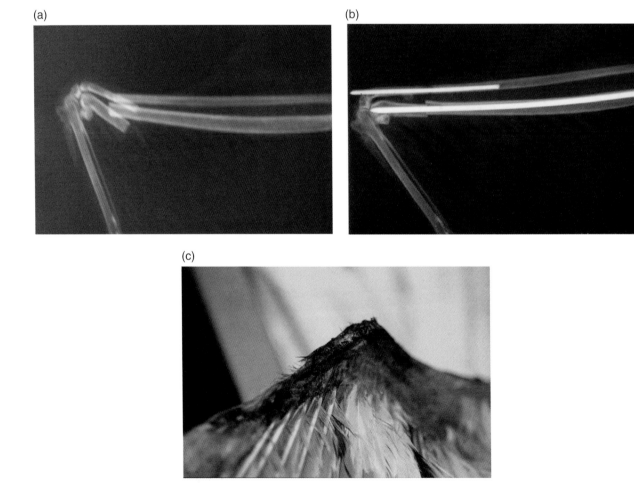

Figure 10.6 Radiographs of a simple transverse distal radius and ulna fracture (a) stabilized with an IM pin (normograde placement proximal to distal in the ulna and retrograde placement distally in the radius) in each bone (b). Due to a limited blood supply to the area, the distal wing necrosed (c).

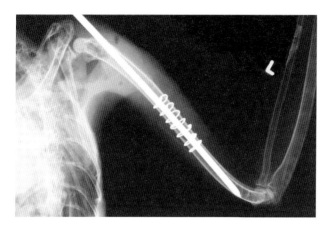

Figure 10.7 Radiograph of a long oblique mid-humeral fracture stabilized with a retrograded IM pin and seven cerclage wires. The IM pin was retrograded out the proximal humerus demonstrating how the pin does not interfere with the joint. The cerclage wires provide torsional stability in long oblique fractures.

IM pin in the proximal tibiotarsus by inserting it at the caudal aspect directing it cranially so it exits the mid-to-cranial tibiotarsus and is not within the joint. For the femur, adduct and extend the hip, and then insert the pin at the caudal aspect directing it cranially so it exits craniolateral and away from the sciatic nerve.

It is not possible to place an IM pin in the tarsometatarsus, carpometacarpus, or phalanges without damaging joints.

Use a pin that fills approximately 60–80% of the medullary canal when used with coaptation, cerclage, or no other fixation. Use a pin that fills approximately 30–60% when using in conjunction with ESF. Insert the pin using either a power drill or a mini or standard Jacob's chuck. Power affords more stability and less wobble during application but keep revolutions per minute below 150 and lavage with cool saline to prevent osteonecrosis. Once through the cortex, the pin should slide easily within the medullary canal. Attempt to place the IM pin without disturbing (opening) the fracture site, especially if the fracture is closed. Fluoroscopy or radiography can be useful. If rotational alignment is difficult to determine, perform an "open but do not touch" approach, where dissection is limited and does not disturb fracture healing. Advance the pin into the other segment until it becomes difficult to advance. To avoid unwanted bone penetration, cut or blunt the trocar tip at the fracture before advancing it into the distal segment. Cut the pin or bend it to incorporate into an IM pin tied-in to external skeletal fixation (IM-ESF).

Orthopedic Wire

Orthopedic wire has little bending strength but considerable tensile strength, which is proportional to its cross-sectional area (r^2). The weakest point of the wire is associated with the method of securing it. It can be used in four methods of application: tension band, cerclage, hemicerclage, and interfragmentary. Tension banding is used to counter the pull of a musculotendinous unit. Cerclage provides centripetal-directed compression to a fracture by encircling an entire bone column, whereas hemicerclage provides compression by encircling only one fragment of the bone and traversing through another. Interfragmentary wiring compresses a fracture by traversing bone tunnels in each segment. Cerclage, hemicerclage, and interfragmentary figure-of-eight wires provide torsional stability.

Several methods are described to oppose the wire ends. Most commonly, a simple twist will suffice. Start the twist by hand, and then, using wire twisters, lift the wire off the bone perpendicularly and continue twisting in the same direction. Twist until it is tight and snug to the entire circumference of the bone, then use wire cutters to transect the remaining wire, leaving at least 1.5 twists (Johnston et al. 2018). While it is tempting to tamp the twist flat, significant loosening will occur and it is not recommended. Instead, if irritation to soft tissues is of concern, when the twist is nearly tight continue twisting while simultaneously laying the twist flush with the bone. Cut the remaining wire after at least 1.5 full twists. Always place at least two wires and space them at least one bone diameter from each other (Figure 10.7).

Bone Plates

Plate fixation is indicated for long bone fractures and is contraindicated with open/dirty fractures and proximal or distal fractures that do not allow at least two bicortical screws in each segment. Hesitation to use bone plates in birds stems from the unique morphologic and physiologic characteristics of avian bone, historically limited implant selection, cost, and technical difficulties associated with plating techniques (Bennett and Kuzma 1992; Gull et al. 2012; Bennert et al. 2016; Darrow et al. 2017). Other disadvantages of plate fixation include extensive tissue dissection requiring a detailed knowledge of musculoskeletal anatomy, potentially prolonged surgery time, and possible need for removal. Primary remiges are attached to the periosteum of metacarpal bones and secondary remiges are attached to the periosteum of the ulna, so periosteal stripping must be avoided. Advantages of plate fixation include neutralization of all forces, anatomic alignment, versatility of application, and early return to function. Decreased postoperative handling (i.e. no pin tract management or fixator removal) may increase safety for the patient and care staff. Plates may increase patient comfort with no external components that could lead to self-trauma. Technologically advanced plates are produced and used with increasing frequency.

Plate fixation has been used successfully in numerous case reports and small case series of various bones in different avian species (Kuzma and Hunter 1991). Prospective studies have demonstrated plates can be applied to the ulna with relative ease and speed, and result in successful healing in a model of radial/ulnar cofractures (Gull et al. 2012; Bennert et al. 2016). Some methods of plate fixation have not had the same success as a result of inappropriate implant selection and application technique, which led to implant bending, loosening, and/or screw pull-out (Christen et al. 2005; Gull et al. 2012). Studies show that locking and nonlocking plates placed on the caudal aspect of the humerus had equal strength and stiffness in bending to an IM-ESF, but plates demonstrated more consistent biomechanical performance (Darrow et al. 2017). Dorsal plate application was significantly weaker than the IM-ESF and caudally applied plates (Darrow et al. 2019). All methods of stabilization were significantly less stiff and weaker than the intact humerus. Both the correct selection of plate and method of application are critical factors for stability.

Several types of nonlocking plates exist, and there are examples of successful use in birds for semitubular plates, dynamic compression plates (DCPs), and veterinary cuttable plates (Figure 10.8). Many sizes of plates are now available including DCPs with as small as 1.1 mm nonlocking screws. Larger thicker plates will afford more strength but may make closure more difficult.

Locking plates pair with screws that interlock into the plate, binding the two components together, functioning as a single construct (Figure 10.9). A major benefit as it relates to thin, brittle, avian bone is that locking plates are less likely to strip threads compared to nonlocking plates during placement (Darrow et al. 2017). As such, locking plates do not rely on friction between the bone and plate for stability allowing for improved preservation of the periosteal blood supply, potentially enhancing the quality of periosteal callus formation (Guerrero et al. 2014). Endosteal callus may also be spared using monocortical screw application; however, given the importance of resisting torsion in the avian wing, bicortical application is preferred by the authors. Very small locking plate systems have been devel-

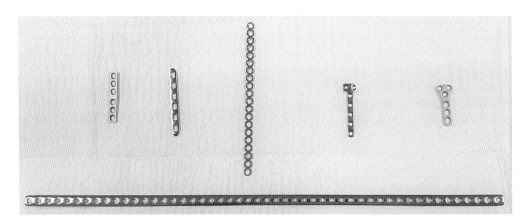

Figure 10.8 Various plate types. From top left to right: 6-hole 2.0 mm dynamic compression plate (DCP), 6-hole 2.0 mm locking compression plate (LCP), 2.0 mm reconstruction plate, 1.5/2.0 mm T-plate, 1.5/2.0 mm T-plate with different conformation, and bottom 50-hole 1.5 mm veterinary cuttable (cut-to-length) plate. The LCP is the only locking fixation pictured here.

(a)   (b)

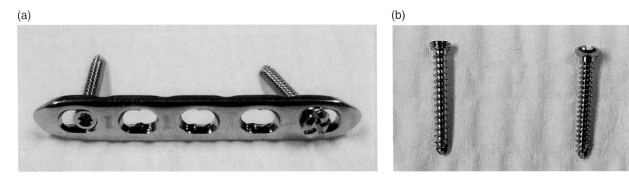

Figure 10.9 Locking and nonlocking screws (a) placed in a 5-hole LCP that accepts both screw types through the advent of a combination ("combi") hole. *Note:* the threads on the head of the locking screw (left screw) interface with the threads in the LCP (b) to create a fixed (90°) angle construct. The nonlocking screw (right screw) can be angled as the smooth head interfaces with the smooth hole in the plate and relies on friction to avoid slippage.

oped suitable for 250–400 g birds. The Advanced Locking Plate System (ALPS) Mini by Kyon (KYON, Zürich, Switzerland) utilizes 3.5 and 4.0 mm wide titanium plates and 1.6 mm titanium locking screws and 1.1 mm nonlocking screws. The Micro-fragment set (DePuy Synthes, West Chester, PA) and Veterinary Orthopedics Implants (VOI, St. Augustine, FL) plates scale down to stainless steel 1.5 mm locking screws. Both systems afford the opportunity to use locking and nonlocking screws. IMEX (Longview, TX) recently developed the VetKISS micro plating system with 1.0, 1.4, and 1.6 mm stainless-steel locking screws (nonlocking screws are not compatible).

Plates may be titanium or stainless steel. Stainless steel has demonstrated success in fracture healing in birds (Gull et al. 2012; Bennert et al. 2016). The ALPS mini-titanium locking system showed equal biomechanical properties to a stainless-steel nonlocking plate (Gull et al. 2012; Bennert et al. 2016; Darrow et al. 2017). A few advantages of titanium implants compared with stainless steel include reduced infection rates (Arens et al. 1996), less thermal transduction, increased osseointegration (allowance of bone and soft tissue in-growth/attachment), and increased resistance to fatigue.

Nonlocking Plate Application

Gather as much information as needed to predict the result of a fracture or angular limb correction, including a thorough examination and quality radiographs or CT images. Three-dimensional (3D) bone models can be printed to allow preoperative plate contouring. Choose a plate whose width approximately matches that of the bone and whose screw size is approximately 30–35% (no more than 40%) of the diameter of the bone. Choose a plate length and number of holes that enables the placement of a minimum of two, ideally three to four, bicortical screws in the proximal and distal fragments (Figure 10.10).

It is very important for nonlocking plates to be well contoured to the bone. Make small changes in contour to avoid cyclical contouring as it will fatigue the metal. A plate is generally placed on the tension side of a bone if possible or a convenient flat aspect of the bone if tension is not readily defined (e.g. place medially where the tibiotarsus is relatively flat) (Figure 10.11). Tension sides are ill-defined in birds, but intuition of flight biomechanics and anatomy can guide placement.

Once the fracture is reduced, apply the plate in a manner that provides an optimal combination of plate contour to the bone and maximizes screw purchase (middle of the bone width through both cortices). The plate can be held carefully to the bone with forceps or an assistant while maintaining reduction. If using an IM pin + plate combination, place the pin first which will help with fracture reduction and alignment. Screw insertion classically begins with both screws farthest from the fracture, then the screws nearest the fracture, and finally fill the middle holes. One screw at a time, pre-drill the hole using an appropriate drill

(a)   (b)   (c)

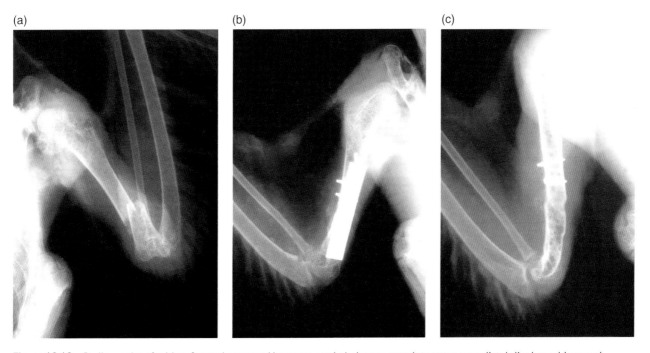

Figure 10.10 Radiographs of a blue-fronted amazon (*Amazona aestiva*) show a complete transverse distal diaphyseal humeral fracture (a). A 7-hole nonlocking plate and two cerclage wires were applied for fissures found at surgery (b). The plate was removed prophylactically (c). Complete osseous union was noted following plate removal (cerclage wires were not removed).

(a)

(b)

(c)

(d)

(e)

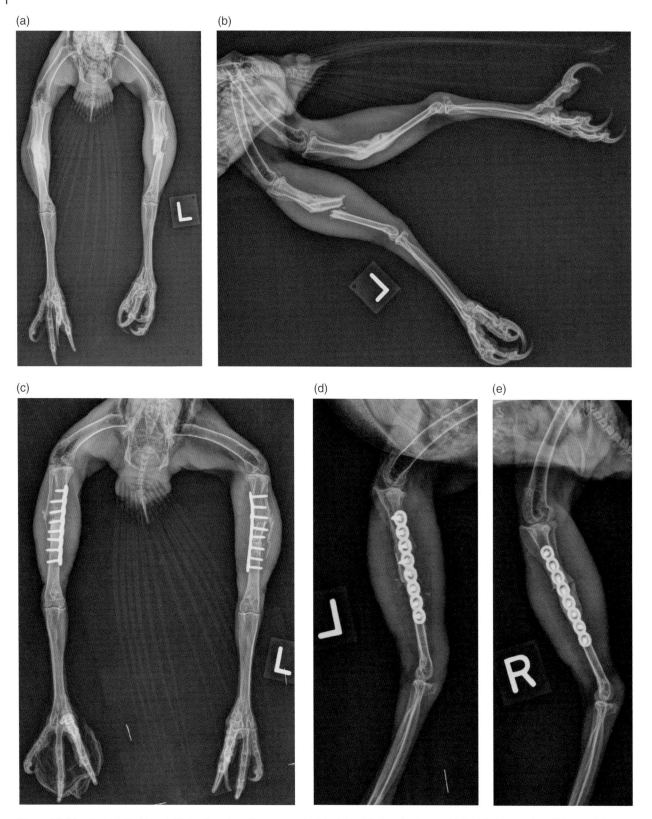

Figure 10.11 A red-tailed hawk (*Buteo jamaicensis*) presented with right-sided malunion and left-sided nonunion tibiotarsal fractures leading to bilateral ALD as shown radiographically (a and b). Single-session bilateral ALD correction was performed and tibiotarsal bones were stabilized with 2.7 mm 8-hole titanium plates from the W. Lorenz Total Mandibular Titanium – Osteosyn System (c–e). Both limbs were healed at 30-day postop with no signs of implant complication. This bird was released.

bit, irrigating with saline to avoid osteonecrosis. Only use a very sharp and straight bit to avoid iatrogenic fractures. With nonlocking plates, the authors prefer to use a tap to create threads in the bone, even when using self-tapping screws. Advance the tap one turn clockwise followed by a quarter turn counterclockwise to clear the flutes. Exact torque values for various screw sizes are not defined in birds and over-tightening will strip the bone threads when using nonlocking screws. In small domestic mammals, a 2.0 mm screw is tightened with two fingers, a 2.7 mm screw with three fingers, and 3.5 mm screw with one hand. This may be too much force for bird bone. The author (BD) has found that for 1.5 mm nonlocking screws, two fingers on the screwdriver shaft, not the handle, is adequate and is likely to avoid stripping. If a screw hole is stripped, it may be possible to use a larger screw, a cancellous bone screw, or fashion a nut from a polypropylene syringe case (Bennett and Kuzma 1992). Polymethylmethacrylate has been infused into the medullary canal to increase screw purchase. In a small case series of wild birds, Kuzma showed successful healing and recovery of flight ability following plate and polymethylmethacrylate (PMMA) application allowing for release in 4/6 animals with a fractured humerus. One bird refractured at the end of the plate and was euthanized three months postoperatively and one bird's malunion did not allow flight. Bandages were applied for two days and flight training began at two weeks allowing for early active rehabilitation.

Locking Plate Application

Apply the locking plate in the same manner as a nonlocking plate with a few exceptions. Contour the plate to fit the bone, but near perfect contour is not required as it does not rely on bone-plate friction. It is usually possible to use both locking and nonlocking screws. Ideally, nonlocking screws are placed first to secure the plate to the bone. Monocortical application of a locking screw may also suffice as one cortex in a locking screw has roughly the same purchase as two cortices with a nonlocking screw. In bones expected to have high torsion, such as the humerus, bicortical application of a locking or nonlocking screw is preferred. Locking plates come with a specific drill guide to ensure that screws are placed perpendicular to the bone and ensures that there is an appropriate interface of the screw with the plate.

Interlocking Nails (ILNs)

Interlocking Nail (ILN) are indicated in femoral, tibiotarsal, and humeral fractures (Figure 10.12). They are avoided in open, infected fractures. An ILN provides excellent resistance to bending and resistance to axial compression, shear, and torsion. An ILN has been used successfully in stabilizing an open comminuted tibiotarsal fracture in a bald eagle (*Haliaeetus leucocephalus*) following vehicular trauma. Callus and clinical union were achieved in four weeks, and the bird was successfully released (Hollamby et al. 2004). Stabilization of a chronic comminuted fracture of the femur of a Bourbon red turkey (*Meleagris gallopavo*) also resulted in complete bony union with return to ambulation (Langley-Hobbs and Friend 2002).

Application of an ILN is technically challenging and should only be undertaken by those with experience. Each nail system comes with its own components, and there are currently three types of nail systems used: the I-Loc ILN (Biometrix, Whippany, NJ), the Original ILN System (Innovative Animal Products, Rochester, MN), and the Targon nail (B. Braun Group, Melsungen, Germany). This text will not cover application due to individual system requirements.

External Skeletal Fixation (ESF)

ESF has become a mainstay of avian orthopedics largely due to the low cost, readily available implants, ease of application, and versatility. ESF is able to counteract all forces

(a)

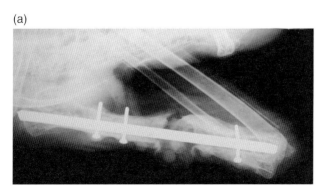

(b)

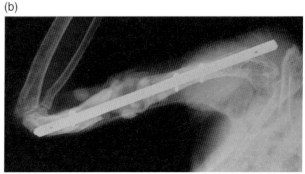

Figure 10.12 Craniocaudal (a) and lateral (b) radiographs of a mid-diaphyseal humeral fracture stabilized with an interlocking nail and two transfixing screws proximally and one screw distally. Antibiotic impregnated beads were inserted near the fracture site to treat local infection.

acting on a fracture, but simple configurations are not overtly strong unless bolstered in some manner (i.e. IM pin, frame geometry, additional connecting bars, etc.). Unless an open approach to the fracture is performed, ESF relies on preserving the biology of the fracture (biologic osteosynthesis), whereas the goal of ORIF is to re-establish alignment and apposition. Thus, healing with ESF will always be secondary, whereas ORIF may be primary or secondary.

ESF affords a variety of configurations. Several factors influence the resulting biomechanics of the ESF construct including frame geometry, number of connecting bars, and number of transfixation pins/wires, as well as type (i.e. threaded, nonthreaded, partially threaded, positive profile threads, and negative profile threads), material, and size. Use positive profile transfixation pins for their high resistance to pullout and lack of stress riser present in negative profile pins. Miniature Interface Fixation Half-Pins (IMEX Veterinary Inc., Longview, TX) are positive profile pins that range in size as small as 0.035″ (1.4 mm) diameter and larger (up to 6.3 mm). Another major advantage of ESF is the opportunity to stabilize a fracture while simultaneously treating soft tissue injuries, preserving the biologic capacity to heal. Disadvantages of ESF include external mechanical components that may interfere with normal function, and cause patient discomfort, require daily care, and require removal under sedation or anesthesia.

Several commercially available systems exist in various sizes, materials, and shapes. The Kirschner–Ehmer (KE) system (Jorgensen Labs, Loveland, CO) was one of the first ESF systems developed. Due to limitations of the KE system, other systems have been developed including IMEX SK system (IMEX Veterinary Inc., Longview, TX) (Figure 10.13). It also comes in three sizes (large, small, and mini). Because it has been shown that clamp components of ESF weaken following use, it is recommended to use new clamps for each patient. The Fessa (Fixateur Externe du Service de Sante des Armees) tubular fixator system (Jorgensen Labs, Loveland, CO) is a reusable and comparatively lightweight commercial ESF system, which comes in two sizes. Transfixation wires are held in place with a hexhead set screw; the 6 mm tube accepts k-wire sizes 0.9 mm (0.035″) to 1.6 mm (1/16″) and 8 mm tube size accepts 1.6 mm (1/16″) to 3.2 mm (1/8″) (Figure 10.14). Armed with knowledge of biology, physiology, and biomechanics, a surgeon is only limited by their creativity. As an example, Montgomery successfully treated a tarsometatarsal fracture in a bald eagle using a externally placed locking plate, which is typically reserved for internal fixation (Montgomery et al. 2011).

ESF allows for adjustments to the construct. Once callus formation is radiographically documented, healing can be

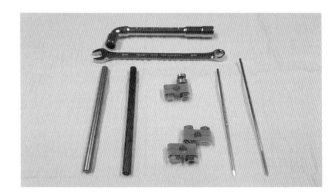

Figure 10.13 Picture of the components of the IMEX SK ESF system. From top left moving clockwise: two 8 mm wrenches, an end-threaded negative profile transfixation pin, a center-threaded positive profile transfixation pin, a single wire clamp and double bar clamp, and two connecting bars (one aluminum and one carbon fiber).

(a)

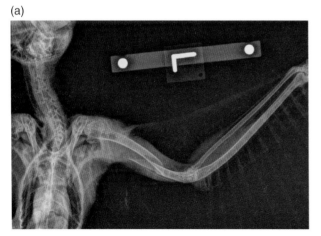

(b)

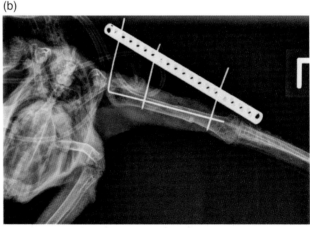

Figure 10.14 Lateral radiograph showing a segmental fracture of the mid-to-distal left humeral diaphysis (a). Post-op lateral radiograph showing excellent reduction of the fracture with the application of a commercially produced IM-ESF (Fessa tubular fixator system, Jorgensen Labs, Loveland, CO) (b). *Source:* Photo courtesy of Javier Nevarez.

accelerated by progressive destabilization of the ESF via hardware removal. The Raptor Center at the University of Minnesota describes destabilization of an intramedullary pin-ESF tie-in construct in the tibiotarsus of raptors (Bueno et al. 2015). Their method included cutting the IM pin tie-in to the ESF around 10 days. Then, after radiographic evidence of callus formation sufficient for stabilization, the IM pin was completely removed (usually around two to three weeks postoperatively). Once continuous callus was observed (four to five weeks), the fixation pins were cut and the entire fixator removed. Documentation of continued healing was again required prior to releasing the raptors to a larger enclosure. To destabilize a type II ESF, cut pins close to the skin on one side and remove one connecting bar converting it to type I ESF and follow the methodology detailed above.

Because the stiffness of transfixation pins is related to the pin radius to the fourth power and proximity of the connecting bar to the third power, keep the connecting bar as close to the skin as possible keeping in mind that additional swelling may occur postoperatively. Do not place an acrylic connecting bar too close to the skin as the exothermic reaction may cause thermal injury. Select transfixation pins that are 20–30% the diameter of the bone. Predrill holes prior to pin insertion using a bit slightly smaller than the pin itself. Insert pins using very slow revolutions to avoid binding soft tissues and thermal osteonecrosis. Positive profile threaded pins are recommended for transfixation pins as they provide the best combination of bending strength and resistance to pull out. If nonthreaded pins must be used, place them angled rather than perpendicular to the long axis of the bone as is done with threaded pins. For example, insert the most proximal pin 70° to the long axis and the next pin distal at 110° so the tips of the pins point toward each other. Inserted in this manner, it is much more difficult to pull the pins out of the bone. This will also increase the pin-bone interface and increase strength and stiffness. As with other types of fixation, attempt to achieve two, ideally three, pins per proximal and distal segment with each pin through both cortices. In the absence of additional fixation, one transfixation pin does not prevent the bone from rotating around the pin.

As with IM pins, if a transfixation pin or wire is too close to a joint, the resulting fibrosis can cause reduced range of motion and osteoarthritis. Place pins no closer than 3× diameter of the pin or 0.5× the bone diameter from joints and fracture edges (Jaeger and Wosar 2018). Other potential complications, while infrequent, include implant loosening, bone resorption, and osteomyelitis. ESF is well tolerated in birds, but self-mutilation and construct mutilation may occur.

Linear ESF

The combination of pins, clamps, and connecting bars create the ESF construct. Veterinarians have attempted to standardize nomenclature, particularly of linear ESF, to better predict each frame's biomechanical properties. The most common configurations of linear ESF are type I (Figure 10.15a), type Ib (Figure 10.15b), type II (and type II hybrid) (Figure 10.15c), type I–II hybrid (Figure 10.15d,e), and type III. Indications for type I are for humeral, ulnar, metacarpal, femoral, tibiotarsal, and tarsometatarsal fractures. When possible a type II or type II hybrid ESF is preferred for tibiotarsal and tarsometatarsal fractures for more stability.

Plan the fixation based on the fracture configuration (bone size, segment size, number of segments), biology (healing potential and surrounding soft tissue status), and clinical factors (perceived patient/caregiver compliance, patient's behavior). Select all components and prefabricate the construct based on the contralateral extremity if possible. Have a plan for the construct based on radiographs but be ready for changes, having extra components sterilized and available for surgery.

Prepare the bird's limb as if an open approach is to be performed using aseptic technique. Identify the proper location within the bone for the fixation pins based on images, palpation, and local anatomy. Place the pins in a location with minimal soft tissue interference using anatomic fascial planes and major vessels, and avoiding muscle bellies where possible. For example, if applying a type I ESF to the femur, insert pins on the lateral to craniolateral aspect of the bone as they will transverse less soft tissue compared to cranial, caudal, or medial placement. Avoid placing pins into the caudolateral surface of the femur because of the sciatic nerve. Make a mini-approach with a stab incision though the skin and blunt dissection with hemostats onto the bone. During pin insertion, attempt to establish and maintain fracture reduction. The skin may move during manipulation, so establish the pin entrance sites while maintaining the skin in its normal position. Use an assistant or overhead traction to create anatomic axial and torsional alignment. Once fixation pins are placed, create axial apposition and, ideally, compression by sliding the pins closer on the frame bar. Only minimal torsional and translational adjustments may be made. The authors prefer to use power when inserting transfixation pins as a hand chuck introduces wobble and some loss of strength at the pin/bone interface. Insert the most proximal and distal transfixation pins first to establish the plane for the remaining transfixation pins. Keep all transfixation elements separated by a distance equal to three pin diameters or one-half the bone diameter from fracture or fissure edges. Once transfixation elements are placed, apply the connecting

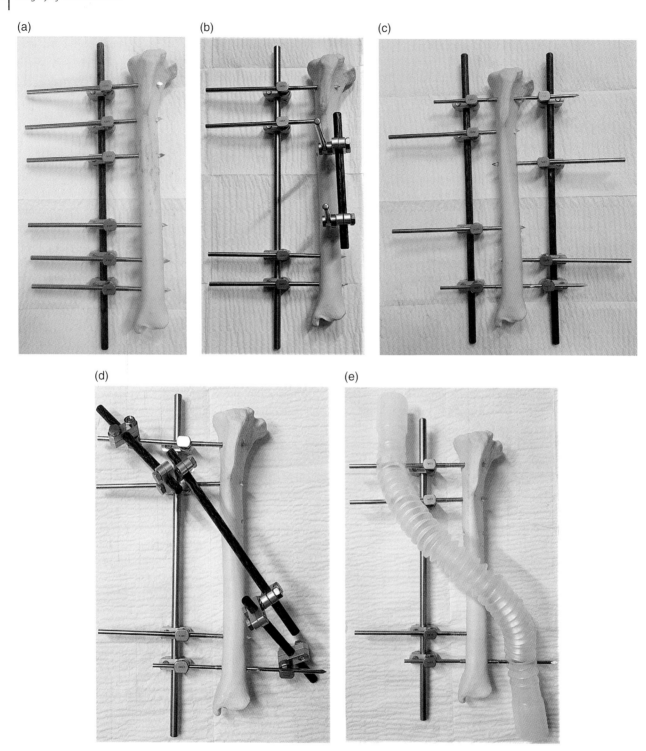

Figure 10.15 Picture of a type I (unilateral, uniplanar) ESF (a), type Ib (unilateral, biplanar) ESF with a longer titanium bar medially and a shorter carbon fiber bar cranially (b), type II hybrid (components of type II and type I, bilateral, uniplaner) ESF (c), and type I-II hybrid constructs with components of a type I SK fixator proximally and type II SK center-threaded pin distally, allowing the application of a second commercial (d) or biphasic connecting bar (e). This hybrid setup (d and e) could be used to stabilize a fracture that requires full load bearing by the construct (i.e. high level of comminution) in a location where a type II construct would not be well tolerated proximally (i.e. femur).

bar. Connecting bars can be stainless steel, aluminum, titanium, or carbon fiber. Carbon fiber is radiolucent allowing better radiographic fracture assessment.

Biphasic ESF

There are several types of commercially produced moldable materials for biphasic ESF. It is important that the chosen material be lightweight, strong, and bind to metal. Some common examples of acrylics include polymethylmethacrylate-based Technovit (Jorvet, Loveland, CO), Jet Denture Repair (Lang Dental Manufacturing Co., Inc., Wheeling, IL), Acrylic Pin External Fixation (APEF) System (Innovative Animal Products, Rochester, MN), and FastFix Putty (Securos, Fiskdale, MA) (Figure 10.16).

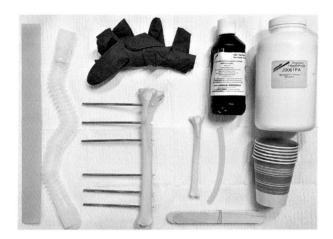

Figure 10.16 Picture of the supplies needed for making an acrylic connecting bar ESF. From left to right – connecting bars of Penrose drain or corrugated tubing, gloves, preplaced transfixation pins in bone, an example of a smaller bone and appropriately sized connecting bar tube, volatile monomer liquid, methylmethacrylate powder, tongue depressors, and paper cups for mixing.

Acrylx (IMEX Veterinary Inc., Longview, TX) is an easy-to-use polymethylmethacrylate-based mixing gun system that allows 2–4 minutes to adjust reduction and alignment, setting completely by 12 minutes (Figure 10.17). The external mold of the connecting system may consist of a variety of materials such as soda straws for small patients, corrugated tubing, or Penrose drains. Resins typically produce a lower temperature exothermic reaction compared to acrylics (Rice et al. 2012). Pierce the center of the tubing onto the transfixation pins ensuring the pin traverses the entire tube diameter. Choose the size of the connecting system that is roughly the diameter of the bone or slightly larger. Fill the mold with the chosen acrylic. If a Penrose drain is used, partially clamp the opposite end of the drain to allow air to escape but to avoid acrylic from leaking out. Do not allow any movement during the setting process. To increase the strength of the adhesion between the transfixation pins and the acrylic, use commercially produced Interface Pins (IMEX Veterinary Inc., Longview, TX) that come with a knurled surface. Alternatively, use a file, rasp, or pliers to create a lightly knurled surface on a nonthreaded pin. The versatility of the biphasic ESF means the surgeon may apply a variety of construct configurations to most fracture types (Figures 10.18 and 10.19).

IM-ESF Tie-In

The IM-ESF tie-in is a widely used fixation in avian fracture stabilization. It is a variation of the ESF with the inclusion of an IM pin that is bent 90° and incorporated into the external fixator. It combines the strength in bending of an intramedullary pin with the rotational stability and versatility of an ESF. Bueno et al. showed successful healing in 84% of treated raptor tibiotarsal fractures with a 59% release rate using a IM ESF tie-in (Bueno et al. 2015). Mean healing

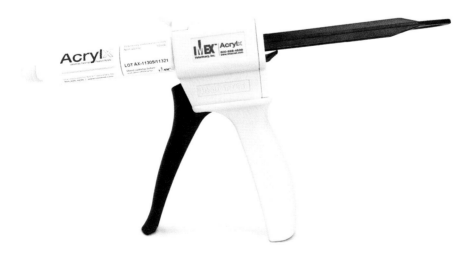

Figure 10.17 Acrylx 2-part resin comes with an applicator, multiuse cartridge, and replaceable nozzles of varying diameters. *Source:* Courtesy of IMEX Veterinary Inc., Longview, TX.

(a) (b) (c)

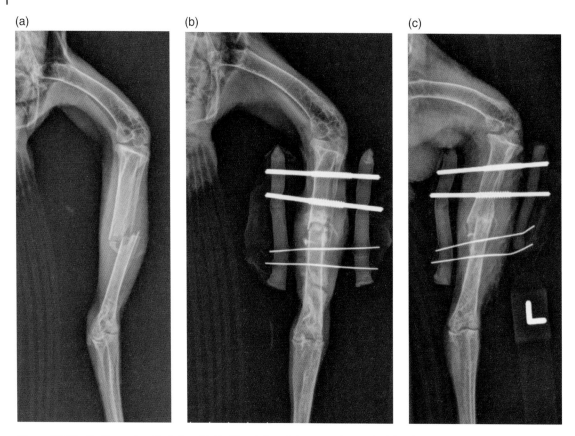

Figure 10.18 Radiographs of adult red-tailed hawk found down on the road with left pelvic limb lameness show a comminuted fracture of the left mid-tibiotarsus with cranial, lateral, and proximal displacement, and fracture of the left fibula (a). The fracture was successfully treated with a biphasic type II ESF as shown by the 3-week (b) and 6.5-week (c) postop radiographs. Note that the distal pins were undersized, and their bending resulted in mild angulation of the tibiotarsus at 6.5 weeks.

time was 38 days. As with ESF, several configurations exist. A study by Van Wettere et al. biomechanically evaluated different configurations on an ostectomized red-tailed hawk (*Buteo jamaicensis*) humerus model with an IM-ESF tie-in construct *in vitro* (Van Wettere et al. 2009) (Figure 10.20). They determined that a standard 1 + 1 configuration was the weakest and least stiff. Both a 1 + 1 variant construct and 1 + 2 construct were stiffer and stronger than the 1 + 1, and there was no difference between the 1 + 1 variant and the 1 + 2 configurations. The 2 + 2 tie-in configuration was significantly stiffer and stronger in both compression and torsion.

An IM-ESF tie-in can be applied to humeral, ulnar, femoral, and tibiotarsal fractures (Figure 10.21). Apply the IM pin first as described. For proximal to mid-diaphyseal fractures, consider not inserting the IM pin completely distal to allow for placement of the transfixation pin distal to the IM pin, avoiding interference. Once the pin is seated, bend the IM pin 90° to be parallel to the transfixation pins. Never bend the pin against the bone as this will compromise its mechanical strength or break bone. Instead, use two wire twisters or, for smaller pins, a Frazier suction tip (Figure 10.22). Some

bones are wider proximally (humerus, tibiotarsus) affording space for safe placement of transfixation pins bypassing the IM pin. Insert the transfixation pins ensuring at least one bicortical pin is placed in the proximal and distal segments. Apply a commercially-produced or acrylic connecting system ensuring that the connecting bar also incorporates the bent IM pin, thus "tying-in" the IM pin.

Ring Fixators and Hybrid Fixators

Ring or circular fixators are rings connected to transfixation wires of small diameter. When placed under tension, transfixation wires can be as stiff as much larger transfixation pins. Because of their bulky design, they are mainly limited to tibiotarsal fractures (Figure 10.23). The main advantage of this system is the ability to stabilize very small fragments. By using smaller wires, dynamization occurs and accelerates healing. Ring fixators are adjustable and applicable for distraction osteogenesis. Distraction osteogenesis has been described to successfully re-establish limb length in two raptor cases (Ponder 2012) and in a yellow-naped Amazon parrot with a chronic nonunion tibiotarsal fracture with substantial bone loss (Johnston et al. 2008).

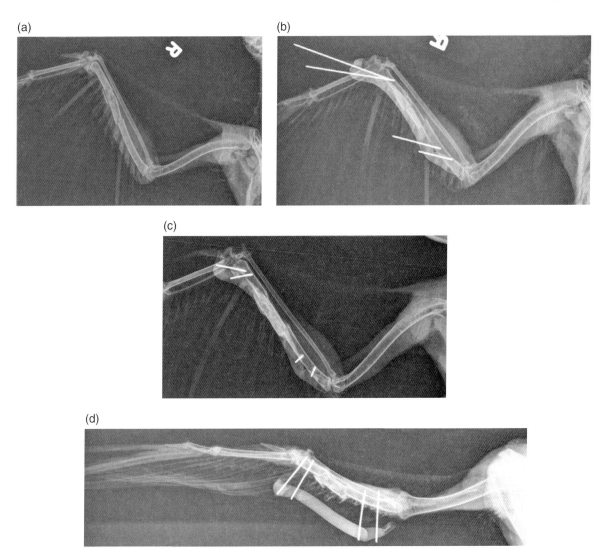

(a)

(b)

(c)

(d)

Figure 10.19 Radiographs of an adult red-shouldered hawk with a complete, severely comminuted mid-diaphyseal right ulna fracture, an intact radius, and mild surrounding soft tissue swelling (a). A type I ESF with a Penrose drain filled with PMMA connecting bar was applied. Radiographs were made post-op (b) and at seven weeks post-op (c and d) with complete osseous bridging noted following treatment with the biphasic ESF.

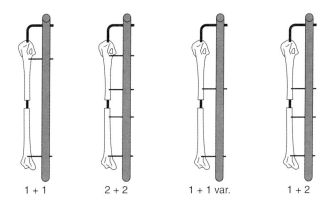

1 + 1   2 + 2   1 + 1 var.   1 + 2

Figure 10.20 Schematic of various configurations of IM-ESF. In terms of biomechanical strength and stiffness, 2 + 2 > 1 + 2 ~ 1 + 1 var. > 1 + 1. *Source:* Van Wettere et al. (2009). Reprinted with permission of Association of Avian Veterinarians.

Ring fixators can be placed in a variety of orientations including hybrid constructs that incorporate both ring and linear components. Place at least two wires in each bone segment (ideally three to four) avoiding critical structures and fissures. When a segment is too short to place three to four wires on two rings, opposing olive wires, which have a larger diameter expansion that abuts the bone, are preferred. Another option is adding a third point of fixation using posts from the single ring to add a wire or transfixing half pin.

When transfixing wires in a short segment of bone, place the first wire at the point closest to the joint using knowledge of anatomy and radiography/fluoroscopy, or a keyhole approach. Use 25-gauge hypodermic needles to locate the joint if needed. This first wire will serve as a reference point

(a)

(b)

(c)

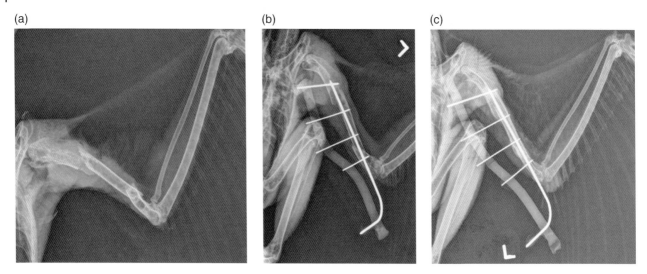

Figure 10.21 Radiographs of a three-year-old Harris hawk (*Parabuteo unicinctus*) that was attacked by a dog show a segmental left humeral fracture with mild surrounding soft tissue swelling suggestive of an open fracture or air from the pneumatic bone (a). An IM pin was placed normograde starting near the elbow. Note that the placement is close to the elbow and could have resulted in ankylosis. The authors prefer to either retrograde the pin proximally or normograde from proximal to distal and to tie-in proximally. Progressive healing of the fracture with stable orthopedic implants was seen at two (b) and four week postoperative (c).

(a)   (b)

(c)

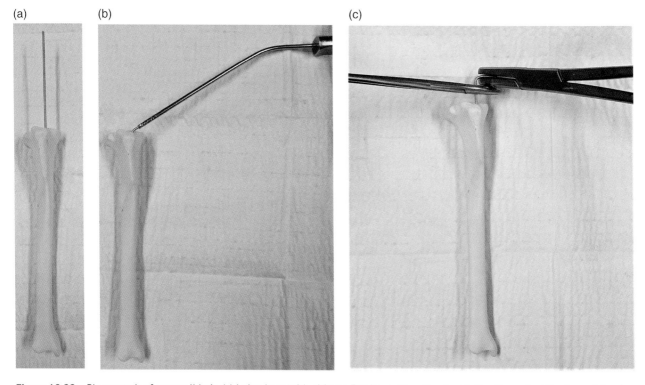

Figure 10.22 Photograph of proper IM pin (a) being bent with either a Frazier suction tip placed directly against the bone (b) or two sets of bending pliers, which will leave a small gap between the bone and the bend to accommodate the wire twisters (c). This gap could be reduced by seating the pin deeper following bending.

for other pins. Place the wire as perpendicular to the long axis of the bone as possible using the capture bolt on the ring as an aiming guide. Affix the ring or partial ring using the system's capture bolts. Once the ring has captured one wire, a second wire can be placed at approximately 45–90° to the first wire on the opposite side of the ring. Tighten the

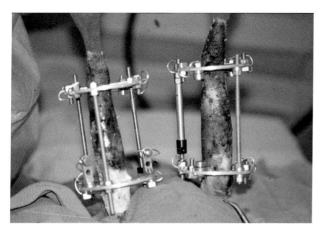

Figure 10.23 Bilateral application of external ring fixators to a bald eagle (*Haliaeetus leucocephalus)* with extensive injuries to both skeletal and soft tissue structures of the tibiotarsi from vehicular trauma. The small transfixation wires can be used even with minimal available bone stock allowing the construct to span large segments and treat concurrent soft tissue injuries. Note, the bird is in dorsal recumbency.

capture bolts moderately, but not yet completely, to hold the ring in place. Importantly, always tighten using two wrenches, one on the nut and one on the bolt for counter pressure to avoid bending the wire.

If enough bone stock is present, place a second ring away from the joint (toward the fracture). The two rings can be fixed using threaded spacers and nuts. Preplace capture bolts before affixing the second ring as there is often limited space between the rings. Alternatively, place only one fixation wire on this ring, on the opposite side of the first ring, as previously described. Add the distal ring(s) in a similar manner. Then apply stainless steel, aluminum, or titanium connecting rods (threaded or partially threaded) to the rings spanning the fracture to serve as platforms for either additional rings or as connecting bars for a hybrid fixator. It may be helpful to tension wires in very large birds (>5 kg). Recommended tension for transfixing wires are published (Jaeger and Wosar 2018). Roughly, tighten with approximately three times the animal's weight (i.e. 30 kg of tension for a 10 kg body weight). When using incomplete rings, it is recommended to not tension more than 30 kg to avoid ring deformation. Completely tighten all connections once appropriate alignment is achieved.

Bone Grafting

Frequently, the situation arises where an osseous defect is large or the biologic healing potential of a fracture is insufficient. For these circumstances, several types of osteogenic materials exist including autogenous grafts,

allografts, and xenografts, in addition to biologic modifiers to provide osteogenesis, osteoinduction, osteoconduction, and osteopromotion. There is a paucity of clinical research in avian bone grafting. Due to the unique avian morphology, autologous cortical and cancellous bone graft is less available. To collect autogenous cancellous bone from the proximal tibiotarsus, make a small approach through the skin over the medial aspect and use sharp and blunt dissection to approach the bone. Create a defect in the cortex and use a house curette to collect the graft, being cautious not to disrupt the trans-cortex.

For a corticocancellous graft, reflect the pectoral muscles from one side of the keel (Figure 10.24). Use an osteotome or appropriately sized biopsy punch to obtain portions of the keel and repeat as needed. Corticocancellous graft may also be collected from ribs. Approach the last ribs cranial to the thigh where they are palpable subcutaneously. Make an incision over the ribs and isolate the appropriately sized segment of a rib or two if needed. Coagulate intercostal vessels along the caudal border of the ribs and elevate the muscles to isolate the segment to be removed. Use heavy scissors or a bone cutter to remove the piece of rib. Once collected, morselize the harvested bone and place it where it is needed. In closed fractures, morselize available cortical bone from unstable fragments found at the fracture site (Martin and Ritchie 1994) or any callus that has formed.

Because of the scarcity of autogenous bone graft, allograft has been used in birds; however, these grafts have limited benefit and may lead to significantly higher occurrence of dehiscence, sequestration, and foreign body reactions than no grafts (MacCoy and Haschek 1988). Demineralized bone matrix (DBM) is one promising option due to both its osteoconductive (when combined with bone chips) and osteoinductive properties. Avian allogenic DBM appears to be safe and improved temporal bone healing in pigeons (Sanaei et al. 2015; Tunio et al. 2015). Intraspecies grafts induce less inflammation than interspecies DBM (Jalila et al. 2004), while xenogeneic sources of DBM did not induce callus, but produced an intense inflammatory reactions (MacCoy and Haschek 1988). Recombinant human bone morphogenetic protein-2 (rhBMP2) was successfully used in a whooping crane (*Grus americana*) in a highly comminuted open proximal humeral fracture with no infection or reported soft tissue reaction (Sample et al. 2008). When using avian DBM, it was shown that the morphology of the product was a significant factor in healing; tubular-shaped product was superior to chips of DBM (Sanaei et al. 2015). Avian DBM is not currently commercially available but can be derived using methods described by the University of Minnesota Raptor Center (Jalila et al. 2004; Sanaei et al. 2015).

(a)

(b)

(c)

(d)

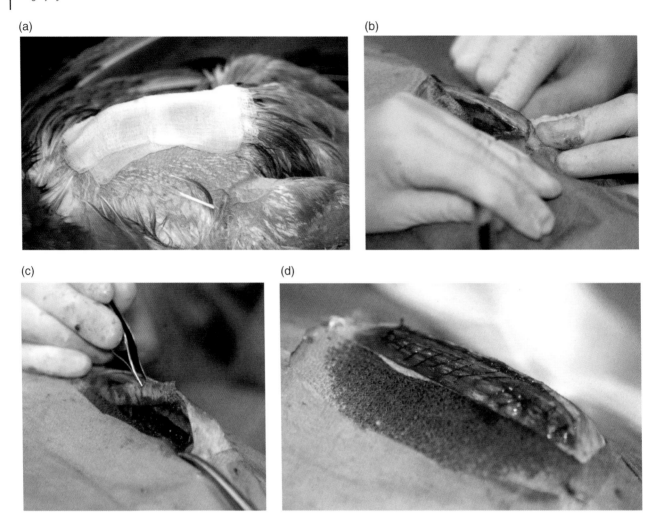

Figure 10.24 Photographs of corticocancellous bone harvest. Aseptically prepare the keel for bone graft harvest (a). Incise the pectoral muscle insertion on one side of the keel and elevate the muscle to expose the keel. Use an osteotome to perform a central block ostectomy leaving intact cortices cranial, ventral, caudal, and dorsal (b and c). Alternatively, use a biopsy punch in smaller birds. Following harvest, appose the pectoral muscles on midline (d) and close the skin routinely.

Fracture Conclusions

The surgeon has many tools available for stabilization. Ultimately, the selection should incorporate patient, surgeon, and owner factors. Table 10.2 lists the authors' recommendations for stabilization of various bones, knowing that each scenario is unique and that no one method is best for all fractures of a specific bone.

Luxation Management Options

Relative to avian fracture fixation, less is defined for avian luxations. Two review articles summarize the knowledge of causes, clinical signs, and treatment of luxations in birds (Azmanis et al. 2014; Gonzalez 2019). Within as little as

three days, significant fibrosis occurs inhibiting reduction of the luxation and predisposing to joint ankylosis. Overall, the most commonly luxated joints are the scapulohumeral and femorotibial joints.

For a luxated joint perform a work-up in a similar manner as for a fracture. Examine the bird as a whole and ensure respiratory and cardiovascular systems are stable. Perform radiography to confirm a diagnosis of joint luxation and rule out fractures and other trauma. Perform distraction views (joint placed in tension) to induce subluxation in mildly affected joints.

External coaptation can be used successfully for management of luxation of coracoid-sternum, shoulder, elbow (mild-to-moderate in severity), carpal, and metatarsophalangeal joints. Joints that usually require surgical intervention include the elbow (severe or chronic

Table 10.2 Fracture stabilization methods.

Bone	Stabilization method
Coracoid	• Body wrap • IM pin • Plate
Humerus	• ESF with IM pin tie-in • Type I ESF • IM pin with torsional support[a] • Plate
Ulna	• ESF with IM pin tie-in • Type I ESF • IM pin with torsional support[a] • Figure-of-eight wrap[b] • Plate
Radius	• Figure-of-eight wrap[b] • IM pin • ESF +/− figure-of-eight wrap if large enough Plate if large
Carpometacarpus	• Figure-of-eight wrap • Type I or type II ESF • IM pin • Carpal splint
Femur	• ESF with IM pin tie-in • Type I ESF • IM pin with torsional support[a] • Plate
Tibiotarsus	• ESF with IM pin tie-in • Type I or type II ESF • IM pin with torsional support[a] • Plate
Tarsometatarsus	• Splint • Type II ESF • Plate

[a] Torsional support to IM pins consists of any single or combination of body wrap, figure-of-eight bandage, cerclage, hemicerclage, antirotational figure-of-eight wire, or stack pin.
[b] Note, if both radius and ulna are fractured, stabilize both bones if synostosis is a concern.

luxations), coxofemoral, stifle, and tarsal joints. The techniques that have been applied include arthroplasty, internal fixation, arthrodesis, and ESF.

Luxation of the Shoulder

Shoulder luxation may involve avulsion of the ventral tubercle of the proximal humerus. Bandage the wing to the body to immobilize the shoulder joint for 10–14 days.

Reluxation can occur with coaptation alone and thus prognosis for flight is guarded. If precision flight is required and the ventral tubercle has avulsed, consider performing open reduction and reattaching the ventral tubercle (Figure 10.25a,b). The authors have not seen reluxation following tubercle pinning. The authors have also had success with a transarticular pin (Figure 10.25c,d). Reduce the luxation, fold the wing to the body, and place a pin from the deltoid crest through the humeral head and into the scapula or coracoid. Immobilize the wing with a body wrap for 10–14 days followed by a figure-of-eight + body wrap bandage if still unstable. This will cause some articular damage and may predispose to developing osteoarthritis.

Luxation of the Elbow

Luxation of the elbow is usually the result of severe blunt trauma with enough force to disrupt the ligamentous support. This type of injury has been reported to occur in as many as 12% of raptor patients (Ackermann and Redig 1997). Luxation most commonly occurs caudodorsal followed by caudal. Ventral luxation occurs only in association with fracture of the radius. The luxation may be mild or severe (Figure 10.26). The wing is generally held with the elbow extended (drooped) and externally rotated. Pain, crepitus, and swelling are noted on palpation. Examine the wing for concomitant soft tissue injury that may affect prognosis. The presence of open wounds and fractures has been associated with a poor prognosis for return to normal function.

For transarticular ESF, place at least two lateral fixation pins proximal and distal to the joint (Figure 10.26f). With the joint in a normal angle, connect the proximal pin of the proximal bone to the distal pin in the distal bone, and the distal pin in the proximal bone to the proximal pin in the distal bone. Maintain the device for two to three weeks to allow scar tissue to stabilize the joint.

To reduce an acute luxation, flex the elbow to counteract the force of the scapulotriceps muscle pulling the ulna caudally. While maintaining flexion, internally rotate the radius and ulna and apply pressure to the dorsal (lateral) aspect of the radial head to force it into apposition with the dorsal (lateral) humeral condyle. Gently extend the elbow – a pop may be palpable as reduction is completed. If the joint is stable following reduction, support the elbow with a figure-of-eight bandage for 10–14 days. Where there is severe ligamentous damage as evidenced by laxity following reduction, apply a transarticular ESF for 5–7 days, followed by 7–10 days of coaptation with a figure-of-eight bandage. Initiate controlled physical rehabilitation following removal of the support. It has been reported that 50% of

(a)　　　　　　　　　　　　　　(b)

(c)　　　　　　　　　　　　　　(d)

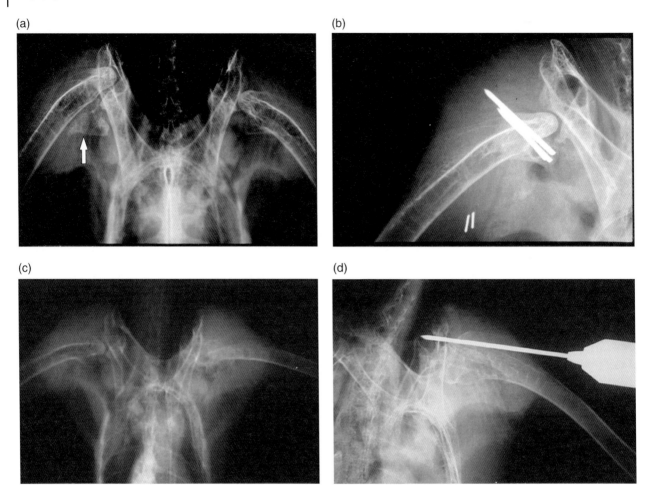

Figure 10.25 Avulsion fracture of the ventral tubercle (arrow) of the proximal humerus resulting in shoulder luxation (a) is stabilized using three diverging K-wires (b). Note that hemostatic clips were used to seal a vessel intraoperatively. Radiographs of a shoulder luxation with no tubercle avulsion (c) followed by reduction and the insertion of a transarticular pin through the deltopectoral crest into the scapula (d). The pin should be maintained for 10–14 days followed by a figure-of-eight + body wrap bandage.

raptors with elbow luxations are released (Martin and Ritchie 1994; Souza et al. 2004)

Commonly, it is not possible to reduce the luxation closed, in which case surgical reduction is indicated. Successful surgical reduction has been described (Ackermann and Redig 1997). Perform a dorsal approach to the elbow. Transect the origin of the supinator if needed to visualize the joint leaving a small amount of the origin to reattach. Assess the transverse radioulnar ligaments as these are often disrupted from the trauma. Use a periosteal elevator to lever the ulnar head into reduction (usually cranial and ventral). Suture the insertion of the triceps tendon to the origin of the extensor digitorum communicus with a monofilament slowly absorbed material to stabilize the joint. Close the incision and apply a transarticular ESF. Remove the ESF after 5–7 days and replace with a figure-of-eight bandage for 7–10 more days. Begin physical therapy at the time of ESF removal.

Luxation of the Carpus

Carpal luxation is generally dorsal. The bird will hold the wing with the carpus extended and externally rotated distally. Reduce the carpal luxation by applying traction and (dorsal) abduction of the distal extremity (Figure 10.27). Toggle the carpometacarpus into reduction and ventrally adduct the carpus. Apply a figure-of-eight bandage to maintain reduction for 10–14 days. With large birds or chronic luxations, open reduction may be indicated. In cases where there is significant laxity following reduction, place a transarticular pin or ESF to maintain reduction. Place a transarticular pin with the carpus in a normal degree of flexion through the major portion of the carpometacarpus into the ulna immobilizing the carpus. This will cause articular damage which may predispose to developing osteoarthritis. Initiate controlled physical therapy after support devices are removed.

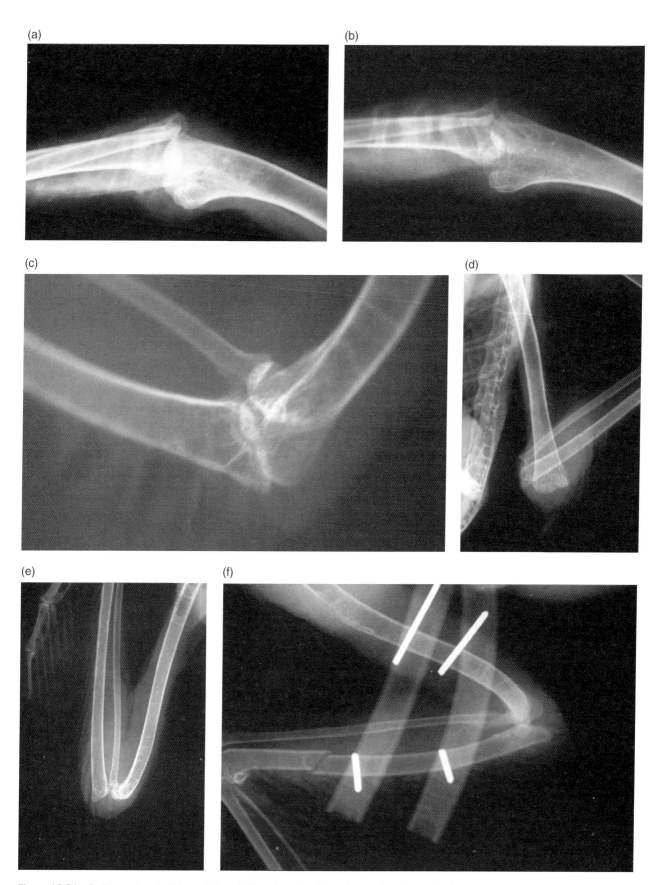

Figure 10.26 Radiographs of mild caudodorsal elbow luxation (a) and normal conformation following closed reduction (b and c). Note that the diagnosis is not always obvious as in this example. Radiographs of a severe caudodorsal elbow luxation (d) followed by normal conformation with closed reduction (e). This patient had a transarticular ESF applied followed by a figure-of-eight bandage (f). Note the iatrogenic fracture of the distal ulna. No additional stabilization was applied since it was maintained in a figure-of-eight bandage.

(a)

(b)

(c)

(d)

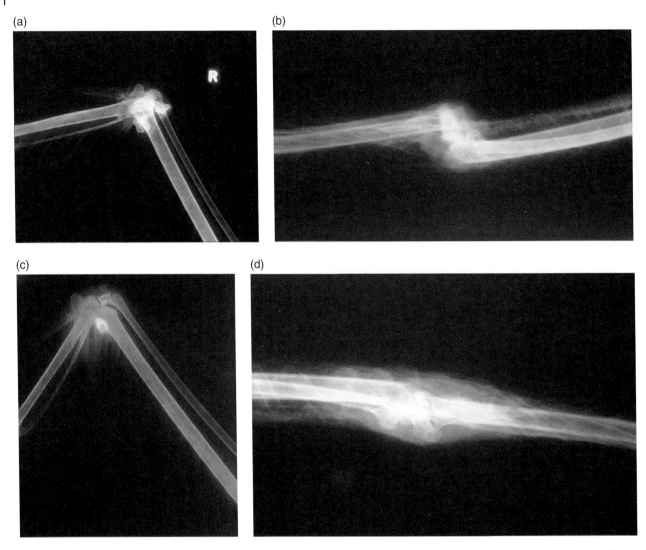

Figure 10.27 Lateral (a) and cranial/caudal (b) radiographs of a dorsal luxation of the carpus. On the lateral view notice that the distal radius is superimposed on the radial carpal bone. Lateral (c) and cranial-caudal (d) radiographs following closed reduction.

Luxation of the Hip

In most psittacines and raptors, the coxofemoral joint is not a tight-fitting ball and socket joint but has a significant amount of cranial to caudal gliding motion with little abduction and adduction. It is a diarthrodial joint supported by a round ligament as well as collateral ligaments. For luxation to occur, both the ventral collateral ligament and the round ligament must be disrupted. In many species, the dorsal rim of the acetabulum is well developed and extends as the antitrochanter to articulate with the broad, flat femoral neck and trochanter. Coxofemoral luxations are generally craniodorsal and the result of traction and rotation trauma such as occurs when the leg is entangled.

Closed reduction and stabilization with slings, splints, and casts have been recommended for smaller birds.

Consider surgical reduction and stabilization for acute coxofemoral luxations in larger birds. Perform a craniolateral approach. The luxation may be reduced and maintained using a transarticular pin (Figure 10.28). Insert the pin through the trochanter into the head of the femur and across the acetabulum with the hip in a normal standing angle. The chuck should be set on the pin at a predetermined length as deep insertion will penetrate the kidney that lies on the medial side of the acetabulum, potentially resulting in intracoelomic hemorrhage. Exact acetabular pin depth would be best determined with CT. In the authors' experience, the medial wall of the acetabulum (Membrana acetabuli) is too thin to support a pin and is likely to damage the kidney. Instead, aim the pin cranially to engage acetabular bone, which causes iatrogenic articular damage. Remove the pin by 5–7 days postoperatively. Support the limb in a spica splint or off-weight bearing

(a)

(b)

(c)

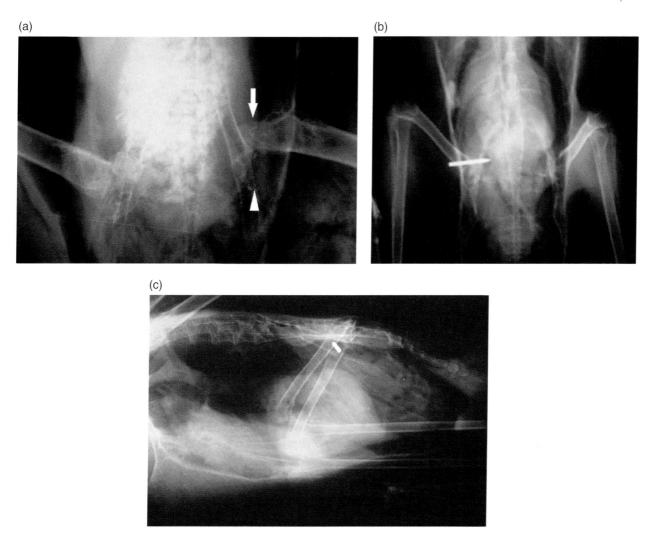

Figure 10.28 Radiographs of a craniodorsal right-sided coxofemoral luxation (a) including the luxated femoral head (arrow) and empty acetabulum (arrowhead). Additional radiographs are shown following open reduction with application of transarticular pin (ventrodorsal (b) and lateral (c)).

sling for another 7–10 days. One author (BD) has placed a toggle pin in a six-month-old red-legged seriema (*Cariama cristata*) (Figure 10.29). The injury to the kidney medial to the acetabulum appeared insignificant. The bird quickly regained ambulation and the joint remained stable for two months before the femoral neck fractured. Toggle pinning is not recommended until further research has been conducted.

Simple capsulorrhaphy is challenging due to the extent of damage following trauma, although successful treatment with suture augmentation of the dorsal capsule was reported in a 240g macaw with a chronic ventral luxation (Martin et al. 1994). Perform a craniolateral approach to the hip. To aid with visualization, transect the iliotrochantericus caudalis at its insertion on the major trochanter. Pass an appropriately sized nonabsorbable or slowly absorbed monofilament suture through the major tro-

chanter and dorsal rim of the ischium, caudal to the acetabulum. Place another suture from the trochanter to the dorsal rim of the ilium, cranial to the acetabulum. Reattach the iliotrochantericus caudalis and close routinely.

In cases of chronic luxation, there may be considerable damage to the femoral head or neck and to the dorsal acetabular rim. Consider a femoral head and neck excision arthroplasty (FHO) for chronic luxations. Perform a craniolateral approach. Remove the head and neck of the femur with an osteotome or sagittal saw. Be sure that no rough edges remain. Note that the femoral neck is short and take care to not remove the greater trochanter. Following FHO, there is a tendency for external rotation of the limb. This can be countered using the support sutures as described in the previous paragraph. These sutures will prevent excessive external rotation of the leg but sutures are not necessary for full recovery. A red-tailed hawk

(a)

(b)

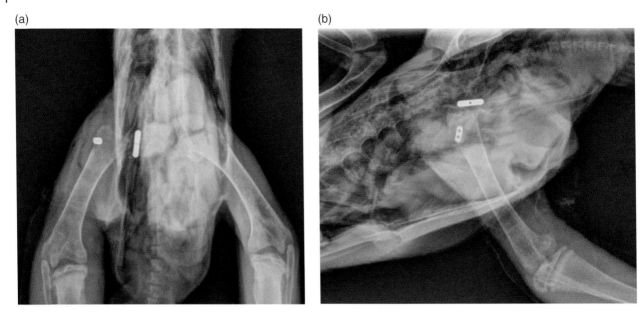

Figure 10.29 Ventrodorsal (a) and lateral (b) radiograph of a toggle pin applied to the right hip of a six-month-old red-legged seriema for the treatment of right coxofemoral luxation. Unfortunately, the femoral neck fractured two months postoperatively.

(*B. jamaicensis*) and Canada goose (*Branta canadensis*) were released or transferred to a wildlife rehab facility to prepare for release only two weeks following FHO (Burgdorf-Moisuk et al. 2011).

Luxation of the Stifle

Stifle luxation occurs following trauma and disruption of the collateral and cruciate ligaments. Not only is a positive drawer sign elicited but also medial and/or lateral collateral instability exists. Surgical repair of the ligaments may be attempted in large birds; however, in most small companion birds, the size of the ligaments precludes surgical apposition. In such cases, transarticular ESF may be used to maintain the stifle in reduction allowing periarticular fibrosis to stabilize the joint (Azmanis et al. 2014). If the injury is severe or articular fractures exist, arthrodesis has been performed in a pet Moluccan cockatoo (*Cacatua moluccensis)* (Rosenthal et al. 1994).

Stifle luxation has also been treated with a lateral extracapsular suture technique in a three-month-old cockatoo (*Cacatua alba*) and a six-year-old African gray parrot (*Psittacus erithacus*) (Chinnadurai et al. 2009; McRee et al. 2017). For this technique, perform a lateral or medial parapatellar approach to the stifle for intraarticular evaluation. If there is an unstable meniscal tear, sharply debride the torn portions being careful to minimize damage to surrounding structures (articular cartilage, collateral ligaments, and remaining cruciate ligament). Close the capsule with an appropriately sized slowly absorbed monofilament suture.

Take care to not over-tighten and induce a patellar luxation (note that not all birds have a patella). To anchor a suture in the distal lateral femoral condyle, place a cortical screw in mono or bicortical fashion in the distal lateral nonarticular surface of the femur to serve as a suture anchor. Alternatively, if the bird is not large enough to accept a screw or a screw is not available, drill a bone tunnel through the distolateral femur from craniolateral to caudomedial. Then drill another small tunnel just large enough to accommodate one or two strands of mono or multifilament slowly absorbed or nonabsorbable suture through the proximal cranial tibiotarsus. Loop the suture around the screw or through the femoral bone tunnel, and then through the tibiotarsal bone tunnel with the medial suture tunneling under (through the stifle joint) or over the patellar tendon. Tie the suture with drawer reduced and the stifle in a standing angle. Ensure the knots are placed as proximal and lateral as possible.

Conjoined femoral and tibiotarsal IM pins may also be used to ankylose a luxated stifle (Bowles and Zantop 2002). This is a useful method in small psittacines. Perform a lateral or medial parapatellar approach to the stifle and examine intra-articular structures and address meniscal damage. Insert an appropriately sized pin (at least 75% of the narrowest intramedullary width, up to 90%) through the craniomedial aspect of the tibiotarsus plateau into the distal medullary canal. High degree of canal filling with IM pins may damage endosteal blood supply resulting in ischemic necrosis. Normograde a pin in a similar manner directed proximally into the femur, starting medial to the patellar tendon, avoiding the insertion of the caudal cruciate ligament. Reduce the luxation. Cut the pins to a reasonable length. Obtain radiographs to confirm the joint is reduced and at an appropriate standing angle (60° is often used). Bend the pins 90° 1–2 cm after they exit the skin so that they cross each other. Apply a binding agent, such as moldable thermoplastic or polymeric resin, over the pins where they cross to secure them together. It must be noted that the IM pins are within the stifle joint and may cause osteoarthritis to develop. In one case, complications with this method required mid-femoral amputation (Harris et al. 2007).

If an arthrodesis must be performed, enter the joint stifle joint with a medial or lateral parapatellar approach and perform an arthrodesis as described below.

Luxation of the Tarsus

Instability of the tarsus is the result of damage to the supporting tendinous and ligamentous structures including the flexor hallucis muscle, gastrocnemius tendon, collateral ligaments, and joint retinaculum. Early surgical intervention is indicated to reduce the risk of developing arthritis and can involve ESF, direct ligamentous repair, arthrodesis, or amputation.

Chronic tarsal luxation has been repaired using collateral ligament augmentation in an adult bateleur eagle (*Terathopius ecaudatus*) (Gjeltema et al. 2017) and should be considered for early surgical intervention as well. Make an incision over the affected medial or lateral collateral ligament. Drill bone tunnels though the cortices of the distal tibiotarsus starting near the joint angling proximally toward the trans cortex. Drill a second bone tunnel starting from the proximal tarsometatarsus distally to the trans cortex of the tarsometatarsus. Incise the skin and bluntly dissect to the bone to expose the exit points of the interosseous tunnels on the contralateral aspect. Pass a single strand of a slowly absorbable or nonabsorbable suture from the entrance points of the tibiotarsus and tarsometatarsus, through the bone tunnels and exiting out the skin. Thread the suture through a stainless steel or acrylic 2-hole (or more) button to function as a stent at each of the exit points. Pass the suture back down the respective bone tunnels. Tighten the suture to snug the buttons against the bone at their respective exit points and tie the strands together with moderate tension and the leg in a standing angle.

More research is needed, but it does not seem that button stents are necessary. As an alternative, create cranial-to-caudal interosseous tunnels in the metaphyseal region just proximal and distal to the intertarsal joint of the side affected. Loop slowly or non-absorbable suture through these tunnels and tie with appropriate tension.

Luxation of the Metacarpophalangeal Joint

A single report describes the extended application (six to nine weeks) of a type I ESF for the arthrodesis of metacarpophalangeal joint following luxation in two raptors (Van Wettere and Redig 2004). Both birds achieved full flight and were released.

Arthrodesis

Arthrodesis is a salvage procedure and is indicated for intractable joint pain, uncontrolled inflammation, and complex injuries. Joint fusion is better tolerated in low motion joints. Follow the basics principles of arthrodesis: careful planning, removal of all cartilage at all sites to be fused down to subchondral bone, close apposition of the joint surfaces, rigid fixation with compression applied across the joint during healing, bone grafting, and careful preservation of the soft tissues surrounding the area. Use a curette or bur to remove the articular cartilage keeping in mind limb-shortening. In dogs, 25% femoral shortening is tolerated though how much limb shortening is tolerated is not defined in birds. After choosing the angle of fixation, cut the bones flat at angles that will allow maximum contact/bone apposition. There are very few reports of arthrodesis in birds.

Luxation Conclusion

As with fractures, the selection of joint stabilization should incorporate patient, surgeon, and owner factors. Table 10.3 lists the authors' recommendations for stabilization of various joints, knowing that no one method is appropriate in all cases.

Angular Limb Deformities (ALD)

Angular Limb Deformities (ALD) involve axial or torsional malalignment. Limb deformities occur for various reasons that are not completely understood with theories ranging from traumatic injuries to developmental and congenital defects. Skeletal malformation may lead to discomfort and strain on adjacent joints. Limb deformities can take a variety of forms. A uniapical deformity is a malformation in a single plane. A biapical deformity is a malformation at two foci that may not be in the same plane. It is very important to classify the type of deformity based on well-positioned radiographs or, ideally, a CT study. A detailed knowledge of anatomy is required before correcting an ALD. If the bird has a normal bone for comparison, it is beneficial to image that side as well for

Table 10.3 Stabilization techniques for luxations.

Joint	Conservative management	Surgical management
Shoulder	• Figure of-eight with body wrap	• Transarticular pin • Pin ventral tubercle
Elbow (minor)	• Figure of-eight wrap	
Elbow (severe)		• Type I or II transarticular ESF (rehab necessary)
Carpus	• Figure of-eight	• Open reduction and Type I or type II ESF if bandaging unsuccessful
Metacarpophalangeal		• Arthrodesis (Type I or type II ESF)
Coxofemoral		• Excision arthroplasty • Polypropylene sutures • Transarticular pin
Stifle		• Extracapsular technique • Type I transarticular ESF • Transarticular pin
Hock		• Extracapsular techniques • Type I or type II transarticular ESF
Metatarsophalangeal		• Tenorrhaphy • Splint • Digit amputation
Perosis	Diet modification	• Tenorrhaphy • Angular limb correction • Arthrodesis

planning. Alternatively, it may be useful to image a similar sized bird of the same species.

The goal for treatment of an ALD is to alleviate pain and restore function. A secondary goal is to prevent further abnormalities including continued exacerbation of the primary lesion and adjacent joints. Many methods have been developed for treating ALD. Selective physeal arrest in growing animals (Zollinger et al. 2005) and corrective osteotomies in skeletally mature animals (Meij et al. 1996) have shown high success in re-establishing skeletal alignment in birds; however, detailed reports on the management of ALD in birds are lacking.

Before attempting surgery, familiarize yourself with the regional anatomy and concepts of ALD correction. Planning an ALD correction can be accomplished in several ways. The simplest approach involves planning an osteotomy at the level of the greatest deformation as determined by imaging. A mathematical approach to performing ALD in humans and small mammals has been developed – the center of rotation of angulation (CORA) method. One method of ALD correction planning uses advances in medical and engineering technology. The authors have used digital imaging and communications of medicine (DICOM) images from CT scanning to print a 3D bone model of a chicken (*Gallus*

gallus domesticus) tibiotarsal ALD and bilateral tibiotarsal ALD in a bald eagle (*H. leucocephalus*). The models allowed unlimited practice operations and precontouring of implants or construction of an ESF system before surgery (Figure 10.30).

Intraoperatively, perform a linear, dome, opening wedge osteotomy, or closing wedge ostectomy. Ensure corrections are appropriate by visualizing the orientation and range of motion of the joints proximal and distal. Fluoroscopy or serial radiographs are helpful to ensure alignment intraoperatively. Once alignment is achieved, apply fixation (ESF, IM-ESF, or plate).

Perosis (Achilles Tendon Luxation)

Limb angulation secondary to Achilles tendon luxation may occur with manganese, biotin, pantothenic acid, or folic acid deficiencies; high protein diets in water fowl; or calcium over supplementation (Coles 2007; Tully 2002); however, not all etiologies have been elucidated. The Achilles tendon (hallucis longus tendon) may luxate medially (most commonly reported) or laterally (Schwahn and Rassette 2013) resulting in angulation (bending and/or rotation) of the distal tibiotarsus causing swelling of the tarsus. This alters the flexor

(a) (b)

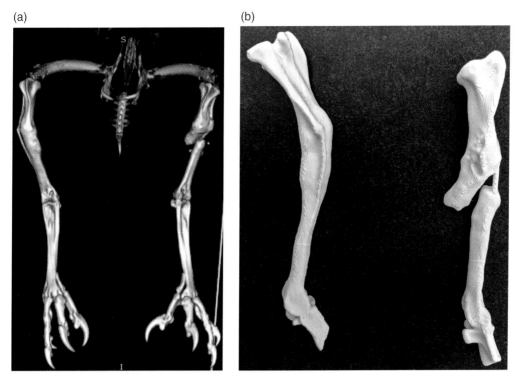

Figure 10.30 CT DICOM images were acquired to make a digital 3-D rendering (a) and 3-D printed bone models (b) for practice surgery and implant selection. The pre- and postoperative radiographs are seen in Figure 10.11.

function of the foot and disables the limb. The tendon may be reducible early on but eventually it becomes nonreducible.

Tenorrhaphy for reducible luxation and potentially ALD correction for severe deformities may be performed. Incise the skin over the caudolateral tarsal joint for a medial luxation. Isolate the tendon and identify the trochlear plantar surface using blunt dissection. Reposition the tendon within the groove in the distal tibiotarsus. Some surgeons advocate deepening the groove. Using a slowly absorbed monofilament material, suture the tendon (approximately ½ thickness) to the lateral periosteum or through a bone tunnel in the lateral epicondyle of the distal tibiotarsus (for a medially luxated tendon). Make this tunnel with either a K-wire or hypodermic needle (Coles 2007; Priyanka et al. 2018). Splint the leg for one to three weeks.

One addition to this technique involves using a hooked K-wire to hold the tendon in place. Following reduction of the tendon, insert a K-wire just lateral to the tendon into the distal tibiotarsus, proximal to the epiphysis. Mold the wire into a hook around the tendon medially, which will serve to hold it in place (Coles 2007).

If it is no longer possible to reduce the tendon, in the authors' experience, it is best to perform an arthrodesis using a transarticular ESF.

Postoperative Care

Postoperative analgesia should be provided and antibiotics may be provided if indicated. Realize that the perioperative period is a very stressful time. Design a recovery enclosure that will limit movement, provide comfort and warmth, and minimize stress to optimize healing. While few studies have focused on rehabilitation, it is well accepted that avian species require early return to function to minimize ankylosis, which can occur very rapidly. Start immediately after surgery. If a limb is bandaged, remove the bandage at a minimum of every two to three days to perform rehabilitation under heavy sedation or anesthesia so the bird does not resist the movement. Be very cautious and support the injured area at all times to prevent disruption of callus or scar tissue.

Passive range of motion involves moving joints as a result of externally applied forces. Active range of motion involves the animal putting a joint through a range of motion under its own power. While active range of motion is best, perform passive range of motion if surgical stabilization is not strong enough for exposure to full physiologic force or an animal is less than willing to move a recently operated limb until adequate healing is documented. In general, at each session, perform approximately 10 repetitions of flexion/extension, holding at each end-point for 10–15 seconds (~5 minutes) for each joint in the affected limb and any other limbs that are idle. Massage the soft tissues to promote elasticity. If not anesthetized, do not perform movements beyond a level of the first signs of discomfort. There are many forms of activities that can be done to promote both active and passive forms of rehabilitation but is beyond the scope of this chapter.

Monitoring for Healing and Complications

Perform a thorough physical examination regularly. Obtain radiographs at two to three weeks post-op, and then every week after that until healing is documented.

Postoperative complications of orthopedic repair include implant failure, malunion, radioulnar synostosis, osteomyelitis/sequestration, muscle atrophy, tendon contracture, propatagial tendon damage, ankylosis, pododermatitis, and others. Implant failure may require revision. Implant migration or radiolucent bone surrounding the implant, often with associated soft tissue swelling, are signs of loose or infected implants. Remove or replace the implant as loose pins and screws may devitalize bone and propagate infection. If necessary, treat a malunion fracture with revision surgery, which requires an osteotomy and application of rigid fixation. To revise a radioulnar synostosis, osteotomize the bridging bone with rongeurs or a bur and fill in the defect with natural tissue (e.g. fat graft) or synthetic material (wax or polypropylene mesh) (Beaufrere et al. 2012).

Open, contaminated fractures are most at risk of developing postoperative infections. When infection is suspected, acquire a sample for culture and sensitivity testing using fine needle aspiration. While awaiting results, provide broad-spectrum antibiotic coverage such as clindamycin or amoxicillin–clavulanate and adjust based on culture and sensitivity (Hawkins et al. 2013). Devitalized or infected bone may cause sequestrum formation. Sequestra are seen on radiographs as normal to sclerotic bone surrounded by a radiolucent halo. There may be a draining tract as the body attempts to extrude the devitalized tissue. Plan surgical excision of the sequestrum with evacuation of all purulence and debridement of devitalized tissue as soon as is reasonable. Provide antibiotics, although alone they will not be curative and the defect will propagate inflammation and impair healing.

Beak Repair

The beak or bill of a bird is an important anatomic structure used for prehension, eating, cleaning/preening, courtship, and feeding offspring. The exact structure and kinesis of the mandibles vary among species, but all consist of a mandible and a maxilla. These bones are covered by a highly keratinized epidermal surface called the rhamphotheca, which is subdivided into rhinotheca (maxilla) and gnathotheca (mandible). The rhamphotheca grows continuously and may even vary in color with seasons. Keratin migrates from vascular beds near the periosteum at the base of the beak and moves rostrally along the beak surface. Any change in rate of production, contour of the pre-maxilla/frontal bone, or inequality results in beak malformation. Large parrots will replace the rhinotheca about every six months and the mandibular keratin every 2–3 months (Lumeij 1994). The opposing edge of the mandible is called the tomium and it is important that this edge remains congruent or the function of the beak may be lost.

Causes of deviations may be related to congenital, traumatic, or nutritional causes. It may be possible to correct small disturbances with routine beak trimming. In young birds, rehabilitative exercises may be applied to counter a mild deviation in the beak. The problem may advance to the point of requiring corrective intervention. Due to the sensitivity of the beak and stress induced during beak trimming and repair, general anesthesia is warranted. An air sac tube is helpful to facilitate the process while avoiding endotracheal tubes and masks. Knowledge of beak repair is limited to only a few small case reports and one recent review (Huynh et al. 2019).

Imaging of the skull and beak can be achieved with radiographs (lateral, ventrodorsal, and right and left obliques). CT is invaluable though windowing must be optimized due to the thinness of the avian skull (Huynh et al. 2019).

Scissor Beak

Scissor beak describes a condition in which the rhinotheca or gnathotheca is deviated to one side. It inhibits prehension and causes abnormal wear – extreme wear on one side and excessive growth on other side. If caught early in a young bird, correct the deformity with gentle pressure applied to the beak in the appropriate direction for 10 minutes, six to eight sessions per day. Once a beak becomes fully calcified, manual adjustments become unfruitful.

Avoid acute correction in parrots, which should have gradual correction (Coles 2007). An approach to redirect the premaxillary growth has been described for scissor beak involving an acrylic ramp fashioned on the gnathotheca (Clipsham technique) (Clipsham 1996) or rhinotheca. Apply a prosthesis to the lateral aspect of the rhinotheca on the side of the mandibular deviation, or the lateral aspect of the gnathotheca to the side of the maxillary deviation. Scarify the keratin with a bur or rasp and clean it to allow the material to adhere. Mold a stainless steel or nylon dental screen mesh to create a ramp to redirect the beak tip to midline. Place a K-wire transversely across the mandible or maxilla to increase the stability of the ramp if needed. Do not place a K-wire in the caudal mandible as it will interfere with or pierce the tongue. Cover the ramp with an acrylic or resin and smooth with a bur. The repair is easiest performed with higher success in young birds with actively developing beaks (Figure 10.31). Correction will often take several weeks to months and may require repeated ramp application with keratin turnover.

A second method for mild scissor beak correction involves a trans-sinus pin and rubber band to apply tension to redirect premaxilla growth (Figure 10.32). Insert a K-wire through the base of the premaxilla. Bend the K-wire to create a hook or loop on both sides. Place an orthodontic rubber band from the hook opposite the maxillary deviation to the rostral aspect of the maxilla (or through a small hole drilled into the distal beak) to pull the beak back into the correct position. The hook on the opposite of the premaxilla serves as a backstop to prevent wire pull-through. Keep the apparatus applied until the deviation is corrected, which is often just a few weeks in young birds.

To surgically correct scissor beak when the mandible appears to be the primary problem, a closing wedge ostectomy on the longer side of the mandible has been described (Coles 2007). The fifth cranial nerve and inferior alveolar artery will be transected during this process. Control hemorrhage with a ligature or judicious use of electrosurgery. To stabilize the fragments, place either an interfragmentary wire and acrylic or an ESF. For interfragmentary wire, elevate a small amount of soft tissue on each side of the osteotomy in the portion of the mandible covered by skin. Make a bone tunnel to fit a small gauge stainless-steel wire (22 or 24 gauge) placed as an interfragmentary wire. Aim for apposition and avoid over-tightening the wire. Alternatively, place a biphasic ESF, though bone purchase of transfixation pins in the beak is very limited and has a higher risk of failure.

In a juvenile mute swan (*Cygnus olor*) with a mandibular malunion causing lateral deviation of its mandible, distraction osteogenesis using a linear ESF was successful in achieving realignment by making small adjustments (Calvo Carrasco et al. 2016).

Mandibular Prognathism

Mandibular prognathism is a condition in which the gnathotheca is deviated rostrally relative to the rhinotheca. Timing and treatment principles are similar to scissor beak. In young birds, apply distraction tension to the distal tip of the rhinotheca for 10 minutes, six to eight sessions per day. In older or more deviated beaks, trim the lower beak and construct an acrylic ramp on the rostral aspect of the rhinotheca to extend beyond the gnathotheca (Figure 10.33). Finally, a modified Doyle technique has been described (Martin and Ritchie 1994). For this technique, place a K-wire through the frontal bone just caudal to the maxilla-premaxilla joint, caudal to the nares. Bend both ends into caudally directed hooks. Place a second K-wire on the dorsal midline of the rhinotheca just distal to the greatest ventral bend. Bend the wire into a cranially directed hook and glue it onto the rhinotheca with acrylic or resin. Connect the frontal and maxillary pins using rubber bands, applying dorsal and caudal tension to the rostral maxilla. Remove the apparatus when correction is observed.

Beak Fractures

Fractures of the beak include simple fractures, depressed fractures, fractures with bone defects, and avulsions. They occur on a roughly equal basis (Huynh et al. 2019). Fractures are met with challenges – fragile blood supply, contamination, and high-stress forces. They are most likely to occur in the mandible and those are easier to stabilize than those of the maxilla with the same principles of anatomic alignment, rigid immobilization, and early return to function. If there is a simple unilateral greenstick fracture of the mandible, nonsurgical conservative management consisting of soft foods may be all that is needed.

To repair defects in the bone, remove debris and any loose tissue fragments. Clean and roughen the rhamphotheca. Manage contaminated wounds open until there is healthy granulation tissue. Once the tissue is healthy, a patch can be applied to protect the wound with less frequent changes to evaluate the wound (Figure 10.34). Granulation tissue forms first and then it becomes firm. The fibrous connective tissue will eventually mineralize and become bone again. Epithelium will migrate over the surface and become new rhamphotheca.

Methods for stabilization include pins and wires, ESF, acrylic/resin fixation, plates, and prosthetics (Huynh et al. 2019). Perform interfragmentary wiring for simple fractures to hold segments in alignment (Figure 10.35). Wires provide poor support against the normal physiologic stresses of the beak and are generally not adequate alone. Most commonly, they are coated with a resin or acrylic creating a type of ESF.

Fractures can be stabilized with pins that bridge the fracture with figure-of-eight or interfragmentary wires, and are then covered with bone cement on both the external and lingual surfaces of the beak. Do not allow the resin/acrylic to seep into any gaps which will cause

(a)

(b)

(c)

(d)

(e)

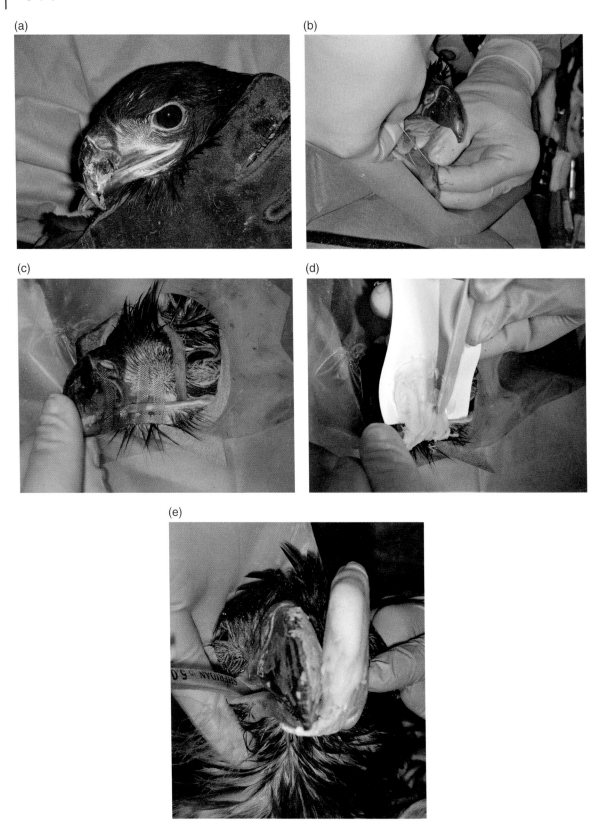

Figure 10.31 Photographs of a juvenile bald eagle (*Haliaeetus leucocephalus*) with moderate-to-severe scissor beak (a) following infection with avian pox. Wires were placed (b) to anchor stainless-steel mesh to the left mandible (c). Acrylic was applied over the mesh using paper as a backstop to make a smooth ramp surface and prevent unwanted mess (d). The final ramp is pictured after being smoothed with a bur (e). Note that the ramp is larger than is typically done as the eagle could open its mouth farther than a psittacine.

(a)

(b)

(c)

(d)

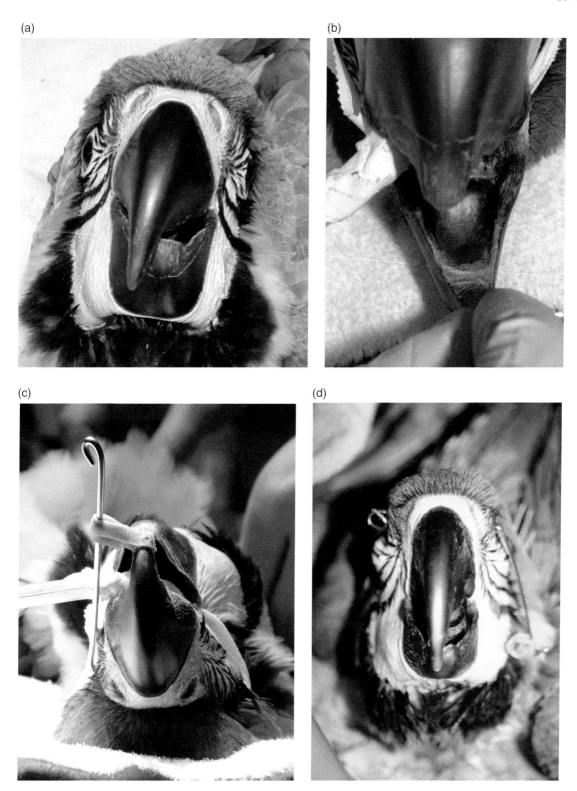

Figure 10.32 Pictures of a blue and gold macaw (*Ara ararauna*) with mild scissor beak whose defect is in the maxilla (a). A dorsal intraoral view shows the angular distortion of the rhinothecal occlusal edge that is already occurring, which will require corrective trimming as well (b). A K-wire was placed through the sinus and bent toward the rhamphotheca on the opposite the deviation. A rubber band was placed from a hook in the pin to the tip of the beak (c) and allowed to gradually correct the deviation (d). *Source:* Photos courtesy of Brian Speer.

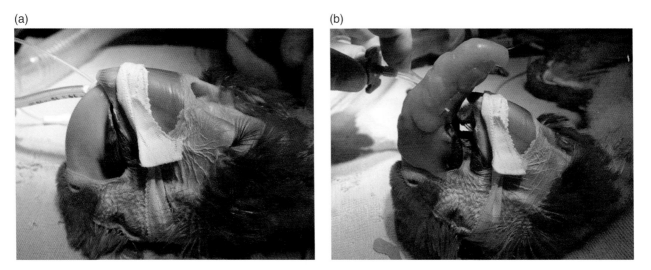

Figure 10.33 Subadult Scarlet macaw (*Ara macao*) with mandibular prognathism (a) corrected with rhinothecal acrylic ramp (b). *Source:* Photos courtesy of Brian Speer.

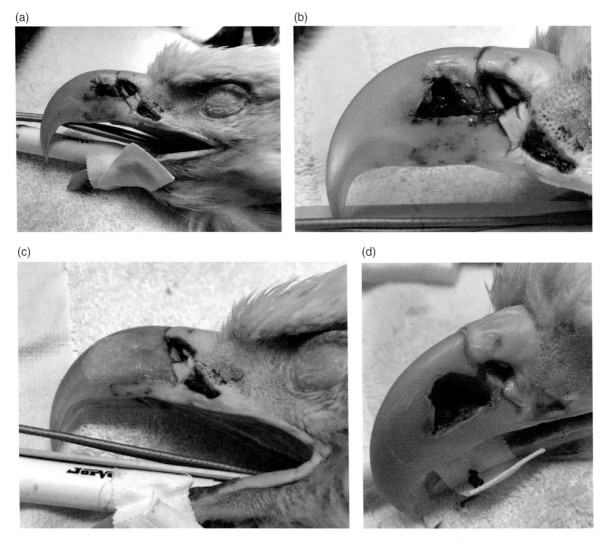

Figure 10.34 Left-sided traumatic beak injury in a bald eagle (*Haliaeetus leucocephalus*) (a) managed as an open wound. The wound was debrided under general anesthesia (b) and a patch of epoxy impregnated gauze was applied to protect the tissues (c). Initially the medial aspect of the right side of the beak across the rostral diverticulum of the infraorbital sinus could be visualized. Three weeks after presentation (d), there was healthy granulation tissue within the wound and the right side of the beak was no longer visible. After 8 weeks (e) epithelium was migrating from the periphery to cover the wound. By 12 weeks (f) the wound had nearly completely epithelialized so the patch was not replaced. (g) At 17 weeks the wound had completely healed, and the bird was released. *Source:* Images courtesy of PAWS Wildlife Center.

(e)

(f)

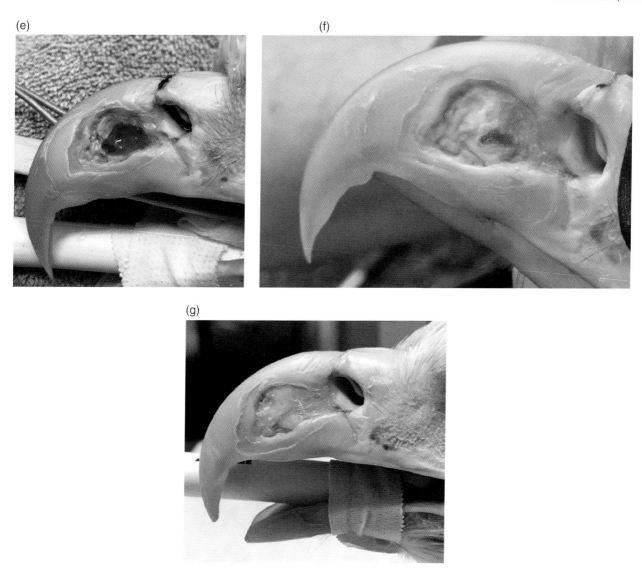

(g)

Figure 10.34 (Continued)

delayed healing. Use multiple layers of material to reinforce the cast, and bur to smooth out the final product covering the mouth to prevent aspiration or ingestion of the dust. Incorporate small wires or other materials into the cast to reinforce the mold, analogous to rebar. Suture overlying soft tissues or glue using cyanoacrylate. Wires and bone cement may still be inadequate to allow healing. The authors have had limited success in treating a mandibular symphyseal fracture ("split mandible") especially in small birds with thin beaks, though Lothamer has reported success using the described technique in two birds (Lothamer et al. 2014).

Employ ESF if a fracture is highly contaminated. Due to the thin bone in the beak, the holding power of pins is minimal. Insert positive profile threaded pins that traverse both sides except caudally, where the tongue will be impeded. Connect the pins with an acrylic bar and consider applying acrylic to the lingual surface of the beak to improve pin security. Feed the bird soft foods only or place an esophagostomy tube to provide food and water.

Finally, a fracture may be stabilized and then protected by bonding the upper and lower beaks with wire and acrylic or resin (Figure 10.36). This prevents the bird from using its beak to eat, bite, climb, etc., all of which can place a lot of force on the fracture allowing it to heal without such stresses. Place an esophageal tube prior to bonding.

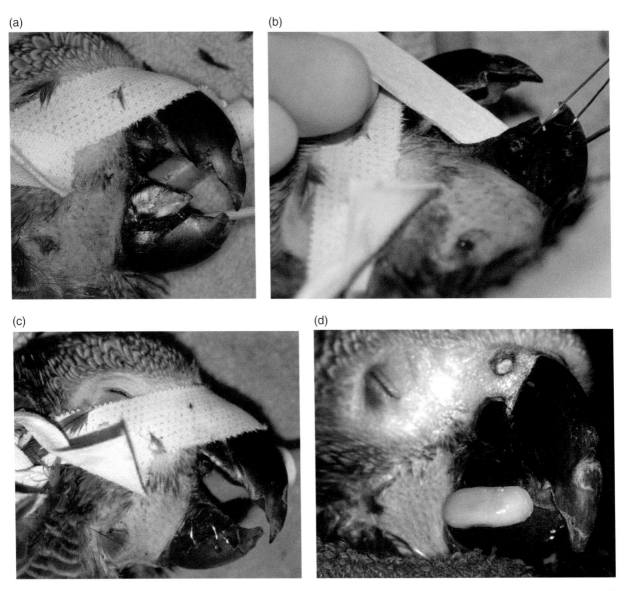

Figure 10.35 Photographs of a right-sided, minimally contaminated mandibular fracture in an African gray parrot (*Psittacus erithacus*) (a) stabilized with interfragmentary wires (b and c) and connected with acrylic (d).

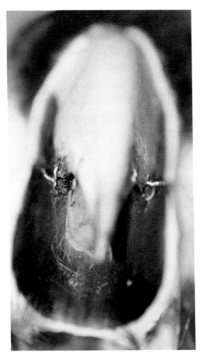

Figure 10.36 Photograph of a scarlet macaw (*Ara macao*) with the upper and lower beak wired together to maintain apposition and alignment preventing the bird from using the beak during healing. Nutrition was administered using an esophagostomy feeding tube.

References

Ackermann, J. and Redig, P. (1997). Surgical repair of elbow luxation in raptors. *Journal of Avian Medicine and Surgery* 11: 247–254.

Arens, S., Schlegel, U., Printzen, G. et al. (1996). Influence of materials for fixation implants on local infection. *Journal of Bone and Joint Surgery British Volume* 78: 647–651.

Azmanis, P.N., Wernick, M.B., and Hatt, J.M. (2014). Avian luxations: occurrence, diagnosis and treatment. *The Veterinary Quarterly* 34: 11–21.

Beaufrere, H., Ammersback, M., Nevarez, J. et al. (2012). Successful treatment of a radioulnar synostosis in a Mississippi kite (*Ictinia mississippiensis*). *Journal of Avian Medicine and Surgery* 26: 94–100.

Bennert, B.M., Kircher, P.R., Gutbrod, A. et al. (2016). Evaluation of two miniplate systems and figure-of-eight bandages for stabilization of experimentally induced ulnar and radial fractures in pigeons (*Columba livia*). *Journal of Avian Medicine and Surgery* 30: 111–121.

Bennett, R.A. and Kuzma, A.B. (1992). Fracture management in birds. *Journal of Zoo and Wildlife Medicine* 23: 5–38.

Biewener, A. and Dial, K. (1995). in vivo strain in the humerus of pigeons (*Columba livia*) during flight. *Journal of Morphology* 225: 61–75.

Bowles, H.L. and Zantop, D.W. (2002). A novel surgical technique for luxation repair of the femorotibial joint in a monk parakeet (*Myiopsitta monachus*). *Journal of Avian Medicine and Surgery* 16: 34–38.

Bueno, I., Redig, P.T., and Rendahl, A.K. (2015). External skeletal fixator intramedullary pin tie-in for the repair of tibiotarsal fractures in raptors: 37 cases (1995–2011). *Journal of the American Veterinary Medical Association* 247: 1154–1160.

Burgdorf-Moisuk, A., Whittington, J.K., Bennett, R.A. et al. (2011). Successful management of simple fractures of the femoral neck with femoral head and neck excision arthroplasty in two free-living avian species. *Journal of Avian Medicine and Surgery* 25: 210–215.

Calvo Carrasco, D., Dutton, T.A., Shimizu, N. et al. (2016). Distraction osteogenesis correction of mandibular ramis fracture malunion in a juvenile mute swan (*Cygnus olor*). *Journal of Avian Medicine and Surgery* 30: 30–38.

Chinnadurai, S.K., Spodnick, G., Degernes, L. et al. (2009). Use of an extracapsular stabilization technique to repair cruciate ligament ruptures in two avian species. *Journal of Avian Medicine and Surgery* 23: 307–313.

Christen, C., Fischer, I., Von Rechenberg, B. et al. (2005). Evaluation of a maxillofacial miniplate compact 1.0 for stabilization of the ulna in experimentally induced ulnar

and radial fractures in pigeons (*Columba livia*). *Journal of Avian Medicine and Surgery* 19: 185–190.

Clipsham, R. (1996). Beak repair, rhamphorthotics. In: *Avian Medicine and Surgery* (eds. R.B. Altman, S.L. Clubb, G.M. Dorrestein and K. Quesenberry), 773–786. Philadelphia, PA: W.B. Saunders.

Coles, B. (2007). Orthopedic surgery. In: *The Essentials of Avian Medicine and Surgery* (ed. B. Coles), 164–182. Ames, IA: Blackwell Publishing.

Comar, C. and Driggers, J.C. (1949). Secretion of radioactive calcium in the hen's egg. *Science (Washington)* 109: 282.

Darrow, B.G., Biskup, J.J., Weigel, J.P. et al. (2017). Ex-vivo biomechanical evaluation of pigeon (*Columba livia*) cadaver intact humeri and ostectomized humeri stabilized with caudally applied titanium locking plate or stainless-steel nonlocking plate constructs. *American Journal of Veterinary Research* 78: 570–578.

Darrow, B.G., Weigel, J.P., Greenacre, C.B. et al. (2019). ex vivo biomechanical comparison of titanium locking plate, stainless steel nonlocking plate, and tie-in external fixator applied by a dorsal approach on ostectomized humeri of pigeons (*Columba livia*). *Journal of Avian Medicine and Surgery* 30: 29–37.

Dumont, E.R. (2010). Bone density and the lightweight skeletons of birds. *Proceedings of the Royal Society of London B: Biological Sciences* https://doi.org/10.1098/rspb.2010.0117.

Gjeltema, J., De Voe, R.S., Minter, L.J., and Trumpatori, B.J. (2017). Intertarsal joint stabilization in a bateleur eagle (*Terathopius ecaudatus*) using a novel application of a braided suture and titanium button system. *Case Reports in Veterinary Medicine* 2017: 1–75.

Gonzalez, M.S. (2019). Avian articular orthopedics. *Veterinary Clinics: Exotic Animal Practice* 22: 239–251.

Griffon, D.J. (2005). Fracture healing. In: *AO Principles of Fracture Management in the Dog and Cat* (eds. A.L. Johnson, J.E. Houlton and R. Vannini), 73–98. New York, NY: Thieme.

Guerrero, T.G., Kalchofner, K., Scherrer, N., and Kircher, P. (2014). The advanced locking plate system (ALPS): a retrospective evaluation in 71 small animal patients. *Veterinary Surgery* 43: 127–135.

Gull, J.M., Saveraid, T.C., Szabo, D., and Hatt, J.M. (2012). Evaluation of three miniplate systems for fracture stabilization in pigeons (*Columba livia*). *Journal of Avian Medicine and Surgery* 26: 203–212.

Harris, M.C., Diaz-Figueroa, O., Lauer, S.K. et al. (2007). Complications associated with conjoined intramedullary pin placement for femorotibial joint luxation in a Solomon

Island eclectus parrot. *Journal of Avian Medicine and Surgery* 21: 299–306.

Hawkins, M.G., Barron, H.W., Speer, B.L. et al. (2013). Birds. In: *Exotic Animal Formulary*, 4e (ed. J.W. Carpenter), 183–437. St. Louis, MO: Elsevier.

Hollamby, S., Dejardin, L.M., Sikarskie, J.G., and Haeger, J. (2004). Tibiotarsal fracture repair in a bald eagle (*Haliaeetus leucocephalus*) using an interlocking nail. *Journal of Zoo and Wildlife Medicine* 35: 77–81.

Huynh, M., Gonzalez, M.S., and Beaufrere, H. (2019). Avian skull orthopedics. *Veterinary Clinics: Exotic Animal Practice* 22: 253–283.

Jaeger, G.H. and Wosar, M.A. (2018). External skeletal fixation. In: *Veterinary Surgery: Small Animal*, 2e (eds. S.A. Johnston and K.M. Tobias), 691–721. St. Louis, MO: Elsevier Health Sciences.

Jalila, A., Redig, P.T., Wallace, L.J. et al. (2004). The effect of chicken, pigeon, and turkey demineralized bone matrix (DBM) implanted in ulnar defects fixed with the intramedullary-external skeletal fixator (IM-ESF) tie-in in pigeons (*Columba livia*): histological evaluations. *Medical Journal of Malaysia* 59: 125–126.

Johnston, M.S., Thode, H.P. III, and Ehrhart, N.P. (2008). Bone transport osteogenesis for reconstruction of a bone defect in the tibiotarsus of a yellow-naped Amazon parrot (*Amazona ochrocephala auropalliata*). *Journal of Avian Medicine and Surgery* 22: 47–56.

Johnston, S.A., von Pfeil, D.J., Dejardin, L.M. et al. (2018). Internal fracture fixation. In: *Veterinary Surgery: Small Animal*, 2e (eds. S.A. Johnston and K.M. Tobias), 654–690. St. Louis, MO: Elsevier Health Sciences.

Kuzma, A.B. and Hunter, B. (1991). A new technique for avian fracture repair using intramedullary polymethyacrylate and bone plate fixation. *Journal of the American Animal Hospital Association* 27: 239–248.

Langley-Hobbs, S. and Friend, E. (2002). Interlocking nail repair of a fractured femur in a turkey. *Veterinary Record* 150: 247–248.

Lothamer, C., Snyder, C.J., Mans, C. et al. (2014). Treatment and stabilization of beak symphyseal separation using interfragmentary wiring and provisional bis-acryl composite. *Journal of Veterinary Dentistry* 31: 255–262.

Lumeij, J.T. (1994). Gastroenterology. In: *Avian Medicine: Principles and Application* (eds. B.W. Ritchie, G.J. Harrison and L.R. Harrison), 482–521. Lake Worth, FL: Winger's Pulbishing.

Maccoy, D.M. (1987). Techniques of fracture treatment and their indications: external and internal fixation. In: *Proceedings of 1st International Conference of Zoological and Avian Medicine*, Oahu, Hawaii, 549–562. Madison, WI: Omni Press.

Maccoy, D. and Haschek, W. (1988). Healing of transverse humeral fractures in pigeons treated with ethylene oxide-sterilized, dry-stored, onlay cortical xenografts and allografts. *American Journal of Veterinary Research* 49: 106–111.

Maccoy, D. and Redig, P. (1987). Surgical approaches to and repair of wing fractures. In: *Proceedings of 1st International Conference of Zoological and Avian Medicine*, Oahu, Hawaii, 564–577. Madison, WI: Omni Press.

Martin, H. and Ritchie, B.W. (1994). Orthopedic surgical techniques. In: *Avian Medicine: Principles and Application* (eds. B.W. Ritchie, G.J. Harrison and L.R. Harrison), 1137–1169. Lake Worth, FL: Winger's Publishing.

Martin, H.D., Kabler, R., and Sealing, L. (1994). The avian coxofemoral joint: a review of regional anatomy and report of an open-reduction technique for repair of a coxofemoral luxation. *Journal of the Association of Avian Veterinarians* 8: 164–172.

McRee, A.E., Tully, T.N. Jr., Nevarez, J.G. et al. (2017). A novel surgical approach to avian femorotibiotarsal luxation repair. *Journal of Avian Medicine and Surgery* 31: 156–164.

Meij, B.P., Hazewinkel, H.A., and Westerhof, I. (1996). Treatment of fractures and angular limb deformities of the tibiotarsus in birds by type II external skeletal fixation. *Journal of Avian Medicine and Surgery* 10: 153–162.

Montgomery, R.D., Crandall, E., and Bellah, J.R. (2011). Use of a locking compression plate as an external fixator for repair of a tarsometatarsal fracture in a bald eagle (*Haliaeetus leucocephalus*). *Journal of Avian Medicine and Surgery* 25: 119–125.

Mueller, W.J., Schraer, R., and Schraer, H. (1964). Calcium metabolism and skeletal dynamics of laying pullets. *Journal of Nutrition* 84: 20–26.

Newberry, R.C., Webster, A.B., Lewis, N.J., and Van Arnam, C. (1999). Management of spent hens. *Journal of Applied Animal Welfare Science* 2: 13–29.

Newton, C.D. and Zeitlin, S. (1977). Avian fracture healing. *Journal of the American Veterinary Medical Association* 170: 620–625.

Orosz, S.E., Haynes, P.K., and Carol, J. (eds.) (1992). *Avian Surgical Anatomy: Thoracic and Pelvic Limbs*. Philadelphia, PA: W.B. Saunders.

Ponder, J.B. (2012). Distraction osteogenesis in two wild raptor species. In: *33rd Proceedings of the Annual Conference of the Association of Avian Veterinarians*, Louisville, KY, 43–44. Red Hook, NJ: Curran Associates.

Ponder, J.B. and Redig, P. (2016). Orthopedics. In: *Current Therapy in Avian Medicine and Surgery* (ed. B.L. Speer), 657–667. St. Louis, MO: Elsevier Health Sciences.

Priyanka, S.S., Chaudhary, R., Niwas, R. et al. (2018). Surgical correction of perosis/slipped tendon in a white pekin duck – case report. *International Journal of Current Microbiology and Applied Sciences* 7: 389–392.

Redig, P. and Roush, J.C. (1987). Orthopedic and soft tissue surgery in raptorial species. In: *Zoo and Wild Animal Medicine* (ed. M. Fowler), 246–253. Philadelphia, PA: W.B. Saunders Co.

Rice, C.A., Riehl, J., Broman, K. et al. (2012). Comparing the degree of exothermic polymerization in commonly used acrylic and provisional composite resins for intraoral appliances. *Journal of Veterinary Dentistry* 29: 78–83.

Rosenthal, K., Hillyer, E., and Mathiessen, D. (1994). Stifle luxation repair in a moluccan cockatoo and a barn owl. *Journal of the Association of Avian Veterinarians* 6: 173–178.

Sample, S., Cole, G., Paul-Murphy, J. et al. (2008). Clinical use of recombinant human bone morphogenic protein-2 in a whooping crane (*Grus americana*). *Veterinary Surgery* 37: 552–557.

Sanaei, R., Abu, J., Nazari, M. et al. (2015). Evaluation of osteogenic potentials of avian demineralized bone matrix in the healing of osseous defects in pigeons. *Veterinary Surgery* 44: 603–612.

Scheelings, T.F. (2014). Coracoid fractures in wild birds: a comparison of surgical repair versus conservative treatment. *Journal of Avian Medince and Surgery* 28: 304–308.

Schwahn, D.J. and Rassette, M.S. (2013). Pathology in practice. *Journal of the American Veterinary Medical Association* 242: 1495–1497.

Souza, M.J., Fields, E.L., and Degernes, L.A. (2004). Thoracic and pelvic limb fracture and luxation management in raptors: a five-year retrospective study. *Journal of Wildlife Rehabilitation* 27: 5–13.

Tully, T.N. (2002). Basic avian bone growth and healing. *Veterinary Clinics of North America: Exotic Animal Practice* 5: 23–30.

Tunio, A., Jalila, A., Goh, Y.M. et al. (2015). Histologic evaluation of critical zize defect healing with natural and synthetic bone grafts in the pigeon (*Columba livia*) ulna. *Journal of Avian Medicine and Surgery* 29: 106–113.

Van Wettere, A.J. and Redig, P.T. (2004). Arthrodesis as a treatment for metacarpophalangeal joint luxation in 2 raptors. *Journal of Avian Medicine and Surgery* 18: 23–30.

Van Wettere, A.J., Redig, P.T., Wallace, L.J. et al. (2009). Mechanical evaluation of external skeletal fixator–intramedullary pin tie-in configurations applied to cadaveral humeri from red-tailed hawks (*Buteo jamaicensis*). *Journal of Avian Medicine and Surgery* 23: 277–285.

West, P.G., Rowland, G.R., Budsberg, S.C., and Aron, D.N. (1996). Histomorphometric and angiographic analysis of bone healing in the humerus of pigeons. *American Journal of Veterinary Research* 57: 1010–1015.

Zollinger, T.J., Backues, K.A., and Burgos-Rodriguez, A.G. (2005). Correction of angular limb deformity in two subspecies of flamingo (*Phoenicopterus Ruber*) utilizing a transphyseal bridging technique. *Journal of Zoo and Wildlife Medicine* 36: 689–697.

11

Approaches to the Caudal Coelom (Abdomen) of Birds

Michael B. Mison and R. Avery Bennett

Anatomy

Birds do not have a muscular diaphragm separating the caudal coelom and its viscera from the cranial coelom and the heart and lungs. Even in avian anatomy, the terminology used often refers to thoracic and abdominal cavities (i.e. thoracic and abdominal air sacs). This chapter describes approaches to the caudal coelom which is equivalent to the abdomen of mammals. The approaches to the cranial coelom are described in Chapter 14. Common approaches to the caudal coelom include the ventral midline approach, midline L approach, midline inverted L approach, midline Y approach, midline inverted T approach, and left or right lateral approaches (Bennett and Harrison 1994; Mison et al. 2016).

The abdominal wall muscles are similar to mammals, but avian species variation exists with regards to the extent of the midventral body wall musculature and the relative thickness (King and McLelland 1984). There is morphologic variation in sternum size among different species that influences access to the coelom (Berger 1956). The linea alba of birds is wide and thin. It is often transparent allowing visualization of internal organs. There is no falciform ligament or omentum in birds.

The intestinal peritoneal cavity is centrally located and contains the intestines and urogenital organs (McLelland 1990a). Its lateral boundary is the caudal thoracic and the abdominal air sac walls on each side. If these are not penetrated, there is no connection to the lungs and fluid irrigation can be safely performed; however, if the air sac walls are damaged, fluid irrigation can enter the lungs with potentially fatal consequences. The liver is not within the intestinal peritoneal cavity, but rather is within the hepatic peritoneal cavity. In order to access the liver, for example to obtain biopsies, the air sac wall surrounding the liver must be incised.

When performing a lateral approach, after incising the body wall, the subpulmonary cavity will be entered. The caudal thoracic air sac wall can be incised to enter the intestinal peritoneal cavity. To reach the reproductive tract, the abdominal air sac wall must also be incised. Fluid irrigation should not be performed using any lateral approach to the caudal coelom as fluid will enter the lung.

Avian skin and subcutaneous tissues differ from those of mammals. In birds, the epidermis is very thin and is diffusely supplied by capillaries in the dermis (Strettenheim 1972). The dermis is firmly attached to the underlying muscle fascia, and there is very little subcutaneous tissue present. Additionally, these tissues are not very elastic.

Patient Preparation

There are many surgical procedures that require an open celiotomy such as surgery of the gastrointestinal, reproductive, and urinary tract, and surgery of the cloaca as well as for obtaining biopsies.

Place the patient in lateral or dorsal recumbency depending on the planned approach. Historically, clear plastic drapes have been recommended for avian celiotomy allowing the anesthetist to be able to visualize the patient in order to monitor thoracic expansion during respiration. Currently, respiratory monitoring using end tidal CO_2 is recommended and does not require being able to actually watch respiratory movements. The anesthetist must be aware that once an air sac is open there will be little resistance to ventilation, and there will be no thoracic expansion with manual ventilation. Once the body wall has been closed, normal resistance and chest expansion will resume.

Create an appropriate sterile field by placing quarter drapes and a patient drape sheet in a standard manner. If a

Surgery of Exotic Animals, First Edition. Edited by R. Avery Bennett and Geoffrey W. Pye.
© 2022 John Wiley & Sons, Inc. Published 2022 by John Wiley & Sons, Inc.

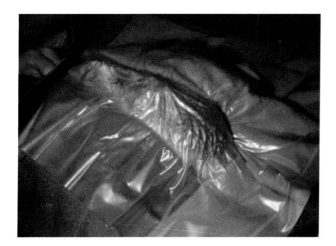

Figure 11.1 A chicken prepared for aseptic surgery. Huck towels have been placed as quarter drapes to isolate the surgical field. A clear plastic drape has been placed over the field and the towels. A large drape sheet will be placed over the plastic drape to create a sterile field of the entire table. A fenestration will be cut in the sheet drape large enough to allow visualization of the patient through the plastic drape.

small clear plastic drape is used, place the quarter drapes around the patient isolating the body but covering the wings and legs allowing visualization of respiratory efforts, and then place the clear plastic drape on top of the quarter drapes (Figure 11.1). Place a patient drape sheet over the plastic drape and cut a fenestration large enough to allow visualization of respiratory movements in order to create a sterile field of the entire table.

A celiotomy can be accomplished using a ventral (midline, transverse, or flap) approach or a lateral (left or right) approach. Use the appropriate approach based on what access is needed. Surgeon's preference and individual bird anatomy and size also determine which approach to use. Note that for a left-handed surgeon, it is difficult to accomplish tasks in the cranial coelom using a left lateral celiotomy because structures such as the ovary are under the ribs. It is difficult to use forceps to reach into the body cavity and under the ribs to manipulate organs. For a right-handed surgeon, a right lateral celiotomy may be difficult for the same reasons. This problem is lessened if the surgeon is on the dorsal side of the patient (legs pointing away from the surgeon), rather than the ventral side.

Skin Incision

In preparation for surgery, pluck body feathers in the direction of their growth. Avoid removing flight feathers, as they are difficult and painful to remove. Take care to avoid tearing the skin while the feathers are being plucked by holding the skin close to the body with the nondominant

hand, pulling them out with the dominant hand. Make skin incisions in the featherless tracts (apterylae) if possible because they have a stronger mesh of collagen fibers.

Bipolar electrosurgery is ideal for skin and abdominal wall incisions to provide hemostasis. It is easier to incise the skin if one arm of the bipolar forceps is bent 45° (Harrison tip bipolar forceps, Ellman International, Inc., Hickville, NY) (Figure 11.2). This modification was developed by Dr. Greg Harrison especially for cutting avian skin. With the bent tip, the current is concentrated into the small point of tip-to-tip contact making it easier to cut the skin with less lateral heat damage. A standard tip can be used but the area of tip-to-tip contact is larger, so the current is spread out decreasing the power creating more lateral heat and making it more difficult to cut the skin. To incise the skin, tent it with atraumatic forceps in the nondominant hand and apply the bipolar forceps to the tented skin with the dominant hand. Activate the current to create a small full thickness defect in the skin (Figure 11.3). Extend the incision by inserting one arm of the bipolar forceps (the straight arm of the Harrison tip bipolar forceps) subcutaneously to the level of the insulation and the other limb (with the bent tip) outside the skin. Lightly oppose the tips, activate the current, and withdraw the forceps with the current on to cut the skin. Repeat this process until the necessary skin incision is complete. If it is not cutting well, oppose the tips looser, which is contrary to the natural response. If they are compressed harder, the gap between the tips is smaller and the current passes from tip to tip without causing change in the tissue. A scalpel can also be used but will not control hemorrhage from dermal vessels.

Once the skin incision has been made, create an incision in the body wall using the bipolar forceps as well. Birds have little subcutaneous tissue that is easily broken down with a moist cotton-tipped applicator. Next, grasp the muscle of the body wall in the bipolar forceps and activate the current, then withdraw the forceps to create a defect in the body wall. Insert one arm of the forceps into the coelom to

(a)

(b)

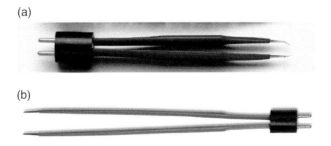

Figure 11.2 The Harrison tip bipolar forceps (a) has a 45° bend on one limb creating a pinpoint focus where the current passes between the tips cutting skin with minimal lateral heat damage compared with the Adson tip forceps (b).

(a)

(b)

(c)

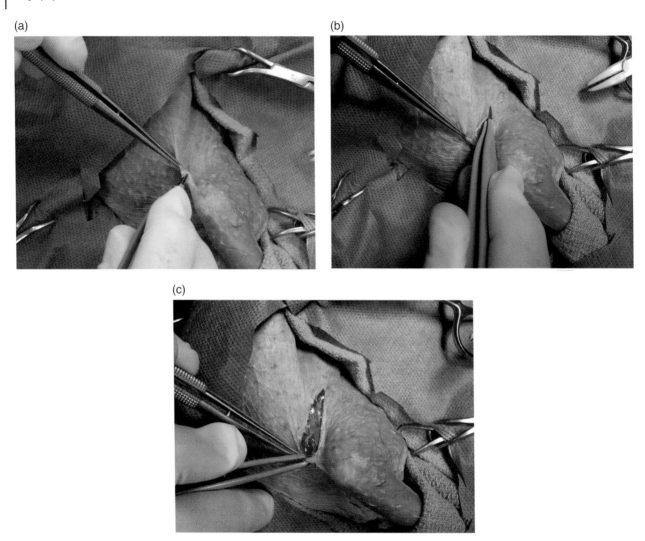

Figure 11.3 To incise avian skin with bipolar forceps, tent the skin with forceps held in the nondominant hand and apply the bipolar forceps with the dominant hand, and then activate the current to create a small nick in the skin (a). Insert the straight arm of the Harrison tip forceps under the skin to the level of the blue insulation (b). Activate the current and withdraw the forceps with the current active to make a linear skin incision with minimal hemorrhage (c).

the level of the insulation on the forceps being careful not to damage internal organs, lightly oppose the tips and withdraw as previously described. Continue this process until the celiotomy incision is the desired length and location.

Left Lateral Celiotomy

A left lateral approach provides access to the majority of abdominal organs including the proventriculus, ventriculus, spleen, colon, heart apex, left liver lobe, left lung, left kidney, left ureter, and left male and female reproductive tracts (Figure 11.4). It does not provide good exposure to the pancreas, duodenum, right liver lobe, right lung, right kidney, and right ureter; however, the right testicle can be

accessed with additional dissection. If access to the right side is needed, consider performing a right lateral celiotomy. The lateral approach often provides the best exposure; however, it is a large approach and often both the caudal thoracic and the abdominal air sacs are entered. Nonetheless, the approach is well tolerated by birds and recovery is rapid. Occasionally, a bird will be lame on the retracted leg for a day or two after surgery, but the lameness resolves quickly with anti-inflammatory medications.

Position the bird in right lateral recumbency with the left leg retracted caudally and externally rotated to expose the left body wall (Figure 11.5). Pull both wings dorsally and secure them to the table with tape in a manner analogous to that used for positioning for a lateral radiograph. Pull the right leg perpendicular to the long axis of the body and secure it to the table. Use a tape stirrup around the left

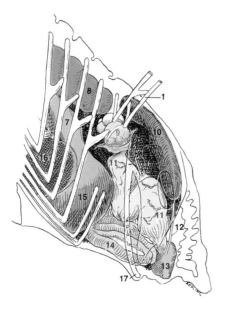

Figure 11.4 A left lateral celiotomy provides exposure to much of the viscera including proventriculus (7), ventriculus (15), spleen, colon, heart apex, left liver lobe (16), left lung (8), left kidney (10), left ureter (12), and left male and female (9) reproductive tracts. *Source*: Bennett and Harrison (1994).

(a)

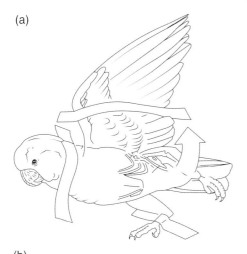

(b)

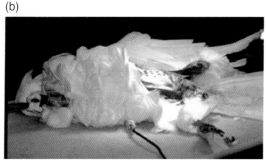

Figure 11.5 Position for left lateral celiotomy (drawing) (a) and an umbrella cockatoo (b). Position both wings dorsally and secure them to the table with tape. Pull the right leg perpendicular to the spine and secure it to the table. Place a tape stirrup around the left tarsometatarsus and retract it caudally and externally rotated. Secure the tape to the table. *Source*: Bennett and Harrison (1994).

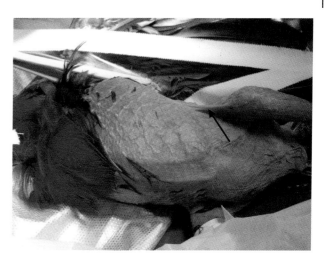

Figure 11.6 When positioned for a lateral celiotomy a fold of skin is created from the stifle to the pectoral muscles called the "knee web" (arrow).

tarsometatarsus to pull the leg caudally and externally rotated and secure it to the table. It is ideal to have an assistant to help retract the leg intraoperatively as the approach progresses. Alternatively, the tape can be secured to the table allowing a nonsterile assistant to reposition the tape and leg from under the drape as needed during the procedure. Pulling the left leg caudally and externally rotated creates a fold of skin from the stifle to the sternum ("knee web") (Figure 11.6).

Palpate the caudal few ribs in a triangle formed by the epaxial muscles dorsally, the pectoral muscle cranioventrally, and the cranial muscles of the thigh caudally. Initiate the incision in the knee web using bipolar forceps as described above. After making a nick incision, insert one limb of the bipolar forceps subcutaneously dorsocranially toward the triangle where the ribs can be palpated and extend skin the incision toward the ribs (Figure 11.3). After making this half of the incision, extend and externally rotate the leg farther using an assistant or by repositioning the tape holding the left leg. Continue the skin incision from the fold of skin to the pubis paramedian approximately midway between the coxofemoral joint and ventral midline. Make the skin incision from the cranial border of the pubis cranially to expose the most caudal three ribs. There is variation in the distance from the last rib to the cranial aspect of the thigh. For example, in cockatoos, there is more space than in macaws. Gently break down the minimal subcutaneous tissue with a cotton tipped applicator exposing the last few ribs and the left lateral body wall (Figure 11.7). Visualize the dorsal termination of the external oblique muscle which is a few millimeters dorsal to the junction of the sternal and vertebral portions of the last rib (i.e. the sharp bend in the ribs). This will also

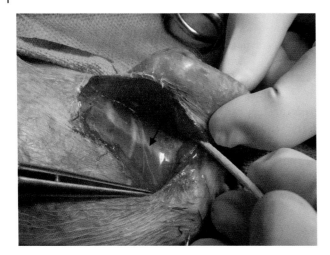

Figure 11.7 After making the skin incision for a left lateral celiotomy identify the dorsal border of the external abdominal oblique muscle (arrow) which is where the body wall incision will be made. Also visible are the last three ribs.

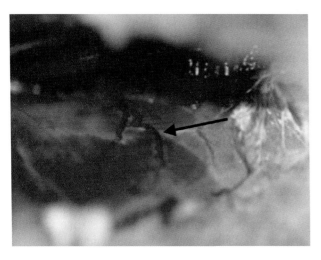

Figure 11.8 Superficial branches of the femoral artery and vein need to be ligated before transection to minimize hemorrhage.

expose the superficial branch of the femoral artery and vein coursing from the area of the coxofemoral joint toward ventral midline (Figure 11.8). These appear to be small vessels but if transected they bleed and can be difficult to control. Coagulate, ligate, or clip these vessels before incising the abdominal musculature.

The intercostal arteries and veins in birds run along the cranial aspect of the intercostal space (McLelland 1990b). Insert one limb of the bipolar forceps under the last rib just dorsal to the junction between the sternal and vertebral portions and advance it to the caudal aspect of the next to the last rib (Figure 11.9). Oppose the tips and activate the current to coagulate the intercostal vessels, and then withdraw with the current activated along the caudal aspect of the last rib as well. This will also create a defect in the muscle cau-

dal to the last rib. Using this bipolar dissection technique will protect underlying structures from an iatrogenic incision. In some birds, it is necessary to cut three ribs to obtain access to the cranial aspect of the reproductive tract and proventriculus. If needed, repeat the process to coagulate the intercostal vessels along the caudal aspect of the next rib cranially. Use heavy scissors to cut the last two or three ribs where the tissue has been coagulated just dorsal to the junction of the sternal and vertebral ribs. Using the opening in the muscle of the body wall just caudal to the last rib, direct the bipolar forceps caudally paramedian toward the pubic bone and extend the incision in the body wall to the cranial aspect of the pubic bone. Place a Heiss or Lone Star retractor between the cut ends of the ribs and evaluate the cranial exposure as well as the location of the caudal aspect of the left lung. If needed, coagulate the intercostal vessels and transect the next cranial rib to increase cranial exposure. It is usually not feasible to transect more than three ribs without cutting into pulmonary tissue. Maintain the retractor to separate the ribs; however, generally body wall muscle contraction provides adequate exposure caudally (Figure 11.10).

After opening the coelom and entering the subpulmonary cavity, visualize the caudal thoracic and abdominal air sac walls. Incise these air sac walls to access the gonad(s) and proventriculus. During the procedure, it is very important to keep the muscles moist. If they desiccate, it will be much more difficult to oppose them during closure. Also take care to not tear the muscles with the retractors.

Once the procedure is complete, release the left leg to help achieve closure. Close the coelomic cavity by apposing the abdominal and intercostal muscles using an appropriately sized slowly absorbed synthetic monofilament suture in a simple continuous pattern (Figure 11.11). The cut ends of the ribs do not need to be united and the air sac walls do not need to be closed. The anesthesiologist can ventilate the patient prior to skin closure to ensure there is no air leakage through the body wall. Close the skin in a Ford interlocking, simple continuous, or simple interrupted pattern. If it is not possible to achieve an airtight body wall closure leave a gap in the skin to prevent the development of subcutaneous emphysema.

Right Lateral Celiotomy

A right lateral celiotomy provides good exposure to the duodenum, pancreas, heart apex, and right hepatic lobe, lung, kidney, ureter, and right male and female (if present) reproductive tracts. It is uncommon to perform this approach, but it mirrors the left lateral celiotomy described above. For a left-handed surgeon, it is much easier to castrate a bird using a right lateral approach than a left.

(a)

(b)

(c)

(d)

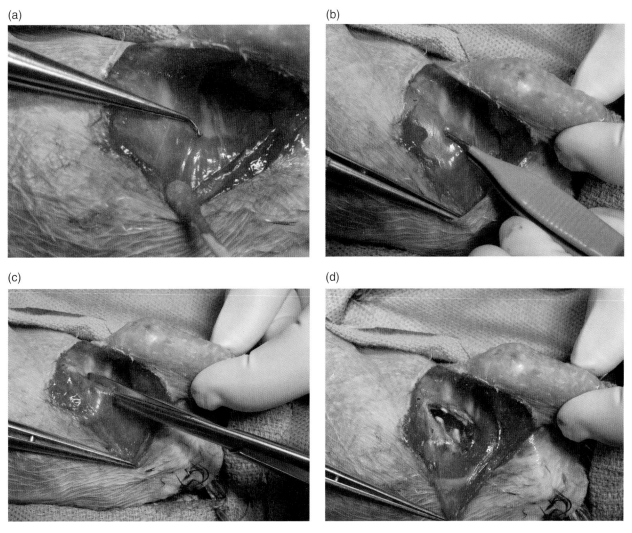

Figure 11.9 Make the incision in the body wall beginning at the last rib. The tips of the forceps are at the eighth rib and the dorsal margin of the external abdominal oblique muscle (a). Insert one limb of the bipolar forceps under the rib and advance it to the caudal aspect of the seventh rib (b). Oppose the tips, active the current, and withdraw the tips to coagulate the intercostal vessels caudal to the seventh and eighth ribs. Use heavy scissors to cut the seventh and eighth ribs where the vessels have been coagulated (c). This will create an opening into the coelom (d).

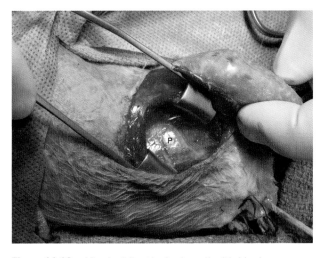

Figure 11.10 After incising the body wall with bipolar electrosurgery a self-retaining retractor has been placed between the cut ribs exposing the caudal thoracic and the abdominal air sac walls. The proventriculus is also visible (P).

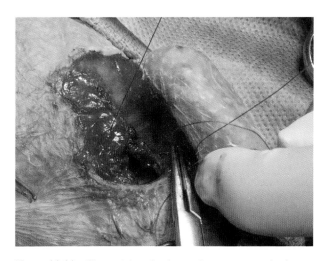

Figure 11.11 Close with a simple continuous pattern in the intercostal and abdominal muscles after releasing the left leg.

(a)

(b)

(c)

(d)

(e)

(f)

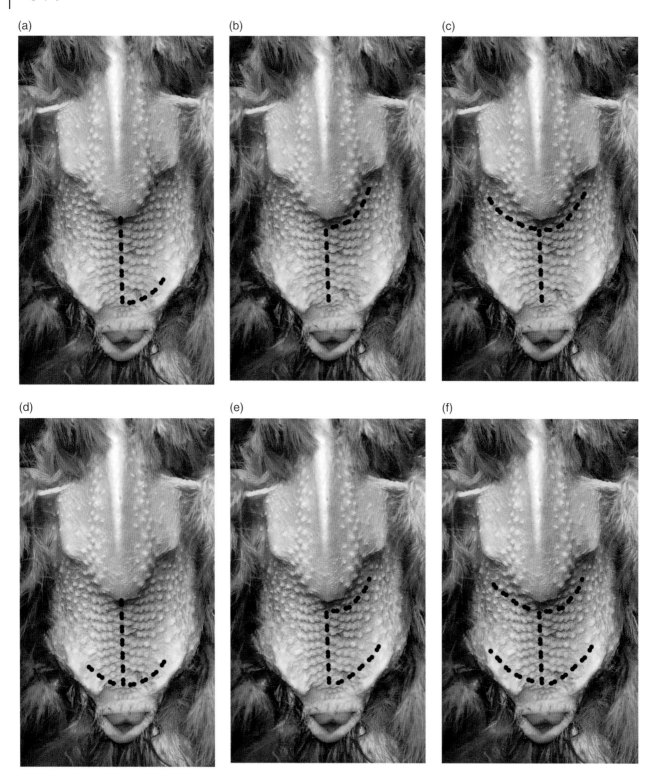

Figure 11.12 A ventral midline celiotomy enters the intestinal peritoneal cavity. Additional exposure can be achieved by making incisions parasternal and/or parapubic to create an L flap (parapubic on one side) (a), an inverted L flap (parasternal on one side) (b), a Y flap (bilateral parasternal incisions) (c) or an inverted T flap (bilateral parapubic) (d), a single French door (parasternal and ispsilateral parapubic) (e), and double French doors (bilateral parasternal and parapubic) (f).

Ventral Celiotomy

A ventral midline celiotomy exposes the intestinal peritoneal cavity. Use this approach for surgical access to the liver, small and large intestines, pancreas, kidneys, ureters, cloaca, and oviduct. To access the liver, the wall of the hepatic peritoneal cavity covering the liver must be incised. Position the patient as for a ventrodorsal radiograph. Place the patient in dorsal recumbency and pull the legs caudally, then secure them in place. Place the wings open on each side and secure them to the table with tape.

Make a ventral midline skin incision using bipolar electrosurgery if it is available. Tent the linea alba to hold it away from underlying viscera, incise the body wall, and extend the incision cranially to the caudal edge of the sternum and caudally to the interpubic space. This can be done with bipolar electrosurgery or small Metzenbaum or microsurgical scissors. Be careful not to damage underlying structures or structures adhered to the inside of the body wall. This will provide access to the intestinal peritoneal cavity and will not enter or damage an air sac wall.

If additional exposure is needed, especially laterally, extend the incision parasternal and/or parapubic to create a flap(s). Make a transverse incision along the caudal edge of the sternum and/or along the cranial edge of the pubis 2 mm or more from the bone leaving an edge to which to suture to for closure. This can be done bilaterally if needed. These incisions effectively create an L, inverted L, Y, inverted T, or French doors pattern (Figure 11.12). When entering the coelomic cavity, avoid traumatizing the duodenal loop and the pancreas that lie ventrally along the midline of the caudal coelom (Figure 11.13). Be especially careful entering the coelom if there is evidence or history of coelomitis which makes visualization of abdominal structures difficult. Additionally, adhesions between the peritoneum and intestine can be present making accidental enterotomy a concern. Increasing the inspired anesthetic gas concentration and manual ventilation are often necessary to maintain the needed depth of anesthesia when multiple air sacs are open. If a large portion of the caudal coelom is open (French doors), it will affect ventilation and depth of anesthesia. It may be necessary to intermittently hold the body wall closed to allow the anesthetist to ventilate the patient several times to provide adequate oxygen and anesthetic gas to the lungs.

Close the body wall in a simple continuous, simple interrupted or cruciate pattern using appropriately sized slowly absorbed synthetic monofilament suture on a taper needle. If a flap approach has been used, place a suture at the apex of the angle of the flap first. This will keep the body wall in proper orientation during closure. Then close the two limbs of the flap incision. Close the

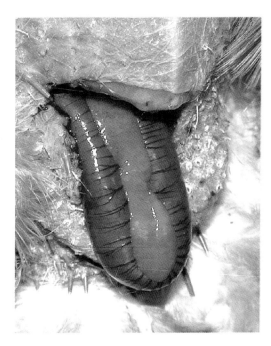

Figure 11.13 Immediately inside the ventral coelomic wall is the duodenal loop and pancreas visible through this transverse abdominal approach.

skin in a simple interrupted, simple continuous, or Ford interlocking pattern.

Transverse Celiotomy

A transverse approach to the coelom provides improved exposure to the lateral aspects of the caudal coelomic cavity. The ventriculus and small intestine are most accessible using this approach. It also provides good access to the site for ventriculotomy to the left of midline. The right liver lobe is larger than the left, but generally the liver can be accessed using a transverse celiotomy only if there is hepatomegaly. Retracting the viscera provides access to the middle and caudal portions of the kidneys as well as the caudal reproductive tract and the cranial aspect of the cloaca.

Place the bird in dorsal recumbency as previously described. Make a transverse incision midway between the caudal extent of the sternum and the vent. The duodenal loop and pancreas lie immediately under the body wall as it is with a ventral midline celiotomy (Figure 11.13). The viscera may be reflected to expose the middle and caudal lobes of the kidneys, the cranial cloaca, and the caudal reproductive tract.

Close the body wall incision using a simple continuous or simple interrupted pattern with a slowly absorbed suture material. Close the skin in a simple interrupted, simple continuous, or Ford interlocking pattern.

References

Bennett, R.A. and Harrison, G.J. (1994). Soft tissue surgery. In: *Avian Medicine: Principles and Application*, 1e (eds. B.W. Ritchie, G.J. Harrison and L.R. Harrison), 1096–1121. Lake Worth, FL: Wingers Publishing, Inc.

Berger, A.J. (1956). Anatomical variation and avian anatomy. *The Condor: Ornithological Applications* 58: 433–441.

King, A.S. and McLelland, J. (1984). Skeletomuscular system. In: *Birds: Their Structure and Function*, 1e, vol. 106 (eds. A.S. King and J. McLelland), 43–49. Philadelphia, PA: Bailliere Tindall.

McLelland, J. (1990a). Peritoneum and peritoneal cavities. In: *A Color Atlas of Avian Anatomy* (ed. J. McLelland), 85–88. London: Wolfe Publishing Ltd.

McLelland, J. (1990b). Respiratory system. In: *A Color Atlas of Avian Anatomy*, 95–119. London: Wolfe Publishing Ltd.

Mison, M., Mehler, S., Echols, M.S. et al. (2016). Approaches to the coelom and selected procedures. In: *Current Therapy in Avian Medicine and Surgery*, 1e (ed. B. Speer), 638–645. St. Louis, MO: Elsevier.

Strettenheim, P. (1972). The integument of birds. In: *Avian Biology*, vol. II (eds. D.S. Farmer and J.R. King), 7. New York/London: Academia Press.

12

Avian Reproductive Procedures
Stephen J. Mehler and R. Avery Bennett

Conditions of the avian reproductive system are some of the most common indications for intracoelomic surgical intervention. Dystocia and egg-related disorders are common in companion birds. Testicular tumors occur with some frequency in birds and vasectomy for prevention of reproduction has been shown to be effective.

The Male Reproductive Tract

The intracoelomic reproductive anatomy of male birds includes the testes, epididymis, and ductus deferens (King and McLelland 1984). Birds have paired testes suspended within the coelom by the mesorchium and are located ventral to the left and right cranial renal division (Figure 12.1). The right testis is slightly cranial to the left. The testes are relatively small in young birds and increase in size in maturity and during the breeding season. The color of the testes (white to yellowish or black) is dependent on the age of the bird and the species. The epididymis is located at the dorsomedial aspect of the testis with the ductus deferens continuing from the epididymis, parallel to the ureters, and terminating at the ureteral ostium in the urodeum. The testicular artery arises from the cranial renal artery and the venous blood returns directly to the caudal vena cava in most birds (Figure 12.2). It is likely that there are many anatomic variations in the vascular supply to the testes. Some species of birds including waterfowl and ratites have a phallus within the cloaca that is not a part of the urinary tract.

Orchidectomy

Orchidectomy in companion bird species is uncommonly performed, but indications include treatment for excessive masturbation, aggression, testicular neoplasia, and orchitis

(Joyner 1994; Speer 1997, 2016; Jenkins 2000). The efficacy of orchidectomy alone on decreasing or abolishing undesirable male sexual behavior is controversial (Mison et al. 2016).

The surgical approach for orchidectomy is either a left lateral approach or ventral midline with transverse parasternal and, if needed, parapubic incisions to create flaps (see Chapter 11). In most cases, the authors prefer the left lateral approach. An air sac separating the right and left testes will have to be incised when approaching the right testicle through a left lateral approach. With gentle traction, pull the left testis ventrally and apply, from the caudal aspect cranially, at least one hemostatic clip dorsal to the testis to control hemorrhage from the testicular blood supply, as close to the vena cava and common iliac vein as possible (Figures 12.3 and 12.4). If the testes are small, it may be possible to remove them with one clip each. Usually, more than one clip is needed to control all of the vessels. After placing the first clip at the caudal pole of the testis, lift the testis and incise distal to and along the clip. Back bleeding from the testis is insignificant. With the caudal pole of the testis elevated, place another clip cranial to the first clip, and then incise along that clip. Repeat this procedure until the entire testis has been removed. Larger clips can also be used but can be difficult to place in the tight space. A right-angled clip applier is ideal for orchidectomy (Figure 12.3a). Identify the right testis through the air sac and incise the air sac. Remove the right testis in a similar manner to the left. Bipolar electrosurgery is preferred over microsurgical scissors to free the testes from the mesorchium. The most common complications of orchidectomy include acute profound life-threatening hemorrhage and incomplete removal of testicular tissue. Bipolar electrosurgery can be used to fulgurate any residual testicular tissue if noted. A vessel sealing device may be useful for castration in birds as well but has not been evaluated.

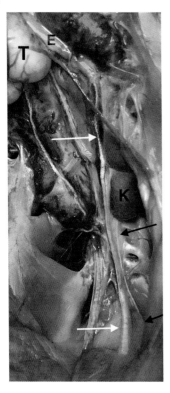

Figure 12.1 Male chicken left reproductive anatomy. Testis (T), epididymis (E), and caudal division of the kidney (K). The ductus deferens is the convoluted line (white arrows) and the fine white line (black arrows) is the urates within the ureter.

Vasectomy

Vasectomy methods are described primarily for population control and scientific research (Samour 2010). It is easier to perform than orchidectomy with fewer complications; however, male birds will retain their secondary sex characteristics, courtship, copulation, and intact male behaviors. Vasectomy can be performed through a craniolateral celiotomy as if approaching the kidney and can be accomplished through a unilateral or bilateral approach. Perform a left craniolateral approach to the coelom and identify the testis and incise the caudal thoracic and abdominal air sacs. The epididymis is dorsal to the testis and can be manipulated to provide access to the ductus deferens as it exits the epididymis. The ureter exits the caudal division of the kidney caudal to this location, so it is relatively safe to grasp the ductus in this location. Be careful not to damage the underlying common iliac vein. Grasp the ductus with thumb or biopsy forceps and pull it off the epididymis. If it does not tear easily, it can be cut being careful not to damage other structures. Remove about 15–10 mm of the ductus. It is not necessary to ligate or clip the severed ends of the ductus deferens. This procedure can also be done with a vessel sealing device. Remove a significant portion of the duct to minimize the

risk of recanalization. Often, both ducti can be accessed through a left lateral approach, but occasionally a right lateral approach is needed to access the right ductus deferens. A ventral midline approach provides access to both ducti as they enter the cloaca where the ductus and ureter diverge before entering into the cloaca separately. Take great care to identify and isolate the highly convoluted ductus deferens separate from the smooth ureter cranial to the cloaca. Usually, pulses of urates can be seen moving in the ureter. The ductus is farthest from the ureter as it exits the epididymis because the ureter does not emerge until the caudal division of the kidney and near the cloaca where they separate again prior to entering the cloaca (Figure 12.5).

Vasectomy can also be accomplished using minimally invasive techniques via the approach used to access the kidneys. Use a 2.7 mm endoscope and operating sheath with biopsy forceps (Karl Storz Veterinary Endoscopy, Inc., Goleta, CA). Grasp the ductus deferens as it exits the epididymis and tear it from the epididymis. Remove 5–10 mm of the ductus by withdrawing the scope/cannula along with the ductus. It is not necessary to ligate or clip the severed ends of the ductus.

Vasectomized birds will still be able to fertilize eggs until any sperm stored in the ductus are no long viable. Reported complications of open vasectomy procedures include recanalization where the cut ends of the ductus heal together and reform a lumen leading to return of fertility and inadvertent laceration of the underlying common iliac vein or the adjacent ureter (Samour 2010).

The Female Reproductive Tract

The anatomy of the female reproductive tract is consistent across the majority of bird species. Right and left ovaries and oviducts are present in the embryologic stages of all birds, but the right regresses leaving only a functional left side in most birds (King and McLelland 1984). Two fully developed ovaries are known to occur in some birds of prey and the brown kiwi (*Apteryx mantelli*). The ovary is attached to the cranial renal division and dorsal body wall by the mesovarian ligament (Figure 12.6). The blood supply to the ovary comes from the ovarian artery, which originates from the left cranial renal artery, or, in rare cases, comes directly off the aorta. Cranial and caudal ovarian veins empty directly into the vena cava in most birds; however, multiple left ovarian veins may drain into the cranial oviductal vein, which then enters the common iliac vein and finally the caudal vena cava. In adult birds, there is rarely a single ovarian artery and vein to ligate. The oviduct is suspended within the coelomic cavity by dorsal and ventral suspensory

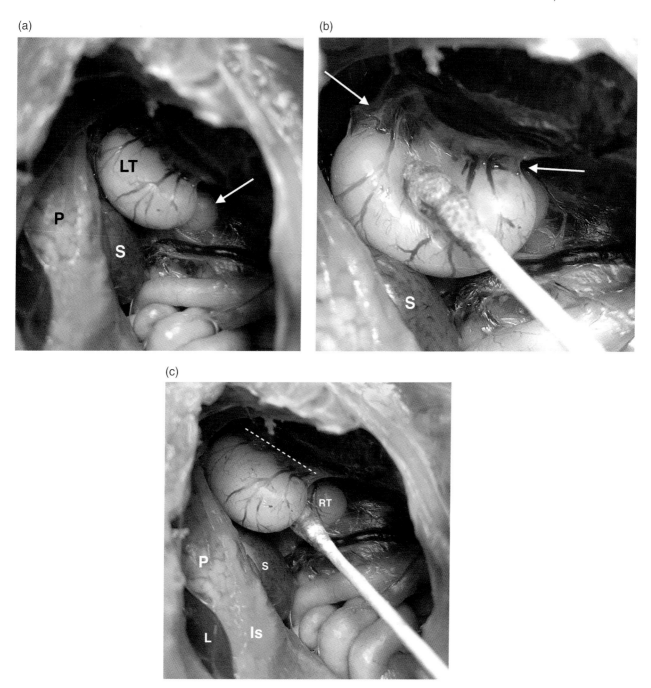

Figure 12.2 Intraoperative view of castration in a rooster. The left testis (LT) is encountered first and the right testicle (arrow) is deeper (a). They are separated by an air sac wall. The proventriculus (P) and spleen are also visible (S). The mesorchium is short and wide (white arrows) (b). Elevate the caudal pole of the kidney (c) and apply clips along the mesorchium (dotted line) from caudal to cranial, one by one until the entire mesorchium has been transected. Right testicle (RT), left liver lobe (L), and isthmus (Is) are also visible.

ligaments and is supplied by numerous arteries. The cranial oviductal artery originates from the left cranial renal artery, supplying the infundibulum and magnum. The accessory cranial oviductal artery arises from the left external iliac artery and supplies the magnum. The middle oviductal artery arises from the left ischiatic artery and supplies the magnum and uterus. The caudal oviductal artery arises from the pudendal branch of the internal iliac artery and supplies the uterus. The vaginal artery also arises from the pudendal artery. The common iliac vein drains the cranial parts of the oviduct, and the internal iliac vein drains the caudal portions of the oviduct and the cloaca.

The ovary is located along the ventral aspect of the left kidney and is tightly adhered by a short mesovarium to the

(a)
(b)
(c)

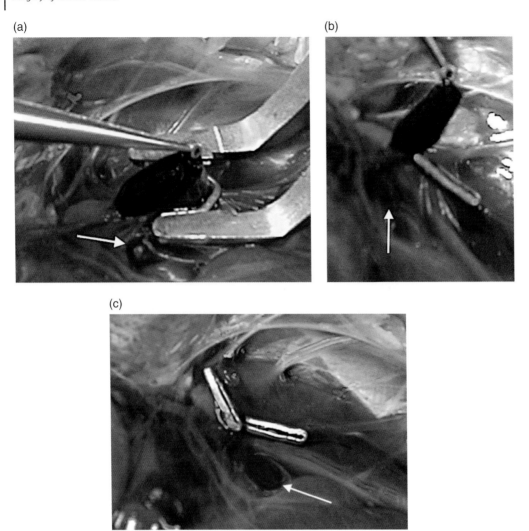

Figure 12.3 Cadaver dissection demonstrating how to perform orchidectomy in a juvenile raptor. Elevate the caudal pole of the testis and apply a clip between the testis and the common iliac vein (a). A right-angled applier makes this easier. Use bipolar electrosurgery or microscissors to transect along the clip (b). The right testis is visible deep to the air sac. Two clips were required to remove the left testis completely (c).

caudal vena cava, left common iliac vein, and cranial segment of the left kidney making dissection and complete surgical removal difficult (Figure 12.7). The ovary is triangular in shape with the base of the triangle cranial and the apex directed caudally along the common iliac vein. The mesovarium is broad and short, with little working space between the wide based ovary and caudal vena cava, left common iliac vein, and cranial portion of the left kidney (Figure 12.6). Efforts to lift the ovary and occlude the ovarian vessels typically result in iatrogenic damage to the left common iliac vein, the renal veins, or the caudal vena cava resulting in severe hemorrhage. It has been suggested that in juvenile birds, the mesovarium is looser, and the vessels not as well developed making ovariectomy potentially easier (Figure 12.8). The kidney and ovary are under the ribs limiting visualization and working space.

Because the right mesonephric duct may persist in many normal adult females, cystic right oviducts are not uncommon (Nemetz 2010). These cystic structures can be a benign and incidental findings or can become large enough that they interfere with other body systems and require surgical removal.

Surgery of the Ovary

Indications for ovariectomy include ovarian neoplasia, cystic disease, oophoritis, and any ovarian disease that cannot be successfully medically managed. Clinical signs of ovarian disease are nonspecific and include coelomic swelling, dyspnea, coelomic effusion, poor or altered reproductive performance, and lethargy (King and McLelland 1984; Speer 1997; Jenkins 2000; Johnson 2000; Mison et al. 2016).

(a)

(b)

(c)

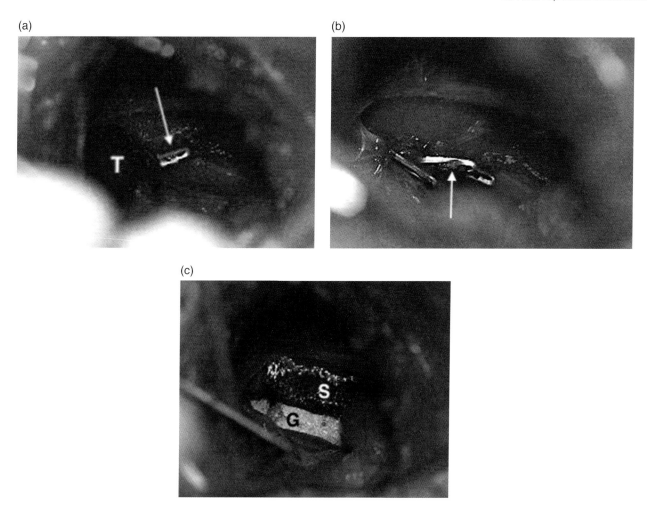

Figure 12.4 Intraoperative image of castration of an umbrella cockatoo. The left testis has been elevated and a clip applied (a) (arrow points at the right testis). The tissue distal to the clip has been incised. A second clip will be applied cranial to the first clip. This process is continued as described for Figure 12.3. After the left testis was removed, there were small remnants of what appears to be testicular tissue (b) (white arrow). This tissue was fulgurated with bipolar electrosurgery. Surgicel™ (S) and Gelfoam™ (G) were applied after bilateral orchidectomy to control any postoperative hemorrhage that might occur (c).

Left-sided lameness or paresis may develop if an ovarian mass compresses the overlying lumbar or sacral nerve plexus. Diagnostics to investigate ovarian disease include radiography, ultrasonography, computed tomography, magnetic resonance imaging, rigid endoscopy, biopsy, and exploratory celiotomy. Although the cause is often unknown, cystic ovarian disease has been reported in numerous avian species. Granulosa cell tumors and ovarian adenocarcinomas are most frequently reported, but carcinomas, leiomyosarcomas, leiomyomas, adenomas, teratomas, dysgerminomas, fibrosarcomas, lipomas, and lymphomatosis have all been identified in bird ovaries (Latimer 1994). A complete ovariectomy is difficult to achieve in adult birds, but even a partial ovariectomy can be palliative in cases where the ovarian disease is compressing air sacs or causing effusion, pain, or dysfunction. In an adult, sexually mature bird, the size and vascularity of the ovary is increased (Figure 12.8). If the indication for ovariectomy is not emergent, attempt to decrease ovarian activity. This can be accomplished with environmental and nutritional cues but is most successfully achieved with medical interventions, like GnRH agonists (Millam and Finney 1994; Scagnelli and Tully 2017).

Ovariectomy is a very challenging surgery and should not be undertaken lightly as fatal hemorrhage is a common complication. The surgical approach for ovariectomy is a left lateral celiotomy (see Chapter 11). If the ovary is significantly increased in size, a ventral midline celiotomy with parasternal and/or parapubic flaps may be required. In most circumstances, removing the oviduct will facilitate visualization of the ovary (Figure 12.8). If large preovulatory follicles or cysts are present that prevent visualization of the ovarian vasculature, it may be indicated to remove the follicles and drain or remove any cysts prior to

(a)

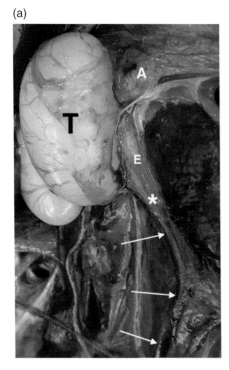

(b)

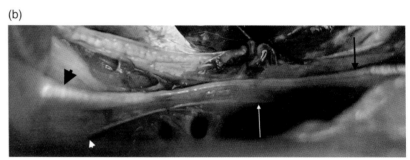

Figure 12.5 To perform a vasectomy using the left lateral approach (a), grasp the ductus deferens (white arrows) as it exits the epididymis (E) (asterisk). Carefully pull on the ductus to break it, and then remove 5–10 mm of the ductus depending on the patient size. Adrenal (A), testis (T). The ureter (white arrow) exits the caudal division of the kidney caudal to the epididymis. (b) At this location, the ductus deferens (black arrow) and ureter (white arrow) are not in close contact. Additionally, as they enter the cloaca, they diverge with the ductus deferens more medial (black arrowhead) than the ureter (white arrowhead).

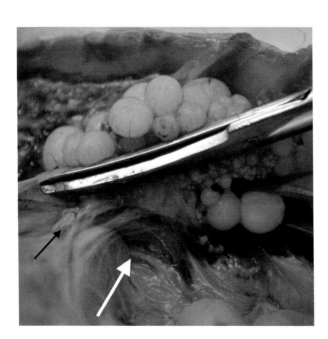

Figure 12.6 The mesovarium is difficult to identify because it is short and broadly attached to the common iliac vein (white arrow). The adrenal gland is visible cranial to the ovary (black arrow).

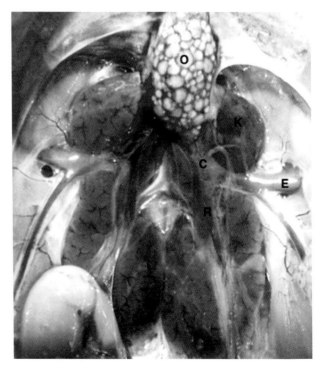

Figure 12.7 Anatomy of the female reproductive tract in a juvenile cockatiel (*Nymphicus hollandicus*). The oviduct has been removed. Ovary (O), common iliac vein (C), external iliac vein (E), renal vein (R), and kidney (K).

(a)

(b)

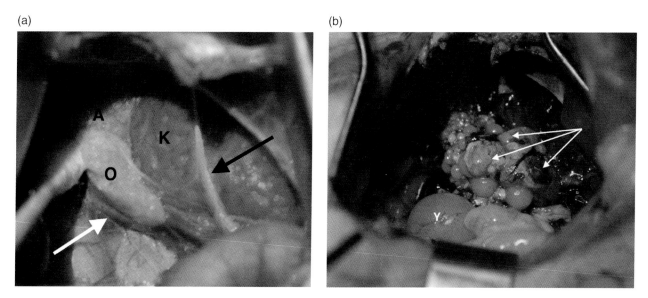

Figure 12.8 Intraoperative anatomy of a juvenile chicken during ovariectomy. (a) Ovary (O), adrenal gland (A), and kidney (K). The black arrow points at the oviduct and the white arrow is pointing at the common iliac vein. Intraoperative view of a mature chicken during ovariectomy after salpingohysterectomy which made it impossible to visualize the ovary. (b) There are many follicles of different sizes. The white arrows are pointing to postovulatory follicles. A large follicle ready to be ovulated is also present (Y).

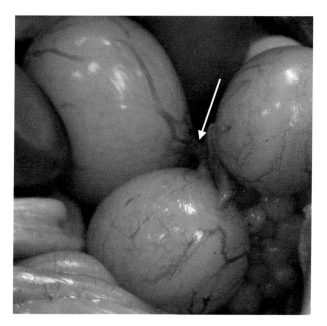

Figure 12.9 Large follicles in a mature bird often obstruct visualization of the ovary. These can be removed by plucking them off by spinning the yolk until the pedicle (arrow) breaks, by ligating the pedicle and transecting distal to it, or by using either bipolar electrosurgery or a tissue and vessel sealing device.

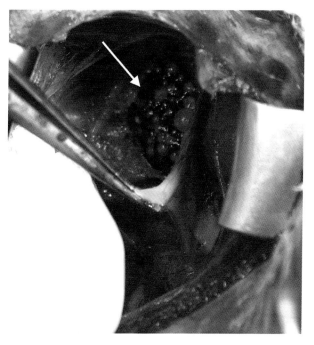

Figure 12.10 Intraoperative view of ovariectomy in an umbrella cockatoo (*Cacatua alba*). The forceps are holding the oviduct allowing visualization of the black ovary (arrow).

attempting to ligate the ovarian vessels (Figure 12.9). Visualize the ovary by retracting the proventriculus and intestines ventrally (Figure 12.10). Grasp the caudal meso-varian ligament with microsurgical forceps and elevate it enough to place a hemostatic clip as proximal on the ovarian vessels as possible. Partially transect the pedicle distal to

the clip. Progressively continue this technique caudal to cranial until all the ovarian vessels are ligated and transected, like the method described above for orchidectomy (Figure 12.11). A right-angled clip applier allows placement of the clips without applying significant back tension on the tissues that often leads to avulsion of the smaller vessels

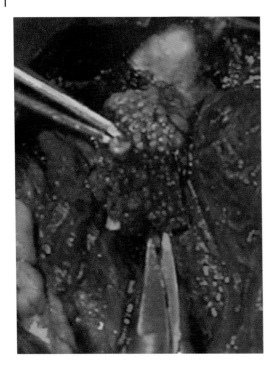

Figure 12.11 In a juvenile bird, the vessels are not well developed and the mesovarium loose making it possible to remove the ovary by carefully incising the mesovarium.

from the larger vessels. Right-angled clip appliers also help prevent deeper structures from being inadvertently damaged when applying clips. If hemorrhage occurs, apply direct and continuous pressure for at least five minutes. Hemostatic aids such as gelatin sponge, oxidized regenerated cellulose, topical thrombin, and thrombin glue may be helpful as well. The clip line should be inspected to ensure that all ovarian tissue has been removed. As well as fatal hemorrhage, failure to remove all of the ovary and its associated disease is a common complication. Use bipolar electrosurgery to fulgurate any ovarian tissue that remains along the clip (Figure 12.12).

A study was performed to determine if ovariectomy can be more easily and safely performed using a vessel and tissue sealing device (Sullivan et al. 2021). Ovariectomy was performed in 10 juvenile (<4 months old) chickens and 10 adult (>18 months old) laying hens using a vessel and tissue sealing device (LigaSure™ and the Small Jaw Open Sealer/Divider handpiece, Medtronic, Minneapolis, MN) (Figure 12.12). All birds survived the surgery and complete removal of the ovary was confirmed at necropsy in 60% of the birds. In the mature birds, it was necessary to remove the oviduct and uterus to gain exposure to the ovary. In two birds, grossly visible ovarian tissue was observed at necropsy and in six more birds microscopic ovarian tissue was identified histologically totalling four adult and four juvenile birds (40%).

Three birds experienced severe hemorrhage. The authors concluded that complete ovariectomy using a tissue and vessel sealing device is possible but still carries the risks of serious hemorrhage and failing to remove the entire ovary.

Surgery of the Oviduct and Uterus (Shell Gland)

Disorders of the oviduct may be incidental findings or the cause of clinical disease. Indications for surgery include ectopic ovulation, cystic hyperplasia of the oviduct, oviductal prolapse, salpingitis, metritis, and oviduct obstruction, rupture, torsion, and neoplasia (King and McLelland 1984; Gorham et al. 1992; Harcourt-Brown 1996; Speer 1997; Jenkins 2000; Johnson 2000; Mison et al. 2016). In birds, ectopic ovulations are typically self-limiting and do not require surgical intervention but can cause severe peritonitis requiring surgical intervention. Diseases of the oviduct often produce vague clinical signs most consistent with a space occupying mass-effect causing compression of the surrounding organs and air sacs, coelomic distension, peritonitis, and ascites. None of these clinical signs are pathognomonic for oviductal disease. Definitive diagnosis is achieved by physical examination, imaging, and either endoscopic or open surgical exploration of the coelom.

Salpingohysterectomy

Salpingohysterectomy is the surgical removal of the entire oviduct and uterus (shell gland) and is indicated for the treatment of oviductal disease that cannot be medically managed such as chronic egg laying, dystocia, chronic infection, and neoplasia (Gorham et al. 1992). In most birds, for left salpingohysterectomy, perform a left lateral celiotomy (see Chapter 11). When the oviduct is significantly enlarged or if more exposure is needed, a ventral midline flap approach may be chosen. In patients with right oviductal disease, perform a right lateral celiotomy or a midventral approach. Incise the caudal thoracic and abdominal air sacs to visualize the ovary and oviduct. With severe and chronic disease, adhesions to the air sacs and surrounding viscera are common, as are adhesions of viscera to the body wall. Use blunt dissection and bipolar electrosurgery to gently break down any adhesions. Be cautious to not inadvertently incise organs that are adhered to the body wall during the approach. In patients with severe oviductal dilation, perform a salpingotomy to remove the contents of the oviduct to achieve visualization of the vessels in the suspensory ligament. The ventral oviductal ligament is relatively avascular and is responsible for the coiling of the oviduct in the coelomic

(a)

(b)

(c)

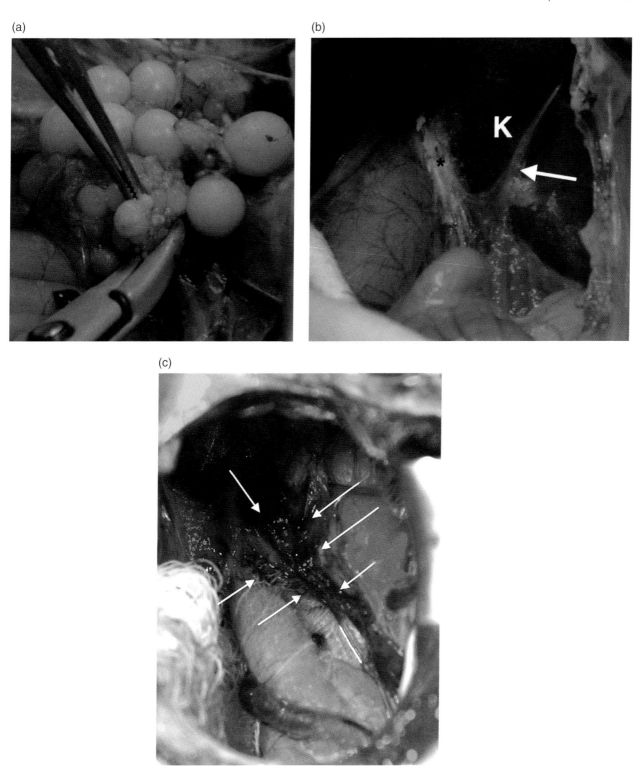

Figure 12.12 LigaSure™ has been evaluated for use for avian ovariectomy. Following removal of the oviduct to provide exposure to the ovary, lift the caudal pole of the ovary and insert the jaws of the handpiece. (a) Activate the current and cutting blade. Repeat the process until the ovary has been completely removed. The ovary has been removed from this juvenile chicken. (b) The kidney (K) and oviduct (arrow) are noted. The site of LigaSure application is marked with an asterisk. The ovary has been removed from this mature reproductively active chicken. (c) The white arrows denote the entire area where the LigaSure was used to remove the ovary. Surgical time was significantly longer in mature chicken partly because of the need to perform a salpingohysterectomy and partly because it required several applications of the sealing device.

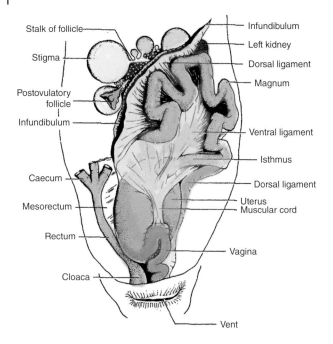

Figure 12.13 Anatomy of the oviduct showing the infundibulum, magnum, isthmus, uterus, and vagina. The ventral ligament is attached to the uterus by a muscular cord that is responsible for the folding of a mature functional uterus. The vagina is closely associated with the cloaca. *Source*: King and McLelland (1984).

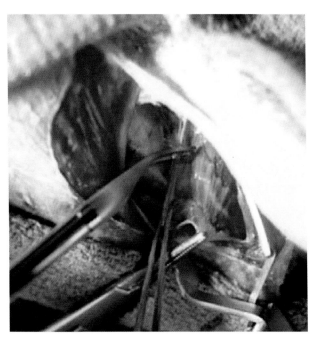

Figure 12.14 Intraoperative image of a juvenile lovebird (*Agapornis* sp.). A hemostat has been applied to the ventral ligament allowing visualization of the vessels in the dorsal ligament. A hemostatic clip is being applied to the cranial oviductal artery and vein. *Source:* Image courtesy of Jeff Jenkins.

cavity (Figure 12.13). Dissect the ventral suspensory ligament first to allow the oviduct to be extended linearly and exteriorized. Identify the dorsal suspensory ligament and the blood supply to the oviduct (Figure 12.14). Identify the infundibulum and gently retract it toward the opening of the coelomic incision. The dorsal ligament at the base of the infundibulum suspends the oviduct and the oviductal branch of the ovarian artery. Apply two hemostatic clips to this vessel and cut between them or use bipolar electrosurgery to coagulate it. After the infundibulum is completely freed, retract the oviduct ventrally and caudally to expose the remainder of the dorsal suspensory ligament. Clip or coagulate branches of the vessels that lie perpendicular to the oviduct and uterus. Keep the dissection as close to the oviduct and uterus as possible because the vessels are smaller there than they are more dorsally. Continue the dissection caudally toward the cloaca, taking care to avoid the ureter. Once the blood vessels in the dorsal suspensory ligament are coagulated and transected, exteriorize the uterus and oviduct in a linear fashion extending the structures completely outside the body wall. Expose and identify the junction of the uterus with the cloaca. Insert a cotton tip applicator through the vent into the cloaca to help delineate its boundaries. Place one or two clips or encircling sutures at

the uterovaginal junction and transect the uterus from its junction with vagina on the cloaca immediately cranial to the clips or sutures. If the uterus is large, a transfixation ligature may be more appropriate.

Endoscopic salpingohysterectomy has been evaluated in juvenile cockatiels with the goal of being able to offer birds for sale that will not experience egg binding or chronic egg laying behaviors, which is a common medical problem in this species (Pye et al. 2001). Because the oviduct and uterus are immature with minimal blood supply, the oviduct was identified using a 2.7 mm scope, cannula, and forceps. The forceps were used to grasp the oviduct which was then just pulled out the defect in the body wall (Figure 12.15). A cotton-tipped applicator was placed in the cloaca and used to push the cloaca toward the opening in the body wall. A hemostatic clip was applied to the oviduct, and it was transected distal to the clip. All 14 birds survived the procedure. One of the authors (R. Plunsky) adopted all of the study birds. When one died, a necropsy was performed. The birds were housed with males. No bird died of reproductive disease, and there was no evidence of any bird having released yolk into the coelom (R. Plunsky, personal communication). This procedure is quick and easy to accomplish.

(a)

(b)

(c)

(d)

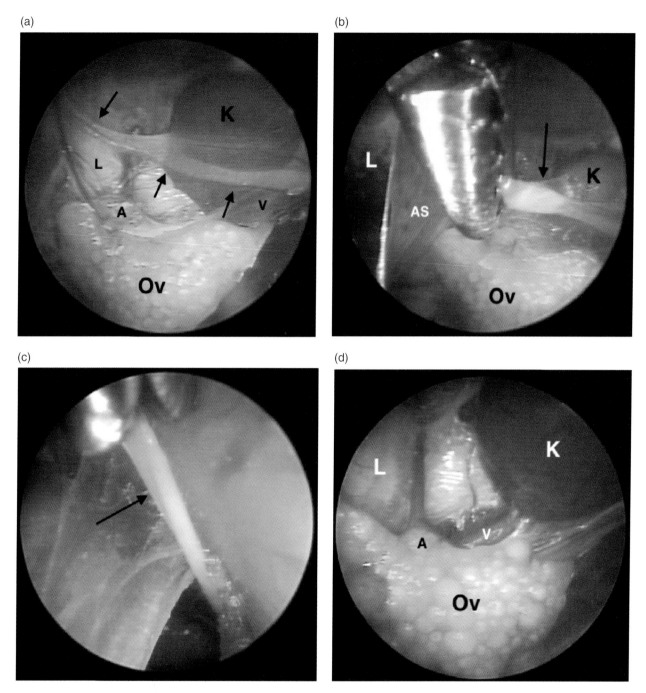

Figure 12.15 Intraoperative image of a juvenile cockatiel (*Nymphicus hollandicus*) undergoing laparoscopic salpingohysterectomy. (a) Adrenal gland (A), kidney (K), lung (L), ovary (Ov), and common iliac vein (V) are labeled. Arrows are point to the oviduct. Use endosurgical forceps to grasp the oviduct (arrow) and pull it to detach it. (b) An air sac wall (AS) is visible. Continue pulling on the oviduct to exteriorize it through the cannula port. (c) Use a cotton-tipped applicator to push the cloaca cranially, place a hemostatic clip at the junction with the cloaca, and then transect distal to the clip. Reinsert the scope to assure there is no hemorrhage. Note the oviduct is no longer present, and there is no visible hemorrhage (d).

Salpingohysterotomy

Salpingohysterotomy is indicated in some patients with egg postovulatory stasis or dystocia, where medical management has failed. As described above, this procedure may precede salpingohysterectomy or may be performed to maintain the bird's reproductive capabilities if the oviduct is otherwise normal. The surgical approach to the oviduct is in part dependent on the location of the egg; a caudal left lateral or ventral midline approach are best. Incise the oviduct in a healthy appearing location, often immediately caudal to the egg. The stretched, friable, and often compromised tissue directly over the egg will have a decreased healing potential and should be spared from surgical trauma. Palpate the egg and gently maneuver it into the incision and then remove it from the oviduct. Close the oviduct in a single layer using a simple continuous pattern with fine, monofilament, synthetic, absorbable suture material on a taper needle (Figure 12.16). Complications of salpingohysterotomy include dehiscence, stricture, and recurrent obstruction.

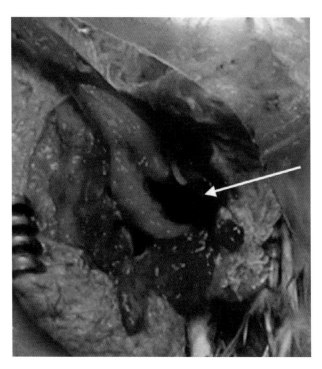

Figure 12.16 A salpingohysterotomy was performed in this love bird (*Agapornis* sp.) to remove an egg that was lodged.

References

Gorham, S.L., Akins, M., and Carter, B. (1992). Ectopic egg yolk in the abdominal cavity of a cockatiel. *Avian Diseases* 36: 816–817.

Harcourt-Brown, N. (1996). Torsion and displacement of the oviduct as a cause of egg-binding in four psittacine birds. *Journal of Avian Medicine and Surgery* 10: 262–267.

Jenkins, J.R. (2000). Surgery of the avian reproductive and gastrointestinal systems. *Veterinary Clinics of North America: Exotic Animal Practice* 3: 673–692.

Johnson, A.L. (2000). Reproduction in the female. In: *Sturkie's Avian Physiology*, 5e (ed. G.C. Whittow), 569–596. San Diego, CA: Academic Press.

Joyner, K.L. (1994). Theriogenology. In: *Avian Medicine: Principles and Application* (eds. B.W. Ritchie, G.J. Harrison and L.R. Harrison), 748–804. Lake Worth, FL: Winger's Publishing.

King, A.S. and McLelland, J. (1984). Female reproductive system. In: *Birds Their Structure and Function*, 2e, 145–165. Philadelphia, PA: Bailliere Tindall.

King, A.S. and McLelland, J. (1984). Male reproductive system. In: *Birds Their Structure and Function*, 2e, 166–174. Philadelphia, PA: Bailliere Tindall.

Latimer, K.S. (1994). Oncology. In: *Avian Medicine: Principles and Application* (eds. B.W. Ritchie, G.J. Harrison and L.R. Harrison), 640–672. Lake Worth, FL: Wingers Publishing.

Millam, J. and Finney, H. (1994). Leuprolide acetate can reversibly prevent egg laying in cockatiels. *Zoo Biology* 13: 149–155.

Mison, M., Mehler, S., and Echols, M.S. (2016). Approaches to the coelom and selected procedures. In: *Current Therapy in Avian Medicine and Surgery* (ed. B. Speer), 638–645. Philadelphia, PA: Elsevier Inc.

Nemetz, L. (2010). Clinical pathology of a persistent right oviduct in psittacine birds. *Proceedings Association of Avian Veterinarians*, San Diego, CA, pp. 73–77.

Pye, G.W., Bennett, R.A., Plunski, R. et al. (2001). Endoscopic salpingohysterectomy of juvenile cockatiels (*Nymphicus hollandicus*). *Journal of Avian Medicine and Surgery* 15: 90–94.

Samour, J. (2010). Vasectomy in birds: a review. *Journal of Avian Medicine and Surgery* 24: 169–173.

Scagnelli, A.M. and Tully, T.N. (2017). Reproductive disorders in parrots. *Veterinary Clinics of North America: Exotic Animal Practice* 20: 485–507.

Speer, B.L. (1997). Diseases of the urogenital system. In: *Avian Medicine and Surgery* (eds. R.B. Altman, S.L. Clubb, et al.), 625–644. Philadelphia, PA: W.B. Saunders.

Sullivan, J.L., Wakamatsu, N., Yin, J.H. et al. (2021). A novel technique for avian ovariectomy using a vessel sealing device in a chicken model. *American Journal of Veterinary Research* 82 (4): 310–317.

13

Surgery of the Avian Gastrointestinal Tract

Michael B. Mison and R. Avery Bennett

Anatomy and Physiology

Major differences exist between the avian (Figure 13.1) and mammalian digestive tract. Mechanical breakdown of ingesta by birds is accomplished by their beak and muscular gizzard. The esophagus is comparatively larger in diameter than in mammals to accommodate swallowing large food items that would be masticated by teeth. The crop or ingluvies is a dilation of the esophagus and functions for food storage. The stomach of a bird is divided into two compartments separated by the isthmus, a cranial proventriculus (glandular stomach) and a caudal ventriculus (gizzard) ending at the pylorus. Carnivorous and piscivorous birds use the stomach for both food storage and digestion. In these species, the proventriculus is large, sac-like, and thin-walled. In contrast, in granivorous species, the proventriculus is relatively small, the isthmus is distinct, and the ventriculus is large and muscular (Figure 13.2).

The proventriculus is the glandular stomach in birds and functions similar to the mammalian stomach. The ventriculus is the muscular compartment that breaks down the ingesta into pieces small enough to pass through the pylorus into the duodenum. Some birds pick up gravel that passes into the ventriculus where it is retained for a variable period. In birds with a distinct ventriculus, it is very muscular and the contractions of the walls grind the food by mashing it with the gravel and stones. The proventriculus and ventriculus act as a unit, propelling ingesta back and forth between the two compartments to optimize acid and enzymatic and mechanical digestion. There are two distinct anatomic forms of the ventriculus that may influence surgical options. Ratites have a large, thin-walled proventriculus that passes dorsal to the ventriculus and empties into the ventriculus at its caudal aspect (Fowler 1991; Lumeij 1994a; Hoefer 1997). In birds that feed on soft food (carnivores and piscivores),

the ventriculus is rounded and uniformly thin-muscled, and may be indistinguishable from the proventriculus. In birds that feed predominantly on harder foods that require more grinding and mixing for digestion (insectivores, herbivores, and granivores), the ventriculus is thick and biconvex (King and McLelland 1984; Degernes et al. 2012). Grit in the ventriculus functions to provide abrasive action for those species that require it (Columbiformes, Galliformes, most Psittaciformes, and Struthioniformes or ratites). Grit in the ventriculus can make surgery more difficult and can potentially contaminate the coelomic cavity when performing a ventriculotomy. The pylorus connects the ventriculus to the duodenum and regulates that passage of food from the stomach into the duodenum. It is poorly developed in many birds but can be a distinct chamber in aquatic species (Duke 1986; Orosz 1997a).

The small intestine absorbs the majority of nutrients. It is similar to mammals but is comprised of a U-shaped duodenum and U-shaped loops of ileum and jejunum attached to the dorsal mesentery with blood vessels and lymphatics within the U (Figure 13.3). Meckel's diverticulum marks the end of the jejunum and the start of the ileum but is not grossly visible in all species.

The large intestine starts with cecal outpouchings. It is short and straight along the dorsal body wall just right of midline. The cecal outpouchings are most prominent in fowl and ostriches and are vestigial in many species.

The terminal part of the digestive tract is the rectum and cloaca, which are involved in excretion of waste and minerals, and hydration. In the cloaca, digestive waste mixes with urinary waste. The reproductive tract also exits into the cloaca. The cloaca is divided internally into three compartments by two mucosal folds: the proximal coprodeum, middle urodeum, and distal proctodeum (Orosz 1997b; Doneley 2011a).

Surgery of Exotic Animals, First Edition. Edited by R. Avery Bennett and Geoffrey W. Pye.
© 2022 John Wiley & Sons, Inc. Published 2022 by John Wiley & Sons, Inc.

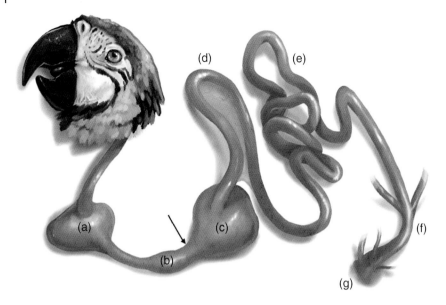

Figure 13.1 Overview of the avian gastrointestinal tract. (a) Crop, (b) proventriculus, (c) ventriculus, (d) duodenum, (e) small intestine, (f) colon, (g) cloaca. The arrow is pointing at the isthmus. *Source*: Image courtesy of Christopher St. Clair.

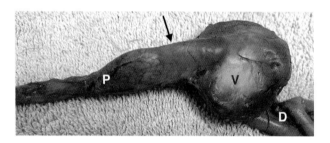

Figure 13.2 The proventriculus (P), isthmus (arrow), and the large and muscular ventriculus (V) of a chicken. Duodenum (D).

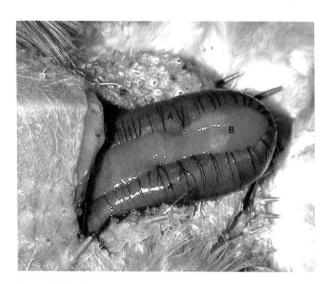

Figure 13.3 A duodenal loop (a) showing pancreas (b) within the loop. The blood supply is in the center under the pancreas that is difficult to directly visualize.

Surgery of the Mouth

Oral papillomas are proliferative, wart-like masses anywhere along the alimentary tract surface of psittacines, such as the oral cavity, crop, proventriculus, intestines, or cloaca. Some researchers have suggested either papillomavirus or herpesvirus may be the etiology (Schmidt et al. 2003; Styles 2004). Oral masses can be removed using cryosurgery, electrosurgery, or chemical cautery (silver nitrate). Because of the viral etiology, recurrence is common.

Surgery of the Esophagus

Indications for esophageal surgery include trauma (fishhooks, traumatic tube feeding, external trauma, and crop burn), retrieval of foreign bodies, placement of feeding tubes, sour crop in raptors, or crop biopsies. For an ingluviotomy, place the patient in dorsal or lateral recumbency. A probe can be introduced per os to aid in delineation of the esophagus. Incise the skin over the left lateral crop wall close to the thoracic inlet. Use stay sutures to isolate the crop wall and incise the crop in a hypovascular section of the wall. Extend the incision as needed. Close the crop with appropriately sized monofilament absorbable suture material in a single or double layer continuous pattern. The crop, being a part of the esophagus, does not have a serosa. An inverting closure is not necessary. Close the skin in a separate layer.

Hand-reared birds fed excessively hot or inadequately mixed food (which leads to hot spots) may suffer crop burns. Birds present with delayed crop emptying or a wet skin patch over the crop. Necrosis may also occur in adult birds following the consumption of caustic substances or if being tube fed a hot diet. Necrosis of the crop wall and skin leads to fistula formation. Delay surgical repair until the necrotic tissue has declared from viable tissue. This usually takes three to five days. The crop wall will have adhered to the skin by the time a fistula has formed. To repair crop burns, surgically separate the skin from the crop wall and debride the necrotic tissues. Close the crop wall as previously described followed by a separate skin closure (Forbes 2002).

Surgery of the Stomach

The left lateral, transverse, and ventral midline with flap celiotomy approaches may be used to access the proventriculus, isthmus, and ventriculus (see Chapter 11). Indications for surgery of the avian stomach include obtaining biopsies, retrieving foreign bodies, relieving complete or partial gastric outflow obstruction, or excising gastric neoplasms or infiltrative intramural lesions. Preoperative fasting is recommended to allow the upper gastrointestinal tract to empty to reduce the likelihood of the patient vomiting/regurgitating and aspirating ingesta. A prolonged fast is not recommended because of the small size and limited hepatic glycogen stores of most avian patients. A three-hour fast is usually sufficient for most companion avian species. Small species may require an even shorter fast. Raptors and waterfowl may require a fast of 12 hours or more. Surgically obtained full or partial thickness biopsies are indicated for conditions where a low-yield diagnosis or treatment is expected with endoscopic methods, or the risk is considered too great to obtain biopsies endoscopically. A technique for obtaining endoscopic biopsies of the proventriculus and ventriculus of pigeons demonstrated that they were not able to obtain acceptable ventricular biopsies (Sladakovic et al. 2017). While they were able to obtain adequate biopsies of the proventriculus by positioning the cup forceps nearly parallel to the proventricular wall, two of the eight pigeons died; one from perforation of the proventriculus and the other from aspiration of the saline used to distend the stomach. A proper work-up is important in determining if there is an indication for biopsy and to target a specific lesion or location for sample collection. Diagnosis of many intramural or invasive mucosal disease processes is facilitated by direct visualization of these organs and appropriate sample collection.

Gastrointestinal foreign bodies are not uncommon in pet birds. Young cockatoos seem to be at a greater risk of foreign object ingestion than other species (Ingram 1990; Adamcak et al. 2000). Although any household items have the potential to become foreign bodies, commonly ingested items include pieces of cage toys, cage hardware, grit, perches, and bedding. Outdoor-housed nonpsittacine birds are more likely to ingest sand, bedding, plant material, and large metallic objects such as screws, coins, and wires. Medical management is frequently recommended as initial therapy for birds with known or suspected partial foreign body obstructions. Consider gastrointestinal obstruction in birds with clinical signs of regurgitation, decreased fecal production, and gastrointestinal dilation (Figure 13.4). Attempts can be made to retrieve gastric foreign bodies endoscopically. Flushing the proventriculus and ventriculus before endoscopic retrieval of foreign materials can aid in visualization. Surgery is indicated in cases of complete gastric outflow obstruction or when endoscopic retrieval is unsuccessful (Hoefer and Levitan 2013).

The isthmus is the most common location for neoplasia of the stomach. Squamous cell carcinoma, adenocarcinoma, adenoma, lymphoma, rhabdomyosarcoma, and leiomyosarcoma are examples of gastric neoplasms that have been reported in birds (Leach et al. 1989; Gibbons et al. 2002; Yonemaru et al. 2004; Maluenda et al. 2010; János et al. 2011; Schmidt et al. 2012; Snyder and Treating 2014). Nonneoplastic lesions of the proventriculus and ventriculus include those associated with macrorhabdosis (budgerigars, cockatiels, parrotlets, and finches), ulcerative proventriculitis, mineralization (cockatiels, budgerigars, lories and lorikeets, macaws), proventricular dilation disease, and cryptosporidiosis (cockatiels, lovebirds, parrotlets, finches). As with any neoplastic conditions, tumor staging is important to help determine treatment options and establish a prognosis. Surgical treatment involves excision of these lesions. The surgical dose can be either palliative (surgical excision to control hemorrhage or to alleviate a neoplastic obstruction by cytoreduction) or curative intent. Curative intent involves excision of the tumor with an acceptable margin of healthy tissue surrounding the tumor to obtain clean surgical margins, which may be difficult in many birds.

Proventriculotomy and Ventriculotomy

Proventriculotomy or ventriculotomy is most commonly indicated for removal of ingested foreign objects that cannot be retrieved with an endoscope or flushing techniques. Ventriculotomy has been considered more likely to leak postoperatively as it is difficult to seal the incision with

(a)

(b)

(c)

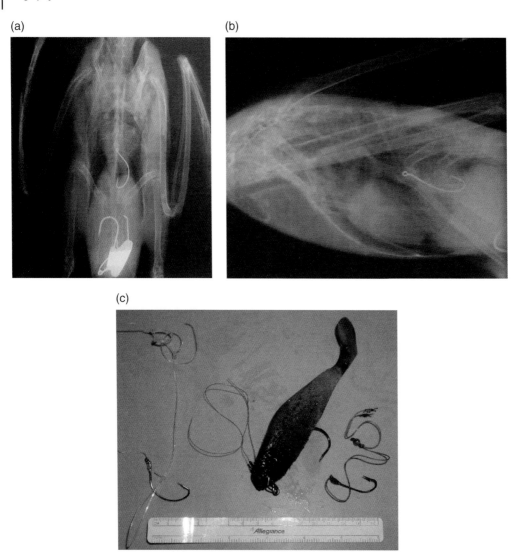

Figure 13.4 (a,b) Orthogonal radiographs of a double-crested cormorant revealing ingested rubber fish lure and hooks. (c) Retrieved rubber fish lure and hooks gastric foreign body.

sutures because birds do not have an omentum; however, this has not been scientifically documented (Ferrell et al. 2003). In many birds, the proventriculus holds sutures poorly, and they can easily tear through during manipulation (Fowler 1991; Lumeij 1994b; Hoefer 1997). Accurately place fine monofilament absorbable suture material to close and consider serosal patching to help create a fibrin seal quickly (Briscoe and Bennett 2011; Simova-Curd et al. 2013).

Proventriculotomy or Ventriculotomy Through the Isthmus

Use a left lateral, transverse, or ventral midline with a parasternal flap celiotomy to access the proventriculus, isthmus, and ventriculus (Figure 13.5). A left lateral approach is commonly used providing good exposure to all three structures (Mison et al. 2016). Identify the ventriculus and place stay sutures in the white tendinous portion of the ventriculus. Use the stay sutures to elevate the proventriculus and bluntly dissect the suspensory tissues (including air sacs) surrounding it to be able to elevate the ventriculus completely outside the coelom. This will bring the isthmus and proventriculus into the field. Avoid placing stay sutures through the proventriculus or in the muscular component of the ventriculus as these tissues are weak and the sutures will likely tear through during retraction (Bennett 1994). Isolate the proventriculus and ventriculus with moistened sponges to minimize contamination. The caudal tip of the left liver lobe lies partially over the isthmus. There are a number of short blood vessels between the tip of the liver lobe and the proventriculus. Carefully, use a moistened cotton-tipped applicator to roll the liver lobe off the isthmus and plan the incision under where the liver lobe is normally

(a)

(b)

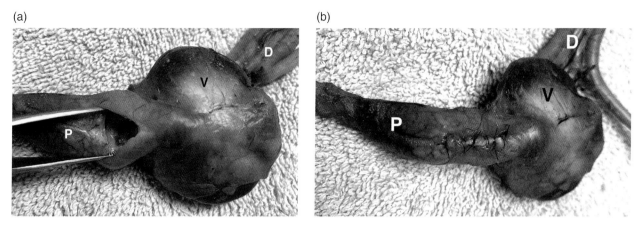

Figure 13.5 For a proventriculotomy, (a) start the incision in a hypovascular area of the isthmus and extend it orad. (b) Interrupted cruciate sutures were used for closure of the proventriculotomy. Proventriculus (P), ventriculus (V), duodenum (D).

(a)

(b)

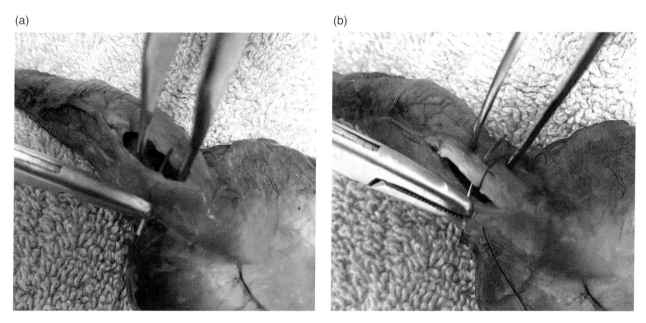

Figure 13.6 Use thumbs forceps for counter pressure to pass sutures to avoid grasping the fragile cut edge of the proventricular wall. On the first side, insert the open forceps into the incision for counter pressure as the needle is passed from the serosal surface into the lumen (a). On the other side, place the open forceps on the serosal surface for counter pressure and pass the needle from the lumen out the serosal surface. Do not use the forceps to hold the wall of the proventriculus (b).

positioned. After closing the proventriculotomy, this piece of liver can serve as a serosal patch to help rapidly create serosal adhesions minimizing the risk of leakage. Make a stab incision in an avascular area of the isthmus using a no. 11 scalpel blade. Avoid using electrosurgery, radiofrequency electrosurgery, or CO_2 laser to create an incision due to the potential for lateral thermal damage that might lead to incisional dehiscence and leakage. Extend the incision orad with fine scissors for a proventriculotomy or aborad for a ventriculotomy. Control gastric contents leakage with cotton-tipped applicators or suction. Use irrigation and suction to carefully evacuate the contents as the air sacs will be open and fluids can enter the lung through the ostium. A rigid endoscope can be used for foreign body retrieval in

selected cases to reduce tissue trauma intraoperatively (Speer 1998; Mison et al. 2016).

Close the gastrotomy with an appropriately sized monofilament rapidly absorbable suture in a simple continuous pattern. A simple continuous pattern creates a better seal than a simple interrupted. It is best not to hold the proventricular wall with thumb forceps because it is fragile and the cut edge is easily macerated. Use the thumb forceps to create counter pressure. Open the jaws of the forceps against the outside of the stomach wall, insert the suture needle into the lumen of the stomach and push the needle through between the jaws of the forceps (Figure 13.6). Once the proventriculotomy is closed, lay the tip of the liver lobe back into its normal position over the proventriculotomy incision. Use fine monofilament absorbable suture on a taper needle to place three to four simple interrupted sutures between the seromuscular layer of the gastric incision and the capsule of the caudal edge of the liver lobe. Place each suture at least 5 mm from the gastric incision to secure the liver lobe over the entire incision. The sutures should not cut into the hepatic parenchyma, which would result in them not holding the liver in place.

Gastrotomy in Carnivores and Piscivores

The stomach of birds that eat whole prey is large, and it is difficult to distinguish the proventriculus from the ventriculus. In these birds, a standard gastrotomy as performed in cats works well. Approach the stomach through a ventral midline celiotomy and identify the stomach on the left side of the coelom. Place stay sutures to aid in manipulation and exteriorization of the stomach. Break down any air sacs or suspensory tissues to exteriorize the stomach. Isolate the stomach from the rest of the coelom with moist gauze before making a stab incision into a hypovascular area of the stomach. Use the stay sutures to help minimize leakage and immediately suction the stomach to remove any contents. After removing the foreign body, close with two layers. The first can be a simple continuous to get good apposition and the second an inverting pattern such as a Connell or Lembert to achieve serosa-to-serosa contact allowing a fibrin seal to develop quickly.

If only one layer can be placed, it is best to use an inverting pattern to allow a seal to form more quickly since birds do not have an omentum. In many avian species, it is often not possible to accomplish a two-layer closure or even a single layer, inverting pattern, but in this group of birds, the stomach is usually large enough to close with an inverting pattern.

Gastrotomy in Ratites

Ratites are notorious for eating anything in sight. Their stomach is usually very large and full of various objects many of which are not food items (Figure 13.7). With the bird in dorsal recumbency, approach the stomach through a ventral midline incision. Once the stomach is located, which is usually easy because it is quite large, bring it up to the ventral body wall incision and exteriorize a portion of the stomach. Much like performing a rumenotomy, suture the exteriorized stomach wall to the surrounding skin circumferentially in a simple continuous pattern creating an area of stomach wall exposed large enough to introduce a hand. Suturing the stomach to the skin surrounding the proposed gastrotomy incision will prevent gastric contents from contaminating the body wall and coelom. Make a stab incision into the stomach and extend the incision large enough to introduce a hand. Using a hand, remove all of the gastric contents including the objects of concern (Figure 13.8). Close the gastrotomy incision with a simple continuous pattern of a rapidly absorbed monofilament material. After the stomach has been closed, thoroughly irrigate the stomach wall that is still sutured to the skin removing as much debris as possible. Once the surface of the stomach is clean, remove the temporary simple continuous suture holding the stomach to the skin and place a second inverting suture layer to

(a)　　　　　　　　　　　　　　　(b)

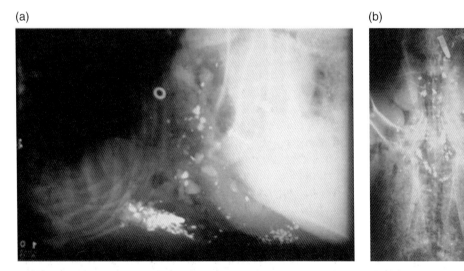

Figure 13.7 Orthogonal radiographs of an ostrich coelom revealing various foreign objects. (a) Lateral coelomic radiograph of an ostrich revealing various gastric foreign objects. (b) VD coelomic radiograph of an ostrich revealing various gastric foreign objects.

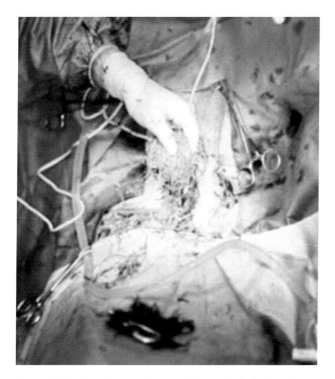

Figure 13.8 The stomach of an ostrich is exteriorized and sutured to the skin in preparation for a gastrotomy. Gastric contents are being removed. After the stomach is empty, close the gastrotomy prior to removing the suture between the stomach and skin to minimize contamination of the coelomic cavity.

achieve serosa-to-serosa contact before replacing the stomach into the coelom.

Ventriculotomy

In addition to being approached through an incision in the isthmus, the ventriculus can also be entered through its caudoventral sac. Use a transverse abdominal or a ventral midline combined with a left parasternal incision approach. The ventriculus has two blind sacs (craniodorsal and caudoventral) covered with relatively thin muscles. The duodenum exits the caudodorsal sac and this area should be avoided unless it is the site of interest. Foreign objects can be retrieved and biopsies obtain using a ventriculotomy of the caudoventral sac. An incision through the overlying thin muscle fibers allows relatively easy entry to the ventricular lumen (Bennett 1994; Ferrell et al. 2003). Meticulous closure is important to minimize the risk of leakage. Do not attempt to repair suspensory ligaments or air sacs. In a study of Japanese quail (*Coturnix coturnix japonica*) undergoing caudoventral sac ventriculotomy through a transverse celiotomy, ventricular mucosal

healing was not complete until 21 days after surgery (Ferrell et al. 2003).

Surgery of the Intestines

Enterotomy is not often indicated in avian patients and has historically carried a poor prognosis. Trauma or accidental incisions during celiotomy because of adhesions are situations where an enterotomy or intestinal resection and anastomosis may be indicated. Midline, flap, or transverse celiotomy can be used to approach the intestine depending on the location of the lesion. Magnification and microsurgical techniques are recommended. Various devices have been used to stop the flow of ingesta during surgery of the intestine of small birds including bobby pins, bulldog clamps, and vessel approximators. Use an appropriately sized monofilament rapidly absorbable suture on a small taper needle in a simple appositional pattern to close an enterotomy (Coles 1997). Because birds lack an omentum, serosal patching using adjacent intestine has been reported to augment intestinal closure creating a mucosa-to-mucosa seal (Briscoe and Bennett 2011). The intact serosa of nearby intestine can be sutured over the repaired intestinal incision in a simple interrupted pattern at 2–5 mm intervals. Place sutures into the intestinal serosal surface approximately 2–5 mm from the sutured incision.

Intestinal resection and anastomosis in birds presents a challenge because the intestines are often in a series of U-shaped loops. A segment of intestine is generally not mobile relative to the remaining intestines as it is in mammals. If the resection is only a few millimeters, the ends can be apposed. If there is a large defect after resecting the lesion, it may not be possible to appose the ends to be anastomosed and the entire loop may need to be resected. The blood supply is within the center of the U-shaped loop. Isolate the vessels near the base of the loop and ligate, seal, or clip the vascular supply. The devitalized section will declare itself quickly. Remove the devitalized segment and perform the anastomosis using an appropriately sized monofilament rapidly absorbable suture material on a fine taper needle in a simple continuous or interrupted pattern. Consider applying a serosal patch as described above.

Surgery of the Cloaca

Cloacotomy

Cloacotomy is indicated for a thorough evaluation of the internal structures for treating cloacal papillomatosis or other masses within the cloaca, or for removal of cloacoliths or eggs

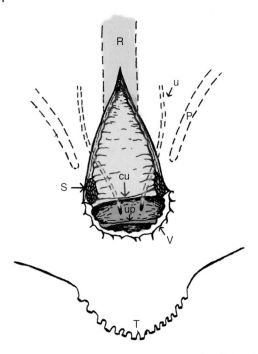

Figure 13.9 Drawing of a cloacotomy visualizing the coprourodeal fold (cu), the uroproctodeal fold (up), and the colonic, ureteral (u) and oviductal openings. R, rectum; P, pubis; V, vent; S, sphincter. *Source:* Dvorak et al. 1998. Reprinted with permission of Association of Avian Veterinarians.

trapped within the cloaca. Through this approach, the surgeon is able to visualize the coprourodeal fold and the uroproctodeal fold, and the colonic, ureteral, and oviductal openings (Figure 13.9). The openings of the vasa deferentia are generally too small to visualize. Insert a moistened cotton-tipped applicator into the cloaca. Using the monopolar electrosurgical wire tip, incise through the skin, the cloacal sphincter, and the ventral cloacal wall from the vent to the cranial extent of the cotton tipped applicator and, thus, the cranial extent of the cloaca. Alternatively, insert one arm of small scissors into the cloaca and cut through the ventral wall including skin, body wall, sphincter, and cloaca all at once, and then control any hemorrhage. Using this technique, the coelomic cavity is not entered. Inspect the urodeum on the dorsal surface to visualize the ureteral openings and urates flowing into the cloaca. It is important to identify the ureteral openings and preserve them.

For closure of the cloacotomy, close the cloacal wall using an appropriately sized monofilament absorbable suture on a taper needle in a simple continuous pattern beginning at the cranial extent of the incision. Appose the cloacal sphincter muscle with a single suture of appropriately sized absorbable material, and then close the skin over the cloaca and sphincter muscle.

Psittacid herpesvirus 1 (PsHV1) causes cloacal papilloma disease (Bonda 1998; Styles 2004). Cloacal examination reveals papillomatous lesions (cobblestone appearance)

that can lead to straining to defecate, urates pasting the vent, and blood on the droppings. A variety of techniques have been reported for the removal of cloacal papillomas including silver nitrate cauterization, cryosurgery, imiquimod application, and cloacotomy for surgical excision (Ramsay 1991; Dvorak et al. 1998). In most cases, the lesions are confined to the proctodeum. There is speculation that there is a correlation between infection with PsHV1 and the development of cloacal adenomas, adenocarcinomas in the pancreas, and carcinomas of the liver and bile ducts (Legler et al. 2008). Consider ruling out these potential concurrent lesions as part of the work up prior to addressing the papilloma disease.

After performing a cloacotomy, identify the ureters and protect them. Excise the papillomatous tissue with electrosurgery or sharp dissection. Bipolar electrosurgery is recommended because the tissue is very vascular and hemorrhage is a serious concern. The lesions typically involve only the mucosa, so full thickness excision is not necessary. After the lesions have been excised, appose the remaining mucosa with monofilament rapidly absorbable suture in a simple interrupted or continuous pattern.

Cloacal mucosal stripping for cloacal papillomas has been reported for the management of circumferential lesions (Antinoff 2000). Perform a cloacotomy and, starting at one side of the incision using electrosurgery (Figure 13.10), carefully dissect the mucosa from the uroproctodeal fold to the mucocutaneous junction from one side of the cloacotomy to the opposite side. Identify the ureteral openings and preserve them during the dissection. Once the mucosa has been removed, appose the caudal edge of the uroproctodeal fold to the skin with a simple continuous pattern using a monofilament rapidly absorbed material. Close the cloacotomy routinely.

There is a risk of stricture following cloacotomy. It usually occurs a week or two after surgery and prevents the bird from being able to void. If this happens, under general anesthesia, carefully work an object into the vent to start to dilate the sphincter. In most cases, a cotton-tipped applicator can be carefully introduced. Swirl it around to dilate the vent until you can introduce a second swab. Stretch the two swabs apart to slowly dilate the sphincter. In one author's experience (RAB), this has only needed to be done once and the strictures have not recurred after dilation.

Cloacopexy

Cloacopexy is indicated for treatment of chronic cloacal prolapse (Figure 13.11). This occurs most commonly in Old World psittacines (primarily cockatoos) and is associated with reduced or lost cloacal sphincter tone. Factors that potentially lead to cloacal prolapse include malnutrition,

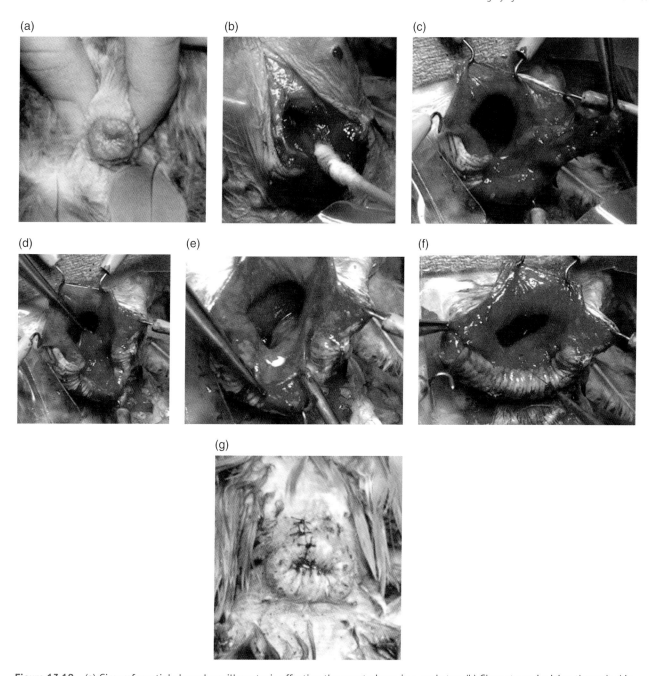

Figure 13.10 (a) Circumferential cloacal papillomatosis affecting the proctodeum in a cockatoo. (b) Cloacotomy, incising through skin, vent sphincter, and cloacal wall in preparation for cloacal mucosal stripping. (c) Starting at one side of the incision and carefully dissect the mucosa off. (d) The affected mucosa has been excised from the uroproctodeal fold to the mucocutaneous junction. The forceps are holding the cranial edge of the remaining mucosa. (e) The caudal edge of the uroproctodeal fold is held in the forceps. Note the white urates that have entered through the ureteral papilla. (f) The mucosa is being apposed to the skin. (g) Closed cloacotomy.

obesity, cloacal papillomas, constipation or diarrhea, coelomitis, coelomic masses, abnormal eggs or chronic egg laying, and sexual behavioral abnormalities (Mison et al. 2016). *Escherichia coli* cloacitis has also been implicated as a cause of straining resulting in tissue prolapse so culture the cloaca, wait three to five days for culture results, so that if pathogens are isolated, the bird may be placed on

appropriate antibiotic therapy prior to surgery. Lavage and lubricate the prolapsed tissues to prevent desiccation and, if necessary, topically apply 50% dextrose on the tissues to reduce swelling. Once reduced, place two simple interrupted sutures equidistant across the cloaca at approximately ⅓ and ⅔ the distance across the opening to prevent immediate recurrence but allowing droppings to pass. Test

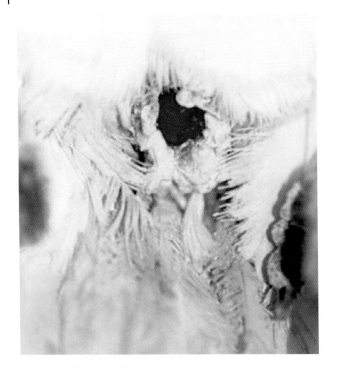

Figure 13.11 Cloacal prolapse in a cockatoo.

the patency by inserting a cotton-tipped applicator or red rubber catheter.

Several procedures have been recommended for the treatment of chronic cloacal prolapse; however, recurrence is observed with all techniques. It appears that permanent adhesions between the cloaca and the body wall are difficult to establish, so it is important to excise the fat on the ventral surface of the cloaca, which can act as a barrier to the formation of adhesions (Figure 13.12). For a rib cloacopexy (circumcostal), make a ventral midline with bilateral parasternal flaps approach to the caudal coelom and locate the serosal surface of the cloaca. Insert an

appropriate structure (gloved finger or a moistened cotton-tip applicator) into the cloaca to define its limits. A circumcostal cloacopexy uses the last rib to which the cloaca is sutured to maintain reduction. In most cases, the cloaca has been stretched and is easy to suture to the last ribs; however, if it does not stretch that far cranially suture it to the cartilaginous border of the caudal sternum. Preplace two sutures on each side around the last rib at the junction of the sternal and vertebral portions of the rib, and then full thickness through the cloacal wall on each of its lateral aspects. Once all four sutures are placed, tighten them to pull the cloaca cranially and secure it to the last rib on each side. This anchors the organ in a reduced position; however, it is unlikely that permanent adhesions will form and recurrence is common if this is the only procedure performed.

Cloacal reduction can be performed if there is excess cloacal tissue. Make an incision in the ventral aspect of the cloaca cranial to the sphincter. Do not cut through the sphincter. Identify the ureteral openings and the entrance of the terminal colon into the coprodeum. These structures must be preserved. Excise excess tissue only from the ventral aspect of the cloaca to avoid damaging vital structures. Close with a simple continuous pattern of a monofilament rapidly absorbed material. Alternatively, leave the incision and use it to create a ventral midline incisional cloacopexy that can be used for an incisional cloacopexy.

In addition to the circumcostal cloacopexy, close the ventral midline body wall incision incorporating the cloacal wall to facilitate formation of adhesions to help reduce the risk of recurrence (Figure 13.12). The incisional cloacopexy involves incorporating the cloacal wall in the closure of the ventral midline celiotomy. Make a partial thickness incision into the ventral cloacal wall exposing the muscle. Place a simple continuous suture incorporating one side of

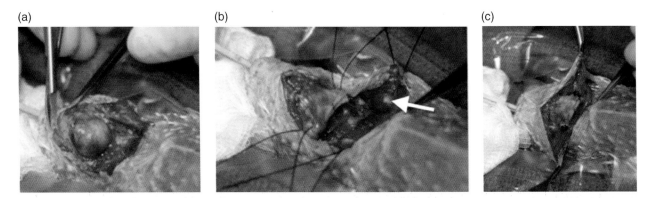

Figure 13.12 (a) Ventral midline and bilateral parasternal flap approach to the caudal coelom. A cotton-tipped applicator has been inserted into the cloaca to define its limits. (b) Preplace sutures placed through the cloaca and around last rib at the junction between the sternal and vertebral portions of the ribs (arrow). (c) Completed rib cloacopexy.

the body wall incision, then the ipsilateral incision in the cloacal wall from cranial to caudal. Repeat that procedure on the contralateral side. Finally, close the ventral body wall over the two continuous suture lines. Much like an incisional gastropexy to prevent gastric dilation and volvulus in dogs, suturing the muscle of the body wall to the muscle of the cloacal wall will create stronger adhesions. If cloacal reduction has been performed, perform an analogous procedure on each side. This will leave the cloaca open after the first two suture lines are placed, but the third line in the body wall only will seal the cloaca.

Be careful not to trap a loop of colon between the cloaca and the body wall (Radlinsky et al. 2004). This can be avoided by inserting a cotton-tipped applicator through the vent into the cloaca and into the terminal colon while the procedure is being performed. After the incisional cloacopexy is complete, remove the cotton-tipped applicator. Birds with colonic entrapment generally do not produce any feces. If the patient has not produced feces in 24 hours after surgery, take the bird back to surgery and open the incision to identify the cause of entrapment.

A report describes using an incisional colopexy for treatment of chronic, recurrent colocloacal prolapse (van Zeeland et al. 2014). It was reported in a sulfur-crested cockatoo and 2.5 years after surgery, there was no recurrence of the prolapse. One month after the colopexy, a ventplasty procedure was performed to reduce the size of the vent. Make a U-shaped incision on the ventral body wall to access the coelomic cavity. Insert a moistened cotton applicator into the cloaca to reduce the colocloacal prolapse and restore normal coelomic anatomy. Perform an incisional colopexy using standard techniques described in mammals.

Ventplasty

Ventplasty is often paired with cloacopexy as an augmentation of the surgical treatment of chronic cloacal prolapse. This procedure reduces the vent size to minimize the risk of recurrence of the cloacal prolapse. Excise the skin over the vent sphincter at both vent lateral commissures exposing the underlying muscle (Figure 13.13). The goal is to remove enough skin that when it is all closed, the new vent opening will be only large enough to allow one cotton-tipped applicator to be inserted. This area is very vascular so bipolar electrosurgery or laser is recommended. Place fine monofilament absorbable suture transversely in the cloacal mucosa from cranial to caudal on both sides of the new opening. Appose the vent sphincter muscle with a synthetic monofilament absorbable suture in a mattress pattern between the cranial and caudal aspects of the sphincter. Appose the skin edges cranial to caudal using a

synthetic absorbable material. Monitor the patient postoperatively to assure that it can still void urine, urates, and fecal material.

Duodenostomy Feeding Tube

A technique for duodenal alimentation in birds has been reported (Goring et al. 1986; Quesenberry 1989). Place a duodenostomy tube to bypass the upper gastrointestinal tract. Approach the duodenum through a ventral midline incision (Figure 13.14). The duodenal loop is immediately inside the body wall. Exteriorize the duodenum and use a through-the-needle catheter. The catheter diameter should be less than $\frac{1}{3}$ the diameter of the intestine. First, pass the needle through the left body wall. With the needle still through the body wall, insert it into the descending loop of the duodenum (the left limb of the loop). Advance the catheter through the needle and into the ascending loop 4–6 cm and withdraw the needle from the intestine and body wall. Remove the stylet from the catheter and advance the catheter until it is into the ascending loop. Place two sutures between the peritoneal surface of the body wall and the intestine to maintain them in apposition while a seal forms to minimize the risk of leakage. Secure the catheter to the outside skin using a finger trap technique and cap the catheter. Direct the catheter caudal to the leg, then under the wing, and bandage or suture it in place. Do not use the tube for 24 hours. It must be maintained at least 10 days to allow a seal to form between the duodenum and body wall before it can be removed. When it is no longer needed, pull the catheter and allow the wound to heal by second intention. In the report using needle catheter duodenostomy, a liquid diet was administered daily for 14 days. Four of the five pigeons had only minor weight loss; however, after oral alimentation was resumed, all five birds exceeded their initial body weight within seven days.

Liver Biopsy

The avian liver consists of the right and left lobes joined cranially on midline. The right lobe is larger than the left. The liver has an elastic capsule of connective tissue. Liver biopsies can be obtained using minimally invasive techniques. The liver can be visualized using a left lateral or ventral coelomic endoscopic approach. In cases of diffuse liver pathology, the caudal edge of the liver is the most accessible site. It is on the ventral floor of the caudal thoracic air sac. Break through this air sac to access the liver. Although these membranes are thin and transparent, it may take repeated attempts using cup biopsy forceps to break through. A single-action endoscopy scissors can be helpful in incising the membranes before using the cup

(a)

(b)

(c)

(d)

(e)

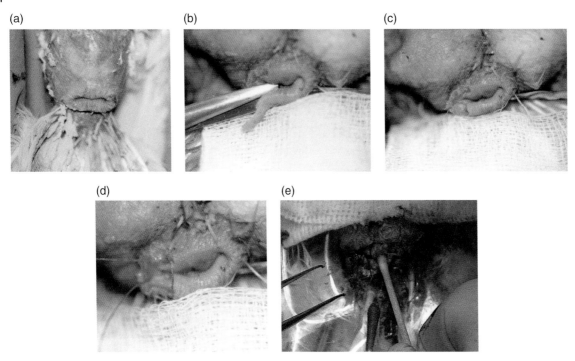

Figure 13.13 (a) Dilated vent in a cockatoo with chronic cloacal prolapse. (b) Excise the skin over the vent sphincter at both lateral commissures of the vent. (c) Underlying sphincter muscle exposed after excision of the skin. (d) Place a mattress suture across the sphincter from cranial to caudal. (e) Completed ventplasty with an opening just big enough to fit one cotton-tipped applicator.

(a)

(b)

(c)

(d)

(e)

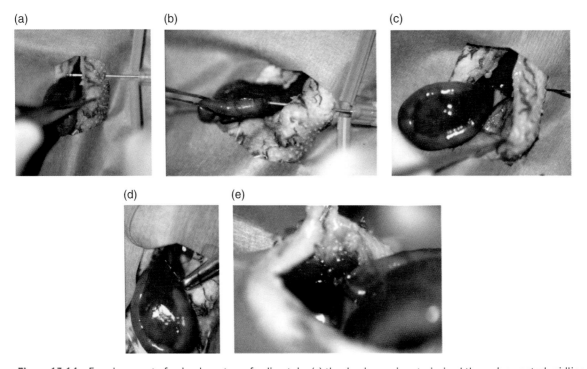

Figure 13.14 For placement of a duodenostomy feeding tube (a) the duodenum is exteriorized through a ventral midline incision. Pass a through-the-needle catheter through the left body wall. (b) With the needle still through the body wall, insert the needle into the descending loop of the duodenum. (c) Advance the catheter through the needle and into the ascending loop 4–6 cm. Withdraw the needle from the intestine and body wall. (d) Place two sutures between the coelomic lining inside the body wall and the intestine. (e) This creates a temporary pexy between the duodenum and body wall to minimize leakage until a seal forms.

(a)　(b)

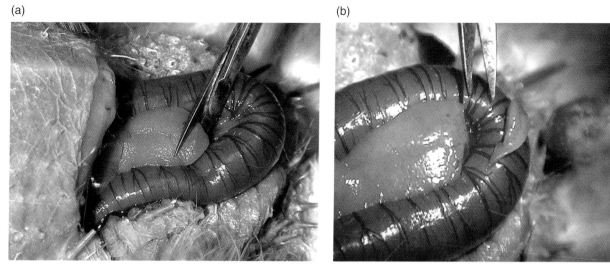

Figure 13.15 Pancreatic biopsy of the caudal edge of the ventral lobe. This section of pancreas can be removed with minimal hemorrhage. (a) Obtaining a pancreatic biopsy of the ventral lobe of the pancreas, (b) Ventral pancreatic lobe biopsy with minimal hemorrhage.

biopsy forceps to collect the liver samples. There is often minor bleeding that is generally self-limiting. For a coeliotomy, traditional methods can be used to obtain biopsies. The coelom can be approached through a ventral midline incision or an incision caudal to the last ribs on either side.

Pancreatic Biopsy

The avian pancreas consists of three lobes. Biopsies can be obtained endoscopically or through a ventral midline celiotomy. After performing a ventral midline celiotomy, identify and carefully exteriorize the duodenal loop (Figure 13.15). This exposes the pancreas within the loop for examination. Any visible or palpable lesions can be biopsied. For diffuse pancreatic disease, the caudal edge of the ventral lobe of the pancreas can be biopsied. Carefully dissect and reflect the pancreas from the duodenal loop to identify the vessels to the pancreas. Biopsy the ventral lobe using a suture fracture technique (Doneley 2011b). Alternatively, place a hemostatic clip proximal to the caudal extent of the pancreas to control hemorrhage, and then transect the piece of pancreas distal to the clip.

Postoperative Management

It is critical to monitor avian patients in the immediate postoperative period including monitoring and supporting body temperature and perfusion parameters. Providing analgesia is also an important component of postoperative care (Hawkins and Paul-Murphy 2011). Signs of pain include abnormal body positions, tucked appearance, aggression, vocalization, reluctance to move or stand, pronounced fear, and self-mutilation. Patients should be placed in a quiet area, but easily visible for proper monitoring.

References

Adamcak, A., Hess, R., and Quesenberry, K.E. (2000). Intestinal string foreign body in an adult umbrella cockatoo (*Cacatua alba*). *Journal of Avian Medicine and Surgery* 14 (4): 257–263.

Antinoff, N. (2000). Treatment of a cloacal papilloma by mucosal stripping in an Amazon parrot. *Proceeding Conference of the Association of Avian Veterinarians*, pp. 97–100.

Bennett, R.A. (1994). Techniques in avian thoracoabdominal surgery. *Association of Avian Veterinarians Core Seminar Proceedings*, pp. 45–57.

Bonda, M. (1998). Western blot immunoassay and immunohistology supporting a papillomavirus as the etiology of a cloacal papilloma/adenomatous polyp in a hyacinth macaw. *Proceeding Conference of the Association of Avian Veterinarians*, pp. 49–54.

Briscoe, J. and Bennett, R.A. (2011). Use of a duodenal serosal patch in the repair of a colon rupture in a female Solomon Island eclectus parrot. *Journal of the American Veterinary Medical Association* 238 (7): 922–926.

Coles, B. (1997). Surgery. In: *Essentials of Avian Medicine & Surgery*, 3e (ed. B.H. Coles), 157–158. London: Blackwell Publishing.

Degernes, L., Wolf, K., Zombeck, D. et al. (2012). Ventricular diverticula formation in captive parakeet auklets (*Aethia psittacula*) secondary to foreign body ingestion. *Journal of Zoo and Wildlife Medicine* 43: 889–897.

Doneley, B. (2011a). Clinical anatomy and physiology. In: *Avian Medicine and Surgery in Practice*, 1e (ed. B. Doneley), 16–19. London: Manson Publishing Ltd.

Doneley, B. (2011b). Surgery. In: *Avian Medicine and Surgery in Practice*, 1e (ed. B. Doneley), 262–263. London: Manson Publishing Ltd.

Duke, G. (1986). Alimentary canal: anatomy, regulation of feeding and motility. In: *Avian Physiology*, 4e (ed. P.D. Sturkie), 269–301. New York: Springer-Verlag.

Dvorak, L., Bennett, R.A., and Cranor, K. (1998). Cloacotomy for excision of cloacal papillomas in Catalina macaw. *Journal of Avian Medicine and Surgery* 12 (1): 11–15.

Ferrell, S., Werner, J., and Kyles, A. (2003). Evaluation of a collagen patch as a method of enhancing ventriculotomy healing in Japanese quail (*Coturnix coturnix japonica*). *Veterinary Surgery* 32: 103–112.

Forbes, N.A. (2002). Avian gastrointestinal surgery. *Seminars in Avian and Exotic Pet Medicine* 11 (4): 196–207.

Fowler, M. (1991). Comparative clinical anatomy of ratites. *Journal of Zoo and Wildlife Medicine* 22: 204–227.

Gibbons, P.M., Busch, M.D., Tell, L.A. et al. (2002). Internal papillomatosis with intrahepatic cholangiocarcinoma and gastrointestinal adenocarcinoma in a peach-fronted conure (*Aratinga aurea*). *Avian Diseases* 46 (4): 1062–1069.

Goring, R.L., Goldman, A., Kaufman, K.J. et al. (1986). Needle catheter duodenostomy: a technique for duodenal alimentation of birds. *Journal of the American Veterinary Medical Association* 189 (9): 1017–1019.

Hawkins, M.G. and Paul-Murphy, J. (2011). Avian analgesia. In: *Veterinary Clinics: Exotic Animal Practice*, vol. 14 (ed. J. Paul-Murphy), 61–80. Philadelphia, PA: Elsevier.

Hoefer, H. (1997). Diseases of the gastrointestinal tract. In: *Avian Medicine and Surgery*, 1e (eds. A.B. Altman, S.L. Clubb, G.M. Dorrestein and K.E. Quesenberry), 419–453. Philadelphia, PA: WB Saunders.

Hoefer, H. and Levitan, D. (2013). Perforating foreign body in the ventriculus of an umbrella cockatoo (*Cacatua alba*). *Journal of Avian Medicine and Surgery* 27: 128–135.

Ingram, I. (1990). Proventricular foreign body mimicking proventricular dilatation in an umbrella cockatoo.

Proceeding Conference of the Association of Avian Veterinarians, pp. 314–315.

János, G., Marosán, M., Kozma, A. et al. (2011). Solitary adenoma in the proventriculus of a budgerigar (*Melopsittacus undulatus*) diagnosed by immunochemistry - short communication. *Acta Veterinaria Hungarica* 59 (4): 439–444.

King, A. and McLelland, J. (1984). External anatomy. In: *Birds: Their Structure and Function*, 1e (eds. A.S. King and J. McLelland), 97. Philadelphia, PA: Bailliere-Tindall.

Leach, M.W., Paul-Murphy, J., and Lowenstine, L.J. (1989). Three cases of gastric neoplasia in psittacines. *Avian Diseases* 33 (1): 204–210.

Legler, M., Kothe, R., Rautenschlein, S. et al. (2008). Detection of psittacid herpesvirus 1 in Amazon parrots with cloacal papilloma (internal papillomatosis of parrots, IPP) in an aviary of different psittacine species. *Deutsche Tierärztliche Wochenschrift* 115 (12): 461–470.

Lumeij, J. (1994a). Gastroenterology. In: *Avian Medicine: Principles and Application*, 1e (eds. B.W. Ritchie, G.J. Harrison and L.R. Harrison), 482–521. Lake Worth, FL: Winger's Publishing Inc.

Lumeij, J. (1994b). Gastroenterology. In: *Avian Medicine: Principles and Application*, 1e (eds. B. Ritchie, G. Harrison and L. Harrison), 509–512. Lake Worth, FL: Wingers Publishing Inc.

Maluenda, A.C., Casagrande, R.A., Kanamura, C.T. et al. (2010). Rhabdomyosarcoma in a yellow-headed caracara (*Milvago chimachima*). *Avian Diseases* 54 (2): 951–954.

Mison, M., Mehler, S., Echols, M.S. et al. (2016). Approaches to the coelom and selected procedures. In: *Current Therapy in Avian Medicine and Surgery*, 1e (ed. B. Speer), 638–645. St. Louis, MO: Elsevier.

Orosz, S. (1997a). The gastrointestinal system. In: *Avian Medicine and Surgery*, 1e (eds. H.L. Hoefer, S. Orosz and G.M. Dorrestein), 412–291. Philadelphia, PA: W.B. Saunders Company.

Orosz, S. (1997b). Urogenital disorders. In: *Avian Medicine and Surgery*, 1e (eds. H.L. Hoefer, S. Orosz and G.M. Dorrestein), 620–622. Philadelphia, PA: W.B. Saunders Company.

Quesenberry, K.E. (1989). Nutritional support of the avian patient. *Proceeding Conference of the Association of Avian Veterinarians*, pp. 11–19.

Radlinsky, M.G., Carpenter, J.W., Mison, M.B. et al. (2004). Colonic entrapment after cloacopexy in two psittacine birds. *Journal of Avian Medicine and Surgery* 18 (3): 175–182.

Ramsay, E. (1991). Cryosurgery for papillomas. *Journal of the Association of Avian Veterinarians* 5 (2): 73.

Schmidt, R.E., Reavill, D.R., and Phalen, D.N. (2003). Integument. In: *Pathology of Pet and Aviary Birds*, 1e, 184. Ames, IA: Iowa State Press.

Schmidt, V., Philipp, H.C., Thielebein, J. et al. (2012). Malignant lymphoma of T-cell origin in a Humboldt penguin (*Spheniscus humboldti*) and a pink-backed pelican (*Pelecanus rufescens*). *Journal of Avian Medicine and Surgery* 26 (2): 101–106.

Simova-Curd, S., Foldenauer, U., Guerrero, T. et al. (2013). Comparison of ventriculotomy closure with and without a coelomic fat patch in Japanese quail (*Coturnix coturnix japonica*). *Journal of Avian Medicine and Surgery* 27 (1): 7–13.

Sladakovic, I., Ellis, A.E., and Divers, S.J. (2017). Evaluation of gastroscopy and biopsy of the proventriculus and ventriculus in pigeons (*Columba livia*). *American Journal of Veterinary Research* 78 (1): 42–49.

Snyder, J. and Treating, P. (2014). Pathology in practice. Adenocarcinoma of the proventriculus with liver metastasis and marked, diffuse chronic-active proventriculitis and ventriculitis with moderate *M.*

ornithogaster infection in a budgerigar. *Journal of the American Veterinary Medical Association* 244 (6): 667–669.

Speer, B. (1998). Chronic partial proventricular obstruction caused by multiple gastrointestinal foreign bodies in a juvenile umbrella cockatoo (*Cacatua alba*). *Journal of Avian Medicine and Surgery* 12 (4): 271–275.

Styles, D. (2004). Psittacid herpesviruses associated with mucosal papillomas in neotropical parrots. *Virology* 325 (1): 24–35.

Yonemaru, K., Sakai, H., Asaoka, Y. et al. (2004). Proventricular adenocarcinoma in a Humboldt penguin (*Spheniscus humboldti*) and a great horned owl (*Bubo virginianus*); identification of origin by mucin histochemistry. *Avian Pathology* 33 (1): 77–81.

van Zeeland, Y.R., Schoemaker, N.J., and van Sluijs, F.J. (2014). Incisional colopexy for treatment of chronic, recurrent colocloacal prolapse in a sulphur-crested cockatoo (*Cacatua galerita*). *Veterinary Surgery* 43 (7): 882–887.

14

Surgery of the Avian Respiratory System and Cranial Coelom

Geoffrey W. Pye

Surgery of the Upper Respiratory Tract

Choanal Atresia Correction

Choanal atresia is a common hereditary disorder seen in African grey parrots (*Psittacus erithacus*) and has also been reported in an umbrella cockatoo (*Cacatua alba*) (Greenacre et al. 1993). Surgical correction of choanal atresia using temporary stents has been described by Harris (1999). Using a 1/8 or 7/64 in. Steinmann pin, hand drill via each naris through the nasal conchae to create a choanal communication between the oral and nasal cavities (Figure 14.1). Using a Steinmann pin reduces hemorrhage compared to a scalpel blade when creating a choanal opening. The pin pushes vessels aside while a blade cuts through them; fatal hemorrhage may occur if a blade is used. Pass each end of a trimmed 8 fr red rubber catheter through a different naris and nasal conchae down through the new choanal opening and out the mouth. The middle of the tube passes across the cere. Placing the catheter helps control any hemorrhage that occurs when creating the choanal communication. At each naris, cut small openings in the tubing to allow mucus to drain. Tie the ends of the tube behind the head and place a chin strap to prevent the tube from slipping over the top of the head. The commissures are soft and will not cut the tube when the bird is eating. With birds that may pull and break the tubing with their feet, cut the catheter tubing near the level of the newly created choanal opening inside the mouth and suture the ends together. Since the tube does not exit the mouth, it is more difficult for the bird to remove it. Leave the tube in place for four to six weeks to allow the formation of a permanent fistula between the nasal and oral cavities. Following removal of the tubes, flush saline through the nares to ensure the communication is patent. Perform twice daily nasal saline flushes for 7–10 days after tube removal to avoid occlusion of the fistula by a buildup of mucus. Closure of the choana can occur following correction with this method. The bigger the connection and the longer the tube is left in place allowing for scar tissue maturation, the better the chances the opening will not close due to contracture.

Formation of a permanent fistula can be performed by surgical removal of tissue in the region of the choanal atresia. When this was attempted without attention to hemostasis, fatal hemorrhage occurred leading to the development of the abovementioned technique. In patients where the new opening closes, consider creating a relatively larger connection surgically. This tissue is highly vascular and so the surgeon must be prepared to control the hemorrhage. Laser ablation of the tissue to create a communication has been successful. Ablate the membrane back to the extent of the nasal bones. If needed, use rongeurs to remove bone to enlarge the opening. Packing the hole and leaving this in overnight can help control hemorrhage.

Sinusotomy

Chronic sinusitis is a common problem in psittacines and can result from the presence of a mass (e.g. granuloma, polyp, or mucocele) (Pye et al. 2000). In these cases, effective resolution relies on removal of the inciting cause. The anatomy of the avian infraorbital sinus is complex with its many diverticula and chambers (Figure 14.2). Magnetic resonance or computed tomography imaging can be used to localize the mass and facilitate surgical planning (Figure 14.3) (Pye et al. 2000).

Approach to the Rostral Diverticulum and Maxillary Chamber

Using a pneumatic bone bur, create an opening in the lateral wall of the upper beak as close to the location of the mass as possible based on the imaging (Figure 14.4). For

Surgery of Exotic Animals, First Edition. Edited by R. Avery Bennett and Geoffrey W. Pye.
© 2022 John Wiley & Sons, Inc. Published 2022 by John Wiley & Sons, Inc.

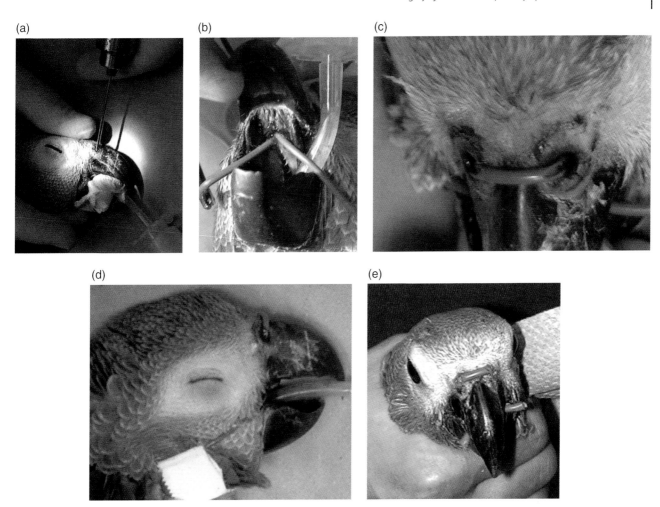

Figure 14.1 Correction of choanal atresia in an African grey parrot (*Psittacus erithacus*): (a) Using a 1/8 inch Steinmann pin, create a communication between the naris and choana into the oral cavity. (b) Pass an 8 fr red rubber catheter as a stent from the nares through the newly created opening in the choana. (c) The midpoint of an 8 fr red rubber catheter passes across the cere, and small openings are made in the tube to allow mucus to drain from the nares. (d) After placement of an 8 fr red rubber catheter, tie the ends behind the head and place a tape chin strap to avoid the catheter slipping over the top of the head. (e) With birds that may pull or break the tubing with their feet, cut the catheter and suture the ends together.

lesions within the beak, curette out the rostral diverticulum. For lesions within the maxillary chamber, remove the septum between the left and right chambers and create an opening in the ventral aspect of the maxillary chamber to allow fluid to drain into the pharynx. For closure, cover the window in the beak with mesh and acrylic (Figure 14.5). The defect will granulate in and the mesh and acrylic will lift off. Ultimately, epithelium and keratin will form as the beak defect grows out. Instill 0.05% chlorhexidine solution or saline into the nares twice daily for 7–10 days. If the lesion is bacterial or fungal, instill appropriate antimicrobial medications into the nares. Fluids instilled into the infraorbital sinus eventually drain through the choana into the pharynx.

Approach to the Preorbital Diverticulum

Make a skin incision caudal to the beak-skull articulation. Using a pneumatic bone bur, create a window in the frontal bone overlying the preorbital diverticulum (Figure 14.6). Curette the lesion out, then place a drain into the diverticulum through an opening in the skin lateral to the incision. Close the skin using a Ford interlocking or simple continuous pattern. Flush the drain with 0.05% chlorhexidine solution or saline twice daily for 7–10 days.

Approach to the Infraorbital Diverticulum

Make a skin incision along the jugal bone and dissect dorsal to the bone to enter the infraorbital diverticulum. This

(a)

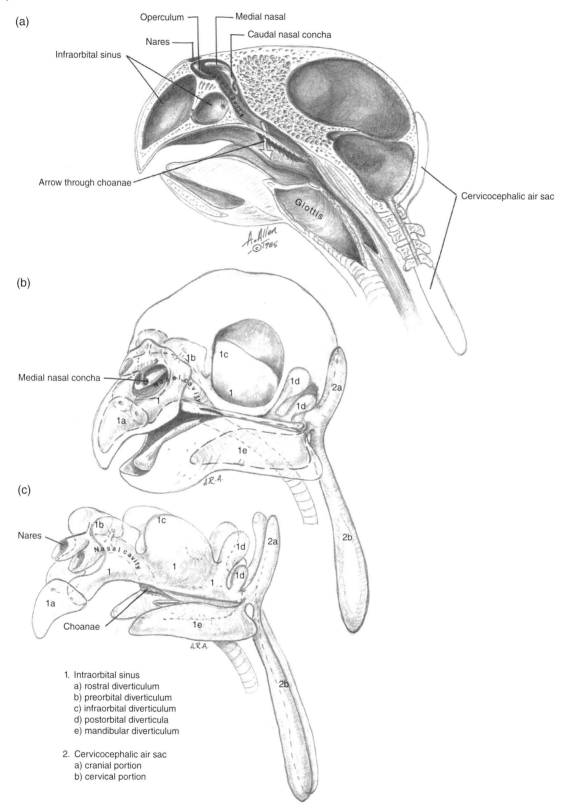

Operculum

Medial nasal

Caudal nasal concha

Nares

Infraorbital sinus

Arrow through choanae

Glottis

Cervicocephalic air sac

A. Allen ©1985

(b)

Medial nasal concha

Nasal cavity

1b

1c

1d

2a

1

1a

1d

1e

A.R.A.

(c)

Nares

Nasal cavity

1b

1c

1d

2a

2b

1

1

1a

1d

Choanae

1e

A.R.A.

2b

1. Intraorbital sinus
   a) rostral diverticulum
   b) preorbital diverticulum
   c) infraorbital diverticulum
   d) postorbital diverticula
   e) mandibular diverticulum

2. Cervicocephalic air sac
   a) cranial portion
   b) cervical portion

Figure 14.2 Knowledge of the anatomy and relationship of the infraorbital sinuses within the skull is essential for performing a sinusotomy. *Source:* McKibben and Harrison (1986). Reprinted with permission of Elsevier.

(a)

(b)

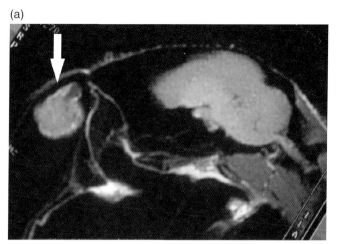
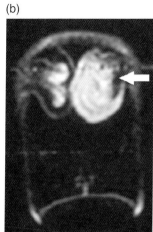

Figure 14.3 (a, b) Magnetic resonance imaging in a scarlet macaw (*Ara macao*) was used to localize a mass (arrow) within the rostral diverticulum of the infraorbital sinuses and facilitate surgical planning.

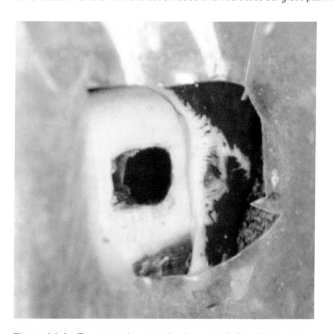

Figure 14.4 To access the mass in the rostral diverticulum (or one in the maxillary chambers) of the avian infraorbital sinuses, create a window in the lateral wall of the upper beak through the rhinotheca and bone into the sinus.

is the largest diverticulum and extends along the length of the jugal bone. Most lesions can be approached dorsal to the jugal bone though some ventral lesions may be more accessible ventral to the jugal bone. Following collection of samples and removal of the lesion, close the skin incision over the jugal bone using a Ford interlocking or simple continuous pattern. If indicated, place a drain to allow access for irrigation and topical administration of antimicrobials. Alternatively, treatments can be injected into the infraorbital diverticulum by inserting a needle dorsal to the jugal bone into the diverticulum.

Approach to the Suborbital, Postorbital, Preauditory, or Mandibular Diverticulum

Place a speculum to open the beak as wide as possible in order to improve the access to these diverticula. Make a skin incision ventral and parallel to the jugal arch. Bluntly dissect the soft tissues to gain access to the sinus. In some cases, the *muscularis adductor mandibulae externus* may need to be transected. Following curettage of the lesion, place a Penrose drain to facilitate drainage. Repair the muscle using three-loop-pulley sutures. Close the skin with a Ford interlocking or simple continuous pattern and anchor the drain by suturing it to the skin.

Following surgery for mass removal from the infraorbital sinuses, treat the bird with standard avian sinusitis therapies. Flush the infraorbital sinus with sterile saline or a 0.05% chlorhexidine solution. Submit the lesion for histopathology and microbial (bacterial and fungal) culture and sensitivity testing so that an appropriate antimicrobial can be used both systemically and locally by flushing the sinuses.

Surgery of the Lower Respiratory Tract

Air Sac Cannula Placement

An air sac cannula can be used to induce and maintain anesthesia during tracheal, syringeal, or oral surgery, or to provide an alternative airway in emergency cases of tracheal obstruction. A cannula can be placed in the clavicular, caudal thoracic, or abdominal air sac. To place a cannula in a caudal thoracic or abdominal air sac position, place the patient in lateral recumbency and extend the uppermost leg at the hip so the foot is next to the head (Figure 14.7). Palpate the depression immediately caudal

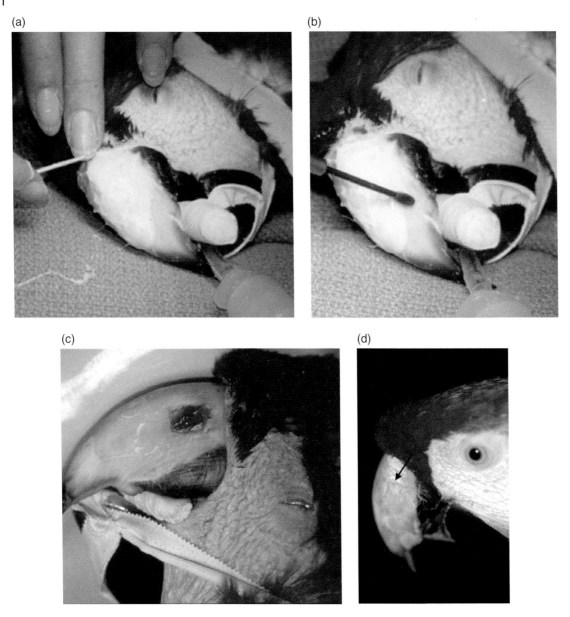

Figure 14.5 The defect in the beak was covered with a dental mesh that was then covered with acrylic (a). Smooth the surface with a bur (b). The defect fills with granulation tissue which is then converted to bone. Epithelium migrates under the patch and it falls off exposing the granulation tissue and the epithelium around the edges (c). Once the surface is completely covered with epithelium (d), the sinus has completely healed (arrow points to location of surgical defect).

to the last rib and ventral to the semitendinosus muscle (*m. flexor cruis medialis*). This depression is the placement point for the cannula. Alternatively, position the uppermost leg caudally and locate the cannula insertion point in the triangular-shaped depression caudal to the pectoral muscle, ventral to the synsacrum, and cranial to the muscle mass of the thigh (Figure 14.8). In psittacines, this entry site is usually between the seventh and eighth ribs.

In the palpable depression, make a small skin incision with a no. 11 scalpel blade. Using microhemostats bluntly penetrate the underlying muscle and air sac. Hold the

hemostats perpendicular to the body wall and use an index finger as a guard to prevent over-penetration (Figure 14.9). As the hemostats penetrate the muscle, followed by the air sac, two "pops" may be felt. Gently open the hemostat jaws sufficiently to allow of insertion the cannula into the air sac and then remove the hemostats. Flow of air through the cannula can be confirmed by using a BAAM (Beck Airway Airflow Monitor, Great Plains Ballistics, Lubbock, TX) or by holding a down feather against the opening. To secure the cannula, place tape tabs on the hub and suture the tabs to the skin. Maintain the cannula until the bird

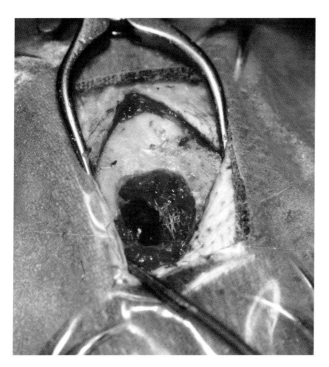

Figure 14.6 To access the preorbital diverticulum of the avian infraorbital sinuses, create a window in the midline of the frontal bone, rostral to the orbit.

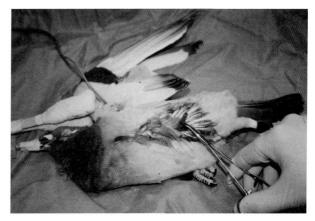

Figure 14.8 Leg caudal positioning of a pigeon (*Columba livia*) for air sac cannula placement in the caudal thoracic or cranial abdominal air sac.

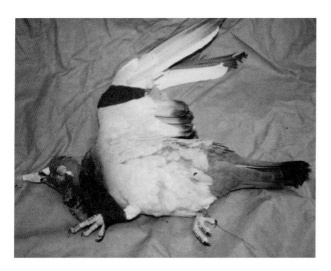

Figure 14.7 Leg cranial positioning of a pigeon (*Columba livia*) for air sac cannula placement in the caudal thoracic or cranial abdominal air sac.

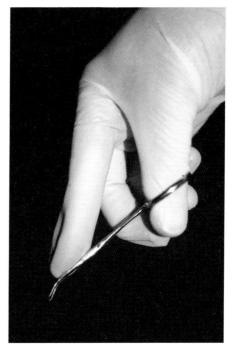

Figure 14.9 Hand position on hemostats to prevent overpenetration when creating an opening in the body wall for an air sac cannula.

breathes easily through the trachea. Test this by blocking the cannula. Remove or replace the cannula within five days of placement due to the risk of bacterial infection and the development of air sacculitis making the tube nonfunctional (Mitchell et al. 1999). Allow the wound to heal by second intention.

For cannula placement in the clavicular air sac, make a small ventral midline skin incision at the thoracic inlet. Reflect the crop to the right, bluntly penetrate the air sac, and insert the cannula. Secure it in place as described above.

Tracheotomy

Tracheotomy is indicated for removal of partial obstructions of either the trachea or syrinx when other methods (e.g. endoscopy, suction) fail. Place a cannula in a caudal air sac to allow for intermittent positive pressure ventilation and anesthesia during the tracheotomy. Correct positioning, magnification, and illumination are important for good visualization. Place the bird in dorsal recumbency, elevate the cranial portion of the body ~45–60°, and allow the head to hang down (Figure 14.10). This positioning aligns the trachea with the eyesight of the surgeon facilitating visualization deep within the trachea and thoracic inlet.

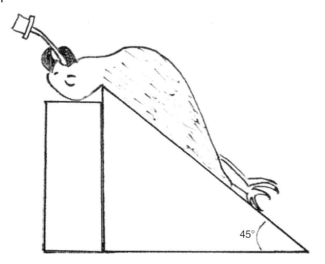

Figure 14.10 Positioning of a bird for tracheotomy to allow the best visualization of structures deep in the thoracic inlet. *Source:* Pye (2000b). Reprinted with permission of Elsevier.

Place an esophageal stethoscope or red rubber tube into the esophagus to allow easy identification during surgery.

With the bird's head toward the surgeon, incise the skin on the ventral midline from cranial to the crop to the keel in order to expose the thoracic inlet (Figure 14.11a). Gently reflect the crop to the right by bluntly dissecting it from the skin and surrounding tissues (Figure 14.11b). A stay retractor (Lone Star Veterinary Retractor System, Jorgensen Laboratories Inc., Loveland, CO) or a Heiss retractor can be used to improve visualization if needed. Identify the trachea and sternotracheal muscles. There are significant blood vessels between the muscle bellies that should be coagulated prior to transection of the sternotracheal muscles (Figure 14.11c). Birds do not have recurrent laryngeal nerves. Place stay sutures around the tracheal rings near the tracheotomy site to help with manipulation of the trachea (Figure 14.12a). Incise the ventral half of the annular ligament between the cartilage tracheal rings (Figure 14.12b). For obstructions in the cervical trachea, incise caudal to the foreign body or granuloma. Remove the foreign body or mass with microforceps or gently curette or excise from the tracheal lining if it is adhered (e.g. granuloma or neoplasia) (Figure 14.13).

For a foreign body or granuloma in the thoracic trachea or the syrinx, bluntly dissect through the interclavicular air sac. Perform a clavicular osteotomy to improve surgical access if needed. Use stay sutures in the trachea or pass a blunt hook caudal to the syrinx at its bifurcation and apply gentle traction to elevate the syrinx toward the surgeon (Figure 14.13). Take care as this can result in avulsion of the bronchi from the lung in Amazon parrots, small macaws, and smaller birds (Bennett and Harrison 1994). A left lateral approach to the syrinx can be considered as an option in these birds. Make an incision in the annular ligament three to five rings cranial to the syrinx as this will facilitate closure of the

tracheotomy. In small birds, the annular ligament may completely tear necessitating an anastomosis. Pass a microcurette or microforceps into the syrinx to remove the lesion. If indicated, use the opportunity to perform local topical treatment with an antimicrobial agent prior to closure of the trachea.

Close the trachea using a simple interrupted pattern. Pass the suture through the annular ligament to encircle one or two tracheal rings on each side of the incision (Figure 14.13). Preplace all the sutures prior to tying as this will make closure easier. Alternate encircling one ring or two rings for each suture so that the tension is not pulling on the one ligament; thereby reducing the risk of pulling off a tracheal ring. To decrease postsurgical tracheal stricture formation, tie the knots on the outside of the trachea and use a fine, monofilament, nonreactive, absorbable suture (e.g. 4-0 to 8-0 polydioxanone suture). There is no need to reattach the sternotracheal muscles or close the clavicular air sac. Close the skin using a Ford interlocking pattern.

Tracheal Resection and Anastomosis

Resection and anastomosis are indicated when partial tracheal obstruction results from stricture formation, a granuloma, neoplasia, localized tracheal collapse, or traumatic avulsion (Figure 14.14). In most avian species, a number of tracheal rings can be resected without creating undue tension following anastomosis; up to 9% of the trachea has been removed in a mallard duck (*Anas platyrhynchos*) (Guzman et al. 2007) and 15 total rings over two surgeries in a blue and gold macaw (*Ara ararauna*) (Jankowski et al. 2010). Place a cannula in a caudal air sac for maintenance of anesthesia during surgery and postoperative ventilation of the patient.

The surgical approach is the same as described for tracheotomy, though in long-necked birds a lateral approach can also be used for cranial tracheal lesions. For thoracic tracheal lesions, place stay sutures in the trachea caudal to the obstruction to prevent the transected caudal portion from disappearing into the cranial coelom. Transect and bluntly dissect away the sternotracheal muscles from the affected portion of the trachea. Incise the annular ligaments of the trachea circumferentially 360° using a no. 11 scalpel blade cranial and caudal to the obstruction. Multiple rings may need to be removed (Figure 14.15). Approximate the cut ends and preplace four to eight evenly spaced fine, monofilament, nonreactive, absorbable suture through the annular ligaments to include one to two craniad and caudad tracheal rings. Alternate encircling one or two rings with each suture to distribute the tension. To facilitate access to the sutures, tie the dorsal sutures first with the knots placed outside the lumen. There is no need to reattach the sternotracheal muscles. Close the skin incsion the same as for a tracheotomy. Remove the air sac cannula when the bird is breathing easily through the trachea. Stricture can occur at the site of the tracheal anastomosis, as early as 7–14 days, though it may take longer.

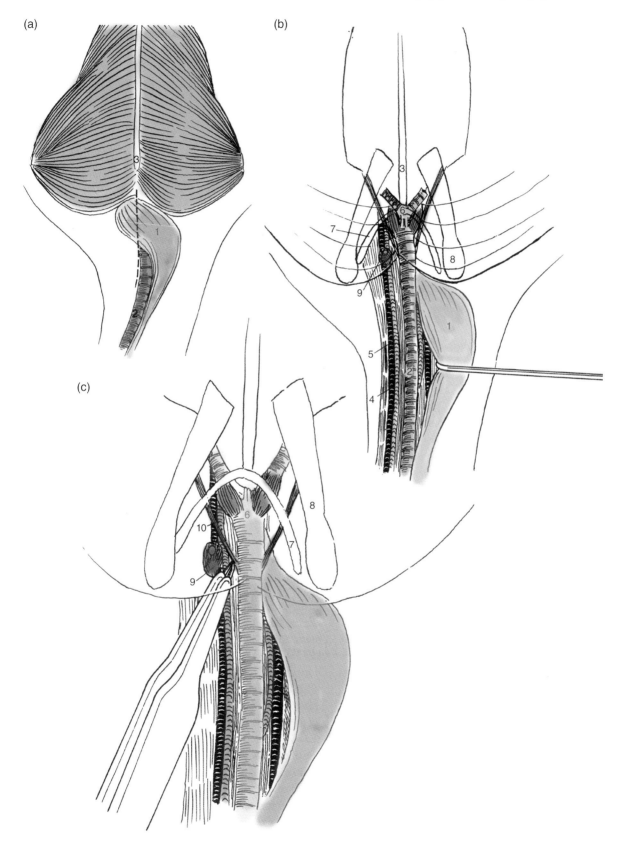

Figure 14.11 For an avian tracheostomy, (a) incise the skin on ventral midline over the crop (1). (b) Gently reflect the crop to the right by bluntly dissecting it from the skin and surrounding tissues to expose the trachea. (2) (c) Identify and coagulate the blood vessels associated with the sternotracheal muscles (10) prior to transection. (1) crop, (2) trachea, (3) sternum, (4) internal carotid artery, (5) jugular vein, (6) syrinx, (7) clavicle, (8) coracoid, (9) thyroid, (10) sternotracheal muscle, (11) esophagus, (12) primary bronchi, (13) pulmonary artery, and (14) aorta. *Source:* Ritchie et al. (1994).

(a)   (b)

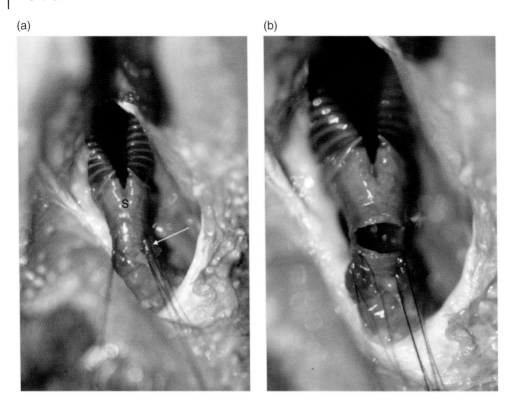

Figure 14.12 For an avian tracheotomy, (a) place stay sutures around the tracheal rings near the proposed tracheostomy site (arrow is pointing at the transected sternotrachealis muscle; S = syrinx) and (b) incise the ventral half of the annular ligament between the cartilage tracheal rings.

An alternative method for management of severe tracheal stenosis has been described in an eclectus parrot (*Eclectus roratus*) (Mejia-Fava et al. 2015). Multiple areas of stenosis were diagnosed in a 25-year-old parrot that responded poorly to endoscopic resection and repeated balloon dilation. Using fluoroscopic guidance, a 4-mm × 36-mm custom-made nitinol wire stent was placed into the trachea and corticosteroid nebulization with or without antibiotics and antifungals was used to treat recurrent bouts of increased respiratory effort. Discontinuation of corticosteroid treatment resulted in relapse within several days. The bird was euthanized 732 days after stent placement due to complications that may have been associated with the stent and/or corticosteroid use, including tracheitis and tracheal malacia.

Lateral Approach to the Syrinx

The lateral approach to the syrinx is used in small birds when traction on the syrinx or trachea may cause avulsion or when there is no other means by which to surgically approach it (Bennett and Harrison 1994). With the bird in right lateral recumbency, incise the skin along the dorsolateral margin of the pectoral muscles overlying the second and third ribs. Transect the attachment of the pectoral muscle to the ribs and reflect the muscle ventrally. Using bipolar forceps, coagulate the intercostal vessels (immediately cranial to each rib) and then remove a portion of each of the second and third ribs to expose the cranial portion of the lung. Using a moistened cotton-tipped applicator gently dissect and reflect this portion of the lung from its attachments. Gently dissect between the jugular vein, pulmonary artery, and branches of the subclavian artery to visualize the syrinx. Using microscissors, incise the syrinx at its junction with the left primary bronchus and remove the mass or foreign body. Do not attempt to close the syringeal incision as the tissues will tear easily; allow it to heal by second intention. Return the lung lobe to its normal position and do not replace the ribs. Pull the pectoral muscle over the defect in the rib cage and suture it in place. Close the skin using a Ford interlocking pattern. This is a very difficult procedure requiring magnification, illumination, and microinstrumentation that should only be used when all other methods have failed (Bennett and Harrison 1994).

Devocalization

Devocalization of birds is considered a cruel and unethical procedure. Attempting to approach the syrinx in psittacines using poultry devocalization techniques is unrewarding and in gallinaceous birds is associated with a high mortality rate (Harrison 1986; Altman 1997).

(a)

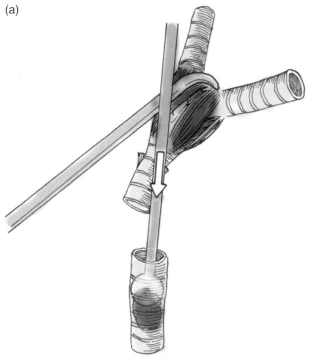

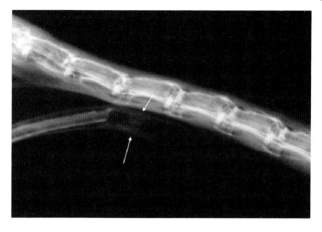

Figure 14.14 This crane had been intubated for anesthesia for a quarantine physical examination two-week prior to the onset of dyspnea. It appears that trauma from the end of the previous endotracheal tube, just aboard to the existing tube, resulted in stenosis (arrows show the stenotic region).

(b)

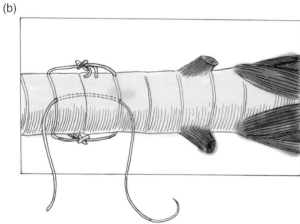

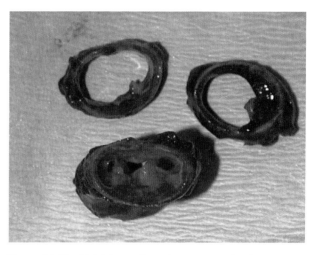

Figure 14.15 Multiple cartilage rings may need to be removed where a tracheal stenosis has formed.

Figure 14.13 (a) To remove a tracheal foreign body, gently remove the foreign body from the tracheal lumen. A blunt hook can be used to elevate the syrinx toward the surgeon if needed. (b) Close the tracheotomy with simple interrupted sutures passed through the annular ligament and encircling one or two tracheal rings on each side of the incision. *Source:* Ritchie et al. (1994).

Lung Biopsy and Partial Pneumonectomy

Endoscopy via a caudal thoracic air sac approach can be used to collect lung biopsies. Alternatively, a direct surgical approach may be used through the third intercostal space (Altman 1997). Incise the skin over the third intercostal space and then bluntly dissect the muscle between the ribs until the lung tissue is exposed. Place vascular clips to allow biopsy of a wedge-shaped piece of lung. For masses of the lung (e.g. fungal granuloma), a partial pneumonectomy can be performed (Bennett and Harrison 1994). Approach the lung through the caudal thoracic air sac or the intercostal space by removing a portion of one or more ribs. The latter approach is similar to that described for the lateral approach to the syrinx. Using moistened cotton-tipped applicators, gently separate the affected part of the lung from the ribs and surrounding structures. Place vascular clips on the viable part of the lung to prevent hemorrhage. Dissect the affected tissue away. If hemorrhage is noted (the avian lung is more vascular and the clotting mechanism less efficient than in mammals), place a piece of oxidized regenerated cellulose (Surgicel™, Johnson & Johnson Medical Inc., Arlington, TX) to aid in hemostasis.

Hyperinflation of the Cervicocephalic Air Sac

Hyperinflation of the cervicocephalic air sac may occur due to an occlusion (e.g. granuloma) to the ostium of the air sac (causing a one way valve effect) or trauma (Bennett and Harrison 1994; Levine 2005). Creation of a communication between the air sac and the skin may resolve this condition (Bennett and Harrison 1994). Make a large skin incision to deflate of the ballooned area and leave it to heal by second intention. The skin heals in three to six days and so the procedure may need to be repeated several times until the condition has completely resolved. Removing a piece of skin and air sac wall may prolong healing and thereby aid resolution of the hyperinflation. A more permanent communication can be created using a Teflon stent (McAllister Technical Services, Coeur d'Alene, ID) implanted in the skin (Harris 1991). The Teflon stent will likely become occluded, though it can take up to one year (R. Avery Bennett, personal communication).

A one-way valve can be implanted connecting the cervicocephalic air sac to the clavicular air sac (Bennett and Harrison 1994). Use a left lateral approach to the thoracic inlet. Place the valve in the hyperinflated air sac and direct it caudally along the esophagus and through the thoracic inlet into the clavicular air sac. To prevent migration, suture the tube to the longus coli muscles. There is no need to suture the air sac around the tube. Alternatively, a cervicocephalic-clavicular air sac two-way shunt can correct cervicocephalic air sac emphysema (Levine 2005). The two-way shunt is created by using the distal end section of a cuff-less small diameter endotracheal tube with an additional side-port created at the other end. Surgery for placement is similar to that of the one-way valve implantation, though in addition to the longus coli muscles anchoring, the tube is sutured to the clavicle and the crop. Muscle fascia and air sacs are closed around the tube using purse string sutures.

Surgery of the Cranial Coelom

Cranial Celiotomy

Cranial celiotomy (thoracotomy) in birds is an extremely challenging and aggressive surgery with likely mortality (Bennett 1999; Pye 2000a). The main indication for this surgery is the removal of masses from the cranial coelom. Place the bird placed in dorsal recumbency. Make a ven-

(a)

(b)

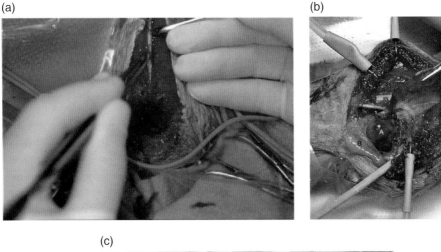

(c)

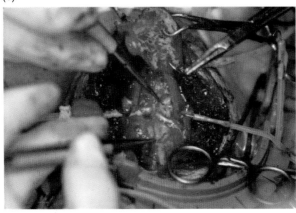

Figure 14.16 For an approach to the cranial coelom, (a) incise the skin over the keel and (b) bluntly dissect the pectoral muscles from both sides of the keel. The mass (A) is visible directly dorsal to the crop (B). (c) Following separation of the coracoids from the sternum and sternal and keel osteotomies, reflect the resulting wedge caudally without fully detaching it.

tral midline incision from the midcervical region to the caudal most aspect of the sternum (Figure 14.16a). Bluntly dissect free the crop and reflect it to the right. Dissect through the clavicular air sac and remove any fat from the thoracic inlet. Perform a midline osteotomy or subtotal ostectomy of the clavicular bones near their attachments to the coracoid bones. Incise the fascia overlying the keel and bluntly dissect the pectoral muscles from both sides of the keel, sternum, and clavicles (Figure 14.16b). Apply bone wax to the sternum to stem hemorrhage from any of the small vessels that were previously attached to the pectoral muscles. Use a stay retractor to retract the muscle and surrounding tissues. Locate the articulations between the coracoids and the sternum. Incise the joint capsules with a no. 11 scalpel blade. Separate the coracoids from the sternum using a Freer elevator. Make two osteotomies in the sternum to create a V-shaped piece and then a third in the keel to meet the point of the V. Expose the cranial coelom by reflecting the wedge caudally, if possible without totally detaching it from the rest of the sternum (Figure 14.16c). Cranial

coelomic masses may surround or incorporate the great vessels exiting the heart and so gently dissect to prevent fatal hemorrhage and blood pressure disturbances. Following removal of the mass, replace and reattach the wedge to the sternum and coracoid using nylon sutures passed through the bone (Figure 14.17a,b). Reattach the left and right pectoral muscles by suturing them to each other across the keel (Figure 14.17c). The clavicles are not replaced (or repaired if an osteotomy is performed). Close the skin using a Ford interlocking pattern.

This approach has been used in three cases of cranial coelom masses (a cockatiel [*Nymphicus hollandicus*] with a carcinoma of air sac origin, an umbrella cockatoo [*C. alba*] with an undifferentiated mesenchymal tumor, and a black-bellied whistling duck [*Dendrocygna autumnalis*] with a cystadenocarcinoma suspected of being air sac origin). In all three cases, this approach provided excellent access to the cranial coelom and the coelomic masses. Unfortunately, the first two birds had masses that involved the great vessels of the heart and died during surgery due to excessive hemorrhage and/or blood

(a)　　　　　　　　　　　　　　　　　　　　(b)

(c)

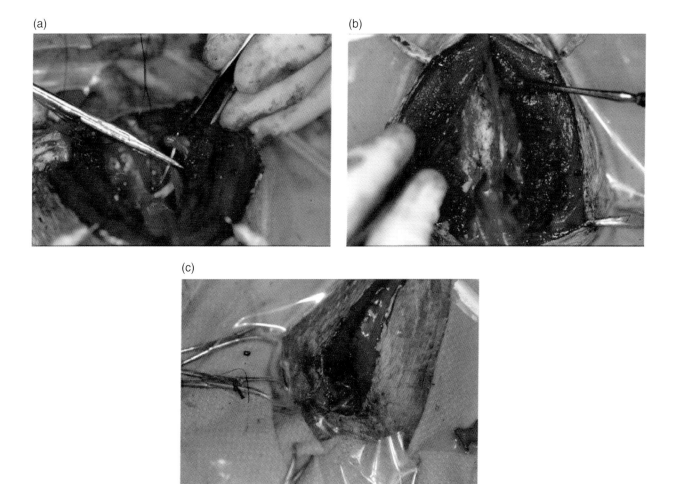

Figure 14.17　To close the cranial coelom, reattach the wedge, by (a) passing suture through the coracoid bone and the sternum to reestablish the joint as well as (b) the sternum caudally, followed by suturing the left and right pectoral muscles to each other across the keel (c).

pressure disturbances. The third bird went into cardiac arrest after successful removal of the mass, but during the closure of the cranial coelomic cavity. It is currently unknown what effect this aggressive surgery would have on the birds' ability to respire normally after surgery. Preemptive multimodal analgesia is a must. This approach could also be used for cardiac surgery.

Bifid Sternum Surgical Management

The surgical management of bifid (cleft) sternum has been reported in African grey parrots and an orange-winged Amazon (*Amazona amazonica*) (Figure 14.18) (Bennett and Gilson 1999; Bürkle and Wüst 2010). Bifid sternum results from a failure of the normal development of the sternum where normally two separate mesenchymal bands arise from each side of the body and migrate toward the midline and fuse from cranial to caudal (Bennett and Gilson 1999). In reported cases in birds, closure of the defect was not possible, but transposition of the pectoral muscles was performed to provide protection to the heart. Make a ventral midline incision from the cranial apex of the sternum to 2 cm caudal to the defect. The heart and liver will be evident directly beneath the skin and so take care when elevating the skin from the heart (Figure 14.19a). If needed, remove portions of the keel to allow transposition of the pectoral muscles over the defect (Figure 14.19b). Elevate the pectoral muscles from the sternum and ribs and then suture them together along the midline in a simple interrupted pattern (Figure 14.19c). Do not attempt to appose the two halves of the sternum. Close the skin over the muscle using a Ford interlocking pattern. Flight does not appear to be compromised by this surgery (Bürkle and Wüst 2010).

In young birds, correction of bifid sternum may be performed by suturing the two halves of the sternum together (Michelle Curtis, personal communication). Incise the skin over the keel of one half of the sternum to prevent accidental trauma to the exposed heart. Carefully dissect the skin from the heart. Once the heart is freed, suture the two halves of the sternum together. At this young age, the cartilaginous halves of the sternum will pull together easily.

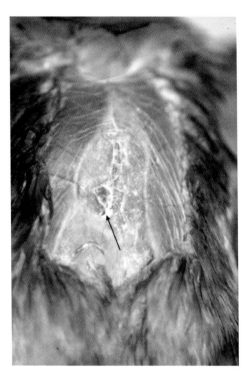

Figure 14.18 Bifid sternum in an African grey parrot (*Psittacus erithacus*). The heart is directly under the skin where there is a superficial lesion (arrow).

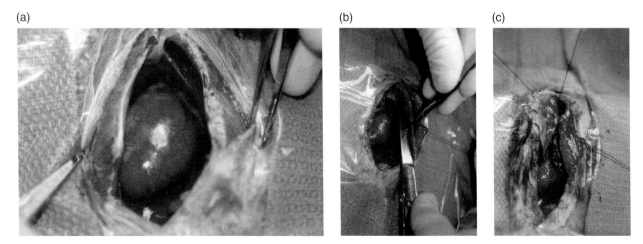

Figure 14.19 To surgically correct bifid sternum in a bird, (a) carefully incise the skin and elevate it from the pectoral muscles, keel, and heart, (b) if needed, remove portions of the keel, and (c) elevate the pectoral muscles from the sternum and ribs so they can be sutured together. Do not attempt to oppose the two halves of the sternum.

References

Altman, R.B., Chubb, S.L., Dorrestein, G.M. and Quesenberry, K. (1997). Soft tissue surgical procedures. In: *Avian Medicine and Surgery* (eds. R.B. Altman et al.), 704–732. Philadelphia, PA: WB Saunders Co.

Bennett, R.A. (1999). Approach to the thoracic cavity of birds. *Exotic DVM* 1: 55–58.

Bennett, R.A. and Gilson, S.D. (1999). Surgical management of bifid sternum in two African grey parrots. *Journal of the American Veterinary Medical Association* 214: 372–374.

Bennett, R.A. and Harrison, G.J. (1994). Soft tissue surgery. In: *Avian Medicine: Principles and Application* (eds. B.W. Ritchie et al.), 1096–1136. Lake Worth, FL: Wingers Publishing Inc.

Bürkle, M. and Wüst, E. (2010). Bifid sternum in an African grey (*Psittacus erithacus*) and an orange-winged Amazon (*Amazona amazonica*). *Proceedings of the Association of Avian Veterinarians*, p. 331.

Greenacre, C.B. et al. (1993). Choanal atresia in an African grey parrot (*Psittacus erithacus erithacus*) and an umbrella cockatoo (*Cacatua alba*). *Journal of the Association of Avian Veterinarians* 7: 19–22.

Guzman, D.S. et al. (2007). Tracheal resection and anastomosis in a mallard duck (*Anas platyrhynchos*) with traumatic segmental tracheal collapse. *Journal of Avian Medicine and Surgery* 21: 150–157.

Harris, J.M. (1991). Teflon dermal stent for the correction of subcutaneous emphysema. *Proceedings of the Association of Avian Veterinarians*, pp. 20–21.

Harris, D. (1999). Resolution of choanal atresia in African grey parrots. *Exotic DVM* 1: 13–17.

Harrison, G.J. (1986). Selected surgical procedures. In: *Clinical Medicine and Surgery* (eds. G.J. Harrison and L.R. Harrison), 577–595. Philadelphia, PA: WB Saunders Co.

Jankowski, G. et al. (2010). Multiple tracheal resections and anastomoses in a blue and gold macaw (*Ara ararauna*). *Journal of Avian Medicine and Surgery* 24: 322–329.

Levine, B. (2005). Cervicocephalic-clavicular air sac shunts to correct cervicocephalic air sac emphysema. *Proceedings of the Annual Conference of the Association of Avian Veterinarians*.

McKibben, J.S. and Harrison, G.J. (1986). Clinical anatomy with the emphasis on the Amazon parrot. In: *Clinical Avian Medicine and Surgery* (eds. G.J. Harrison and L.R. Harrison), 47. Philadelphia, PA: W.B. Saunders.

Mejia-Fava, J. et al. (2015). Use of a nitinol wire stent for management of severe tracheal stenosis in an eclectus parrot (*Eclectus roratus*). *Journal of Avian Medicine and Surgery* 29: 238–249.

Mitchell, J. et al. (1999). Air sacculitis associated with the placement of an air breathing tube. *Proceedings of the Association of Avian Veterinarians*, pp. 145–146.

Pye, G.W. (2000a). Surgery of the avian respiratory system. *Veterinary Clinics of North America: Exotic Animal* 3: 693–713.

Pye, G.W. (2000b). Surgery of the avian respiratory system. *The Veterinary Clinics of North America Exotic Animal Practice* 3: 704.

Pye, G.W. et al. (2000). Magnetic resonance imaging in psittacines with chronic sinusitis. *Journal of Avian Medicine and Surgery* 14: 243–256.

Ritchie, B.W., Harrison, G.J., and Harrison, L.R. (1994). *Avian Medicine: Principles and Application*, 1108. Lake Worth, FL: Wingers Publishing, Inc.

15

Minimally Invasive Surgery Techniques in Exotic Animals

Stephen J. Mehler and R. Avery Bennett

Introduction

Minimally invasive diagnostic and surgical procedures in veterinary medicine are currently being provided at many academic institutions and private practices around the world. Laparoscopy, thoracoscopy, and endoscopy procedures are currently a growing part of exotic animal practice and their increased usage is inevitable. This chapter will summarize the principles and instrumentation used during laparoscopy and thoracoscopy, as well as the common indications and contraindications in exotic animal practice.

Laparoscopy and thoracoscopy are defined as the minimally invasive exploration of the abdominal, thoracic, and coelomic cavity, and their organs with a rigid endoscope (Monnet and Twedt 2003; McCarthy and Monnet 2005). Both are indicated for many diagnostic and surgical procedures. Currently, diagnostic indications with examination and biopsy of viscera are the most common uses of these techniques; however, therapeutic interventions are a rapidly growing set of indications for laparoscopy and thoracoscopy. Specimens acquired by endoscopic biopsy are generally superior to percutaneous biopsy methods due to direct visualization of the structure of interest and the relatively larger sample size that can be obtained. In addition, due to the magnification and intense lighting provided by the endoscope, small lesions not easily seen by other diagnostic methods such as ultrasound are more apparent. For these reasons, laparoscopy and thoracoscopy are particularly useful in exotics. Laparoscopy and thoracoscopy have been used to perform a variety of surgical procedures in animals. The number and type of procedures that can be performed by minimally invasive techniques in exotic animals are only limited by imagination, innovation, and instrumentation.

Instrumentation

The basic equipment includes a rigid endoscope, a video camera, a high definition monitor, a light source, a light cable, a tower (cart), trocar-cannula units, a high flow CO_2 insufflator, and various forceps and accessory instruments (Chamness 2005). The most commonly used endoscope in small animal laparoscopy and thoracoscopy is a 5 mm zero degree rigid endoscope; however, smaller scopes are recommended for most birds, small reptiles, rabbits, ferrets, and guinea pigs and other rodents. Rigid scopes of 1.9 or 2.7 mm diameter and 0° or 30° lenses are ideal for exotic pets (Taylor 2006; Divers 2010a; Mehler 2011). The 1.9 and 2.7 mm scopes are often used with a 3.5 mm sheath that also has two-valved connections for ingress and egress of fluid or gas as well as an instrument channel. A zero-degree scope provides the surgeon with a visual field that is in line with the true field. This type of endoscope makes orientation and manipulation of instruments easier. It also maximizes light transmission when compared to endoscopes with an offset viewing angle. The most common angled endoscope used is 30°. This type of endoscope enables visualization over or under organs and widens the area of visualization. Regardless of type, the endoscope must be attached to a high-quality cool light source via a light cable. A high-intensity xenon light source is recommended because it gives the truest organ colors. Halogen is less expensive and still provides adequate illumination of body cavities. At the end of the eyepiece of the endoscope, a video camera unit is connected to a high-definition monitor. This projects the image at the tip of the endoscope onto a video monitor located across from the surgeon. The camera can be sterilized using low-temperature hydrogen peroxide gas plasma or it can be placed into a plastic disposable sterile camera bag.

A CO_2 insufflator is used to create the pneumoperitoneum required to perform laparoscopy in small mammals. It is usually not necessary for thoracoscopy in mammals or for coelioscopy in birds and reptiles. In reptiles, insufflation improves visualization in some cases. In birds, coelom portals usually enter an air sac so the use of CO_2 is contraindicated. Most CO_2 insufflating systems have a standard means of delivering CO_2, an adjustable flow rate, and a constant or intermittent pressure reading. It is recommended to keep intra-abdominal pressure (IAP) between 8 and 15 mmHg (Monnet and Twedt 2003; McCarthy and Monnet 2005; Twedt and Monnet 2005; Chamness 2005). Insufflate to the lowest pressure that will allow the procedure to be performed efficiently and safely. Generally, this results in a pressure of about 8–12 mmHg in small mammals and 5–8 mmHg in reptiles (Divers 2010a,b,c; Mehler 2011; Proença and Divers 2015; Sladakovic and Divers 2016).

Trocar-cannula units are used to gain access to the body cavity, provide a means to insufflate with gas, and act as portals for the endoscope and accessory instruments. Remove the trocar after access is made into the cavity and place an endoscope or instrument into the remaining cannula. The cannula maintains access into the cavity and prevents unnecessary trauma to the body wall from repeated removal and insertion of instruments. During procedures, they also protect the scope against bending as the surgeon attempts to manipulate the scope into position. These units come with sharp or blunt trocars and the diameter corresponds to the size of the instruments to be used. There are a variety of types of cannulae subdivided into closed and open. Closed cannulae have valves within the tube that prevent leakage of gas when instruments are being switched out and are used for laparoscopy. Open cannulae do not have valves and can be used for laparoscopy, but leakage of the CO_2 can prolong the procedure time since it is necessary to stop and reinsufflate periodically. They are most commonly used for thoracoscopy and coelioscopy when there is no need for insufflation. Cannulae can also be rigid or soft. Rigid cannulae are the most commonly used for laparoscopy and provide protection to the endoscope. Soft cannulae are generally used during thoracoscopy. Threaded cannulae can be helpful during laparoscopic and thoracoscopic procedures because they engage the soft tissues more securely and are less likely to slip out of the body cavity like the traditional "top heavy" cannulae.

Various accessory instruments are required depending on the procedure to be performed. A blunt-tipped palpation probe is essential for moving and palpating organs. Most probes have centimeter markings etched on them so the surgeon can estimate the size of organs and lesions. For biopsies, oval biopsy cup forceps (liver, spleen, pleura,

lymph nodes, and masses), cup biopsy forceps (pancreas), and core biopsy needles (kidney, deep tissue) are recommended. Various grasping forceps, retractors, needle drivers, and scissors are other essential instruments. Clip applicators and stapling devices are generally 5 or 10 mm in diameter requiring corresponding cannulae. Stapling equipment designed specifically for minimally invasive surgery (MIS) is available. Suction and irrigation devices are also useful in MIS to be utilized for dissection of tissues as well as local irrigation of tissues, and to remove blood or other fluid from the surgical site.

The basic principles of laparoscopy and thoracoscopy involve gaining access to a cavity through small incisions, creating a workspace, and maneuvering within that cavity using instruments activated extracorporeally. Placement of endoscope and instrument portals varies with each procedure. In general, the endoscope is placed in direct line with the organ of interest, and the instrument portals are placed to each side of the endoscope to create a triangle that points toward the organ of interest (Figure 15.1). Placement of instruments too close to the area of interest can severely limit maneuverability within the cavity and prohibit completion of the procedure.

Most instruments have a capability for monopolar electrosurgery at their tip. Electrosurgery is useful for cutting tissue and for providing hemostasis. Bipolar electrosurgery

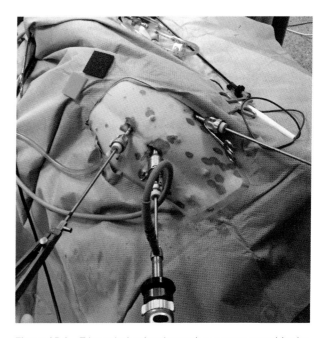

Figure 15.1 Triangulation involves using a scope portal in the center and two instrument portals, one on each side of the scope portal. Triangulation is very helpful for MIS. The scope is used to visualize the action of the two instruments entering from each side to perform intracorporeal procedures. *Source:* Image courtesy of Phillipp Mayhew.

is essential for surgery in small exotic pets. The forceps contain both electrodes in the jaws so there is no need for a ground plate. The forceps are insulated except for the tips. They are most useful for hemostasis within body cavities as the current passes between the tips of the electrodes rather than through the patient. Bipolar electrosurgery instruments are available to be used through 5 mm and larger cannulae. Vessel sealing devices (LigaSure™ – Covidien, Mansfield, MA) and the Harmonic Scalpel® (Harmonic Scalpel-Ethicon, Somerville, NJ) are examples of such devices available for MIS use in exotic animals. While LigaSure is a type of bipolar electrosurgery, the Harmonic Scalpel is not. The Harmonic Scalpel converts mechanical energy to heat energy and the heat seals and cuts tissue. These instruments are approved to ligate vessels up to 7 mm (LigaSure) and 5 mm (Harmonic Scalpel) in diameter.

Positioning of the surgical team and equipment is an acquired skill that can be perfected with experience. Ideal team positioning will be different for every procedure. The position of the tower and monitor is important in order to facilitate the procedure. It should always face the frontal plane of the surgeon and ideally the endoscope should be directed toward the monitor and the monitor positioned so the surgeon can view it looking straight ahead. If the tower is to the side or behind the surgeon, it makes instrument operation difficult, similar to performing surgery in front of a mirror. For advanced procedures where both sides of the patient need to be accessed, a circulating assistant should be available to move the tower to keep it positioned in front of the surgeon. The ideal situation is to have two or more monitors available in the operating room and the surgeon can look at whichever monitor is in the best position.

Patient Positioning

Patient positioning includes the recumbency of the animal (dorsal, sternal, lateral, or lateral oblique) and whether the head will be tilted down (Trendelenburg position), tilted up (reverse Trendelenburg position), or remain neutral. The effect of positioning can greatly improve the working space by allowing gravity to assist with retraction of viscera. Reverse Trendelenburg is useful for access to the stomach, liver, and gallbladder. Most simple procedures such as liver biopsies can be done without tilting the patient. The head-down or Trendelenburg position is 10–30° from horizontal; however, 10–20° is usually adequate for most procedures in small mammals and is indicated for performing laparoscopic cystotomy in rabbits, guinea pigs, iguanas and

ferrets, as well as for abdominal orchidectomy in rabbits and rodents (Mehler 2011; Sladakovic and Divers 2016).

In order to visualize organs and maneuver within the abdomen a pneumoperitoneum must be created, except in birds and some reptiles. This is achieved by insufflating the abdomen with CO_2 gas. CO_2 is considered to be the safest gas for abdominal insufflation because it reduces the risk of gas embolization. Pneumoperitoneum inflates the body wall off the organs creating a workspace. Since it is expected that pneumoperitoneum will increase intraabdominal pressure (IAP) and reduce the excursions of the diaphragm in mammals, laparoscopy with pneumoperitoneum is most commonly performed under general anesthesia with assisted or controlled patient ventilation. In birds, a pneumoperitoneum is not created. The extensive air sac system provides a space within which to work. In reptiles, once the coelom is open, room air enters creating pneumocoelom providing some space within which to work; however, insufflation expands the space and is recommended in most cases. Insufflation is of some, but limited, value in chelonians because the shell limits distention.

Increasing IAP has several effects on the patient's cardiovascular and respiratory systems (Freeman 1999; Monnet and Twedt 2003; McCarthy and Monnet 2005). The hemodynamic disturbances related to an increase in IAP reported in mammals are decreased cardiac output (Q), elevation of abdominal arterial pressure, and increased systemic and pulmonary vascular resistance. The decrease in Q is proportionate to the increase in IAP. When IAP is greater than 20 mmHg, Q may become severely compromised. With large increases in IAP (>30 mmHg) the caudal vena cava is compressed and venous return (cardiac preload) is decreased. There is no insufflation device currently available that accurately regulates the pressure within the abdomen of smaller exotic patients. Most insufflation units measure CO_2 flow in l/min and it would be ideal to be able to deliver CO_2 in ml/min in small patients. Because of this, set the high limit of the pressure sensor to 8 mmHg in patients less than 5 kg and 8–12 mmHg in patients >5 kg.

Laparoscopy

Patient Preparation

Patients should be clipped/plucked and prepared for aseptic surgery as for an open procedure. The surgeon should be prepared, and the clients should be aware that if complications occur or if it is warranted, traditional open surgery may be performed. If the patient has a urinary bladder, it should be emptied in order to prevent iatrogenic penetration of the urinary bladder during trocar placement and to provide more working space within the abdomen or coelom.

In general, dorsal recumbency is used for most diagnostic procedures. In mammals and most reptiles, left lateral recumbency will provide adequate visualization for evaluation of the liver, gallbladder, right limb of the pancreas, duodenum, right kidney, and right adrenal gland. Although right lateral recumbency is not generally used due to the location of the spleen in mammals, it is the preferred recumbency for many techniques in avian species because it allows visualization of the female reproductive tract as well as most other viscera (Divers 2010e; Mehler 2011). Ventral recumbency is rarely used, but is used for some thoracic techniques in mammals.

The most common location for the camera portal in mammals in dorsal recumbency is on or immediately caudal to the umbilicus (Monnet and Twedt 2003; McCarthy and Monnet 2003; Mehler 2011; Sladakovic and Divers 2016). In birds, place the camera portal on ventral midline if in dorsal recumbency or immediately caudal to the last rib just dorsal to the junction of the sternal and vertebral portions of the rib for a left lateral approach. In species that have ribs to the level of the lateral pelvis, use an intercostal approach. Modify approaches for the individual patient, species, and organ of interest in order to provide adequate working space.

Before the endoscope and instrument portals can be placed into the abdomen of a mammal and some reptiles, a pneumoperitoneum must be created. Initial insufflation can either be provided using a Veress needle, which is a closed technique, or by placing a cannula through a mini-celiotomy (Hasson technique), which is an open approach. They both have advantages and disadvantages, which are important to consider for each case. The Veress needle consists of an inner blunt obturator spring-loaded within an outer sharp cutting tip needle. The obturator retracts as the cutting needle is advanced through the tissues, and then the blunt obturator advances beyond the sharp tip after entering the abdominal cavity, thereby protecting abdominal organs from the sharp tip of the outer needle. The Veress needle can be placed either on ventral midline or in the caudal abdomen to the right of midline to avoid the spleen and falciform ligament. Once the surgeon is confident that the needle is in the abdomen, initiate insufflation with CO_2. Some surgeons perform a test injection of saline through the Veress needle or use the hanging drop technique to verify intraperitoneal cavity placement prior to insufflation. The injection should be easy with no resistance. To test using the hanging drop technique, fill the needle hub with saline and lift up on the body wall. The negative pressure created should pull the saline in the hub

into the abdominal cavity. Once insertion into the peritoneal cavity is confirmed, attach the tubing connected to the automatic CO_2 insufflator to the hub of the Veress needle. Keep the pressure below 15 mmHg, with 8–12 mmHg usually being adequate for most procedures in small mammals. Following abdominal insufflation, blindly insert a sharp trocar-cannula system through the abdominal wall in the predetermined location for the endoscope. The main advantage of the Veress needle technique is that it is usually quickly performed; however, gas introduction is slower, and it requires blind introduction of the first trocar, which carries the risk of inadvertent iatrogenic penetration of abdominal viscera. Accidental insufflation of the spleen, falciform, or subcutaneous tissue can lead to complications requiring conversion to an open procedure.

In most cases, the authors prefer to make a mini-open approach into the abdominal cavity, place a blunt tipped trocar-cannula system, and then insufflate the abdomen via the cannula (Hasson technique). Make a stab incision through the skin and subcutaneous tissue, and grasp and elevate the linea alba or fascia. Place sutures at each end of the proposed incision through the linea alba and external rectus sheath and use them to elevate the body wall. Make a stab incision through the linea alba into the peritoneal cavity and advance a blunt trocar-cannula system into the abdominal cavity. Aim the trocar laterally and ventrally toward the right side of the patient in order to avoid the spleen. The cannula should slide into the abdomen with a slight twisting motion without resistance. Once positioned, remove the blunt trocar from the cannula, infuse CO_2 into the abdomen, and observe the degree of abdominal distention. The abdomen should distend evenly without a sudden increase in pressure. Uneven insufflation or very high pressure may indicate that the subcutaneous space or an organ is being insufflated. Once the abdomen is sufficiently distended, safely place the rigid endoscope connected to the camera into the abdomen. Keep the stay sutures in place because they can be used to help reduce the size of the incision if it exceeds the outer diameter of the cannula. If the incision is too large, gas will escape, and it will not be possible to adequately insufflate. The stay sutures can be tightened around the cannula to minimize gas leakage. There is a short learning curve with the Hasson technique; however, it is less likely the abdominal viscera will be punctured and insufflation of the subcutaneous space instead of the abdominal cavity is less likely to occur.

One author (RAB) prefers to use a threaded cannula instead of a trocar-cannula. Make the incision in the body wall only 2–3 mm. Insert the tip of the threaded cannula into the incision and twist clockwise to thread the cannula into the incision. This will gradually widen the incision to accommodate the cannula. Once the cannula is removed, the incision will be very small. In humans, surgeons do not close an incision for a 5 mm cannula.

Both techniques for initial insufflations have similar complications: iatrogenic damage to organs (usually the spleen or small intestine), introduction of CO_2 into the subcutaneous tissues, and fatal gas embolism if CO_2 is infused into a mass, vessel, or organ (Monnet and Twedt 2003). Maintaining an airtight seal at the portal sites will allow for constant and appropriate insufflation, thereby providing good visualization and allowing a safer and faster procedure.

Often, the endoscope will become blurred on initial entrance into the abdomen due to condensation on the lens from a temperature change, or from contamination from blood, fat, or other fluid while passing through the cannula. The endoscope should be removed and wiped with a warm saline-soaked gauze square or a commercially available sterile anti-fog solution.

Perform a general exploratory to identify any relative contraindications to laparoscopic intervention (e.g. adhesions, large masses, and iatrogenically damaged viscera). Instrument portals can then be safely introduced using direct internal visualization with the scope and camera. The easiest way to locate a cannula site is to depress the body wall repeatedly over the potential site until the location can be visualized with the endoscope within the abdominal cavity (Figure 15.2). The light source can be used to illuminate the body wall from within in order to help avoid blood vessels. Make a small skin incision, paralleling tension lines, slightly larger than the cannula to be used. Advance the sharp trocar-cannula unit with a rotational advancement, alternating the trocar in a clockwise and counterclockwise motion while applying gentle pressure (pushing alone does little to advance the trocar). The camera should always follow and visualize the trocar point as it enters the body cavity (Figure 15.2). Instruments should never leave or enter the abdomen without being directly visualized. Additionally, if not in use, instruments should not sit unobserved within the abdomen. Once the endoscope and accessory portals are in place perform a complete exploration of the abdomen. A palpation probe and fan retractor can help maneuver organs as needed.

Following completion of the laparoscopic procedure, evacuate the CO_2 from the body cavity by stopping the insufflation and opening the valves on the cannulae. As inflation decreases, remove the cannulae and allow the remaining gas to escape from the incisions. Gently press on the abdomen to release trapped pockets of gas. Residual peritoneal CO_2 is a cause of extreme postoperative pain in humans, but has not been observed or reported in animals. Close the small incisions routinely. If stay sutures have been placed across the incision, they can be used to close the incision. Infiltrate the cannula sites with bupivacaine (1 mg/kg) for additional analgesia.

Many endosurgeons prefer using a single incision, single port called a Sils™ Port (Medtronic, Minneapolis, MN) (Figure 15.3) for procedures that require multiple instruments. This device was originally designed for trans-anal minimally invasive procedures so it will fit into a human anus. It contains a tube for insufflation, a scope port, and two instrument ports. The port is designed to give surgeons the ability to use two instruments through adjustable cannulae within a low-profile blue soft port. The disadvantage of the Sils Port is that all cannulae are parallel so triangulation is not possible. It takes practice to learn to use this port with all instruments parallel to each other.

(a)   (b)

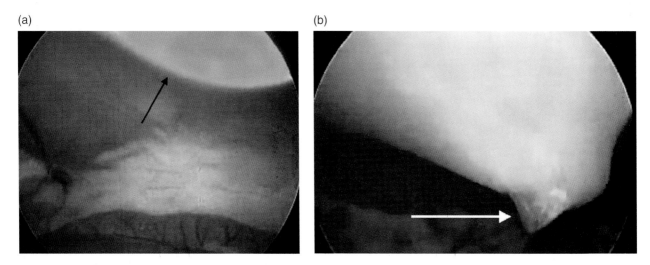

Figure 15.2 Use a finger to push on the body wall while visualizing internally with the scope (a) to identify where the next portal will be placed (arrow). Continue observing the location and use a trocar stylet to insert the cannula (b). The tip of the cannula is visualized (arrow) as it is advanced into the insufflated abdomen.

(a)

(b)

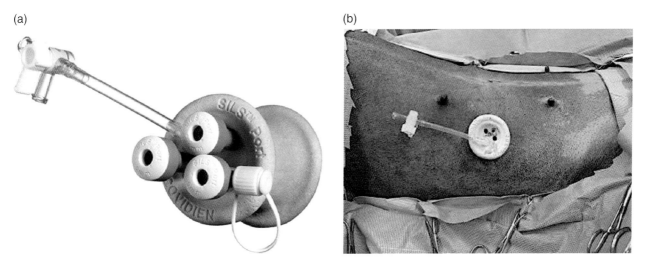

Figure 15.3 A Sils™ Port (Medtronic, Minneapolis, MN) (single incision, single port) is used for procedures that require multiple instruments (a). It contains a tube for insufflation, a scope port, and two instrument ports. It is designed to give surgeons the ability to use two instruments through adjustable cannulae within a low-profile blue soft port. A Sils™ Port placed for a laparoscopic spay and gastropexy (b).

(a)

(b)

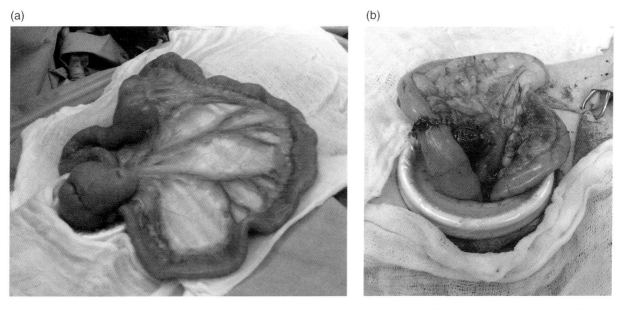

Figure 15.4 Exteriorize the mass (a) and perform an intestinal resection and anastomosis (b). Replace the intestine into the abdomen and close. *Source:* Images (a) and (b) courtesy of Philipp Mayhew.

The Alexis® Wound Protector/Retractor (Applied Medical, Rancho Santa Margarita, CA) was developed to protect the edges of an abdominal incision from contamination and desiccation in an effort to reduce incision site infection. It has gained popularity in veterinary MIS for scope-assisted procedures (Figure 15.4). There are two firm plastic rings connected by a sleeve of plastic. After insufflating the abdomen and inserting the scope, place a second portal on midline in a location that will allow an endo-Babcock forceps to retrieve the organ of interest. After having grasped the organ, enlarge the portal enough to allow insertion of

one of the rings of the Alexis Retractor. Pull up on the outer ring to tighten the plastic sleeve and roll up the sleeve on the outer ring until it is tight against the skin and body wall. The tension from the rings will maintain circumferential retraction allowing the organ, for example intestine, to be exteriorized. Following completion of the procedure, replace the organ and remove the retractor.

The Alexis Retractor is available in various sizes and is relatively inexpensive. They protect the incision from contamination and keep the tissues moist. They are commonly used in animals for MIS gastrointestinal procedures.

Complications

General complications of laparoscopy include iatrogenic damage to abdominal organs, portal site seroma or abscess formation, and tumor seeding of portal sites. Complications specific to each procedure are discussed below.

Coelioscopy in Birds and Reptiles

Avian Coelioscopy

Left, right, ventral, and clavicular endoscopic approaches to the avian coelom have been described (Pye et al. 2001; Divers et al. 2007; Divers 2010c). Familiarity with avian anatomy and the disease of the patient will determine which approach is appropriate for each case. As previously discussed, the left approach to the avian coelom is most frequently utilized for open and closed procedures. Position the bird in right lateral recumbency as if a left celiotomy is to be performed, except pull the left leg and secure it to the table over the head or neck (Figure 15.5). This exposes the entry site located caudal to the last rib and just ventral to the flexor cruris medialis muscle. Make a 2–4 mm skin incision at this point and use a hemostat to bluntly dissect into the left caudal thoracic or abdominal air sac. Place the scope inside a cannula or sheath and advance it into the incision as the hemostat is removed. In most birds, use a 1.9 or 2.7 mm scope within the 3.0 mm sheath. Correct placement of the scope is confirmed by

identifying the lung cranially and the caudal edge of the liver and proventriculus ventrally (Figure 15.6). Normal air sac membranes are transparent and visceral structures are readily observed through them. Blind advancement of

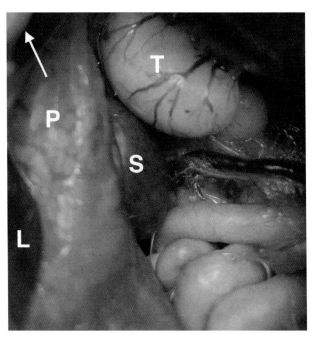

Figure 15.6 Once the coelomic cavity has been entered identify the liver (L), proventriculus (P), and lung (arrow, not visualized in this image). The spleen (S) and left testis (T) are also visible.

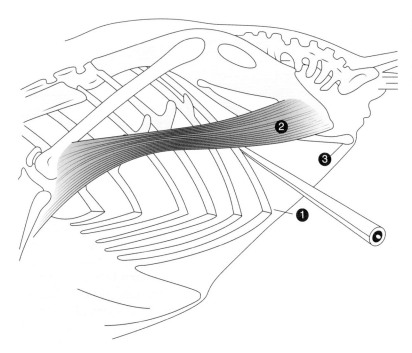

Figure 15.5 The entry point for avian endoscopy with the leg pulled over the head. Pull the leg cranially and identify the entry site at the junction of the caudal edge of the (1) eighth rib and the (2) flexor cruris medialis muscle. (3) The pubic bone serves as an additional landmark. (*Source:* Taylor (1994). Figure 13.3).

the telescope through thickened and opaque air sacs is dangerous and may lead to inadvertent puncture of coelomic viscera. Blunt dissection through diseased air sacs followed by slow and gentle advancement of the telescope is preferred. Repair of the penetrated air sacs is not necessary. Close the muscle and skin in two separate layers.

Positioning for the right approach is analogous to the left. The pancreas is best visualized from the right by looking ventral and cranial and sweeping caudal and ventral to identify the duodenum. The ventral approach allows the best access to both liver lobes. The ventral approach also allows for exploration of the hepatoperitoneal cavity in birds with ascites without entering the air sac system. Position the bird in dorsal recumbency and enter on the ventral midline, just caudal to the keel.

The clavicular approach is rarely used; however, some practitioners prefer it (Divers 2010c). Identify and preserve the crop by performing a larger, 1 cm incision, in the midventral cranial coelomic inlet (analogous to the thoracic inlet of mammals). Upon entering the clavicular air sac, carefully advance the telescope. This approach provides visual access to the syrinx, heart, and great vessels, and has been useful for the identification, sampling, and treatment of cranial coelomic masses.

Reptile Coelioscopy

Given the diversity in body shape, and the visceral anatomy and distribution in reptiles, there is not a specific set of body positions and port placements described for all species. In general, insufflation is useful in reptiles, including chelonians, but as mentioned, use a lower flow rate and maintain intracoelomic pressure lower than what is reported in small animals (Divers 2010d; Mehler 2011). Increased intracoelomic pressure in reptiles compresses the lungs because there is generally no diaphragm. Ventilation must be assisted during MIS in reptiles.

It is difficult to perform complete coelioscopy in snakes because of the elongation of the coelomic viscera; however, if there is a focal area of interest, a ventrolateral entry point for a scope in a sheath with an instrument cannula can be used. Place the sheathed scope through a small skin incision made at the junction of ventral most row of lateral scales and the scutes.

In laterally compressed lizards, such as chameleons, use lateral recumbency and use dorsal recumbency for dorsoventrally compressed species. In iguanas and some monitor lizards, dorsal or lateral recumbency can be used. In round-bodied lizards (iguanas and most monitor lizards), most of the coelomic structures can be visualized with the patient in left or right lateral recumbency. In these species, the best portal site for a sheathed scope is caudal to the

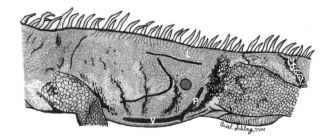

Figure 15.7 Landmarks for scope portal placement (blue dot) for a lateral approach in a green iguana. The best portal site for a sheathed scope is caudal to the last rib (arrows), ventral to the lumbar musculature (L), and cranial to the femur. Avoid the pelvic vein (P) and ventral abdominal vein (V). *Source:* Image courtesy of Ariel Schlag.

last rib, ventral to the spine, and cranial to the femur (Figure 15.7). Incise the skin and use a hemostat to bluntly dissect through the body wall musculature and enter the coelomic cavity. Replace the hemostat with a sheathed 1.9 or 2.7 mm telescope. Visualize the organs in a systematic manner evaluating for abnormalities.

In chelonians, supported lateral recumbency or dorsal recumbency is used to access the left or right prefemoral or axillary fossa. In an attempt to increase the intracoelomic working space in chelonians, encourage the patient to urinate by placing them in shallow warm water bath before premedication and anesthetic induction, or drain the bladder percutaneously or with retrograde catheterization. For a prefemoral approach, in dorsal recumbency, retract the hind limb caudally (Figure 15.8). Make an incision in the skin large enough for the appropriate sized sheath or cannula in the center of the prefemoral fossa and use a hemostat to bluntly dissect down to the fascia of the body wall. The body wall and coelomic membrane are thick and fibrous in some species of chelonians. Take care while advancing a hemostat or cannula obturator into the coelomic cavity.

Specific Laparoscopic Techniques

Liver Biopsy

Laparoscopic liver biopsy is technically easy to perform and provides adequately sized and lesion-specific tissue samples for histopathologic analysis and other tests (culture and heavy metal analysis). Evaluation of coagulation parameters prior to liver biopsy is recommended; however, coagulation status does not necessarily predict bleeding following biopsy. Abnormal coagulation profiles are not an absolute contraindication to laparoscopic liver

(a)

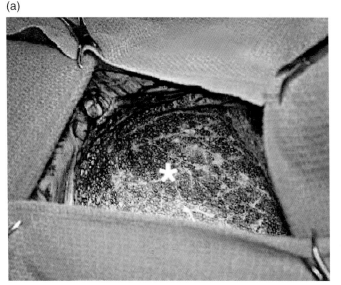

(b)

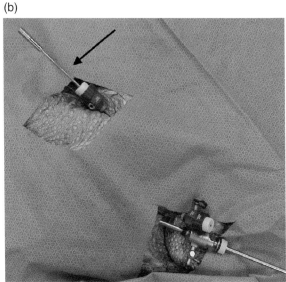

Figure 15.8 For coelioscopy in chelonians, pull the hind limb caudally to allow access to the prefemoral fossa (a). The * denotes the location for the scope portal. (b) In this alligator snapping turtle, a scope portal has been placed in the right prefemoral fossa and an instrument portal in the left axillary fossa with a blunt probe (arrow). *Source:* Mehler (2011). Cranial is to the left.

biopsy. Knowledge of abnormal parameters will allow the surgeon and anesthetist to be prepared for bleeding (e.g. hemostatic aids, vessel sealing devices, and blood products). Use an oval cup biopsy forceps following exploration of the liver with a palpation probe. Take biopsies from the edge of the liver and take both normal and abnormal appearing tissue (Figure 15.9). Monitor the biopsy sites for bleeding. Magnification of bleeding can make hemorrhage look more significant than it actually is. Where hemorrhage is a concern, use the palpation probe to apply pressure, or hemostatic agents such as an absorbable gelatin sponge or an absorbable cellulose-based product can be placed into the biopsy site. Take several biopsies depending on the tests required. A technique that allows for one large piece of liver to be removed instead of many small pieces involves the use of a pre-tied loop of suture or an extracorporeal slipknot placed around the peripheral edge of a liver lobe and tightened securely. The ligature will incorporate all vessels while cutting through the parenchyma. Then transect the piece of liver distal to the suture. Confirm hemostasis prior to completion of the procedure. This can also be accomplished using a tissue and vessel sealing device.

A ventral approach is used for liver biopsy in birds. Incise any air sacs prior to biopsy. The hepatoperitoneal membranes covering the liver are the walls of the air sac. Incise them using endo-scissors or cup biopsy forceps. Attempts to biopsy the liver through the wall of the air sac can lead to excessive hemorrhage and damage to surrounding structures. Once the incision through the air sac membranes is

large enough for the biopsy forceps to pass through them, collect the liver samples.

Pancreatic Biopsy

Chronic pancreatitis in cats has been diagnosed using laparoscopy and it may be useful in other species if the patient is suspected to have chronic pancreatitis (Monnet and Twedt 2003). Take specimens from the edge of the pancreas away from the pancreatic ducts. A recent study evaluating laparoscopic pancreatic biopsies in normal dogs found no postoperative complications or secondary pancreatitis. Biopsy of the avian pancreas has been described and is useful in diagnosing pancreatitis, neoplasia, and pancreatic insufficiency (Speer 1997; Doneley 2001).

Renal Biopsy

Biopsy of the right kidney is technically easier than the left in most mammalian species given the increased mobility of the left kidney and the location of the spleen. Laparoscopy permits direct visualization of the biopsy site as well as monitoring of hemorrhage. A palpation probe is needed to stabilize the kidney and tamponade hemorrhage if necessary. Make a small (1–2 mm) incision in the skin to directly advance a core biopsy needle into a location allowing direct access to the kidney using endoscopic guidance. It should be placed caudal to the last rib to prevent iatrogenic pneumothorax from leakage of the pneumoperitoneum through the diaphragm. As with

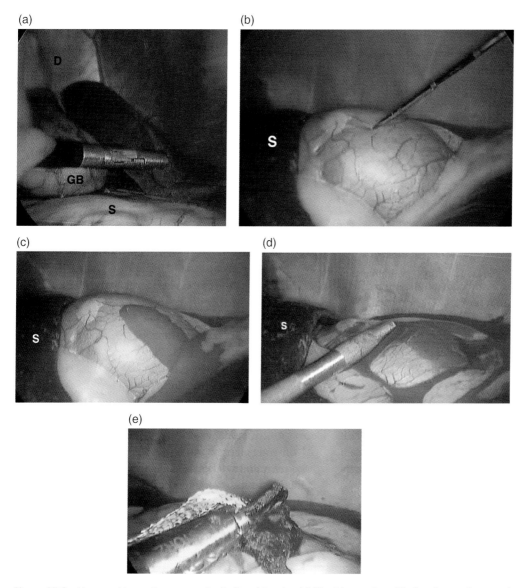

Figure 15.9 Use cup biopsy forceps to obtain liver biopsies (a). The biopsy site will often hemorrhage and may seem serious but keep in mind the image visualized has been magnified. Hemorrhage is typically self-limiting. Alternatively, a hemostatic agent such as Surgicel™, can be applied to the site to aid in hemostasis. Use a core needle biopsy instrument for renal biopsies directed into a representative site of renal cortex, not into the medulla (b). Hemorrhage can be serious (c) and can be controlled by direct pressure from a blunt probe (d) or a hemostatic agent such as Surgicel (e) *Source:* Images courtesy of Philipp Mayhew.

renal biopsies taken using an open approach, take the biopsy samples from the cranial or caudal pole of the kidney (Figure 15.9). Do not direct the needle into the corticomedullary junction so as to avoid the arcuate vessels. Moderate hemorrhage is expected. Allow the site to bleed for three to five seconds, and then provide pressure to the site with the probe to reduce the amount of blood that collects under the renal capsule. The bleeding biopsy site can also be plugged with a hemostatic agent. Take two to four biopsies. This technique has been used mainly to diagnose renal neoplasia in small mammals, but can be used to diagnose renal tubular and glomerular disease and to monitor the response to treatment of these diseases.

Intestinal Biopsy

In most species of exotic animals, place the patient in dorsal recumbency and insert the endoscope through a portal immediately caudal to the umbilicus. Establish two instrument portals to be able to run the bowel by first locating the cecum or ileum and running it orad or by finding the pylorus and running it aborad. Intestinal

(a) (b)

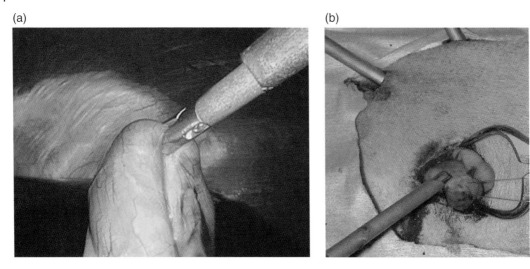

Figure 15.10 Obtain gastrointestinal biopsies using a scope-assisted technique. Identify the segment of bowel to be biopsied and grasp it with endo-Babcock atraumatic forceps (a). Enlarge the incision of the instrument portal that was used to grasp the segment of bowel and exteriorize the segment (b). After obtaining the sample, replace the bowel into the abdomen. In order to continue, the enlarged portal must be tightened around the cannula to achieve insufflation. Identify the next segment and exteriorize it through the same portal incision. *Source:* Reprinted with permission from Twedt and Monnet (2005). Notice the triangulation of the cannulae. Once the intestine has been exteriorized, immediately place a stay suture (shown) to maintain control of it after the endo-Babcock has been removed.

biopsy, in most cases, is an endoscope-assisted procedure. After the location of bowel to be biopsied is determined, enlarge the instrument portal with a number 11 scalpel blade under visualization with the endoscope, and then exteriorize the bowel (Figure 15.10). Place stay sutures through the submucosa to allow an assistant to hold the section of bowel outside the abdominal cavity. Take the biopsy and close the enterotomy created as would be done in an open abdominal procedure. Lavage the biopsy incision and replace the bowel into the abdomen. Temporarily occlude the enlarged portal incision with a finger and re-insufflate the abdomen. Alternatively, replace the cannula into the incision and use a towel clamp or purse string suture to temporarily close the skin and body wall around it to create a seal. Locate the next intestinal site to be biopsied and exteriorize it through the same body wall incision. Turn off the insufflation while working outside the body to prevent wasting gas. Alternatively, use an Alexis Wound Protector/Retractor.

Other Diagnostic Techniques

Lymph nodes can be biopsied using a punch or cup biopsy instrument, or using a combination of sharp and blunt dissection with electrosurgery or a tissue and vessel sealing instrument. Collection of abdominal effusion from small pockets within the abdomen can also be performed for culture and cytologic examination. Use laparoscopic suction/irrigation instruments or an endo-needle on a syringe for collection of effusion under laparoscopic guidance.

Feeding Tube Placement

Several techniques for placing feeding tubes in small animals have been described and are readily applied to exotic animals. Place a gastrostomy tube by identifying and grasping the body of the stomach with the scope and exteriorizing a small part of it through the left abdominal wall by enlarging the instrument port. Place stay sutures to hold the bubble of stomach outside the body wall. Place a purse string suture where the tube will be inserted. Make a stab incision into the stomach in the center of the purse string suture and insert the tube into the stomach. Tighten the purse string suture and secure it. Place sutures between the stomach and the body wall to create a gastropexy and then secure the tube to the skin with a finger trap suture.

Postpyloric feeding tube placement is also an endoscope-assisted procedure performed by using laparoscopy to exteriorize the section of bowel, and then placing the tube into the intestine outside the body cavity. Identify the segment of intestine into which the tube will be placed and exteriorize it by enlarging an instrument portal. Place a purse string in the intestine, make a stab incision, insert the tube, tighten the purse string suture, and place sutures between the intestine and the body wall to create an enteropexy.

Intestinal foreign bodies can be removed by identifying the object and exteriorizing the object by enlarging an instrument port. Then perform an enterotomy to remove the object, close the enterotomy routinely, and replace the intestine into the abdominal cavity.

Ovariectomy/Ovariohysterectomy

Ovariectomy and ovariohysterectomy can be performed in dorsal recumbency in small mammals and most reptiles. For mammals in dorsal recumbency, place the endoscope portal at or caudal to the umbilicus on midline. A one, two, or three instrument portal technique can be used (Mehler 2011; Divers 2015; Proença 2015). One author (SJM) prefers a two instrument portal technique for ovariectomy/ovariohysterectomy (Girolamo and Mans 2016). Place the instrument portals on midline, cranial and caudal to the camera portal, or at the level of the umbilicus on each side at the lateral margin of the rectus abdominis. Reflect the intestine

and omentum covering a uterine horn, grasp the horn, and elevate it to expose the ipsilateral ovary. Ligate the ovarian pedicle either with endoscopic clips, suture ligatures, bipolar or monopolar electrosurgery, or a tissue-sealing device depending on the size of the vessels (Figure 15.11). The other author (RAB) prefers a one instrument portal technique. Grasp the ovary and elevate it ventrally to the body wall. Pass a suture on a large needle percutaneously to hold the ovary against the body wall rather than holding it up with an instrument (Figure 15.11). With the ovary maintained in position with the suture, seal and transect the ovarian vessels and the tip of the uterine horn.

If the method used to control hemorrhage does not transect the tissue, use endoscopic Metzenbaum scissors to transect the pedicle distal to the site of hemostasis. Visualize the entire ovary to ensure that no ovarian tissue is left. As in the open procedure, break down the mesovarium

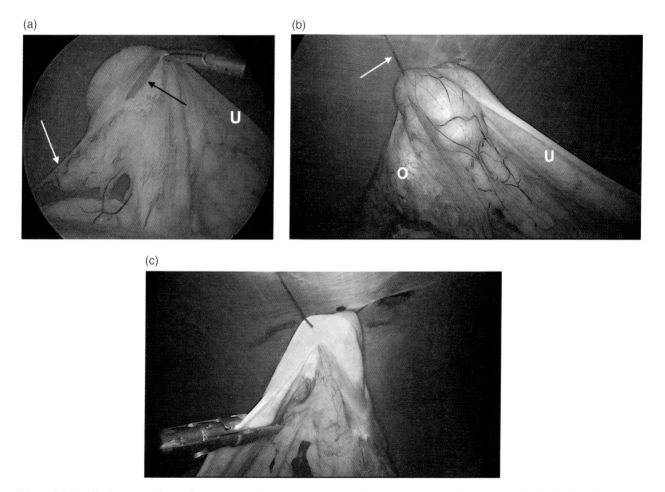

(a)

(b)

(c)

Figure 15.11 For laparoscopic ovariectomy using a three-port technique, grasp the proper ligament of the ovary with endo-hemostats and lift it ventrally up to the body wall (a). While maintaining this position use a second instrument portal to introduce a tissue sealing device and transect the suspensory ligament (white arrow), and then the more caudal vascular bundle and the tip of the uterine horn (U). *Source:* Image courtesy of Ameet Singh. The black arrow is directed at the ovarian bursa. Alternatively, use a two port technique and use a percutaneous suture to hold the ovary against the ventral abdominal wall (b). Then use a vessel-sealing device to seal the ovarian vessels, ligaments, and the tip of the uterus (c). *Source:* Images courtesy of Philipp Mayhew.

(a)

(b)

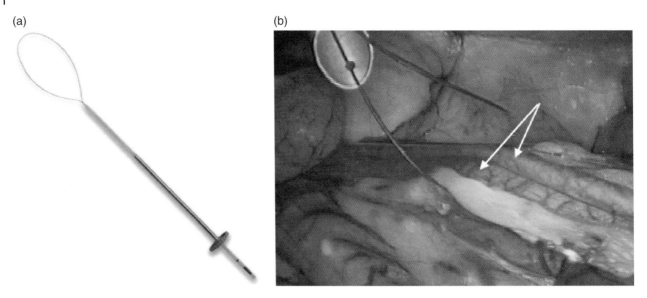

Figure 15.12 Surgitie™ (Medtronic) is a suture loop on a stick that will pass through a cannula (a). For an ovariohysterectomy, pull the two uterine horns (arrows) through the loop and advance the loop to the cervix (b). *Source:* Reprinted with permission from Twedt and Monnet (2005). Once in place, break the stick where indicated and pull the suture line which will cinch down the loop. The premanufactured knot will not loosen.

with scissors and electrosurgery or tear it with forceps. The hysterectomy can be accomplished using a pre-formed suture loop brought into the abdomen through one of the cannulae. Pull the ovaries, uterine horns, and body of the uterus through the suture loop to the level of the cervix (Figure 15.12). Tighten the loop and cut distal to the knot with endo-suture scissors. Transect the uterus cranial to the loop with endo-Metzenbaum scissors. Inspect all three pedicles for bleeding. Remove the ovaries and uterus through an instrument portal. Often, these tissues are too large to pull through an instrument cannula and the entry needs to be enlarged in order to remove them from the abdomen.

Alternatively, a laparoscopic-assisted hysterectomy technique can be performed by enlarging a caudally placed instrument portal enough to exteriorize the uterus and ovaries prior to ligating the uterine body. Ligate the uterine vessels and body of the uterus and transect the uterus as in an open procedure. Endoscopic ovariohysterectomy is difficult in hind-gut fermenting species with a large cecum and/or colon because the reproductive tract is covered by the gastrointestinal tract. In general, laparoscopic ovariectomy is easier to perform than ovariohysterectomy, and ovariectomy has not been associated with any postoperative reproductive complications such as pyometra. Without a functioning ovary, pyometra cannot occur, and it nearly eliminates the risk of developing uterine disease such as uterine cancer (Griffiths 1975). Especially in rabbits and rodents, endoscopic ovariectomy is preferred to endoscopic ovariohysterectomy.

Avian Salpingohysterectomy

Place the bird in right lateral recumbency for an endoscopic salpingohysterectomy. Salpingohysterectomy in birds has been described utilizing a three-port technique but a two-port technique and a single port technique have also been used in clinical cases (Pye et al. 2001; Divers et al. 2007; Divers 2010e). Using the technique described previously for access to the left coelomic cavity in birds, insert a sheathed a 1.9 or 2.7 mm scope into the left caudal thoracic or abdominal air sac. Place an instrument cannula cranial to the pubic bone midway between its ventral and dorsal border. Advance a cannula into the caudal aspect of the left abdominal air sac under endoscopic guidance. Once inside the abdominal air sac, remove the trocar. Place a second instrument cannula immediately caudal to the last rib, at the ventral border of the flexor cruris medialis muscle and cranial to the scope cannula and direct it in a caudoventral direction. Rotate the telescope to image the caudal coelomic cavity. Use a grasping instrument to manipulate the oviduct ventral to the ureter and kidney. Use scissors connected to an electrosurgery unit to transect the uterus at the level of its junction with the cloaca. Electrosurgery has not been proven to seal structures with a lumen, so use this technique with caution especially if the bird is reproductively active and the opening from the cloaca into the uterus might be large. Manipulate the oviduct and uterus cranial and ventral to expose and tighten the ventral and dorsal suspensory ligaments. Use the electrosurgery-activated endoscopic scissors to coagulate and transect the ligaments and the vasculature within the dorsal suspensory ligament. Coagulate the vessels in the dorsal ligament where they are smaller, as close to the oviduct and uterus as possible. If the cranial oviductal vessels are greater than 1–2 mm, it is recommended to convert to an open procedure to finish the salpingohysterectomy as electrosurgery units may not be able to adequately seal vessels of that size; however, a 5 mm vessel sealing device (LigaSure®) can be used through an appropriately sized cannula to complete the procedure in a minimally invasive fashion. After the caudal, middle, and cranial oviductal vessels are sealed and transected, remove the oviduct and uterus through an instrument cannula and inspect the surgical site for hemorrhage. If needed, apply hemostatic agents along the dorsal oviductal pedicle where the oviductal vessels were transected. Close the skin incisions routinely.

In juvenile birds, use a single-port entry and identify the oviduct as it crosses the cranial pole of the kidney. Grasp the oviduct and then gently exteriorize the oviduct and uterus. There is no need to ligate the oviductal or suspensory ligament vessels (Figure 15.13) (Pye et al. 2001). Once exteriorized, place a single hemostatic clip on the uterus where it enters the cloaca and transect. It is important to note that salpingohysterectomy may not cease ovulation in all birds and does not stop hormone related behavioral or medical conditions.

Endoscopic ovariectomy has been performed, but there is a high risk of fatal hemorrhage associated with this procedure (Divers 2005). A single-entry (one large incision) technique, telescope-assisted, is preferred by the authors for left ovariectomy in birds. Use the left coelomic cavity approach for positioning and patient preparation as described previously for salpingohysterectomy in birds. Identify the ovary by retracting the proventriculus lateral and ventral. Grasp the mesovarium with endo-Babcock forceps or curved laparoscopic forceps. Elevate the ligament and apply a hemostatic clip using a laparoscopic clip applier as proximal on the mesovarium as possible. Partially, transect the pedicle distal to the clip with laparoscopic scissors. This technique is progressively continued from caudal to cranial until all of the ovarian vessels are ligated and transected. The clip line should be inspected to ensure that all ovarian tissue has been removed. In larger birds, a 5 mm vessel-sealing device (LigaSure) is preferred for ovariectomy. Common complications include fatal hemorrhage and failure to remove all of the ovary and its underlying disease.

Endoscopic Avian Vasectomy

Endoscopic vasectomy in pigeons has been described for population control (Heiderich et al. 2015). Position the bird in right lateral recumbency. Secure the wings dorsally over the back. Retract the left leg caudally and secure it to the table with tape. Remove feathers from the left flank. Make a 3–5 mm skin incision caudal to the last rib, cranial to the iliotibialis cranialis muscle, and ventral to the synsacrum. Bluntly insert a hemostat into the left abdominal wall to enter the caudal thoracic or the abdominal air sac. Insert the telescope into the abdominal air sac. Grasp the ductus deferens near the caudal division of the left kidney with endo-Babcock forceps. Gently retract the biopsy forceps to separate the duct from the ureter (Figure 15.14). Tear the duct until at least 1 cm of duct is removed from the patient. Repeat the same procedure on the right side.

Chelonian Oophorectomy/Ovariectomy/ Ovariosalpingectomy

Female chelonian sterilization techniques have been described using an endoscopic-assisted technique and an intracorporeal three-port technique (Innis 2010; Proença and Divers 2015). In sexually immature chelonians, the underdeveloped ovary is tightly adhered to the dorsal aspect of the caudolateral coelom. This makes visualization of both ovaries from a single prefemoral approach difficult, so perform the procedure using both prefemoral fossae. Position the patient in lateral recumbency to remove one ovary, and then rotate the patient into the opposite recumbency to complete the procedure. The left prefemoral fossa approach allows visualization and access to the left ovary. The patient can also be placed in dorsal recumbency with both prefemoral fossae exposed eliminating the need for rotating the patient; however, it is usually more difficult to visualize the ovaries with the patient in dorsal recumbency because the viscera lay on top of the ovaries. In most cases, insufflation is not required but is useful to create a larger working space. Make a single incision large enough to allow insertion of the scope and two instruments or, in larger specimens, make three separate cannula incisions in the prefemoral fossa or place a Sils Port. Grasp the ovary and retract it ventrally using forceps. Use endoscopic scissors connected to electrosurgery to coagulate vessels and dissect the ovary free from the mesovarium. Close the prefemoral body wall incision(s) separate from the skin incision(s). Repeat the procedure on the other side. In sexually mature chelonians, endoscopic ovariectomy is difficult to accomplish.

Cryptorchid and Abdominal Castration

Laparoscopy provides excellent visualization and removal of intra-abdominal cryptorchid testes and, in rodents and rabbits, an abdominal approach for castration. Place small

(a)

(b)

(c)

(d)

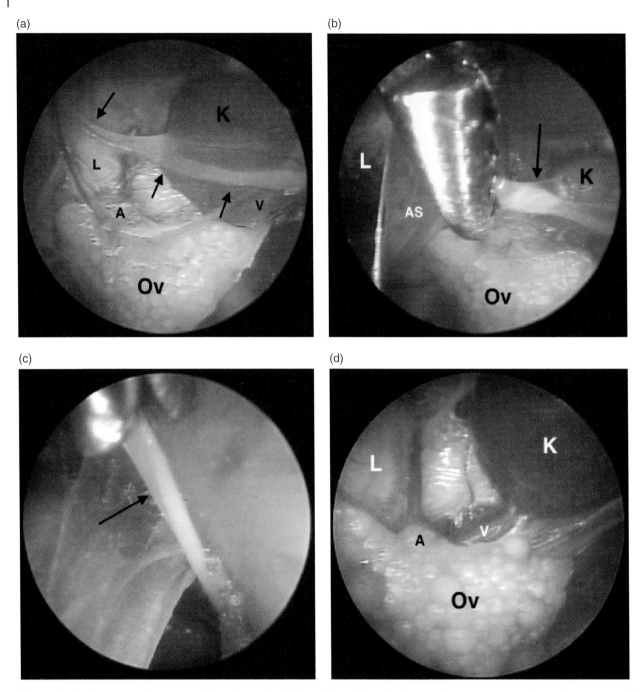

Figure 15.13 Intraoperative image of a juvenile cockatiel (*Nymphicus hollandicus*) undergoing laparoscopic salpingohysterectomy (a). Adrenal gland (A), kidney (K), lung (L), ovary (Ov), and common iliac vein (V) are labeled. Arrows are point to the oviduct. Use endosurgical forceps to grasp the oviduct (arrow) and pull it to detach it (b). An air sac (AS) wall is visible. Continue pulling on the oviduct to exteriorize it through the cannula port (c). Use a cotton-tipped applicator to push the cloaca cranially, place a hemostatic clip at the junction with the cloaca, and then transect distal to the clip. Re-insert the scope to assure there is no hemorrhage. Note the oviduct is no longer present, and there is no visible hemorrhage (d).

mammals in reverse Trendelenburg dorsal recumbency so the viscera fall cranially providing better access to structures in the caudal abdomen. Locate the endoscope portal cranial to the umbilicus and place one or two instrument portals as described for ovariohysterectomy (Divers 2010b;

Mehler 2011). If a scope-assisted technique is used, only two portals are needed. Identify the internal inguinal rings first. If the vas deferens and testicular vessels are observed entering the internal ring (Figure 15.15), then the testis is not in the abdomen. If the vas deferens and testicular

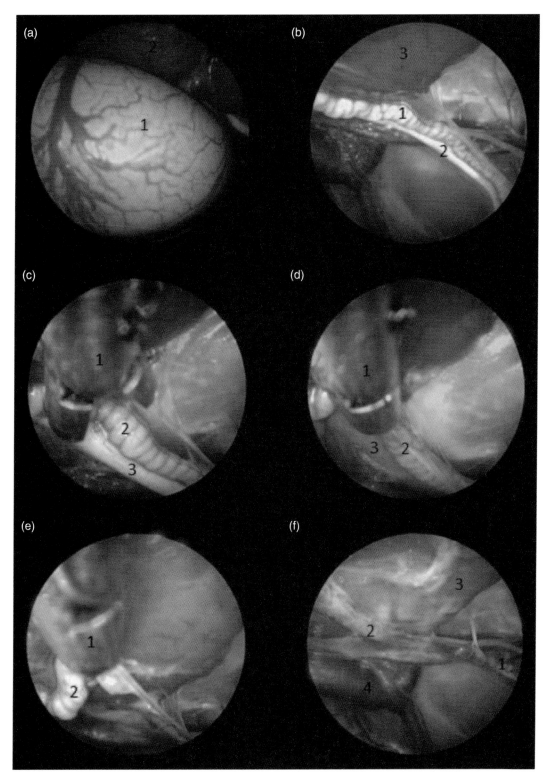

Figure 15.14 Endoscopic view during vasectomy of a male pigeon. (a) left testis (1), kidney (2); (b) ductus deferens (1), ureter (2), kidney (3); (c) biopsy forceps (1), ductus deferens (2), ureter (3); (d) separate the ductus deferens (2) from the ureter (3) with biopsy forceps (1); (e) withdraw the biopsy forceps (1) to remove the ductus deferens (2); and (f) the remaining part of the ductus deferens (1), ureter (2), kidney (3), blood vessels (4). *Source:* Reprinted with permission from Heiderich et al. (2015).

(a)

(b)

(c)

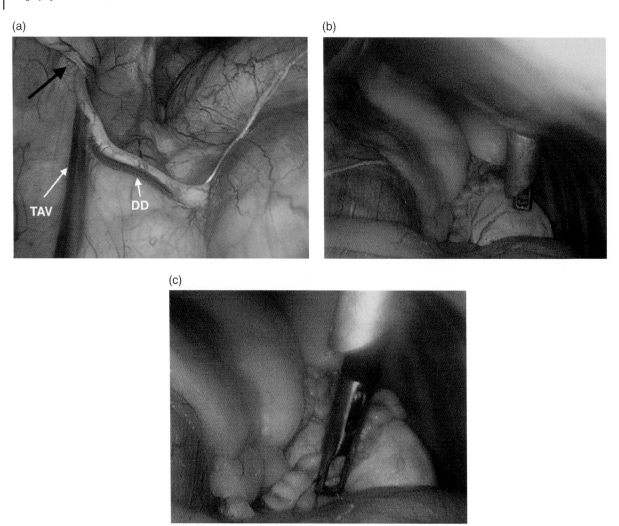

Figure 15.15 Intraoperative view of internal inguinal ring (a). *Source:* Image courtesy of Philipp Mayhew. The black arrow is pointing at the internal inguinal ring. TAV, testicular artery and vein; DD, ductus deferens. Identifying the cryptorchid testis. The endo-Babcock is pressing on the retained testis (T) and the ductus deferens is clearly visible (arrow) (b). The endo-Babcock forceps are holding the ductus (c) and will be used to stabilize the testis while the vascular bundle is coagulated and transected with a tissue-sealing device.

vessels are not in the inguinal ring, the testis can be located anywhere from the internal inguinal ring to the caudal pole of the kidney. Once the cryptorchid testis is located, place a ligature around the spermatic cord or seal it with a tissue-sealing device, and then transect distal to the ligature. This will leave the testis unattached within the abdomen. Often, a cryptorchid testis is small enough to be removed through the cannula, but other times enlarge the instrument port incision enough to remove the testis from the abdomen. For laparoscopic castration in rabbits and rodents, identify the vas deferens dorsal to neck of the urinary bladder and ventral to the colon. Grasp it with endoforceps and apply gentle traction to the vas to find the testis within the abdomen or to pull it into the abdomen if it is within the scrotum. Ligate the vascular pedicle and vas deferens with vascular clips,

pretied suture loops, or a tissue-sealing device. Repeat the procedure for the other testis and remove them as described by enlarging the instrument portal.

For the scope-assisted technique, only two portals are needed, the midline umbilical telescope portal and one instrument portal. Identify the vas deferens dorsal to neck of the urinary bladder and ventral to the colon. Grasp it with endoforceps and apply gentle traction to the vas to find the testis within the abdomen or to pull it into the abdomen if it is within the scrotum. Enlarge the midline portal incision in a caudal direction to expose the caudal peritoneal cavity, the isolated vas deferens, and the testis. A traditional open technique can be applied for ligation and transection of the testicular vessels. Repeat the procedure on the contralateral testis.

Endoscopic Avian Orchidectomy

Endoscopic avian orchidectomy has been described using a double-port technique, a single-entry (one larger incision) technique, and a two-portal technique has also been performed in pigeons but not in clinical patients (Pye et al. 2001; Divers et al. 2007; Divers 2010d; Mehler 2011). Use the left coelomic cavity approach described previously for salpingohysterectomy in birds. Use a polypectomy snare connected to a radio frequency electrosurgery generator to remove the testes from their attachments. Once a testis has been snared and elevated from the kidney, activate the radiofrequency generator and coagulate the vascular pedicle of the testis. Quickly remove the snare, insert an endo-hemostat into the cannula, and grasp and remove the testis. In larger birds, use a 5 mm vessel-sealing device through an appropriately sized cannula to complete the procedure. Place the jaws of the device on the mesorchium to seal vessels and cut through the seal zone. After removing the testis, evaluate the orchidectomy pedicle for hemorrhage and for any remnants of testicular tissue. Close the port sites and turn the bird over into left lateral recumbency to repeat the procedure on the right side.

Endoscopic Green Iguana Orchidectomy

A technique for endoscopic orchidectomy in green iguanas has been described (Divers 2010d; Mehler 2011). Place the patient in left or right lateral recumbency and place a cannula on ventral midline at or immediately caudal to the umbilical scar to be used as the scope portal. Place the first instrument cannula at any intercostal space or immediately caudal to the last rib ventral to the epaxial musculature to facilitate triangulation (Figure 15.16). The precise insertion site is determined by visualizing the location of the testis with the scope. Place the second instrument cannula in the paralumbar fossa, immediately cranial to the femur (Figure 15.7). Insert endoscopic forceps into the intercostal/

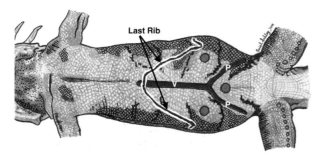

Figure 15.16 Sites for instrument and scope portals (blue dots) for castration in a green iguana. Landmarks are the last rib (arrows), pelvic veins (P), and ventral abdominal vein (V). *Source:* Courtesy of Ariel Schlag.

paracostal cannula and grasp the testis and apply lateral traction to expose the mesorchium and the vascular pedicle. Insert an endoscopic scissor attached to a monopolar electrosurgery generator in the caudal or paralumbar cannula. Activate the generator while cutting the mesorchium with the endoscissors. Remove the testis through the instrument cannula enlarging it if needed. Remove all instruments and telescopes and reposition the patient into the opposite recumbency. Repeat the procedure on the other side.

Endoscopic-Assisted Chelonian Orchidectomy

Minimally invasive orchidectomy has been described in turtles and tortoises (Innis et al. 2013; Proença et al. 2014; Proença and Divers 2015; Girolamo and Mans 2016). Place the patient under general anesthesia. Place the patient in left lateral recumbency and extend the hind limb caudally to expose the prefemoral fossa. Aseptically prepare the prefemoral fossa and surrounding shell.

Incise the skin of the prefemoral fossa in a craniocaudal direction 50–75% of the craniocaudal length of the prefemoral fossa. Bluntly dissect the subcutaneous tissues and incise the aponeurosis of the tendinous parts of the ventral and oblique muscles. Make a 3–5 mm incision in the coelomic membrane to permit insertion of the telescope. Confirm entry into the coelom and not into the urinary bladder. Enlarge the coelomic membrane incision. Apply a ring retractor to improve exposure. Using a single prefemoral celiotomy incision permits the use of multiple instruments through a single incision.

After endoscopic examination of the coelomic cavity, identify the left testis and grasp it with the endo-Babcock forceps. Elevate the testis to expose the mesorchium. Use hemostatic clips and laparoscopic scissors or a bipolar vessel sealing device to dissect the testis free in a caudal to cranial direction. Once freed from the mesorchium, remove the testis through the prefemoral incision. Insert the scope and identify the right testis. If the right testis cannot be isolated from the left approach, close the left prefemoral celiotomy in a routine manner, and repeat the procedure from the right prefemoral fossa.

Cystotomy

Laparoscopic cystotomy is an endoscope-assisted procedure that is indicated primarily in mammal and reptile species prone to cystic calculi formation. Use the scope to identify the urinary bladder within the abdomen or coelom and then place an instrument port caudal to the apex of the bladder. Use endo-Babcock forceps to hold the bladder while the instrument port is enlarged enough to exteriorize the bladder and stone(s). Perform a cystotomy extracorporeally and

(a)

(b)

(c)

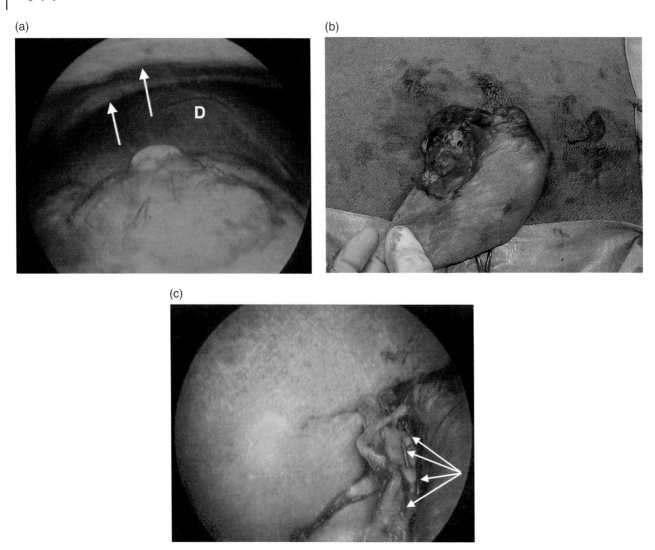

Figure 15.17 Intraoperative thoracoscopic view of a primary lung tumor (a). D – diaphragm; arrows are pointing at ribs. The lobe was grasped with endo-Babcock forceps, and then exteriorized through a mini-thoracotomy caudal to the scope portal (b). A thoracoabdominal (TA) stapler was used to seal the lung lobe which was transected distal to the staples. The stump was replaced and evaluated endoscopically (c). Arrows are pointing at the staples. The TA stapler fires two rows of staggered staples.

remove the stones. Close the bladder, replace it into the abdomen or coelom, and then close routinely.

In large mammals with a few small stones, rigid cystoscopy is often feasible for cystic calculi removal. Use the laparoscope to locate the bladder and place an instrument cannula directly over the bladder closer to the trigone than the apex. If the instrument cannula is placed too close to the apex or cranial to it, the bladder will not be able to be exteriorized. Use atraumatic grasping forceps (endo-Babcock) to pull the bladder to the body wall and enlarge the instrument port under laparoscopic guidance to allow the bladder to be exteriorized. Exteriorize the apex of the bladder and stabilize it with stay sutures. Remove the laparoscope and cannula and place them into the bladder through a stab incision. Remove the scope leaving the

cannula and place a urinary catheter retrograde from the urethra into the bladder. Flush sterile saline into the bladder forcing the calculi out of the bladder and into the cannula. Replace the scope into the bladder and cranial urethra to be sure all of the stones have been removed. After all of the stones have been expelled out of the cannula, close the bladder incision with a simple interrupted or cruciate suture and replace it into the abdomen.

Thoracoscopy

In general, small mammal thoracoscopy is easier to perform than laparoscopy because there are fewer organs to maneuver around and pneumothorax is easier to induce than pneumoperitoneum. This is not true in patients with a coelom because there is no definitive separation between the thorax and abdomen and, therefore, no difference in intracavitary pressures. Thoracoscopy has many advantages over open thoracotomy. The biggest differences are decreased pain, more rapid recovery, shortened hospital stay, and a more rapid return to normal activity (McCarthy and Monnet 2005). Thoracic surgery patients must be intubated and ventilated throughout the procedure. Patients can be placed in dorsal, slightly oblique dorsal, or lateral recumbency as determined by the procedure to be performed. The thoracic cavity can be accessed through a lateral intercostal, a transdiaphragmatic/paraxiphoid, or a cranial (thoracic inlet) approach. The lateral intercostal and paraxiphoid approaches are the most useful in small animal thoracoscopy. Portal sites are chosen on a case-by-case basis. Prepare the area for thoracoscopy as wide as or wider than that for open thoracotomy in order to provide enough space to triangulate portals and to place a chest tube. As for laparoscopy, clients should be aware that if complications arise or if it is warranted, traditional open surgery might be performed.

For procedures that involve only one side of the thorax, use a lateral intercostal approach with the patient in lateral recumbency as described below for thoracoscopic-assisted partial lung lobectomy. For procedures involving both sides of the thorax, it is best to use a paraxiphoid approach. Place the first trocar next to the xiphoid process (paraxiphoid) and into the thoracic cavity. Insert the cannula either to the left or right of midline in the angle between the xiphoid and last rib where it attaches to the sternum to avoid the caudal mediastinum. Use a scalpel to make a small incision through the skin, subcutaneous tissue, and body wall, then enlarge the hole with a hemostat and penetrate the ventral diaphragm and pleura. Insert a blunt trocar-cannula unit directed cranially, and slightly laterally and ventrally to avoid the mediastinum. Once the trocar is in place, allow air to enter the chest cavity creating a pneumothorax. Insert the scope into the thorax and explore the hemithorax. Under direct visualization with the camera, place the first instrument portal into one hemithorax and an instrument can then be inserted into the hemithorax to break down the mediastinum which will allow access to the other hemithorax. It is ideal to use a coagulating or vessel-sealing instrument to break down the mediastinum. Once both sides of the thorax are exposed, place a second instrument portal into the opposite hemithorax. In some cases, a third instrument portal will be required for appropriate visualization and to complete the procedure. Creating bilateral pneumothorax will improve the working space and exposure to thoracic organs.

Methods for increasing the working space during thoracoscopy include creating a bilateral pneumothorax, one-lung ventilation or single bronchus intubation, and endobronchial blockade. Creating bilateral pneumothorax is done routinely during thoracoscopic procedures. Using endobronchial blockade devices or one bronchus intubation for one-lung ventilation is becoming more common in veterinary endosurgery and increases the working space within the thorax while maintaining adequate ventilation of the rest of the lung. Use a flexible endoscope to guide an endobronchial tube into the bronchus of the lung on the side opposite to where the lesion is located. Ventilate the unaffected lung during the procedure at a higher frequency to provide normal minute ventilation. The affected lung is not ventilated providing more working space. Endobronchial blockers are placed into the bronchus of the lung with the lesion so that it alone does not expand during ventilation providing more working space. One-lung ventilation and endobronchial blockade require an experienced anesthesia team and advanced monitoring equipment.

When the procedure is complete, irrigate and suction the thoracic cavity. Make sure there are no air leaks or hemorrhage and place a chest tube under thoracoscopic visualization. Secure the chest tube in place in a routine fashion for postoperative control of the pleural space.

Complications of thoracoscopy include iatrogenic damage to viscera (lungs and heart), vessel laceration (intercostal and internal thoracic vessels as well as the great vessels), portal site seroma formation, and, rarely, tumor seeding of portal sites.

Thoracoscopic Procedures

Thoracoscopic Lung Lobectomy, Partial Lobectomy, and Lung Biopsy

For multiple lung lobe lesions or diffuse disease, position the patient in dorsal recumbency and use a paraxiphoid approach with the remaining portal sites determined by the location of the area of interest. If the side of the diseased lobe can be determined prior to surgery lateral recumbency is preferred. Small peripheral lesions or pieces of tissue for evaluating chronic diffuse lung disease can be removed with a loop suture or the lung can be exteriorized for extracorporeal removal.

If diffuse lung disease is present or if the lesion is located within the periphery of a particular lung lobe, a thoracoscopic-assisted lung biopsy or partial lobectomy can be performed in lateral recumbency with the affected side up. For a cranially located lesion, place the telescope portal in the caudal thorax immediately dorsal or ventral to the costochondral junction and place the telescope in the cranial thorax ventral to the costochondral junction for a caudal lesion. Place the instrument portal 1–3 intercostal spaces cranial to the lesion if in a caudal lung lobe and 1–3 intercostal spaces caudal to the lesion if in a cranial lung lobe, while visualizing placement with the scope (Figure 15.17). This is done to account for the space between the lung and the relatively fixed thoracic cage. Place the instrument portal directly over the lobe for the right middle lung lobe. Grasp the periphery of the lung lobe with an endo-Babcock or other atraumatic forceps and enlarge the instrument portal incision, full thickness and parallel to the ribs, being careful not to damage the intercostal neurovascular bundle located on the caudal aspect of the ribs in mammals. After enlarging the incision, partially exteriorize the lung lobe and obtain a biopsy with a guillotine suture fracture technique. The thoracoabdominal (TA™) stapler (Covidien, Mansfield, MA) is useful for partial and complete lung lobectomy. The TA stapler is available in three staple line lengths and two sizes of staples. The TA 55 and 90 mm long staple lines place two staggered rows of staples in the tissues. After application of the staples, transect the tissue distal to the lines of staples. The TA 30 mm V3 has a shorter staple line but applies three staggered rows of smaller staples to the tissue and is superior for sealing bronchi and pulmonary vasculature. These staples can be applied across a lung lobe for a partial lobectomy or across the hilus for a complete lobectomy (Figure 15.17). Alternatively, sutures can be used as they would be for an open thoracotomy partial or complete lung lobectomy. Return the lung pedicle to the thorax after the sample has been collected and check the suture or staple line for any evidence of hemorrhage or air leakage using the endoscope. Place a chest tube under thoracoscopic guidance and close the thorax routinely.

Small masses located away from the hilus are easily removed. Large masses located at the hilus can be difficult to completely visualize, which can restrict appropriate placement of instruments, laparoscopy clips, or suture loops. Lateral recumbency usually provides the best access. Use the basic principles of triangulation with the endoscope and two instrument portals placed in locations depending on the lobe to be removed. Place pretied loops of suture and/or clips over the vein, artery, and bronchus without dissecting them out individually. After the vessels and bronchus are securely ligated, transect the pedicle distal to the clips or sutures. The lobe can be removed through a minithoracotomy by enlarging one of the instrument portals. Lymph nodes should be evaluated prior to completion of the procedure and removed or biopsied if indicated. Place a chest tube and close the ports as previously described.

Hilar Lymph Node and Mediastinal Mass Biopsy and Removal

The hilar lymph nodes can be visualized if they are enlarged. When the lungs partially collapse, the lymph nodes can usually be seen between the lung lobes after gentle manipulation of the lungs with a blunt probe. They can be biopsied with cup biopsy forceps or removed with a combination of sharp and blunt dissection, and hemostasis. Mediastinal masses in rabbits and ferrets can be visualized and biopsied using the above techniques.

Nephrectomy in a Rabbit

One author (SJM) has performed a nephrectomy in a rabbit with renal carcinoma. The technique used was similar to what has been described in dogs (Mayhew et al. 2013). Position the rabbit in near lateral recumbency with the affected kidney up and a small foam wedge placed under the epaxial musculature. Use a three-port technique. Establish the camera portal 1 cm caudal to the umbilicus using a modified Hasson technique for placement of a 5 mm blunt-tipped trocar-cannula. Establish pneumoperitoneum and maintain IAP at 8–12 mmHg. A 5 mm 0° telescope is placed into the camera portal to guide subsequent instrument port placement. Place two additional instrument portals, the first just caudal to the last rib in the cranial abdominal quadrant on the affected side and the second in the caudal abdominal quadrant just cranial to the pelvic limb. Use a 5 mm trocar-cannula assembly in the cranial instrument portal and a 5 mm trocar-cannula assembly in the caudal portal. Insert a blunt probe and endo-Babcock or Kelly forceps into the instrument portals to allow manipulation and mobilization of the kidney. Incise the peritoneum along the lateral margin of the kidney and caudally over the cranial aspect of the ureter using a vessel-sealing device. Identify the ureter as early as possible to allow circumferential dissection around its cranial end, which is subsequently used for retracting the kidney during dissection of the renal hilus. Individually seal the renal artery and vein, and transect with a vessel-sealing device or laparoscopic scissors. Transect the remaining attachments of the kidney to the surrounding retroperitoneum with the vessel-sealing device. Once the kidney is completely dissected free, apply mild traction on the cranial aspect of the ureter to facilitate dissection of the caudal section of ureter to its insertion into the bladder. At a point close to the bladder, double occlude the ureter with laparoscopic hemostatic clips and transect with laparoscopic scissors. Remove the resected specimen through the most caudal instrument portal using a specimen retrieval bag after enlarging the portal incision enough to allow the kidney to be removed. Close portal sites with simple interrupted or simple continuous monofilament absorbable sutures in the body wall making sure to incorporate the external muscle fascia. Close the skin with an intradermal layer of absorbable suture material.

Summary

Endoscopic and endoscopic-assisted procedures currently performed in exotics include but are not limited to exploratory laparoscopy coelioscopy/thoracoscopy, procurement of thoracic and abdominal organ biopsies, intestinal foreign body removal, cystotomy, and sterilization procedures. The techniques described above offer a less-invasive approach to diagnostic and therapeutic modalities that decrease postoperative pain, lessen hospitalization times, and offer a faster return to normal function.

References

Chamness, C.J. (2005). Introduction to veterinary endoscopy and endoscopic instrumentation. In: *Veterinary Endoscopy for the Small Animal Practitioner*, 1e (ed. T.C. McCarthy), 1–20. St. Louis, MO: Elsevier Saunders.

Divers, S. (2005). Minimally invasive endoscopic surgery in birds. *Journal of Avian Medicine and Surgery* 19: 107–120.

Divers, S.J. (2010a). Endoscopy equipment and instrumentation for use in exotic animal medicine. *Veterinary Clinics of North America: Exotic Animal Practice* 13: 171–185.

Divers, S.J. (2010b). Exotic small mammal diagnostic endoscopy and endosurgery. *Veterinary Clinics of North America: Exotic Animal Practice* 13: 255–272.

Divers, S.J. (2010c). Avian diagnostic endoscopy. *Veterinary Clinics of North America: Exotic Animal Practice* 13: 187–202.

Divers, S.J. (2010d). Reptile diagnostic endoscopy and endosurgery. *Veterinary Clinics of North America: Exotic Animal Practice* 13: 217–242.

Divers, S.J. (2010e). Avian endosurgery. *Veterinary Clinics of North America: Exotic Animal Practice* 13: 203–216.

Divers, S.J. (2015). Endoscopic ovariectomy of exotic mammals using a three-port technique. *Veterinary Clinics of North America: Exotic Animal Practice* 18: 401–415.

Divers, S.J., Stahl, S.J., Wilson, G.H. et al. (2007). Endoscopic orchidectomy and salpingohysterectomy of pigeons (*Columba livia*): an avian model for minimally invasive endosurgery. *Journal of Avian Medicine and Surgery* 21: 22–37.

Doneley, R.J. (2001). Acute pancreatitis in parrots. *Australian Veterinary Journal* 79: 409–411.

Freeman, L.J. (1999). *Veterinary Endosurgery*. St. Louis, MO: Mosby.

Girolamo, N. and Mans, C. (2016). Reptile soft tissue surgery. *Veterinary Clinics of North America: Exotic Animal Practice* 19: 97–131.

Griffiths, C.T. (1975). Effects of castration, estrogen, and timed progestins on induced endometrial carcinoma in the rabbit. *Gynecologic Oncology* 3: 259–275.

Heiderich, E., Schildger, B., Lierz, M. et al. (2015). Endoscopic vasectomy of male feral pigeons (*Columba livia*) as a possible method of population control. *Journal of Avian Medicine and Surgery* 29: 9–17.

Innis, C.J. (2010). Endoscopy and endosurgery of the chelonian reproductive tract. *Veterinary Clinics of North America: Exotic Animal Practice* 13: 243–254.

Innis, C.J., Feinsod, R., Hanlon, M. et al. (2013). Coelioscopic orchiectomy can be effectively and safely accomplished in chelonians. *The Veterinary Record* 172: 526.

Mayhew, P.D., Mehler, S.J., Mayhew, K.N. et al. (2013). Experimental and clinical evaluation of transperitoneal laparoscopic ureteronephrectomy in dogs. *Veterinary Surgery* 42: 565–571.

McCarthy, T.C. and Monnet, E. (2005). Diagnostic and operative thoracoscopy. In: *Veterinary Endoscopy for the Small Animal Practitioner*, 1e (ed. T.C. McCarthy), 229–278. St. Louis, MO: Elsevier Saunders.

Mehler, S.J. (2011). Minimally invasive surgery techniques in exotic animals. *Journal of Exotic Pet Medicine* 20: 188–205.

Monnet, E. and Twedt, D.C. (2003). Laparoscopy. *Veterinary Clinics of North America: Small Animal Practice* 33: 1147–1158.

Proença, L. (2015). Two-portal access laparoscopic ovariectomy using LigaSure atlas in exotic companion mammals. *Veterinary Clinics of North America: Exotic Animal Practice* 18: 587–596.

Proença, L.M. and Divers, S.J. (2015). Coelioscopic and endoscope-assisted sterilization of chelonians. *Veterinary Clinics of North America: Exotic Animal Practice* 18: 555–570.

Proença, L.M., Fowler, S., Kleine, S. et al. (2014). Single surgeon coelioscopic orchiectomy of desert tortoises (*Gopherus agassizii*) for population management. *The Veterinary Record* 25: 404.

Pye, G.W., Bennett, R.A., Plunski, R. et al. (2001). Endoscopic salpingohysterectomy in juvenile cockatiels (*Nymphicus hollandicus*). *Journal of Avian Medicine and Surgery* 15: 90–94.

Taylor, M. (1994). Endoscopy evaluation and biopsy techniques. In: *Avian Medicine: Principles and Application* (eds. W. Ritchie, G.J. Harrison, and L.R. Harrison), 327–354. Lake Worth, FL: Wingers Publishing, Inc.

Sladakovic, I. and Divers, S.J. (2016). Exotic mammal laparoscopy. *Veterinary Clinics of North America: Exotic Animal Practice* 19: 269–286.

Speer, B.L. (1997). A clinical look at the avian pancreas in health and disease. *Proceedigns of the Annual Conference on Association of Avian Veterinarians*, Association of Avian Veterinarians: Reno, NV, pp. 57–64.

Taylor, W.M. (2006). Endoscopy. In: *Reptile Medicine and Surgery*, 2e (ed. D.R. Mader), 549–563. Philadelphia, PA: W.B. Saunders.

Twedt, D.C. and Monnet, E. (2005). Laparoscopy: technique and clinical experience. In: *Veterinary Endoscopy for the Small Animal Practitioner*, 1e (ed. T.C. McCarthy), 357–385. St. Louis, MO: Elsevier Saunders.

16

Orthopedic Surgery in Small Mammals

Michael S. McFadden

Anatomy and Physiology

Small mammals commonly kept as pets include ferrets (*Mustela putorius furo*), rabbits (*Oryctolagus cuniculus*), small rodents (mice [*Mus musculus*], rats [*Rattus norvegicus*], chinchillas [*Chinchilla lanigera*], guinea pigs [*Cavia porcellus*]), sugar gliders [*Petaurus breviceps*], and hedgehogs [*Atelerix albiventris*].

Fortunately, for veterinarians attempting orthopedic procedures in these species, the principles used for dogs and cats are easily adapted to small mammals, especially larger species such as rabbits and ferrets. Many of these small mammals have similar anatomy and physiology, and information used in dogs and cats can be readily adapted for use in these species with ease compared to other exotics such as birds or reptiles.

Ferrets have a long slender elongated body with a lightweight, strong, flexible skeleton. Their skeleton is very similar to dogs and cats with the exception of the spine. Ferrets have 15 thoracic vertebrae and 5–7 lumbar vertebrae (Powers and Brown 2012).

Rabbits have a lightweight skeleton surrounded by very well-developed, powerful muscles that make them prone to fractures. The skeleton of rabbits represents only 7–8% of their body weight compared to 12–13% in cats, while their muscle mass accounts for 50% of their body weight (Abdalla et al. 1992). The hind limb musculature alone can account for up to 13% of the body mass, giving rabbits the strong powerful hind limbs needed to accelerate quickly and maintain high speeds to avoid predators. If patients are not appropriately restrained and supported, their powerful hindlimbs can kick with sufficient force to cause fracture and/or luxation of the lumbar spine and damage to the spinal cord. The number of thoracic and lumbar vertebrae in rabbits varies, and the spinal cord extends into the sacral spinal canal (Vella and Donnelly 2012; Vennen and Mitchell 2009).

Variations in the musculoskeletal system of hedgehogs include fusion of the distal radius and ulna, and the complex system of muscles involved in positioning the spines. The frontodorsalis muscle, panniculus carnosis muscle, caudodorsalis muscle, and orbicularis muscle function to allow the hedgehog to roll into a ball and have the entire body protected by spines except for a 1 cm diameter ventral opening (Abou-Madi et al. 2004).

Small rodents and rabbits have been extensively used in biomedical research. Textbooks detailing their anatomy have been published and are recommended to clinicians interested in specific anatomic variations in these species (Popesko et al. 1992a,b).

Diagnostics

The diagnostic work-up for small mammal patients with orthopedic disease is similar to that for dogs and cats. Diagnostic imaging studies such as radiographs, computed tomography (CT), and magnetic resonance imaging (MRI) have all been used in small mammals to assess bone density as well as evaluate the skeletal system for any fractures (pathologic or trauma induced) or luxations. Standard radiographic equipment can be used; however, dental radiography units may be helpful in smaller rodents to get adequate detail of the extremities. In recent years, CT has become more available in general practice settings and has the added benefit of allowing 3D reconstructions. In some cases, 3D bone models can be made from the CT scans and used as aids for complex fractures or limb deformities.

Joint fluid aspirates and cytologic evaluation have been used in exotic companion mammals with joint disease and should be evaluated on any swollen or painful joint. Aseptic preparation of the skin over the joint of interest is critical to prevent iatrogenic introduction of skin microflora. Assessment of joint fluid includes color, turbidity, volume, viscosity, protein concentration, total cell count, and a

Surgery of Exotic Animals, First Edition. Edited by R. Avery Bennett and Geoffrey W. Pye.
© 2022 John Wiley & Sons, Inc. Published 2022 by John Wiley & Sons, Inc.

differential cell count. This can help differentiate degenerative joint disease, immune-mediated arthritis, and septic arthritis. Normal joint fluid should be clear, viscous, and poorly cellular (limited to small amounts of mononuclear cells). There should be a dense eosinophilic background and cells will often be in a linear arrangement referred to as "windrowing." Inflammatory joint fluid is often turbid, has decreased viscosity, and contains increased amounts of neutrophils/heterophils and mononuclear cells. In many cases of septic arthritis, infectious agents are not seen on cytologic examination of joint fluid. Culture is recommended for any abnormal joint fluid samples. Many exotics have very small volumes of joint fluid available for diagnostics, even in an effusive joint. If there is only a small volume of fluid available, a small amount of sterile saline can be aspirated into the syringe after slides for cytology have been prepared. The saline and any remaining joint fluid in the needle and hub can be submitted for culture and sensitivity testing.

Bone biopsies from exotic animals can be collected in a similar fashion to mammals using bone biopsy instruments, such as a Jamshidi bone marrow biopsy needle (Becton, Dickinson, and Company, Franklin Lakes, NJ) of appropriate size for the lesion and patient. In smaller species, hypodermic needles can be used. If these are used gently rotate the needle while it is in the lesion to cause the sample to break off inside the needle. Remove the sample with a smaller needle or expel it from the lumen with air or saline. Submit the bone for histopathology and/or for culture and sensitivity testing in cases of suspected osteomyelitis.

Joint Disease

Elbow luxations are common in ferrets and rabbits (Ritzman and Knapp 2002; Ertelt et al. 2010). They can occur spontaneously or be secondary to trauma. Affected ferrets will have a forelimb lameness and a swollen painful elbow joint palpable during an orthopedic examination. Closed reduction should be attempted under heavy sedation or general anesthesia. In dogs, closed reduction followed by splinting the leg with the elbow in extension is often successful because they have a well-developed anconeal process. When the elbow is in extension, the anconeal process engages the supratrochlear foramen of the humerus helping to maintain the elbow in reduction. Ferrets and rabbits do not have a well-developed anconeal process and closed reduction with external coaptation alone often results in re-luxation. Additional stabilization with a transarticular pin or a transarticular external skeletal fixator is often required (Figure 16.1).

(a)　　　　　　　　　　　(b)

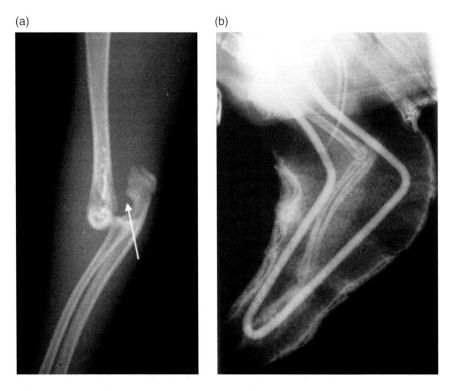

Figure 16.1 Luxation of the elbow in a rabbit (a). It was successfully reduced, closed, and placed in a lateral splint (b). Note the small anconeal process (arrow). *Source:* Images courtesy of R. Avery Bennett.

(a)   (b)

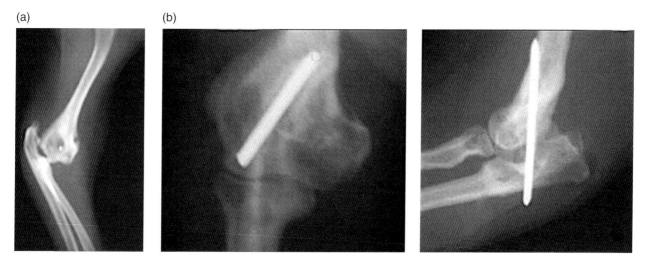

Figure 16.2 A pre-operative radiograph showing an elbow luxation in a ferret. Note the small anconeal process (a). A lateral and cranial-caudal postoperative radiographs showing proper placement of a transarticular pin following reduction (b). *Source:* Images courtesy of R. Avery Bennett.

To place a transarticular pin, once reduction is achieved, place the elbow in 100–110° of flexion and insert a pin at the caudal aspect of the ulna, through the semilunar notch, and into the distal humerus (Figure 16.2). Use external coaptation for additional support. After two to three weeks remove the transarticular pin but maintain the external coaptation for two to three weeks after pin removal (Zehnder and Kapatkin 2012).

Unlike dogs, cranial cruciate ligament injury is uncommon in ferrets. Few anecdotal reports exist and surgery is rarely required. Diagnosis is similar to dogs by documenting cranial translation of the tibia (cranial drawer). Like cats with a documented cranial cruciate ligament tear, ferrets can be managed without surgery often responding to cage rest, analgesics, and anti-inflammatory medications.

Stifle joint instability also occurs in rabbits. There is a single report of bilateral cranial cruciate ligament rupture in a rabbit (Zuijlen et al. 2012). A female intact Lotharinger presented for a right hind limb lameness. Cranial drawer was present and extraarticular stabilization was performed. The rabbit presented again four months later with a left hind limb lameness due to a ruptured cranial cruciate ligament and the procedure was repeated on the left stifle. Long-term follow-up showed the rabbit had normal behavior with no pain on palpation or manipulation of either hind limb. There are also anecdotal reports of successful conservative management of cranial cruciate injuries in rabbits.

Splay leg is an inherited congenital developmental condition seen in young rabbits ranging in age from a few days to a few months. It can also be seen in older sedentary rabbits. Affected animals are unable to adduct their hind limbs or ambulate normally. The condition may affect any or all limbs. In young developing rabbits, the hind limb anatomy is altered, which leads to changes in the angles of inclination of the proximal femur, subluxation of the coxofemoral joints, valgus deformities, and patellar luxations (Fisher and Carpenter 2012). The etiology behind this condition is not completely understood, but both genetic and environmental factors may play a role (Vennen and Mitchell 2009; Fisher and Carpenter 2012). The role of appropriate nest box flooring has been shown to affect the incidence; therefore, young rabbits should be raised on nonslip flooring (Owiny et al. 2001). Euthanasia is recommended if more than one limb is affected which is often the case. Amputation can be performed if the condition involves a single leg. Early identification of the problem and treatment using splints and hobbling can be attempted to restore more normal anatomy but is rarely successful.

A traumatic shoulder luxation was also treated nonsurgically by the author (Figure 16.3). Under heavy sedation, the shoulder was reduced and placed in a Velpeau sling to hold the carpus, elbow, and shoulder joints in flexion and to prevent weigh bearing on the affected limb. The sling was removed after four weeks and the shoulder was stable.

Trauma

Fractures in small mammals are often due to inappropriate handling, cage trauma, and bite trauma. Dogs and cats are often presented after vehicular trauma. This is less common in small mammal exotic patients, but still possible, especially in scenarios where wildlife is presented for care.

(a)　　　　　　　　　　　　　　　　　　　　　　　(b)

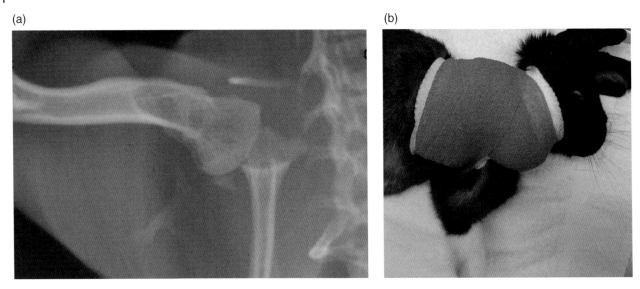

Figure 16.3 A radiographic image showing a traumatic lateral shoulder luxation in a domestic rabbit (a). Following closed reduction a Velpeau sling was placed (b) to hold the joint in reduction. Radiographs were made after splint placement to ensure the shoulder remained in reduction. After four weeks the sling was removed and the joint maintained reduction.

Bone Composition and Bone Healing

Bone Composition

The basic composition of bone is similar across taxa. Bones are a mixture of cells (osteocytes, osteoblasts, and osteoclasts) and calcium hydroxyapatite ($Ca_{10}[PO_4]_6[OH]_2$). The inorganic components give bone its strength and rigidity (Dunning 2002). The amount of calcium can vary among species and ultimately affects bone strength, stiffness, and density.

In mammals, there is considerable variation in arrangement of the bone cortices. Lower mammals such as opossums have bone that is rudimentary in appearance (Foote 1911). Incomplete lamellar bands surround the cortex followed by incomplete Haversian systems. Internal circumferential lamellae are present but not complete. In rats, there is a wide distinct band of external circumferential lamellae followed by a second, wide band of incomplete Haversian systems. The internal circumferential lamellae are poorly defined. In rabbits, external circumferential lamellae are present in some areas and indistinct in others. A wide, central ring exists that is composed of both incomplete Haversian systems and well-developed Haversian systems. Well-developed internal circumferential lamellae surround the medullary canal. Higher mammals, such as mink, skunks, felids, and canids, have well-developed external and internal circumferential lamellae with a mixture of complete and incomplete Haversian systems. The proportion of complete Haversian systems increases in these species. Periosteum covers the outer cortex of all bones and a layer of endosteum covers the surface of the medullary canal. In mammals, the periosteum and endosteum contain osteogenic cells responsible for growth, repair, and remodeling (Dunning 2002; Bliss and Todhunter 2018).

Bone Healing

Bone healing has been referred to as either direct bone healing (primary) or indirect bone healing (secondary) (Moreno et al. 2018). These models are taught as the basics in most veterinary orthopedics courses and are based on mammals. Many small mammal species such as rodents and rabbits are commonly used in research and much of what is known about bone healing is due to research in these species.

Indirect bone healing occurs through the formation of a callus. When the fracture occurs, a hematoma develops at the fracture site. Cytokines are released from platelets and other cells within the hematoma and recruit pluripotent mesenchymal cells from the periosteum, endosteum, and surrounding soft tissues. These cells differentiate into fibroblasts, chondroblasts, and osteoblasts that produce fibrous tissue, cartilage, and woven bone, respectively. This results in the formation of a callus that bridges the fracture gap and continuously reorganizes into progressively stiffer tissue until a bony callus bridges the fracture. The later stages can be evaluated radiographically, and clinical healing is complete when the bony callus bridges the fracture gap.

Primary or direct healing occurs through contact healing or gap healing. Contact healing requires a gap <0.01 mm and absolute stability with no interfragmentary motion. Lamellar bone is directly deposited in the normal axial direction of the bone. This process is started by the formation of cutting cones at the ends of osteons with osteoclasts lining the tip of the cutting cones and osteoblasts at the base. These cutting cones advance across the fracture line at a rate of 70–100 μm/d. This is also known as Haversian remodeling and results in new Haversian systems crossing the fracture line. Gap healing occurs when the fracture gap is <1 mm and >0.01 mm, and there is no motion at the fracture site. The fracture gap fills directly with intramembranous bone. The newly formed lamellar bone is oriented perpendicular to the long axis of the bone and is later reorganized through Haversian remodeling. When direct bone healing is evaluated radiographically to assess for healing, there is minimal to no callus present. The fracture lines that are present after the initial stabilization become less distinct over time and eventually disappear. Direct bone healing is commonly seen in mammals after anatomic reduction and rigid fixation of fractured long bones.

Principles of Fracture Stabilization

The principles of fracture repair are similar regardless of species (see Chapters 7 and 10). While techniques vary significantly, fractures are manipulated and stabilized with the ultimate goal of re-establishing the anatomy regarding apposition of the fracture fragments, alignment of the limb, restoration of the limb length, and maintenance of soft tissue support. When choosing which methods are used, veterinarians must take into account the soft tissue surrounding the fracture as well as ensuring that forces acting on the fracture (and its stabilization) are adequately counteracted. The methods for fixation vary and fall into two main categories, surgical and nonsurgical techniques. In some cases, the options available are limited due to the size of the patient, the anatomy, the skill of the veterinarian in orthopedic surgery, and expense.

External coaptation refers to the use of a splint, bandage, or cast to immobilize the fracture. Internal fixation refers to the use of orthopedic implants such as intramedullary (IM) pins, orthopedic wires, bone plates and screws, and interlocking nails. External skeletal fixation (ESF) refers to the use of fixation pins that are inserted percutaneously through the cortices of the bone and then connected externally to a bar or acrylic. Minimally invasive osteosynthesis is also becoming more common in veterinary orthopedics and can be applied in select exotic mammal cases. In all cases of fracture stabilization, it is important to restrict the animal's activity until the fracture has healed based on radiographs.

Fractures

Fractures are common in exotic small mammals due to their small size and delicate skeletons. Falls, being stepped on, bites from other animals, and getting limbs caught in cages are all common traumatic injuries that can lead to fractures. Fracture management in exotic small mammals is based on the same principles used in other animals. In addition, many exotic small mammals, particularly rabbits, have been extensively used as models for fracture stabilization and bone healing in humans, and some controlled studies have been performed specifically investigating fracture management in these species (Ritzman and Knapp 2002; Barron et al. 2010; Zehnder and Kapatkin 2012). As with any animal that has sustained a traumatic injury, systemic life-threatening problems should be identified and addressed before moving to the orthopedic injuries. Any signs of shock should be treated, neurologic injuries assessed, and appropriate pain management administered. Keep in mind that most exotic small mammals are prey species that respond to stress and pain stimuli in a different manner than predator species such as dogs and cats. It is very important to minimize anxiety and stress, and to anticipate analgesic needs even though they may not be overtly showing signs of pain (Zehnder and Kapatkin 2012). Any obvious fractures can be stabilized with a simple bandage or splint while a systemic evaluation is performed. Once the patient is stabilized, a systematic orthopedic examination can be completed and radiographs of any areas of instability, pain, crepitus, swelling, or other signs consistent with an orthopedic injury can be performed.

The methods of fracture fixation selected should be based on the availability of the fixation system, costs, surgeon's experience, species, and patient size. As previously mentioned, there is considerable variation in bone structure among species. Some mammals have well-developed Haversian systems, while others, especially rodents, have primitive bone systems. These differences may affect how bone heals and may play a role in how the fracture is best managed.

External coaptation is an important aspect of fracture management in exotic small mammals, especially in species that are too small for commercially available orthopedic implants. Although external coaptation does not provide the most rigid stabilization and there are some potential pitfalls, many fractures are successfully treated

(a)   (b)

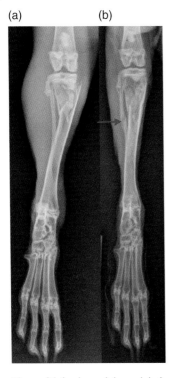

Figure 16.4 A cranial-caudal view of a proximal tibia fracture in a juvenile domestic rabbit showing the fracture before (a) and after (b) treatment with external coaptation. Note the healing fibular fracture (red arrow) not present on the initial radiograph. Since the bandage did not provide rigid stabilization, stress caused the fibular fracture.

with bandages, splints, and casts (Figure 16.4). Basic principles of external coaptation can be applied to exotic small mammals. The joint proximal and distal to the fracture must be immobilized. There are many different types of materials that can be used to provide rigid fracture stabilization (Figure 16.5). There are also a number of potential complications associated with external coaptation that should be considered including delayed union, nonunion, and malunion. Splints and bandages can also lead to bandage morbidity causing extensive wounds that may be more devastating than the fracture. External coaptation also results in joint ankylosis. Care must be taken during splint application to supply adequate padding to avoid pressure sores and to prevent any constriction of the extremity that can affect venous drainage or perfusion to the distal limb; however, if too much padding is applied, it will allow movement at the fracture site that can delay bone healing (Figure 16.6). It is also important to consider proper limb alignment and joint angles when bandaging. Rigid immobilization in an extreme extended or flexed position for long periods of time can lead to long-term joint abnormalities. Similarly, if the limb is excessively internally or externally rotated while applying bandage material it can lead to long-term changes in limb function. Take care when

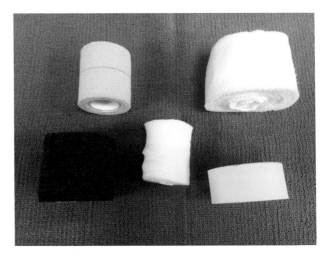

Figure 16.5 Bandaging materials commonly available in most veterinary clinics. Cast padding, conforming gauze, self-adhering bandages, and a variety of tape can be used to construct a proper bandage.

applying the layers of the bandage and alternate clockwise and counterclockwise application of layers to ensure that the limb is not inadvertently externally or internally rotated. Apply the bandage with the limb in a normal standing angle allowing early use of the limb (Figure 16.7), which can be challenging in small mammals.

Frequent bandage changes are important to identify developing wounds early so they can be treated and the bandage can be altered to prevent additional problems. In most cases, bandages can be changed once a week as long as the owners are diligent and prevent wetting, soiling, or chewing of the bandage. Bandage changes are often performed under sedation or general anesthesia as manipulation of the affected limb during the bandage change can lead to disruption of the callus and de-stabilization of the fracture in the early stages of healing. The owners must carefully monitor their pet to ensure that there are no sudden changes in comfort or pain associated with the bandage, and they must be instructed to keep the bandage clean and dry at all times.

IM pinning can be done in most exotic small mammals. Kirschner wires (K-wires) are available as small as 0.028 in. (0.071 cm), making IM pinning possible in very small patients. When placing IM pins and not other IM devices, 70% of the medullary canal should be filled (Johnston et al. 2018); therefore, a 0.028″ K-wire can be inserted into a medullary canal as small as 1–2 mm. In very small patients, hypodermic needles and spinal needles (longer) or the stylet of a spinal needle can be used as IM pins. IM pins stabilize against bending force. External coaptation, cerclage wire, hemi-cerclage wire, anti-rotational figure-of-eight wire, and simple ESF frames can be added to IM pins to counteract all forces acting on the fracture

(a) (b)

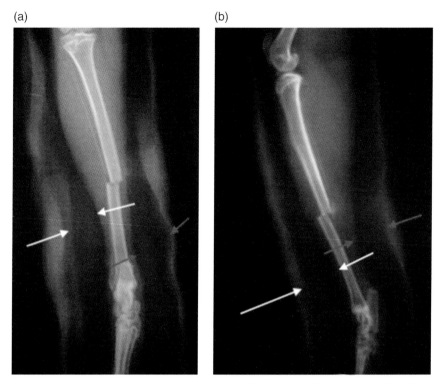

Figure 16.6 Craniocaudal (a) and lateral (b) radiographic images of a fractured tibia and fibula in a guinea pig treated with external coaptation. There is excessive padding (arrows) that can allow excess movement which can delay or prevent healing. A splint should have enough padding to protect soft tissue but not enough to allow for excess motion. *Source:* Images courtesy of Karen Rosenthal.

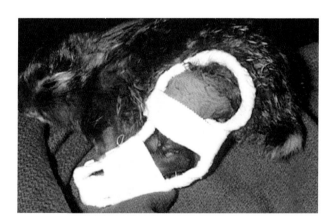

Figure 16.7 A modified Schroeder–Thomas splint applied to stabilize an open fracture of the distal tibia in a rabbit. The splint should be fabricated to conform to the normal standing angles of the patient's limb as shown. The wound is not covered to allow management of the wound without having to change the splint. *Source:* Image courtesy of R. Avery Bennett.

(Figure 16.8). Decrease the pin diameter if other IM devices, such as fixation pins for an ESF, are used to accommodate them (Figure 16.9).

Bone plates have been used in many small mammals. Due to patient size, 1.5/2.0 mm veterinary cuttable plates

are most commonly used. Other plates such as 2.0/2.7 mm veterinary cuttable plates and 2.0 mm dynamic compression plates or limited contact dynamic compression plates can also be used. More recently, small locking plates have become available and are especially useful in small exotics. Their size and locking constructs are especially adapted to small, thin, brittle, or weak bone. Many manufactures produce 1.5 mm locking plates that allow threads cut into the screw head to engage threads within the screw holes. Special drill guides are used to ensure the screw holes are in the proper orientation to allow the screw head to lock into the plate (Figure 16.10). The VetKISS Microplating System (IMEX veterinary, Longview, Texas) is the smallest veterinary locking plate system and is available in 1.0, 1.4, and 1.6 mm plate sizes. The plates are cut to length to minimize inventory and reduce costs associated with the system (Figure 16.11).

ESF are versatile and can be adapted to many different species and fracture configurations. Because of their relative low cost and equipment requirements compared with plating systems, ESF are one of the most commonly used methods for fracture fixation in exotic companion mammal orthopedics (Figure 16.12). It is important to remember the principles for insertion of fixation pins to achieve the best results and limit patient morbidity. In general, two

(a)

(b)

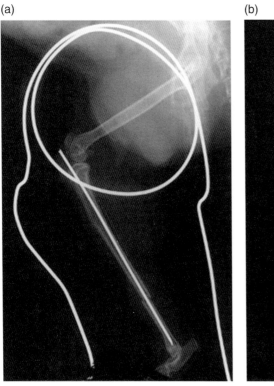

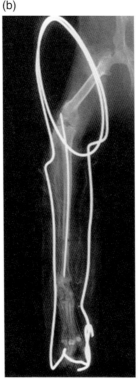

Figure 16.8 Lateral (a) and craniocaudal (b) radiographic images of a chinchilla with a distal diaphyseal fracture of the tibia treated with an IM pin. A single IM pin does not stabilize against rotation so a modified Schroeder–Thomas splint was applied to provide rotational stability. Note the IM pin occupies about 70% of the medullary canal, and the joints are maintained in normal standing angles to minimize ankylosis. *Source:* Images courtesy of R. Avery Bennett.

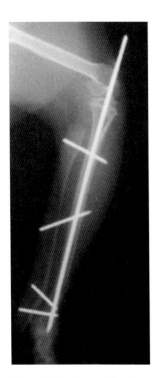

Figure 16.9 A lateral radiographic image of a chinchilla with a distal diaphyseal fracture of the tibia treated with an IM pin. A type I ESF was applied to provide rotational stability. When creating this type of construct, only fill about 50% of the medullary canal with the IM pin to allow space for insertion of the fixation pins. *Source:* Image courtesy of R. Avery Bennett.

to four ESF pins are placed in each fracture fragment. The addition of each pin increases the stability of the construct up to four pins. Any additional pins increase morbidity without any increase in stability. Fixation pin diameter should be approximately 25% of the bone diameter and placed away from important neurovascular structures. "Safe zones" for fixation pin placement have been described for dogs and cats in order to avoid vital structures (Marti and Miller 1994a,b). These anatomic locations to avoid when placing fixation pins are similar to those in exotic small mammals. Ideally, ESF are avoided in the femur and humerus because the added muscle mass penetrated by the fixation pins in these areas can lead to significant morbidity.

Commercially, available ESF systems can be used in many exotic small mammals (Acrylx™ ESF Acrylic, IMEX, Longview, TX,). Where the patients are too small for these systems, ESF can be constructed from spinal needles or hypodermic needles as fixation pins and acrylic for a connecting bar.

Repair of Specific Fractures

Prior to attempting surgical stabilization of fractures, carefully review the regional anatomy (Johnson 2014).

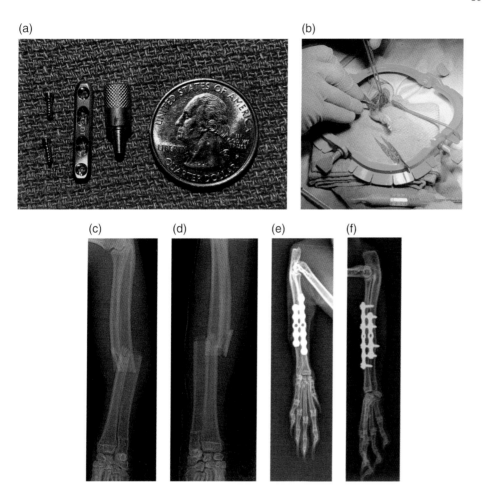

Figure 16.10 A 4 hole 1.5 mm locking plate, locking screws, and drill guide placed next to a US quarter for size comparison (a). Implants provided by VOI. *Source:* Veterinary Orthopedic Implants, St. Augustine, FL. Intraoperative image of application of a Kyon mini APLS bone plate with 1.0 mm self-tapping screws (Kyon Veterinary Surgical Products, Boston, MA, main@kyon.us) in a Guinea pig with a tibial fracture (b). *Source:* Image courtesy of Michael Karlin. A 9-month-old male mini-lop eared rabbit presented with mid-diaphyseal fractures of the radius and ulna (c, d). The fractures were stabilized with two 1.5 mm double-threaded locking adaptation plate (Veterinary Orthopedic Implants) (e, f). *Source:* Images courtesy of Andrew Levien.

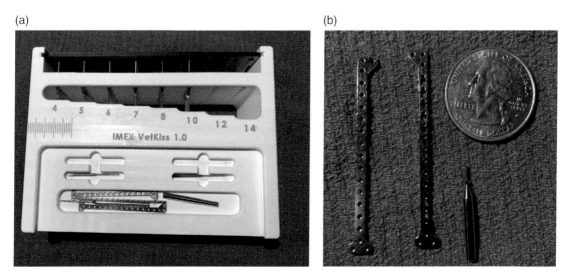

Figure 16.11 (a) The IMEX 1.0 VetKISS microplating system and (b) cut-to-length plates and locking screw placed next to a US quarter for size comparison. *Source:* Image (a) courtesy of IMEX Veterinary, Longview, Texas.

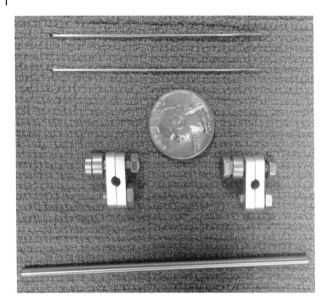

Figure 16.12 An IMEX mini SK External skeletal fixator with 1.6 mm half pins, Mini SK single clamps, and stainless steel connecting rod next to a US quarter for size comparison. *Source:* IMEX Veterinary, Longview, Texas.

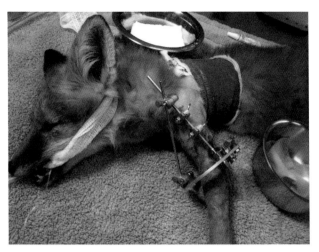

Figure 16.13 A hybrid external skeletal fixator placed on a distal humeral fracture in a juvenile red fox. This patient was caught in a trap causing extensive soft tissue injuries. The ESF allowed continued wound management and fracture stabilization simultaneously.

Fractures of the Humerus

Fractures of the thoracic limb can involve any bone from the scapula to the digits. Scapular fractures are usually managed conservatively (coaptation) unless the articular surface of the glenoid cavity is involved, in which case, anatomic reduction is preferred to minimize the changes to the articular surface that can lead to secondary degenerative joint disease. For these types of fractures, open reduction and stabilization with screws, pins, or wire are recommended.

Humeral fractures can occur at the proximal physis, diaphysis, and distal metaphysis. Because the humerus is located adjacent to the thoracic cavity, careful assessment of the thoracic cavity should be performed and radiographic evaluation of the thorax is recommended with most humeral fractures. Rib fractures, pulmonary contusions, and pneumothorax are commonly associated with trauma to the thoracic limb. Reduce and stabilize proximal physeal fractures with cross pins to minimize disruption of bone growth. Diaphyseal fractures are common and can pose a challenge to even experienced orthopedic surgeons. Avoid using external coaptation, if possible, because it is difficult to adequately immobilize the shoulder joint (the joint proximal to the fracture) and malunions are common.

Prior to attempting surgical stabilization of humerus fractures, carefully review the regional anatomy. Along the medial diaphysis there are many important neurovascular structures, including the brachial artery and vein, and the median, ulnar, and musculocutaneous nerves. Laterally, the radial nerve courses across the distal diaphysis (Johnson 2014). Diaphyseal fractures can be stabilized with bone plates or ESF. Bone plates can be applied to the medial, lateral, or cranial surface of the bone. Application can be challenging due to the shape of the humerus. If ESF is chosen, be careful to avoid the previously mentioned neurovascular structures when the fixation pins are placed (Figure 16.13).

Fractures of the Radius and Ulna

Radius fractures are commonly reported in exotic companion mammals. Because there is minimal soft tissue coverage over the distal radius, open radius fractures are common. In general, the radius is the primary weight bearing bone in mammals and fractures of the ulna are not specifically addressed unless the articular surface of the elbow is involved or if there is a displaced fracture of the olecranon. These ulnar fractures can be managed with bone plates or a pin and tension band wire. Radial fractures can be stabilized using external coaptation, bone plates, or ESF. In toy breed dogs, much like exotic small mammals, there is a higher incidence of nonunions for distal radial and ulnar fractures because of the minimal soft tissue coverage and poor extraosseous blood supply. External coaptation is not recommended for these types of injuries. IM pinning of the radius cannot be performed without passing into the carpus or elbow and, therefore, is not recommended. Plates are a recommended method of managing these and can be applied to the cranial or medial surface of the radius.

Although applying bone plates on the medial aspect can have a biomechanical advantage, cranial application is easier. Type Ib ESF are most commonly used for radial fractures, although type Ia or type II ESF could be used (see Chapter 10).

Fractures of the Metacarpal Bones

Metacarpal fractures are less commonly seen in exotic companion mammals than dogs and cats. Most of these injuries can be managed with splints or soft padded bandages. Internal fixation is usually not possible due to the small size of the bone. Digit amputation may be necessary in patients with chronic pain or arthritis secondary to articular damage or ligamentous injuries.

Fractures of the Pelvic Bones

Pelvic fractures can appear dramatic and daunting on radiographs because multiple fractures are often present; however, in most cases, only fractures of the weight-bearing axis need to be stabilized. These include acetabular fractures, fractures of the ilium, and fractures or luxations of the sacrum or sacroiliac joint. Fractures of the pubis are rarely stabilized unless there is an avulsion of the prepubic tendon and herniation of the urinary bladder. Ischial fractures are rarely addressed. Although surgery may be the preferred treatment, most small mammals with pelvic fractures can be managed conservatively. Malunions that form can lead to narrowing of the pelvic canal and dystocia or chronic constipation. Ilial body fractures should be stabilized with bone plates or interfragmentary wires in exotic small mammals. Acetabular fractures can be stabilized with bone plates, pins and polymethylmethacrylate, or, in situations where the patient is too small for implants or the fracture is comminuted and anatomic reduction is not possible, a femoral head and neck excision arthroplasty (FHO).

Fractures of the Femur

Femoral fractures can involve the capital physis, femoral neck, diaphysis, distal metaphysis, or distal physis. Most cases of capital physeal or femoral neck fractures in exotic small mammals are best managed with FHO with a good prognosis due to patient size. External coaptation of diaphyseal fractures is to be avoided due to the significant displacement that is often seen with femoral fractures and the inability to immobilize the hip joint. Diaphyseal fractures of the femur can be managed with plates, ESF, IM pins, or

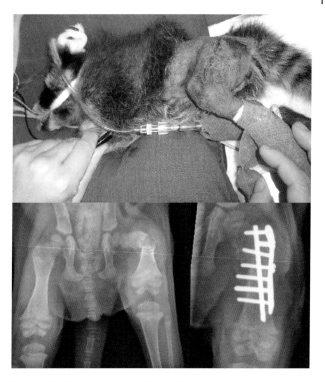

Figure 16.14 A pre- and postoperative femur fracture in a juvenile raccoon stabilized with a 1.5 mm/2.0 mm veterinary cuttable plate and IM pin (0.0062″ K-wire).

a combination of implants. Care must be taken when placing IM pins to avoid the sciatic nerve as it courses close to the trochanteric fossa. Bone plates are applied to the lateral surface of the femur to avoid neurovascular structures on the medial side and also to take advantage of the biomechanical advantage of plating the tension surface of the bone (Figure 16.14). Place ESF fixation pins through the lateral aspect of the femur. One disadvantage of ESF in the femur is the high morbidity associated with pin placement through the musculature of the thigh. Stabilize distal metaphyseal and physeal fractures with cross pins (Figure 16.15).

Fractures of the Tibia and Fibula

Tibial fractures, like radial fractures, are commonly open due to the minimal soft tissue covering most of the medial aspect of the tibia. Tibial fractures can be treated with external coaptation, IM pins, bones plates, ESF, or interlocking nails. IM pins and interlocking nails can be inserted in a normograde fashion through a small medial parapatellar incision. Insert the pin at a point on the tibial plateau just inside the medial cortex and halfway between the patellar ligament and the medial collateral ligament. Bone plates and ESF fixation pins are placed medially to avoid the musculature on the lateral aspect of the tibia. Careful

(a)   (b)   (c)

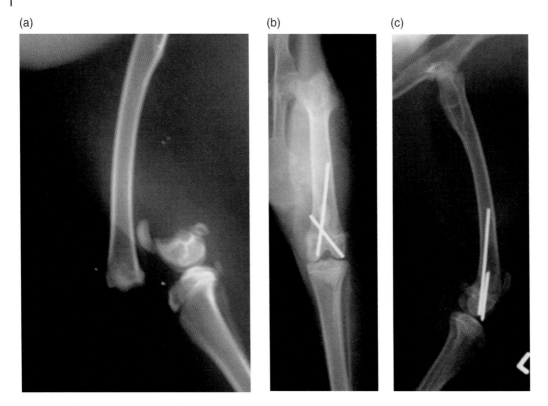

Figure 16.15 Lateral radiographic image of a raccoon with a distal Salter–Harris I femur fracture (a). The fracture was reduced and stabilized using cross pins (b, c). *Source:* Images courtesy of R. Avery Bennett.

dissection is needed to avoid the medial saphenous artery, vein, and nerve as they cross the medial tibial diaphysis. Metatarsal and digit fractures are managed in a similar fashion to metacarpal fractures.

Complications associated with fracture repair can occur due to inappropriate choice of implants, improper placement of the implants, poor owner compliance with postoperative instructions, or, in some cases, bad luck. Delayed unions, nonunions, and malunions can occur. Depending on the severity of the complication, treatment may not be required, the fracture stabilization may need revision, or, in the worst case, amputation may be indicated. In general, exotic small mammal patients tolerate amputation well and techniques for amputations are adapted from dogs and cats. Leaving a stump generally leads to repetitive trauma and should be avoided if possible. Forelimb amputations should be done at the shoulder joint or, preferably, done in addition to the removal of the scapula so there are no bone prominences to rub on the substrate after the scapular musculature has atrophied. Hind limb amputation should be done at the level of the proximal femoral diaphysis with the end of the femur covered by muscles or by disarticulation of the coxofemoral joint.

References

Abdalla, K.E.H., Abd, E.-N., Ibrahim, M. et al. (1992). Comparative anatomical and biochemical studies on the main bones of the limbs of rabbit and cat as a mediclegal parameter. *Assiut Veterinary Medical Journal* 26: 142–153.

Abou-Madi, N., Scrivanim, P.V., Kollias, G.V. et al. (2004). Diagnosis of skeletal injuries in chelonians using computed tomography. *Journal of Zoo and Wildlife Medicine* 35: 226–231.

Barron, H.W., McBride, M., Martinez-Jimenez, D. et al. (2010). Comparison of two methods of long bone fracture repair in rabbits. *Journal of Exotic Pet Medicine* 19: 183–188.

Bliss, S. and Todhunter, R. (2018). Tissues of the musculoskeletal system. In: *Veterinary Surgery: Small Animal*, 2e (eds. K. Tobias and S. Johnston), 1764–1797. St Louis, MO: Elsevier.

Dunning, D. (2002). Basic mammalian bone anatomy and healing. *Veterinary Clinics of North America: Exotic Animal Practice* 5: 115–128.

Ertelt, J., Maierl, J., Kaiser, A. et al. (2010). Anatomical and pathophysiological features and treatment of elbow luxation in rabbits. *Tierärztliche Praxis. Ausgabe K, Kleintiere/Heimtiere* 38: 201–210.

Fisher, P. and Carpenter, J. (2012). Neurologic and musculoskeletal disease. In: *Ferrets, Rabbits, and Rodents: Clinical Medicine and Surgery*, 3e (eds. K. Quesenberry and J. Carpenter), 245–256. St. Louis, MO: Elsever.

Foote, J.S. (1911). The comparative histology of femoral bones. *Transaction of the American Microsopical Society* 30: 87–140.

Johnson, K. (ed.) (2014). *Piermattei's Atlas of Surgical Approaches to the Bones and Joints of the Dog and Cat*, 5e. Philadelphia, PA: Saunders.

Johnston, S.A., Dirsko, J.F., Dejardin, L.M. et al. (2018). Internal fracture fixation. In: *Veterinary Surgery: Small Animal Eselvier*, 2e (eds. S.A. Johnston and K.M. Tobias), 1907. MO: St. Louis.

Marti, J.M. and Miller, A. (1994a). Delimitation of safe corridors for the insertion of fixation pins in the dog – Part 1: Hindlimb. *Journal of Small Animal Practice* 35: 16–23.

Marti, J.M. and Miller, A. (1994b). Delimitation of safe corridors for the insertion of fixation pins in the dog – Part 1: Forelimb. *Journal of Small Animal Practice* 35: 78–85.

Moreno, M.R., Zambrano, S., Dejardin, L.M. et al. (2018). Bone biomechanics and fracture biology. In: *Veterinary Surgery: Small Animal*, 2e (eds. S.A. Johnston and K.M. Tobias), 1857–1866. St. Louis, MO: Eselvier.

Owiny, J.R., Vandewoude, S., Painter, J.T. et al. (2001). Hip dysplasia in rabbits: association with nest box flooring. *Comparative Medicine* 51: 85–88.

Popesko, P., Rajtova, V., and Horak, J. (eds.) (1992a). *A Colour Atlas of the Anatomy of Small Laboratory Animals: Rat, Mouse, and Hampster*, vol. 2. Bratislava: Wolfe Publishing.

Popesko, P., Rajtova, V., and Horak, J. (eds.) (1992b). *A Colour Atlas of the Anatomy of Small Laboratory Animals: Rabbit and Guniea Pig*, vol. 1. Bratislava: Wolfe Publishing.

Powers, L. and Brown, S. (2012). Basic anatomy, physiology, and husbandry. In: *Ferrets, Rabbits, and Rodents: Clinical Medicine and Surgery*, 3e (eds. K. Quesenberry and J. Carpenter), 1–12. St. Louis, MO: Elsever.

Ritzman, T. and Knapp, D. (2002). Ferret orthopedics. *Veterinary Clinics of North America: Exotic Animal Practice* 5: 129–155.

Vella, D. and Donnelly, T. (2012). Basic anatomy, physiology, and husbandry. In: *Ferrets, Rabbits, and Rodents: Clinical Medicine and Surgery*, 3e (eds. K. Quesenberry and J. Carpenter), 157–173. St. Louis, MO: Elsevier.

Vennen, K. and Mitchell, M.A. (2009). Rabbits. In: *Manual of Exotic Pet Practice* (eds. M. Mitchell and T. Tully), 375–405. St. Louis, MO: Saunders.

Zehnder, A. and Kapatkin, A. (2012). Orthopedics in small mammals. In: *Ferrets Rabbits, and Rodents: Clinical Medicine and Surgery*, 3e (eds. K. Quesenberry and J. Carpenter), 472–484. St. Louis, MO: Elsevier.

Zuijlen, M., Vrolijk, P., and van der Heyden, M. (2012). Bilateral successive cranial cruciate ligament rupture treated by extracapsular stabilization surgery in a pet rabbit *(Oryctolagus cuniculus)*. *Journal of Exotic Pet Medicine* 19: 245–248.

17

Rabbit Soft Tissue Surgery

R. Avery Bennett

Introduction

The blood volume of a rabbit is 5.7% of the total body weight, which is less than that of dogs (10%) and cats (8%) (Vargas 2013). Loss of 15–20% of blood volume causes cardiovascular compromise and a loss of more than 20% results in critical or fatal consequences. Venous access is essential for all rabbits undergoing any but the most minor procedures to provide intraoperative fluid support as well as in the event of an emergency. If an intravenous catheter cannot be placed, place an intraosseous catheter. Subcutaneous fluid administration will not allow for fluid resuscitation.

While rabbits do have different blood types, typing is not routinely performed making preoperative cross-matching essential prior to performing any surgery where major blood loss might be anticipated. Cross-matching should be performed prior to administering blood from another rabbit. If rabbit blood is not available, consider a colloid or blood substitute.

Careful anesthetic monitoring of the patient's status during surgery is vital. If possible, body temperature, electrocardiogram, ventilation, end-expiratory CO_2, blood pressure, SpO_2, and blood gas levels should be monitored and appropriate measures taken if clinically important alterations occur. If direct blood pressure monitoring is available, rabbits have a medial saphenous artery that is easily catheterized.

Celiotomy

The basic principles of celiotomy in other species apply to rabbits; however, rabbits are especially prone to developing postoperative gastrointestinal (GI) ileus and intraabdominal adhesions. In humans, postoperative adhesions occur commonly and are usually associated with discomfort and pain, which is likely the same in rabbits. Adhesions can cause dysfunction and require intervention. To reduce the risk, minimize manipulation of abdominal structures, especially the GI tract. Manipulation of structures causes trauma to their serosal surface predisposing to adhesion formation. Gentle tissue handling is essential. It is better to use instruments than fingers. Use powderless gloves or wash the power off gloves before touching organs as talc is irritating. Instilling antibiotics into the abdomen has not been shown to be beneficial in any species and most antibiotics are irritating, so this practice is contraindicated in rabbits. Desiccation of the serosal surfaces also predisposes to adhesion formation. Keep all visceral surfaces moist by frequently irrigating and covering viscera with moist sponges. Fat necrosis and hematomas from incomplete hemostasis during surgery will also predispose to adhesion formation and have been reported to occur in the broad ligament of the uterus following hysterectomy in rabbits (Varga 2016). Tissue distal to ligatures will necrose, so it is important to minimize the amount of tissue left distal to any ligatures. Use the smallest minimally reactive suture possible on an atraumatic small needle. Catgut suture is not recommended for use in rabbits.

It is best to prevent formation of adhesions because surgical lysis creates additional irritation, inflammation, and recurrence. Various medications have been studied to prevent adhesion formation including verapamil with and without recombinant tissue plasminogen activator, such as pentoxifylline, diltiazem, melatonin, NSAIDs, and others (Vargas 2013). Currently, intraabdominal topical agents are not recommended. Postoperative NSAID therapy is the only medication routinely recommended to reduce the risk of adhesion formation. Following surgical lysis of adhesions, pentoxifylline (2.5 mg/kg q12h for six treatments) has been shown to reduce recurrence of adhesions (Steinleiter et al. 1990).

Surgery of Exotic Animals, First Edition. Edited by R. Avery Bennett and Geoffrey W. Pye.
© 2022 John Wiley & Sons, Inc. Published 2022 by John Wiley & Sons, Inc.

Engage the peritoneum and the external rectus sheath when closing the body wall if the incision was not in the linea alba to reduce adhesions. In dogs and cats, if the incision was not in the linea alba, it is recommended to only suture the external rectus sheath because suturing the peritoneum has been associated with increased adhesion formation. A study in rabbits showed a decreased risk of adhesion formation if the peritoneum was sutured closed during closure of the body wall (Whitfield et al. 2007).

The omentum of rabbits is smaller and less flexible than that of dogs and cats (Vargas 2013). It may not reach to all areas of the abdomen to help seal incisions.

GI Surgery

The general principles of GI surgery in other species apply to rabbits. The submucosa is considered the holding layer and must be engaged during closure of an enterotomy or gastrotomy. Because of the propensity to develop GI stasis and adhesions, it is best not to use clamps, even those

considered atraumatic, to hold back ingesta. Use an assistant's fingers if possible.

Anatomy

The cardia and pylorus of rabbits are well developed and the stomach is never empty even after days of anorexia. Rabbits are not able to vomit or eructate. Everything must exit through the pylorus. The orad duodenum has a larger diameter for 1–2 cm aborad to the pylorus where it narrows and maintains that diameter throughout the small intestine to the ileocecocolic junction (Figure 17.1). The ileum opens into the sacculus rotundus, a spherical thick-walled enlargement, through the ileocolic valve, another location of a narrower lumen. The cecum is very large with a nearly transparent, thin wall. The fusus coli is a thick, muscular area of the colon with a narrower lumen between the orad and aborad colon. The orad and aborad colon are separated by the fusus coli and are functionally and morphologically distinct from each other. These three locations are common sites of intestinal obstruction.

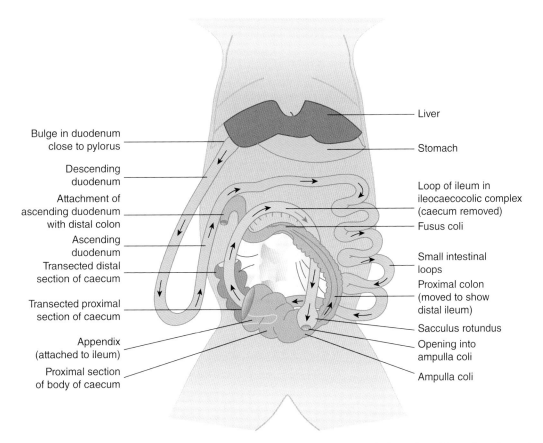

Figure 17.1 Image of the gastrointestinal track of a rabbit. Approximately 1–2 cm aborad from the pylorus the duodenum narrows. This is a common site for an obstruction. With obstruction at this location, the course of the disease is very acute, and patients decline rapidly without intervention. The ileocolic valve is another location where foreign objects can become lodged. With obstruction at this location, there will be many gas distended loops of small intestine and a more gradual progression of disease. A third location for obstruction is the fusus coli where the diameter narrows. It is uncommon for obstruction to occur at this location, but fiber and other materials may accumulate and cause a partial or complete obstruction. *Source*: Harcourt-Brown et al. (2016b).

Gastric Surgery

Indications for gastric surgery in rabbits include neoplasia (most commonly lymphoma), severe ulcers not responsive to medical management, and removal of duodenal tricho-bezoars that can be massaged orad into the stomach. The orad duodenum is wider for about 2 cm aborad to the pylorus, which is a common site of obstruction due to trichobezoars. If possible, manipulate the object orad and remove it through a gastrotomy. Gastrotomy is considered to have fewer potential complications than enterotomy and, in rabbits with small diameter, thin-walled intestine, this is especially valid.

Gastric surgery in rabbits is similar to that in other species. Isolate the area with saline moistened laparotomy pads. Use stay sutures to manipulate the stomach and control contamination. The incision can usually be closed with two layers: simple continuous oversewn with an inverting pattern. Because the submucosa is the holding layer, it is vital to engage it during closure. In most cases, it is not feasible to differentiate mucosa from submucosa, so full thickness sutures are recommended by the author.

Intestinal Obstruction

The stomach contains ingested material including food, hair, and other items as well as cecotropes and fecal material since rabbits are coprophagic. The pH of the stomach of rabbits is very low (1–2). Rabbits are not able to open their mouth very far and chew ingested grasses until the particle size is small so that foreign body ingestion/obstruction is rare; however, they will ingest materials such as carpet fiber that can cause problems.

The most common cause of intestinal obstruction is a trichobezoar (Harcourt-Brown 2016). It is theorized that hair ingested while grooming leaves the stomach and in the colon is molded into a hair pellet, the same way fecal pellets are formed. The pellet is then ingested by the rabbit, and because it has been so densely packed in the colon, it is not broken down in the stomach. The pellet then leaves the stomach and may pass through the intestine again, but if it is large enough, it can cause intestinal obstruction. Intermittent obstruction also occurs commonly in rabbits if an object causes signs of obstruction, but then moves aboard relieving signs of obstruction, and then it obstructs again farther aborad. This can happen repeatedly before the object passes into the aborad colon and out or fails to pass in which case clinical signs fail to resolve. If it makes it past the fusus coli, it will be passed into the feces. Other small objects like locust seed, dried corn kernels, and carpet fiber have been reported to cause intestinal obstruction in rabbits (Harcourt-Brown 2016).

Intestinal obstruction is difficult to differentiate from GI ileus especially if the obstruction is at the ileocolic valve or fusus coli compared to the orad duodenum because the process is more insidious with a more aborad obstruction. Table 17.1 summarizes the differences between GI stasis, a foreign body that is moving through the intestine causing intermittent obstruction, and complete intestinal obstruction. Orad duodenal obstruction has an acute course. Rabbits can be eating and behaving normally and dead in as little as 6–8 hours (Harcourt-Brown 2016). It appears to be a common cause of acute death in rabbits.

Dogs and cats with intestinal obstruction present with intractable vomiting, anorexia, lethargy, depression,

Table 17.1 A summary of the differences between gut stasis, a moving foreign body, and complete intestinal obstruction. *Source*: Harcourt-Brown (2016b).

Feature	Intestinal obstruction	Moving foreign body	Gut stasis
Speed of onset	Rapid: owner often says rabbit was "fine" a few hours before	Rapid	Slow: owners often can't say when signs began
Demeanor of rabbit at outset	Depressed, immobile, may hide in corners, may show signs of colic	Variable	Progressively quieter; becomes more depressed when anorexia has been present for 2–3 d (unless another condition is making rabbit ill)
Palpation of stomach	Large, balloon-like structure behind ribs on left-hand side	Dilated stomach is often palpable	Stomach is not palpable or can be felt as small, hard mass
Abdominal radiology	Gastric dilation; may or may not be distended loops of intestine (depending on site of obstruction); no gas in ileocaecocolic complex	Gastric dilation; distended loops of intestine usually visible, unless they are filled with fluid; large amount of gas in ileocaecocolic complex once foreign body passes through	Small stomach with or without impacted contents and halo of gas, depending on stage of gut stasis; gas in caecum is common; may be large amounts of caecal gas in later stages
Blood glucose	High >20 mmol/l	Raised 15–25 mmol/l	Low, normal, or slightly raised (>15 mmol/l); low or within normal range in early stages

dehydration, and abdominal pain. Rabbits are not able to vomit and mask signs of illness making it more difficult to diagnose an obstruction. Early clinical signs in rabbits include anorexia, behavior changes, hiding, nonresponsive signs of pain including frequently changing their position, pressing the abdomen on the floor, and potentially a bloated appearance. Perform a complete physical examination paying attention to processes that predispose to GI ileus such as dental disease, respiratory disease, and difficulty grooming. Early in the course, the only physical abnormality may be a bloated abdomen which could be from obstruction or ileus.

Rabbits with intestinal obstruction typically have very elevated blood glucose, as high as 500 mg/dl (>20 mmol/l) (Harcourt-Brown 2016), compared with a moderately elevated glucose (<250 mg/dl: 15–25 mmol/l) in rabbits with ileus. If a rabbit has a normal or slightly elevated glucose, then surgery is not indicated. Rapidly increasing blood glucose is an indication for surgical intervention, likely for an intestinal obstruction.

Serial abdominal radiographs are indicated in all rabbits with suspected GI stasis or intestinal obstruction (Figure 17.2). In rabbits with intestinal obstruction, the amount of gas in the stomach rapidly increases especially with duodenal obstruction. If the object is more aborad, the intestine orad to the obstruction will also be distended with gas. If there is gas throughout the GI tract into the colon, it indicates the object has recently passed into the colon and surgery is not indicated.

Rabbits with intestinal obstruction show an initial response to treatment for ileus including fluid resuscitation, motility stimulants, and syringe feeding. In some, these treatments may result in the object moving, resolving the problem. If the object does not move, the patient status will continue to deteriorate. If the obstruction is in the orad duodenum, in many ways, the pathophysiology is similar to that of gastric dilation and volvulus in dogs. The stomach rapidly becomes distended with gas compromising venous return to the heart and potentially compressing the thorax resulting in respiratory compromise.

In rabbits with rapidly worsening gastric tympany, urgent surgical intervention is indicated. Prior to surgery decompression is essential. In many rabbits, it is possible to pass in orogastric tube under sedation. This will allow gas to escape, but the diameter of the tube that can be passed in a rabbit is narrow and very easily clogged. Trocarization is an alternative, but there is a risk of gastric perforation resulting in contents free in the abdomen, a life-threatening complication. If an orogastric tube can relieve some of the tympany and the patient can be stabilized, then perform surgery as soon as possible.

If the distention cannot be relieved and the patient does not respond to fluid resuscitation and prokinetic medications, consider performing a gastrostomy to allow gastric contents to be removed.

Gastrostomy

A gastrostomy can be performed under local anesthesia with or without sedation especially in compromised patients. With the rabbit in right lateral recumbency, inject local anesthetic caudal to the last rib at the gastric distention. Block the skin and muscle and allow at least 10 minutes for the anesthetic to take effect. Make a 2–3 cm incision through the skin, a grid approach through the muscle of the body wall, and incise the peritoneum. The distended stomach is easy to identify and exteriorized. Place a simple continuous suture circumferentially between the stomach and body wall to create a seal. Incise the portion of the stomach in the center of the suture to create the stoma. Through this stoma gas, fluid and even food material can be evacuated, and it will continue to serve as an outlet for fluid and gas as they continue to be produced. This procedure can keep the stomach decompressed and allow the patient to be stabilized for anesthesia and surgery. Once the patient is stable, perform a celiotomy and surgically relieve the obstruction, take down the gastrostomy and close the stomach, and then close the left body wall incision used to create the gastrostomy.

Surgical Management of Intestinal Obstruction

Perform a celiotomy from the xiphoid to the mid-abdomen. Extend the incision as needed but keep the incision small to decrease the risks of adhesions and postoperative ileus. Exteriorize a portion of the small intestine and trace it orad and aborad to identify the object (Figure 17.2). Determine if it is possible to massage it orad into the stomach or into the colon in patients with ileocolic or fusus coli obstructions. If it can be manipulated into the stomach, perform a gastrotomy to retrieve the object. If it can be passed into the aborad colon, it will be passed with feces. A technique for manipulating an object into the aborad colon has been described with specific reference to anatomic structures encountered (Harcourt-Brown 2016).

If it is not possible to manipulate the object into the stomach or aborad colon, perform an enterotomy. Carefully, isolate the area with moistened laparotomy sponges. Make the incision in a healthy segment of intestine through which it is possible to remove the object. Close the incision with a simple interrupted pattern because the wall is thin and typically distorted by a simple continuous pattern. Use a fine (6-0 or smaller) rapidly absorbed material on a fine atraumatic needle. If the mucosa everts, trim it to minimize the amount exposed reducing adhesion formation.

(a)

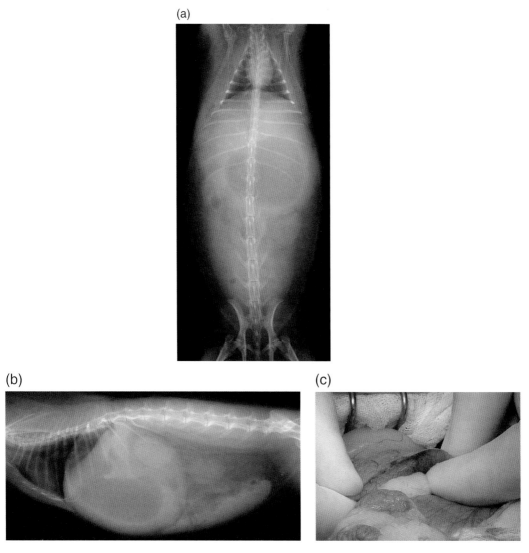

(b)　　　　　　　　　　　　　　　(c)

Figure 17.2　Ventrodorsal (a) and lateral (b) images of a rabbit with a duodenal obstruction. At surgery, the obstructing ball of hair and fiber was removed (c). Note the stomach is severely distended with gas and fluid, but the small intestines are normal. *Source:* Images courtesy of Karen Rosenthal.

Place full-thickness sutures to ensure the submucosa is engaged. Consider closing a longitudinal enterotomy transversely so as not to reduce lumen diameter. The author does not recommend injecting saline into the intestine to test for leaks. Use gas or ingesta within the intestine to distend the site of the incision to check for leaks. Do not over-inflate or apply supraphysiologic pressure, it is always possible to create a leak through needle holes. If possible, place the omentum over the enterotomy and tack it in place creating an omental patch. If there is concern for the integrity of the intestine, place a serosal patch using another segment of intestine. Carefully, lavage the segment to minimize contamination before replacing it into the abdomen. Close the celiotomy routinely.

Liver Lobe Torsion

Liver lobe torsion is considered rare in any species; however, it occurs relatively frequently in rabbits (Stanke et al. 2011). Early reports identified liver lobe torsion as an incidental finding at necropsy (Weisbroth 1975). In recent years, a number of reports document liver lobe torsion in rabbits with as many as 16 cases at one institution in a five years period (Graham et al. 2014). Lop-eared rabbits appear to be overrepresented with 13 of 16 in that report being lops and other reports in lops (Wenger et al. 2009; Stock et al. 2019). The caudate lobe is most commonly affected (62–63%), but torsions of the right lateral, left lateral, right medial, and quadrate lobes have been reported. Two rabbits were diagnosed with two liver lobe torsions (Graham et al. 2014). The caudate lobe has a narrow attachment to the dorsal liver hilum which is speculated to predispose this lobe to torsion (Graham and Basseches 2014). It has also been speculated that gastric dilation secondary to GI ileus stretches the triangular ligament predisposing to liver lobe torsion because many cases have had a history of GI stasis (Graham et al. 2014).

Clinical signs of liver lobe torsion and GI stasis are similar; anorexia, lethargy, decrease production and soft feces, inappropriate urination and defecation, hunched posture, and hiding behavior (Taylor and Staff 2007). Most cases have been initially diagnosed and treated for GI stasis. While in one study three of seven rabbits survived with medical management, liver lobe torsion is generally considered a surgical emergency (Graham et al. 2014).

Physical examination may reveal abdominal pain, dehydration, increased intestinal gas, tachypnea, decreased gut sounds, hypothermia, dull mentation, and a palpable cranial abdominal mass or liver edge. Other than a palpable mass effect or liver edge in the cranial abdomen found in 19% of rabbits in one study (Graham et al. 2014), these findings are the same as in a rabbit with GI stasis.

The clinical pathologic findings in rabbits with liver lobe torsion include anemia, elevated liver enzymes, and elevated BUN and creatinine. Red cells may show evidence of fragmentation (Graham et al. 2014). These findings are consistent with liver lobe torsion and not GI stasis, underscoring the importance of hematologic evaluation as soon as possible after presentation. In one report of three rabbits with liver lobe torsion, two were managed medically and died; however, the third was taken to surgery urgently and survived suggesting early surgical intervention is important (Sanders et al. 2009).

Radiographs are not helpful in arriving at a diagnosis, but ultrasound has been very accurate. In 14 of 14 rabbits with liver lobe torsion, the diagnosis was made using ultrasound and color flow Doppler showing a decrease or lack of blood flow to an abnormal portion of the liver (Graham et al. 2014). In that study, no contrast enhancement was used while in a case report contrast-enhanced ultrasound showed a complete lack of perfusion in an abnormal right liver lobe (Stock et al. 2019). Ultrasonographic findings include heterogenous liver parenchyma, an abnormally large liver lobe, rounded liver margins, hyperechoic hepatic mesentery, anechoic free abdominal fluid, and decreased intestinal motility (Wenger et al. 2009; Stock et al. 2019).

Liver lobectomy has been associated with an excellent prognosis for long-term survival, and there are no reports of a second occurrence, though in one report, two rabbits had two lobes torsed. In the report of 16 rabbits, nine underwent surgery and all nine survived long term (Graham et al. 2014). The other seven rabbits were

managed medically with fluid therapy, antibiotics, nutritional supplementation, analgesics, and prokinetic medications, and three survived long-term. On follow-up examination, all three had normal or improved liver enzymes. The authors also reported a patient with what they believed to be a chronic liver lobe torsion found incidentally on ultrasound examination that they have followed for years. Others have reported chronic liver lobe torsion as an incidental finding characterized by an atrophied lobe (Weisbroth 1975).

While liver lobe torsion in rabbits is considered a surgical emergency, it is important to stabilize the patient prior to surgery as best as possible with IV fluids, antibiotic therapy, and analgesics. There are reports of rabbits dying during anesthetic induction and preparation for surgery underscoring the importance of early diagnosis and preoperative stabilization (Sanders et al. 2009; Graham et al. 2014).

Perform a standard ventral midline celiotomy and identify the affected lobe. The site of torsion is typically very tight and narrow. Place a single or double encircling ligatures, hemostatic clips, thoracoabdominal stapler, or tissue-sealing device at the location of the torsion and transect the parenchyma distally allowing removal of the affected lobe. It is essential not to try to untwist the lobe as this can result in release of toxins that are thought to predispose to disseminated intravascular coagulation. No intraoperative or postoperative complications have been reported and surgery carries an excellent prognosis.

Urinary Tract Surgery

Normal urine production in rabbits is 130 ml/kg/d and maintenance fluid rate is 100 ml/kg/d (Jenkins 2012; Klaphake and Paul-Murphy 2012; Keeble and Benato 2016). Rabbits have a limited ability to concentrate urine, so dehydration quickly results in prerenal azotemia (Klaphake and Paul-Murphy 2012).

Anatomy

The kidneys are retroperitoneal and the right kidney is consistently larger than the left. It is located at the level of the first lumbar vertebra (Keeble and Benato 2016). The left kidney is slightly more caudal. The hilum is a slight depression on the medial aspect where the vessels and ureter connect. The renal capsule is continuous with the renal pelvis. Rabbits have a single papilla at the vertex of the renal pyramid. The ureters are also retroperitoneal and a continuation of the renal pelvis. The cranial aspect of the ureter receives blood from the cranial ureteral artery, a branch of the renal artery, and the caudal aspect from the caudal ureteral artery, a branch of the vesicular artery. The bladder wall is thin with a capacity of 60 ml in a 4 kg rabbit (Keeble and Benato 2016). In female rabbits, the urethra is very short and ends at the external urethral orifice in the floor of the vagina.

Urolithiasis

Calcium metabolism in rabbits is different from that of many mammals. Dietary calcium absorption is independent of vitamin D_3 and excess calcium is eliminated by urinary excretion as calcium carbonate. The fractional excretion of calcium in rabbits is 40–60% compared to <2% in most mammals (Keeble and Benato 2016). It is normal for rabbits to have amorphous calcium carbonate crystals resulting in turbid to creamy urine. This material is radiopaque (Figure 17.3). Ammonium magnesium phosphate crystals are also normally present in rabbit urine. It may be difficult to distinguish this sludge from calculi radiographically. There are numerous theories regarding why stones form, but little scientific research has been conducted to define the pathophysiology in rabbits. High dietary calcium levels, dehydration, genetic predisposition, metabolic disorders, bacterial or parasitic infections, limited exercise, and obesity have been implicated (Martorell et al. 2012; Keeble and Benato 2016; Tahas et al. 2017). Uroliths in rabbits are usually composed of calcium carbonate and have been reported in all parts of the urinary tract.

Rabbits may be asymptomatic or have clinical signs of hyporexia, weight loss, lethargy, hematuria, hunched posture, stranguria, bruxism, and perineal urine scald (Martorell et al. 2012; Keeble and Benato 2016). Radiographs may be helpful for diagnosing urolithiasis; however, ultrasound examination is recommended to confirm the presence and location of uroliths. Urethral catheterization (3.5 or 5 fr for males and 5 or 8 fr for females) is fairly easy to perform because of the large diameter of the urethra in both males and females.

Administration of 2% lidocaine gel into the urethra and systemic midazolam have been recommended (Klaphake and Paul-Murphy 2012).

Medical management with fluid diuresis and administration of an alpha-adrenergic antagonist such as prazosin (0.25 mg/rabbit q12h [Keeble and Benato 2016]) may be effective in moving renal and ureteral stones out the urinary tract (Markovich and Labato 2014; Milligan and Berent 2018). Typically, attempt medical management for two to three days depending on the patient's clinical status, which has been effective in 10–13.5% of cats with ureterolithiasis (Markovich and Labato 2014; Milligan and Berent 2018). Administration of a diuretic agent such as mannitol or furosemide has also been recommended (Markovich and Labato 2014). Voiding urohydropropulsion can be effective for removing sand, sludge, and small stones from the urinary bladder and urethra of rabbits (Klaphake and Paul-Murphy 2012).

There is no scientific evidence that therapies directed to prevent calculi formation are effective; however, a calcium restricted diet, removal of any dietary supplements containing vitamin D, encouraging water intake, increasing activity, and weight reduction are commonly recommended.

After surgery, always perform imaging to confirm all stones have been removed. If there are stones remaining, consider going back in to remove them; however, if they are not obstructing, depending on the patient's status, it might be better to postpone the second procedure for a day to allow the patient to recover from anesthesia.

Nephrolithiasis

Nephrectomy

Nephrectomy as a treatment for nephrolithiasis and ureterolithiasis has been reported (Rhody 2006; Klaphake and Paul-Murphy 2012; Tahas et al. 2017); however, in light of the fact that the pathophysiology of stone formation in

(a)

(b)

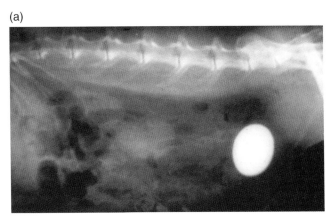
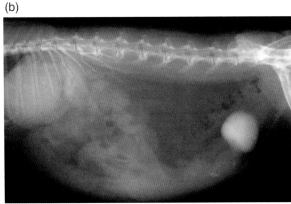

Figure 17.3 Lateral radiograph of a rabbit with a single cystic calculus (a) and a different rabbit with calcium carbonate sludge in the bladder (b).

rabbits is not understood, it is best to preserve any functioning kidney and perform nephrectomy only for end-stage disease (see Section "Nephrotomy").

Nephrotomy

Nephrotomy is recommended for removal of nephroliths that cause progressive loss of renal parenchyma due to increasing stone size, cause obstruction at the ureteropelvic junction resulting in hydronephrosis, or are a nidus for continued bacterial infection not responsive to medical management (Milligan and Berent 2018). Surgery is not indicated for small stones not causing clinical problems or renal compromise. Much of the literature cites a 1977 study in dogs evaluating the effect of nephrotomy on renal function (Gahring et al. 1977). They reported 40–53% reduction in glomerular filtration rate (GFR) when the nephrotomy was closed with chromic gut suture and minimal reduction in GFR with sutureless closure (holding the halves together allowing a clot to form) at 21 days, but a similar reduction in GFR immediately postoperative. More recent studies have shown increased GFR (Stone et al. 2002) or no change in GFR following either bisectional or intersegmental nephrotomy in dogs and cats (Zimmerman-Pope et al. 2003; King et al. 2006; Bollinger et al. 2005).

Check clotting times prior to surgery. With the rabbit in dorsal recumbency, perform a ventral midline celiotomy and open the peritoneum freeing the kidney from surrounding tissues. Identify the renal artery and vein and occlude flow using vascular clamps, Rummel tourniquets, or the fingers of an assistant to minimize hemorrhage. Make a sagittal incision on the middle of the greater curvature of the kidney down to the stone. Quickly remove the stone and collect diagnostic samples. Pass a 3.5 fr catheter to flush debris from the renal pelvis and ureter down into the urinary bladder. Hold the two halves of the kidney together for five minutes. Then place a simple continuous rapidly absorbed suture in the renal capsule only, not through the parenchyma. Release the vascular occlusion and make sure hemorrhage is controlled.

A lateral approach to the kidney for nephrotomy to retrieve a nephrolith has been described (Martorell et al. 2012). This approach is minimally invasive and does not allow evaluation of other parts of the urinary system and abdomen; however, if no other abnormalities are noted on ultrasound or CT, a complete exploratory celiotomy may not be necessary. The approach is analogous to that used for adrenalectomy (Adin and Nelson 2018). Make an approximately 4 cm incision through the skin and subcutaneous tissues parallel and caudal to the last rib. Identify the muscle of the body wall and use a grid approach to dissect through the external and internal abdominal oblique

muscles and the transversus abdominis to enter the peritoneal cavity. Exteriorize the retroperitoneal kidney and apply digital pressure to the vessels. Exposure is limited and it is not feasible to apply clamps or tourniquets. Perform a nephrotomy as described above to remove nephroliths. Following closure of the renal capsule, replace the kidney and close the three muscle layers of the body wall individually with an absorbable monofilament material in a simple continuous pattern. The advantages of this lateral approach are that it is minimally invasive, the GI tract is not manipulated, and exposure of the kidney is better (Martorell et al. 2012).

Pyelotomy

Pyelotomy is indicated for removal of smaller nephroliths because it does not impact renal function. There is no need to occlude blood flow. There must be pelvic dilation, and the stones must be small enough to be removed through the renal pelvis. The normal renal pelvis is too small to identify and access surgically. The renal pelvis is not accessible through the ventral aspect.

Perform a routine ventral midline celiotomy and free the kidney from the peritoneum so it can be reflected medially to expose the renal pelvis on the dorsal aspect of the kidney. Identify the white fibrous renal pelvis and the ureter exiting. Make a stab incision with a #11 blade longitudinally toward the ureter. Urine should be seen exiting the incision confirming it has been made in the correct location. Extend the incision so it is long enough for retrieval of the stone(s). Collect the appropriate samples and irrigate the renal pelvis and ureter. Close the incision with fine monofilament rapidly absorbable material in a simple continuous pattern. Inspect the closure for leaks, then replace it to its normal position. Perform a nephropexy placing 3-4 sutures between the renal capsule and the body wall to prevent renal torsion.

Ureterolithiasis
Tube Nephrostomy

Tube nephrostomy is indicated to divert urine in an unstable patient directly from the kidney to relieve the pressure caused by ureteral calculi and minimize subsequent damage caused by hydronephrosis. Often, one kidney has already lost function and the second ureter becomes obstructed with uroliths rapidly resulting in azotemia. Nephrostomy tubes can be placed percutaneously with ultrasound and fluoroscopic guidance (Infiniti Medical, www.infinitimedical.com) or intracorporeally. In a study of 153 cats, nearly half had complications including poor drainage, urine leakage, and tube dislodgement (Kyles et al. 2005); however, tube placement can result in life-saving urine diversion.

Make a lateral approach to the kidney as described by Martorell (2012) and localize the kidney. Insert an 18 ga Teflon catheter into the greater curvature directed toward the renal pelvis. Urine will flow freely out the catheter if it is properly placed. Pass a hydrophilic guide wire through the catheter into the renal pelvis and remove the catheter. Enlarge the opening if needed using a dilator then insert the nephrostomy tube into the renal pelvis. Place sutures between the renal capsule and body wall to secure the kidney in place. Close the body wall around the tube and stabilize it with sutures to the body wall. Close the subcutaneous tissues and skin routinely. Secure the nephrostomy tube to the body wall with a finger trap suture. Once the tube is no longer needed, during the definitive surgery to remove the ureteroliths, remove the tube and place a suture in the renal capsule.

Percutaneous placement is similar. Use fluoroscopy to direct the Teflon catheter into the renal pelvis. Inject contrast to confirm placement. Place a hydrophilic guide wire through the catheter and remove the catheter. Advance a dilator over the guide wire to enlarge the opening, and then place the nephrostomy tube. Secure it in place with a finger trap suture.

Ureterotomy

Ureterotomy to remove stones requires microsurgical techniques. It is vital to preserve the blood supply to the ureter contained in periureteral fat. Palpate the ureter to identify the location of the stone and open the peritoneum to isolate the section of ureter. Use a #11 blade to incise onto the stone in a location that will allow its removal, which is usually in the distended more proximal part. Remove the stone and collect diagnostic samples before irrigating the ureter in both directions to remove debris and ensure patency. Consider passing a temporary stent (ureteral catheter or strand of suture) from the kidney into the urinary bladder before closing the ureterotomy. This stent can be removed after the ureter is closed or left in place two to three days while the incision forms a fibrin seal. If it is to be left in place, advance the catheter through the bladder and out the urethra so it can be retrieved later. Connect the catheter to a closed collection system. If it is not necessary to stent the ureter, after closing the ureterotomy, remove it through a tiny incision into the bladder.

Consider closing a small ureterotomy transversely to effectively widen the ureter. If the incision is long, this technique may not be feasible. Close with a fine (6-0 to 8-0) monofilament rapidly absorbed material in a simple continuous or interrupted pattern. Complications include ureterotomy site edema, reobstruction from nephroliths, missed ureteroliths, urine leakage, and site stricture (Milligan and Berent 2018). Reduce the risk of stricture formation by making the incision longitudinally, handling tissues gently, and using microsurgical techniques.

Ureteral Stenting

Placing a double pigtail ureteral stent as an alternative to ureterotomy has been reported in dogs and cats with excellent outcomes (Milligan and Berent 2018) (Infiniti Medical, www.infinitimedical.com). A stent immediately relieves the obstruction with a decreased risk of stricture, recurrence of obstruction, and urine leakage. This has become the treatment of choice for dogs with ureteroliths. There are no reports of ureteral stenting in rabbits; however, these were developed for cats and stent sizes are applicable to rabbits.

Subcutaneous Ureteral Bypass (SUB) Device

A subcutaneous ureteral bypass (SUB) device is a ureteral replacement consisting of a locking loop nephrostomy tube, a cystostomy tube, and a subcutaneous port that connects them (Milligan and Berent 2018) (Norfolk Vet Products, www.norfolkvetproducts.com). Urine flows from the kidney to the subcutaneous port and then into the bladder bypassing the ureter, so there is no need to address the cause of the obstruction. Device mineralization requiring replacement occurred in 13% of 134 cats in one study (Berent et al. 2011). This device has become the treatment of choice for cats with ureteral obstruction. While there are no reports of using SUB devices in rabbits, the sizes available are applicable to rabbits. Compared with stents, they are easier to place, have lower incidence of postoperative dysuria, have a lower incidence of reobstruction, and have a low postoperative mortality rate. In dogs, there was a 50% device mineralization rate causing SUB occlusion which is why ureteral stenting is preferred in dogs. It is unknown which procedure might be better in rabbits; however, rabbits appear to be more prone to developing concretions on sutures which may cause SUB device occlusion. Until there is more information, either of these techniques might provide an alternative to ureterotomy in rabbits.

Ureteroneocystostomy

In a rabbit with ureteroliths causing obstruction near the urinary bladder, nephrectomy was elected, and the rabbit did well (Tahas et al. 2017); however, ureteroneocystostomy could have preserved the kidney. For ureteroliths close to the bladder, consider performing an ureteroneocystostomy. Isolate the ureter at the location of the stone and ligate it proximal to the stone. Ligate the ureter remnant as close to the bladder as possible, then excise the segment containing the stone. Perform a cystotomy and use a hemostat to penetrate the bladder wall near the apex. Grasp the suture on the ureter and pull the ureter into the urinary bladder. Transect the ureter proximal to the ligature to remove the damaged portion. The ureter will be dilated because of the obstruction making it easier to perform the ureteroneocystostomy. Spatulate the ureteral opening and pass a 3.5 fr catheter retrograde. Suture the ureter to the bladder mucosa with 5-0 or 6-0 monofilament rapidly absorbable simple interrupted sutures. Make sure urine is flowing freely into the bladder prior to closing the cystotomy.

Cystolithiasis

Cystotomy

Prior to surgery, place a urethral catheter to minimize the risk of stones migrating into the urethral and to allow retrograde irrigation of the urethra intraoperatively to assure urethral patency. This is especially important in rabbits because their urethra is relatively wide. Prepare and drape the catheter and the genitalia into the surgical field. With the patient in dorsal recumbency, perform a ventral midline celiotomy from xiphoid to pubis if a complete exploratory is indicated or a caudal (umbilicus to pubis) celiotomy if there is no other abdominal pathology. The caudal celiotomy will not provide access to the kidneys and ureters.

Exteriorize the bladder and place stay sutures, one at the apex and one on each side of the proposed incision. Isolate the bladder with saline moistened gauze and make a cystotomy incision in a hypovascular region of the ventral bladder cranial to the trigone. Remove stones with a gall spoon, curette with its edge dulled, or forceps being careful not to damage the bladder mucosa or push stones into the urethra. The catheter will help prevent larger stones from migrating. While flushing saline through the catheter withdraw it to force any urethral stones back into the bladder. Attempt to remove additional stones. Then advance a catheter antegrade through the urethra flushing stones out. Repeat this process of retrograde flushing, removing any stones from the bladder, and antegrade flushing until no stones remain.

Obtain a mucosal culture sample by excising 1–2 mm of mucosa from the edge of the incision. Close the cystotomy with a simple continuous or interrupted pattern of a rapidly absorbed material. The bladder regains near-normal strength in 10 days (see Chapter 2). Rabbits form calculi on suture more so than other mammals; however, if absorbable suture is used the concretions resolve at seven days postoperative (Keeble and Benato 2016). Because the holding layer is the submucosa and it is very difficult to differentiate mucosa from submucosa, the author recommends taking full thickness bites. Using a rapidly absorbed material, the suture will be absorbed and not become a nidus for stone formation. If needed, a second inverting pattern can be applied to create a better seal. An inverting pattern creates serosa-to-serosa

contact quickly creating a fibrin seal. Pass the urethral catheter and fill the bladder to check for leaks at the incision. If saline leaks around the catheter, and the incision and needle holes does not leak, there is no need to overfill the bladder for leak testing. If it is difficult to control leaks, consider leaving a urethral catheter for 1–2 days postoperatively allowing a fibrin seal to form.

Transvesicular Percutaneous Cystolithotomy (TPC)

In rabbits, more than one cystic calculus is uncommon (Capello 2004a) making transvesicular percutaneous cystolithotomy (TPC) an excellent minimally invasive method for removing stones. With the rabbit in dorsal recumbency, pass a urethral catheter and instill saline to distend the urinary bladder until it is easy to palpate. It needs to be large enough to displace the cecum and intestines laterally. Make a 2 cm incision through the skin and subcutaneous tissues. Make a corresponding incision through the linea alba being careful not to incise the urinary bladder. Place a stay suture in the urinary bladder and exteriorize a small amount (Figure 17.4). Place 4-6 sutures between the bladder and body wall circumferentially to hold the bladder in place and minimize the risk of urine spilling into the abdomen. Make a 1–2 cm incision into the bladder and retrieve the stone(s) with a gall spoon. If there are multiple stones, it is best to use an endoscope to ensure all stones have been removed from the bladder and urethra. Use a urethral catheter to flush until all stones and debris have been removed. Once the stone(s) has been removed, close the bladder with interrupted or cruciate sutures. Use the urinary catheter to fill the bladder to check for leaks before removing the

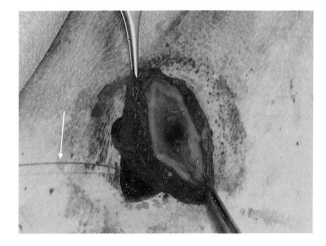

Figure 17.4 Transvesicular percutaneous cystolithotomy for removal of a single stone. The urinary bladder has been sutured to the body wall to prevent bladder contents from entering the abdomen (arrow points to a suture tail). After the procedure is complete, remove the sutures, close the bladder wall, replace the bladder into the abdomen, and close the body wall routinely.

sutures between the bladder and body wall. Replace the bladder into the abdomen and close the body wall, subcutaneous tissues, and skin.

Urethrolithiasis
Tube Cystostomy

Tube cystostomy allows diversion of urine from the bladder bypassing the urethra for management of urethral obstruction when the patient needs to be stabilized before anesthesia. This can be done with sedation and local anesthesia percutaneously or through a mini-laparotomy. The bladder should be enlarged because of the obstruction making it easy to palpate. Make a mini-laparotomy at the level of the middle of the bladder (the bladder will shrink once the urine has been removed). Place a stay suture in the bladder to be able to exteriorize it slightly. Place a purse-string suture in the bladder, make a stab incision into the bladder, suction all of the urine, and insert a Foley catheter. Tighten the purse-string and inflate the balloon of the catheter. Place four sutures between the bladder and body wall to hold it in place (cystopexy) and close any gaps in the subcutaneous tissues and skin. Secure the catheter using a finger trap suture and connect it to a closed collection system. Once the patient is stable and a definitive surgery is undertaken to relieve the obstruction, remove the catheter and close the defects in the bladder wall and the body wall.

Percutaneous cystostomy tube placement is performed using fluoroscopy. With the bladder distended place an 18 ga intravenous catheter into the urinary bladder. Remove the stylet and place a hydrophilic guide wire through the catheter into the bladder. Remove the catheter and pass a cystostomy tube (Infiniti Medical, www.infinitimedical.com) over the guide wire and advance it into the urinary bladder. Confirm placement by injecting contrast into the bladder.

Urethrotomy

Urethral calculi appear to occur more commonly in male rabbits (Keeble and Benato 2016). Because of the large diameter of the urethra, most urethral stones migrate to the urethral opening which has the narrowest diameter in both sexes. These stones are typically very large (as large as 2 cm diameter (Vannevel 2002)) but do not cause complete urethral obstruction, patients often present with a chronic history (Vannevel 2002; Capello 2004a) (Figure 17.5). Some have theorized these stones actually enlarge while at the distal urethral opening because they are so large (Vannevel 2002). In some cases, it might be possible to retrohydropulse the stone into the bladder and perform a cystotomy, preferred over urethrotomy. It is vital to pay attention to bladder distention during retrohydropropulsion to avoid rupture. Retrohydropropulsion is safer to perform if there is a tube cystostomy or cystotomy so excess urine has an exit. Urethral calculi in the distal urethra are usually very large and adhered so it is not feasible to retrohydropulse them.

Urethrotomy at the urethral opening is easily performed. In female rabbits, if the stone is palpable, stabilize the stone between the thumb and first finger of the nondominant hand and incise onto the stone from cranial to caudal through the vagina and the urethra enough to allow removal of the stone. The urethra can be sutured closed, followed by the vaginal wall and skin. Alternatively, the incision can be left to heal by second intention (Weber et al. 1985). If it is not sutured, urine will pass through the incision for a couple of days, but the mucosa quickly heals. If the incision is

(a)

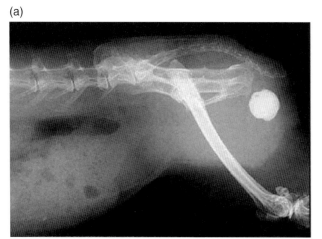

(b)

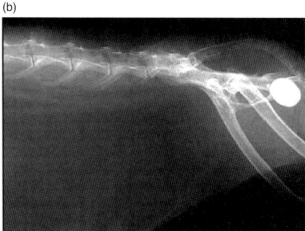

Figure 17.5 Radiographs of a male (a) and female (b) rabbit with a distal urethral calculus. These become very large and can be removed by urethrotomy which can be closed primarily or allowed to heal by second intention. *Source:* Images courtesy of Capello (2004a).

closed and there is urine leakage, it will collect in the tissues potentially causing necrosis (Vannevel 2002). If this occurs, remove all sutures and manage the wound open allowing it to heal by second intention or perform an urethrostomy once the tissues are healthy.

In male rabbits, make a skin incision lateral to the penis and dissect through the subcutaneous tissues onto the stone in the urethra (Capello 2004a). Stabilize the stone with the nondominant hand and incise the urethra over the stone making the incision large enough to remove the stone. Pass a catheter from the penis through the urethrotomy and into the proximal segment of urethra flushing any debris from the urethra. The urethra can be closed primarily over the catheter with fine monofilament rapidly absorbable suture in a simple continuous pattern. Alternatively, allow the incision to heal by second intention. Partial closure is contraindicated because urine will potentially collect in the tissue resulting in necrosis and dehiscence.

Renal Biopsy

Biopsy of the kidney is indicated to determine a diagnosis and prognosis for nephropathies and masses. Clotting times must be evaluated because excessive hemorrhage can be life-threatening. Renal biopsies can be obtained using a core biopsy needle with ultrasound guidance, but some are reluctant to use this methodology because it is not possible to control hemorrhage. Alternatively, biopsies can be obtained using laparoscopy or laparotomy and a 16–18 ga spring-loaded core biopsy needle (see Chapter 15). Pathologists need nephrons from the cortex, so aim the needle across the renal cortex and not toward the renal pelvis. Hemorrhage can be controlled by applying pressure with a cotton-tipped applicator (laparotomy) or laparoscopic blunt probe.

Nephrectomy

Nephrectomy is indicated for renal neoplasia, severe renal trauma resulting in hemorrhage and/or uroabdomen, abscessation, and end-stage renal pathology. Embryonal nephromas are benign tumors and common in rabbits of all ages often diagnosed at necropsy (Klaphake and Paul-Murphy 2012). Carcinomas, leiomyomas, and lymphosarcoma have been reported in rabbit kidneys. Prior to removing a kidney, it is vital to determine if the contralateral kidney is functioning enough to maintain life. Elevated blood urea nitrogen and creatinine indicate neither kidney is functioning enough to support life, and nephrectomy is contraindicated. In a study of dogs undergoing unilateral nephrectomy, 67% developed azotemia (Gookin et al. 1996). Excretory urography is not quantitative but can be helpful in determining if there is some

renal function. If the kidney shows contrast enhancement, even if delayed and weakly enhancing, it indicates there is functional renal parenchyma. GFR can be determined using scintigraphy. It is the most accurate and provides the percent renal function attributable to each kidney, but it is not readily available. In a case report, urine protein:creatinine ratio and gamma-glutamyltransferase index were used to confirm the contralateral kidney was functioning adequately to allow nephrectomy (Tahas et al. 2017).

Nephrectomy in rabbits is performed as in other species. Identify the renal artery and vein, and the ureter on the ventral aspect by dissecting through the perirenal fat. Isolate, ligate, and transect the renal artery and vein. In most cases, ligate the artery first; however, if nephrectomy is for treatment of cancer, ligate the vein prior to manipulating the tumor and potentially sending tumor cells out through the renal vein. Historically, it is recommended to dissect the ureter to the bladder wall and ligate and transect it at the level of the bladder. With laparoscopic nephrectomy, this has been challenged because it is difficult to dissect it to the bladder and leaving some ureter has not cause the creation of ureteroceles. Laparoscopic nephrectomy has been successfully performed in a rabbit (S. Mehler 2019, personal communication).

Partial Cystectomy

For bladder tumors (Keeble and Benato 2016; Cikanek et al. 2018), traumatic rupture of the bladder, bladder wall necrosis from eversion or inguinal herniation, and for polypoid cystitis, partial cystectomy is indicated. Polypoid cystitis has been diagnosed in two rabbits (Di Girolamo et al. 2017) but was not treated with partial cystectomy; however, in dogs, partial cystectomy is typically part of the treatment. There are reports of inguinal herniation of the urinary bladder in both male and female rabbits (Grunkemeyer et al. 2010; Thas and Harcourt-Brown 2013). There are also reports of transurethral bladder eversion in male and female rabbits (Pompeu et al. 1995; Greenacre et al. 1999; Szabo 2017). With either, damage to the bladder may necessitate partial cystectomy. It has been reported that as much as 70% of the bladder can be resected without compromising function as long as the trigone is preserved (Keeble and Benato 2016).

Remove the affected portion of bladder being careful to preserve the trigone. If needed, place urethral and ureteral catheters to ensure they are not damaged during the resection and closure. A single-layer closure is adequate, either simple continuous or interrupted, using a rapidly absorbed material full thickness. If a large segment of bladder is resected, consider placing a urethral catheter for 1–2 days to allow a fibrin seal to form.

Transurethral Urinary Bladder Eversion and Prolapse

Transurethral urinary bladder eversion and prolapse has been reported in both male and female rabbits (Greenacre et al. 1999; Szabo 2017). It has also been reported in humans, mares, cows, bitches, and queens typically post-partum multiparous, and secondary to tenesmus from cystitis in a mare and a queen. In the male rabbit, it was theorized that the wide diameter of the male rabbit urethra allowed for eversion and prolapse of the bladder, but the underlying cause was not determined (Szabo 2017).

Clean the exposed bladder mucosa and apply 50% dextrose if there is edema preventing reduction. Position the patient in dorsal recumbency and prepare for draping in the genitalia. Perform a caudal ventral midline celiotomy and use a combination of traction from intra-abdominal and pushing externally to invert the bladder and reposition it into the abdomen. Evaluate the bladder and perform a partial cystectomy if indicated. Perform a temporary cystopexy placing absorbable sutures between the bladder and the body wall. If a permanent cystopexy is indicated, make corresponding incisions in the seromuscular layer of the bladder wall and the internal abdominal oblique, and suture bladder wall to body wall as is done for a gastropexy.

Inguinal Urinary Bladder Herniation

Inguinal herniation of the urinary bladder has been reported in both male and female rabbits (Grunkemeyer et al. 2010; Thas and Harcourt-Brown 2013). Presenting complaints are often vague including lethargy and hyporexia. On physical examination, a swelling is present in the inguinal region or, in males, in the inguinal canal or scrotum. Diagnosis is confirmed using imaging with ultrasound or excretory urography. In the reported cases, all were treated by making an incision over the external inguinal ring, reducing the bladder into the abdomen and closing the external inguinal ring. In one rabbit, the bladder and intestine were both herniated (Thas and Harcourt-Brown 2013).

With the rabbit in dorsal recumbency, pass a urethral catheter to drain the urine from the bladder. Make an incision in the inguinal region over the swelling being careful not to cut into the bladder or other structures within the hernia sac. In many cases, it is necessary to enlarge the external inguinal ring to be able to replace the bladder into the abdomen. In intact males, the spermatic cord passes through the inguinal canal. To create a secure closure, it is beneficial to remove the testis. Incise the tunic opening the peritoneal cavity. Replace the bladder into the peritoneal cavity and close the external inguinal ring with slowly absorbed monofilament suture keeping in mind the external pudendal vessels also pass through the inguinal canal. In a report of six male rabbits with inguinal hernias, two had recurrence, one immediately postoperatively and the other 18 months later (Thas and Harcourt-Brown 2013).

Alternatively, perform a caudal midline celiotomy and close the internal inguinal ring following reduction of the herniated bladder. Replace the bladder using a combination of traction and external pressure. In most cases, it is not necessary to make an inguinal incision. Blocking the entrance of viscera into the inguinal canal appears to be more effective than stopping them from coming out the external ring once they have begun migrating through the canal. Another reported advantage of an abdominal approach is the ability to evaluate both inguinal canals as small hernias may not be detected on physical examination (Smeak 2018).

Postoperative Considerations

Potential complications following urinary tract surgery in rabbits include obstruction due to tissue swelling, blood clots, debris, stricture, and adhesions. It is important to diurese the patient for at least 24 hours after surgery to help flush out blood and debris from the bladder, as well as to potentially improve renal function and resolve azotemia. Monitor urine output, body weight, and cardiovascular parameters to make sure the patient is not being overhydrated. Administer antibiotics if appropriate. Trimethoprim/sulfamethoxazole (30 mg/kg PO q12h) and enrofloxacin (20 mg/kg PO q24h) have been recommended for rabbits with urinary tract disease (Keeble and Benato 2016). Prokinetics are also recommended.

Reproductive Tract Surgery

Neutering is the primary reproductive surgery performed in rabbits. In a retrospective review of 10 cases of dystocia presenting over a 20 years period at one institution, seven were treated and only one required surgery with the other six managed medically and/or with assisted vaginal delivery (Gleeson et al. 2019). Fetal macrosomia with or without uterine inertia was the most common cause. The one rabbit that underwent a Cesarean section was a wild rabbit, and it survived to discharge.

Pyometra has been described in rabbits and is often associated with *Pasteurella multocida* infection (Harcourt-Brown 2016). Rabbits with pyometra often present with vaginal discharge as well as lethargy, anorexia, abdominal distention, and a palpable uterus. As in other species, pyometra is considered a surgical emergency once the patient is stable.

Rabbits have a relatively high incidence of ectopic pregnancy (Bergdall and Dysko 1994). The ectopic fetus usually attaches to the peritoneum and develops but does not survive. It becomes mummified. They can be an incidental finding. Surgical removal of ectopic mummified feti is recommended.

In female rabbits, the indications for prophylactic neutering include preventing reproduction, false pregnancy, and territorial and aggressive behaviors. A clear connection between estrogen and the development of mammary adenocarcinoma has not been established, but it has been suggested that ovariectomy may decrease the risk of developing mammary neoplasia in rabbits (Szabo 2016). Uterine adenocarcinoma is very common in rabbits with as many as 60% of 4 year old and 75% of 7 year old rabbits having uterine cancer (Greene 1941) (Figure 17.6). Many rabbits are asymptomatic so abdominal ultrasound should be performed prior to spaying female rabbits over 2 years of age. The most common presenting complaint is hematuria or hemorrhagic vaginal discharge. It is difficult for owners to determine from where the blood is originating, and they often assume it is from the urinary tract. Uterine adenocarcinoma is often multicentric with polypoid masses into the uterine lumen. It can spread within the abdomen and metastasize to lungs, brain, skin, and bone (Harcourt-Brown 2016). Abdominal palpation may reveal abdominal masses. Abdominal ultrasound easily confirms the diagnosis. Ovariohysterectomy is often curative in patients without metastasis or invasion into viscera. Mammary

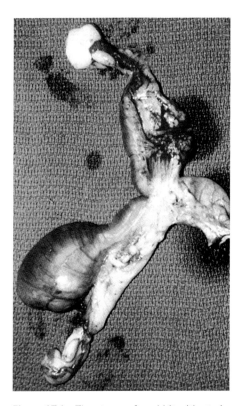

Figure 17.6 The uterus of a rabbit with uterine adenocarcinoma. If it has not metastasized, ovariohysterectomy is often curative.

adenocarcinoma seems to occur concurrently with uterine adenocarcinoma, but a pathophysiologic connection has not been established (Harcourt-Brown 2016; Szabo 2016); however, ultrasound evaluation of the uterus is recommended in any rabbit presenting with mammary neoplasia. Because of the high risk of developing uterine adenocarcinomas, juvenile ovariectomy is recommended.

Elective early neutering of male rabbits is not typically indicated for medical reasons. It is more commonly performed to prevent unwanted behaviors. Indications for orchiectomy include preventing reproduction, decreasing aggression toward other rabbits, decreasing urine spraying and marking behaviors, and decreasing humping behavior. Orchiectomy is also indicated to treat testicular tumors, testicular torsion, cryptorchidism, and inguinal hernias. Benign interstitial cell tumors are the most common type of testicular tumor and may be associated with mammary development in male rabbits (Maratea et al. 2007). Testicular torsion can occur in rabbits of any age. Presentation is acute with anorexia, depression, and pain. The affected testis is typically enlarged, firm, painful on palpation, and in an abnormal location. Orchiectomy for testicular torsion should be performed as soon as possible. As in other species, cryptorchid testes are at high risk of developing neoplasia, and orchiectomy is recommended. When repairing an inguinal hernia, it is possible to spare the testis, but closure of the inguinal canal is more easily accomplished following orchiectomy because the spermatic cord passes through the inguinal canal.

Anatomy of the Female Reproductive Tract

The female reproductive tract is bilaterally symmetrical having two ovaries and a bicornuate uterus; however, there is no uterine body, and each uterine horn has its own cervix. The two cervices are adjacent and enter a long, flaccid, muscular vagina that may be seen to contract intraoperatively (Figure 17.7). The ovaries are elongated, and the oviduct is long and encircles the ovary from caudal to cranial with the infundibulum at the cranial end of the ovary. It is red compared to the ovary and surrounding fat. Rabbits deposit large amounts of fat in the mesovarium and mesometrium as they approach 1 year of age. Ovulation is induced and postpartum estrus occurs shortly after parturition. Developmental abnormalities have been reported including absent uterine horns, rudimentary vagina, and absent cervix (Thode and Johnston 2009). Uterine and myometrial venous aneurysms occur in rabbits and have reportedly ruptured with fatal consequences (Harcourt-Brown 2016).

Ovariectomy

Following ovariectomy, the mammalian uterus atrophies and developing uterine disease is very rare. In a study to

(a)

(b)

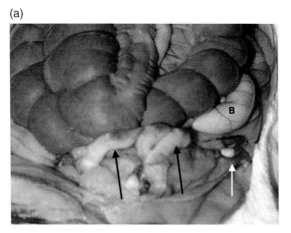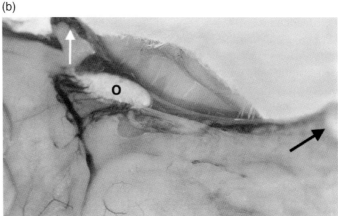

Figure 17.7 The abdominal anatomy of a female rabbit after removal of the body wall (a). Note the uterus (black arrows) and ovaries (white arrow left ovary) are caudally located and the cecum occupies a majority of the abdomen. The cecum is green because the cecal wall is so thin, the green ingesta can be seen (B = urinary bladder). The anatomy of the ovary (b) with the long oviduct (white arrow) encircling the ovary (O) and the large amount of fat deposited in the mesovarium and mesometrium. The black arrow points to the end of the uterine horn.

determine the influence of estrogen on the development of uterine adenocarcinoma in rabbits, 102 rabbits were ovariectomized, and strings impregnated with 3-methylcholanthrene and beeswax were implanted in the right uterine horn to induce adenocarcinomas, and stings with beeswax only were implanted in the left uterine horn serving as a control (Griffiths et al. 1975). They concluded that ovariectomy (castration) strongly inhibited carcinogenesis and that effect was reversed when estrogen was supplemented proving a strong correlation between estrogen and the development of uterine carcinomas. This study suggests that ovariectomy prevents the development of uterine adenocarcinoma without a need to remove the uterus. The authors were unable to find evidence that ovariectomy is therapeutic in rabbit with uterine adenocarcinoma. Until studies have been conducted to determine if ovariectomy results in resolution of uterine adenocarcinomas, ovariohysterectomy is recommended in rabbits with uterine carcinomas. In all rabbits over 1 year old ovariohysterectomy has been recommended in case the patient might have uterine adenocarcinomas (Harcourt-Brown 2016; Vargas 2013; Szabo 2016). Alternatively, an ultrasound examination of the uterus to rule out the presence of uterine disease can be performed and, if not present, ovariectomy can be recommended.

Goebel reported that laparoscopic ovariectomy was performed in 700 rabbits <9 months age and none developed uterine disease (Vargas 2013). He also reported that in another population age 9–18 months, the uterus was evaluated, and if there was evidence of uterine disease, ovariohysterectomy was performed. In this anecdotal report, 50% of rabbits had evidence of uterine disease (not specified) and the others received ovariectomy. Of those (no numbers

reported) only one developed uterine disease (not specified), three years later. This anecdotal evidence suggests that perioperative ultrasound or visual examination of the uterus in rabbits over 9 months age should be performed, and if there is evidence of uterine pathology, an ovariohysterectomy should be performed. If the uterus is normal, the patient is a candidate for ovariectomy.

Ovariectomy is easier to perform with fewer complications. Harcourt-Brown suggested following ovariohysterectomy, there is risk of adhesions between the uterine/vaginal stump and the colon and/or urinary bladder (Harcourt-Brown 2016). Additionally, she reports granulomas at the stump can obstruct ureters, cause urinary incontinence, and can even cause a rectal stricture. Further, she reports that fat necrosis from the mesometrium is "unavoidable" and, if there is infection, can result in abscess formation that can spread. She also reports that if the uterus is completely removed ligating the vagina, urine can leak into the abdomen causing a "local peritonitis" that "may be life-threatening or may cause adhesions and tissue reactions involving ureters, bladder or rectum"; however, these are not documented in the scientific literature and uroabdomen after ovariohysterectomy has not been reported in rabbits. All of these potential complications can be avoided by performing ovariectomy, rather than ovariohysterectomy.

Laparoscopic ovariectomy in rabbits is analogous to that performed in dogs. Use a 5 mm scope, a 5 mm tissue-sealing device, and a two or three port approach. Be careful not to leave an isolated piece of oviduct that encircles the ovary because an isolated piece of oviduct will secrete fluid and potentially form a cyst. McLean et al. demonstrated that a tissue-sealing device was effective for sealing the tip of the uterus for ovariectomy but was not effective in sealing the cervical–vestibule junction for ovariohysterectomy (McLean et al. 2020).

Alternatively, ovariectomy can be performed through a mini-celiotomy. Make a 2 cm incision midway between the umbilicus and pubis. Use a finger to exteriorize an ovary. It is recommended to not use an instrument such as a spay hook as these can cause iatrogenic damage to the cecum with potentially life-threatening consequences. There is a small weak suspensory ligament that can be broken to allow the ovary to be exteriorized a little more if needed. Place a clamp proximal to the ovary and its encircling oviduct. Use a ligature or hemostatic clip proximal to the clamp, transect distal to the clamp, and remove the ovary. Release the clamp and inspect for hemorrhage. Because rabbits are prone to developing adhesions and fat necrosis, minimize the amount of tissue distal to the ligature and only place a single secure ligature. Remember, tissue distal to the ligature is devitalized.

Ovariohysterectomy

Make a 2–3 cm incision midway between the umbilicus and pubis. A celiotomy in this location allows the ovaries and uterus to be exteriorized but keeps other viscera, especially cecum and colon, within the abdominal cavity. Keep in mind that rabbits may develop adhesions postoperatively so handle tissues gently and minimize the amount of devitalized tissue distal to ligatures left in the abdomen. Use a finger or blunt instrument to exteriorize the uterus and ovaries. The uterus is coiled in the caudal abdomen and both the mesometrium and mesovarium are fat ladened in rabbits over 1 year old (Figure 17.8). Identify the ovarian vessels within the mesovarium and create a window to allow placement of a hemostat proximal to the ovary and oviduct. Place a second clamp proximal to the first to crush the fat allowing placement of a more secure

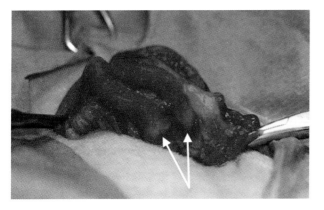

Figure 17.8 Intraoperative image of a rabbit ovariohysterectomy. Note the coiled uterine horns located in the caudal abdomen. The two cervices are clearly visible (arrows).

ligature. Consider transfixing if there is a lot of fat. Transfixation will also allow the tissue to be transected closer to the ligature minimizing the amount of devitalized tissue left distal to the ligature. Break the round ligament and the broad ligament to the level of the vagina. Ligate any large vessels. The cervices are firm and the vagina is thin, flaccid, and caudal to them (Figure 17.9).

The uterine vessels are farther from the cervices and vagina than in dogs and cats (Figure 17.10) and the mesometrium often contains a lot of fat. The author recommends ligating them on each side separate from the ligature on the vagina. It may be helpful to carefully dissect fat if the vessels are not visible.

Opinions differ on whether the cervices should be removed during hysterectomy. It has been anecdotally reported that if the cervices are left, they can develop aneurysms that can rupture with fatal consequences. Others consider the cervices a barrier to bacteria and urine entering the abdomen from the vagina and recommend they may not be removed (Harcourt-Brown 2016). The author has routinely ligated through the vagina removing the cervices with no incidence of uroabdomen or septic peritonitis because the ligature prevents it. A literature search failed to yield any reports of these complications following ovariohysterectomy in rabbits with a ligature placed at the vaginal vestibule. Place a transfixation ligature through the vestibule close to the cervices. Because this tissue is thin, it is not necessary to apply a clamp to crush the tissue. A clamp will also flatten the vaginal tissue making it more difficult to place a secure ligature. Transect the tissue just distal to the ligature.

Anatomy of the Male Reproductive Tract

It is commonly stated that, unlike other mammals, the inguinal canal of male rabbits remains open; however, the inguinal canal remains open in all mammals, both males and females, unless it is surgically closed as with an inguinal herniorrhaphy. Structures pass through the internal inguinal ring, through the inguinal canal, and out through the external inguinal ring. In females, the tunica vaginalis, the round ligament of the uterus, the ilioinguinal nerve, and the external pudendal artery and vein pass through this canal, and in males, the spermatic cord with its contents, the ilioinguinal and genitofemoral nerves, and the external pudendal vessels pass. In rabbits, the testes are able to pass through the inguinal canal partly because they are long and narrow. Inguinal hernias occur when abdominal viscera pass through the canal into the inguinal region of females and into the scrotum of males. Because of the relatively large inguinal canal of rabbits, they are used in research for herniorrhaphy in humans. Excluding these studies, a literature search of inguinal hernias in rabbits only revealed reports of urinary bladder herniation through

(a)   (b)

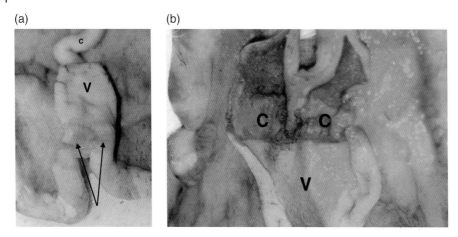

Figure 17.9 The junction of the two uterine horns with the vaginal vault (a). The reproductive tract has been reflected caudally and the colon (C) can be seen. Each cervix (arrows) and the vagina (V) have been opened (b) demonstrating the internal structures. The vagina (V) can often be seen contracting during ovariohysterectomy. There is no evidence to support that ligating through the vagina will result in urine or bacteria entering the abdomen. Cervices (C).

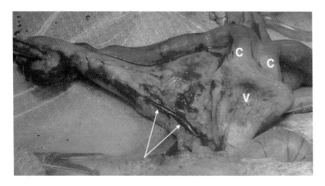

Figure 17.10 The uterine blood vessels (arrows) are located farther from the uterus than in dogs and cats. The author recommends ligating them separate from the encircling ligature. Cervices (C) and vaginal vault (V).

the inguinal canal (see Section "Inguinal Urinary Bladder Herniation"). The author was unable to find reports of other organs herniated; however, it has been suggested that intestinal herniation, entrapment, and incarceration are likely to occur if one does not close off the inguinal canal during orchiectomy in rabbits (Redrobe 2000; Capello 2005; Richardson and Flecknell 2006; Harcourt-Brown 2016; Szabo 2016). If this were a significant problem, it is logical there would be many reports of intestinal incarceration in inguinal hernias in rabbits following orchiectomy.

There are anatomic reasons inguinal hernias are as uncommon in rabbits as they are in other mammals. First, the testes are very long, thin, and tubular making it easy for them to pass through the canal (Figure 17.11). In other species, the testes pass through the canals into the scrotum when they are small. The testes then grow within the scrotum and become large and round, unable to pass through the canal back into the abdomen. Second, there is a large fat pad within the abdomen blocking viscera from entering the

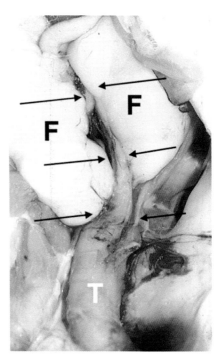

Figure 17.11 While male rabbits have a large inguinal canal that allows the testes to move into and out of the abdomen, the inguinal fat (F) inside the abdomen and the epididymal fat within the vaginal tunic prevent herniation of abdominal viscera. Arrows show the spermatic cord as it passes through the inguinal canal. The testis within the tunic is labeled T. It is evident the fat prevents visceral herniation.

narrow inguinal canal. The testes can be retracted from the scrotum into this inguinal fat. The spermatic cord consists of the vaginal tunic which surrounds the contents including the ductus deferens, the testicular vessels, and the cremaster muscle. It is contraction of the cremaster that pulls the testes into the abdomen. The vaginal tunic is an extension of the vaginal process of the peritoneum. Its contents are within the peritoneum. Ligating the tunic, therefore, effectively cuts off this extension of the peritoneum at the level it is ligated, often at the external inguinal ring. There is also an accumulation of fat within the tunic proximal to the head of the epididymis blocking other viscera from entering. Remembering that all that is required to be removed it the testis, leaving this epididymal fat within the canal also blocks any viscera from migrating into the scrotum.

The author has been unable to find any studies evaluating the incidence of inguinal herniation in rabbits that have had orchiectomy with or without surgical closure of the inguinal canal. Reports of inguinal hernias in rabbits are anecdotal and rare, apparently no more common than in other mammals. Therefore, the reported requirement to close off the inguinal canal in rabbits having orchiectomy is unsubstantiated.

The testes of rabbits typically descend at 10–12 weeks of age, and if they have not by 6 months old it is unlikely they will (Harcourt-Brown 2016). There are two relatively hairless scrotal sacs, one on each side of the penis (Figure 17.12). The testes are relatively long with a narrow diameter and a prominent tail of the epididymis. The scrotal skin is very thin, easily damaged, and tightly attached to the tail of the epididymis. The appearance of the penis of an intact rabbit is longer and pointed with a slight curve while that of an orchiectomized male is small, short, flaccid, and difficult to exteriorize.

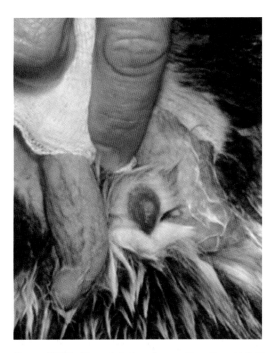

Figure 17.12 The genital anatomy of a male rabbit. The finger is pushing to extrude the penis. There is a scrotal sac on each side of the penis and the spermatic cord extends cranial to the penis.

Approaches for orchiectomy in rabbits have been described as prescrotal, inguinal, scrotal, and abdominal. The author prefers not to make an incision in the thin, sensitive, delicate scrotal skin. It is usually too thin to suture and those who recommend scrotal incisions recommend they not be sutured (Harcourt-Brown 2016). A prescrotal approach involves making a single midline longitudinal or transverse skin incision cranial to the penis (Figure 17.13). It is necessary to move the skin from side to side to be able to access the spermatic cord on both sides through a single incision. This can be technically challenging, but both testes can be removed through a single incision in this thicker, more resistant skin. Alternatively, make an incision over the spermatic cord cranial to the penis on each side. This is technically easier and the author's preferred approach for novices. Because the testes can be pulled into the abdominal cavity, they can be removed using a caudal abdominal approach. A testicular and incisional local anesthetic is recommended for orchiectomy in rabbits.

Open Orchiectomy

The main disadvantage of open orchiectomy is opening the peritoneal cavity to the outside environment. The main advantage is the blood vessels are easily isolated and ligated alone, not along with the tunic and its other contents, resulting in a more secure ligature. The author ligates the ductus deferens with the testicular vessels, still a very small bundle. There is very little need for dissection of subcutaneous tissues.

Palpate the spermatic cord in the inguinal area adjacent to the penis and make a 1 cm skin incision. Bluntly dissect down to the spermatic cord but do not isolate the spermatic cord. Instead, incise the tunic and pull the contents (ductus deferens and testicular vessels) out of the incision until the testis is completely exteriorized (Figure 17.14). There is no need for additional dissection. The testis will be attached to the tunic and scrotum by the ligament of the tail of the epididymis and the scrotum will be turned inside out. Place a mosquito hemostat onto the tunic at its attachment to the epididymis and carefully peel the epididymis off the tunic. Once this is done, the scrotum can be returned into its normal location. Leave the hemostat attached to the tunic because there is a small vessel in the cremaster muscle within the tunic and the hemostat will crush it minimizing the risk of postoperative hemorrhage. Place a ligature around the ductus deferens and testicular vessels, and then transect distal to the ligature. Double ligate if additional security is desired. After the testis has been excised, remove the hemostat on the tunic and inspect for hemorrhage from the tip of the tunic. If hemorrhage is observed from the cremaster vessels, place a ligature around the tip of the tunic to prevent a scrotal hematoma. Close the subcutaneous

(a)

(b)

(c)

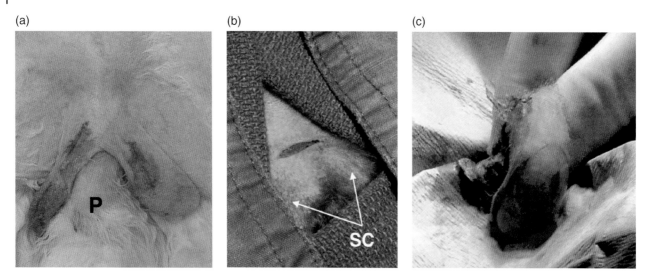

Figure 17.13   For orchiectomy in a rabbit, the skin incision can be made cranial to the penis over the spermatic cord on each side (a) (penis = P) or a prescrotal incision cranial to the penis at the level of the external inguinal rings (arrows, SCs = spermatic cords) either transverse (b) or longitudinally, or through the thin scrotal skin (c) (not recommended by the author).

(a)

(b)

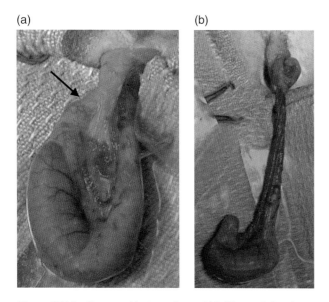

Figure 17.14   Open orchiectomy in a rabbit. The tunic has been incised and the testis exteriorized (a). The ligament of the tail of the epididymis must be torn to allow the scrotal skin (arrow) to return to its normal position (b). Then ligate the vascular bundle and ductus deferens.

tissues with a simple continuous monofilament rapidly absorbed material. The skin may be closed with an intradermal suture or tissue adhesive, or left to heal by second intention. Repeat the procedure on the other side. Orchiectomized rabbits should be considered fertile for 4 weeks following surgery (Harcourt-Brown 2016).

Closed Orchiectomy

The primary advantage of the closed technique is that the peritoneum is not opened and, potentially beneficial in

rabbits, the ligature around the spermatic cord at the external inguinal ring effectively closes the ring. The main disadvantage is the ligature is placed around a large bundle of tissue (the spermatic cord and all of its contents). Additionally, the tunic is adhered to the subcutaneous tissue and must be dissected free from the scrotum and all attachments up to the external inguinal ring. In dogs and cats, this dissection is not difficult as the attachments are loose and relatively easy to "strip down"; however, in rabbits, it is much more difficult to isolate the testis within the tunic proximally upto the external ring.

Make an incision as described above on each side of the penis in the inguinal skin. Dissect down to the spermatic cord, and then dissect around it circumferentially. Apply traction to the isolated segment of spermatic cord and continue to dissect distally to free it from the subcutaneous tissue and scrotum until the entire testis within the tunic has been exteriorized (Figure 17.15). This dissection is time-consuming, difficult, and risks tearing scrotal skin. Once the testis within the tunic has been exteriorized to the level of the external inguinal ring, place two hemostats across the spermatic cord to crush the bulky bundle. Place a ligature in the more proximal area crushed by the hemostat. A second ligature may be placed for added security if desired. Transect distal to the ligature(s). The ligature will close the inguinal canal at the external inguinal ring. Close the subcutaneous tissues and skin as described above.

It has been reported that rabbits having had a closed orchiectomy are prone to scrotal swelling and edema with fluid accumulation in the scrotum (Capello 2005; Harcourt-Brown 2016). This usually resolves in 5–6 days or less if massage and warm compresses can be applied.

(a)

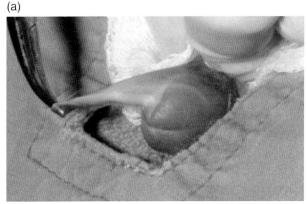

(b)   (c)

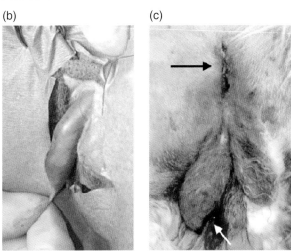

Figure 17.15 Closed orchiectomy in a rabbit. The ligament of the tail of the epididymis must be broken down to be able to exteriorize the testis within the tunic (a). This is more difficult in a rabbit compared to dogs and cats. Then the testis within the tunic can be exteriorized for ligation of the spermatic cord (b). Be careful not to tear the scrotal skin (c) (white arrow points at the tear). Note the skin incision is prescrotal and longitudinal (black arrow).

Because of the difficult dissection and the perceived need to close off the inguinal canal, some recommend an "open-to-closed" technique (Capello 2005; Harcourt-Brown 2016; Szabo 2016). The peritoneal cavity is opened, but the tunic is ligated at the external inguinal ring after open orchiectomy, effectively closing off the canal.

Make the skin incisions as described above. Isolate the spermatic cord circumferentially as for a closed orchiectomy. Do not dissect out more of the cord. Rather, make an incision in the tunic as for an open orchiectomy. Perform the orchiectomy as described above for the open technique. After the testis has been remove, place a ligature circumferentially around the tunic where it was isolated in the initial approach effectively closing the inguinal canal. This ligature can also be preplaced before opening the tunic. The tunic does not need to be removed distal to the ligature because it has subcutaneous attachments that will provide blood supply.

Abdominal Orchiectomy

Because the testes can be accessed within the abdomen, orchiectomy can be accomplished using a caudal abdominal approach. This technique is commonly used in a laboratory animal setting (Hoyt 1998). One author reports it as being more painful because it requires a celiotomy (Szabo 2016) but provides no data to support that claim.

Perform a 2–3 cm caudal abdominal celiotomy about 1 cm cranial to the pubis (Figure 17.16). Exteriorize and caudally reflect the urinary bladder to expose the ducti deferentia as they enter the urethra. Apply traction to a ductus while pushing the testis into the inguinal canal until it can be exteriorized through the celiotomy. At this point, the procedure is analogous to an open orchiectomy. The testicular vessels can be ligated along with or separate from the ductus deferens on each side. The ligament of the tail of the epididymis must be detached from the tunic, and the scrotum with be inverted until it has been detached. If there is hemorrhage from the tunic where it was detached, it can be controlled with a ligature or other means. Once both testes have been removed, close the celiotomy routinely. It must be noted that the inguinal canal remains open using this approach unless the surgeon closes the internal inguinal ring, which is not typically done.

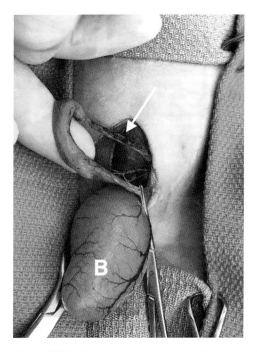

Figure 17.16 Because the testes move freely into the abdomen, a caudal abdominal approach can be used for orchiectomy. Reflect the urinary bladder caudally (B) and identify the ductus deferens as it enters the neck of the bladder. Because the tunic is still attached to the scrotal skin, it must be detached (hemostat) or ligated and transected. Then ligate the vascular supply and ductus deferens together (arrow) to allow excision of the testis.

Thoracic Surgery

Endotracheal intubation and positive pressure ventilation are essential. Do not ventilate to pressures greater than 20 cm H_2O. Mechanical ventilators are available that can accommodate small tidal volumes and are recommended. Nonrebreathing systems are commonly used in rabbits and many do not have a manometer, so the anesthetist does not know to what pressure they are ventilating. Anesthetists are more likely to ventilate to pressures that are too high rather than too low. The lungs should only be inflated to a level that prevents atelectasis, not so the lungs billow out of the chest and become pale to white in color. During surgery, having the patient on a mechanical ventilator can be problematic. When dissecting near vital structures, the surgeon does not want lungs inflating unexpectedly. If the patient is on a mechanical ventilator, make sure the anesthetist knows how to efficiently switch from mechanical to manual ventilation at the request of the surgeon.

Thymoma and Thymic Lymphoma

In rabbits, the thymus persists in adults and is easily identified cranial and ventral to the heart on both the right and left sides. Thymomas arise from the thymic epithelial cells and can be subdivided based on the epithelial component of the mass (Morrisey and McEntee 2005; Bennett 2009; Kunzel et al. 2012; de Mello Souza 2013). They are considered histologically benign; however, clinically they are considered benign or malignant based on their invasiveness and prognosis for surgical excision (Bennett 2009; de Mello Souza 2013). Thymic lymphoma and thymic carcinoma have been reported in rabbits but are considered rare (Wagner et al. 2005; Pilney and Reavill 2008; Huston et al. 2012). Metastasis of thymoma has not been reported in rabbits; however, renal metastasis of thymic carcinoma was reported in a rabbit (Wagner et al. 2005). Thymomas occur most commonly in older rabbits (6–10) and recent reports indicate they are relatively common (Bennett 2009; Andres et al. 2012; Kunzel et al. 2012; Dolera et al. 2016). In three rabbits, a genetic basis for thymoma was identified and was associated with immunodeficiency and hemolytic anemia (Weisbroth 1994). A paraneoplastic exfoliative dermatitis has been associated with thymomas in other species and a presumptive diagnosis was made in five rabbits (Florizoone 2005; Rostaher Prelaud et al. 2013). Hypercalcemia and myasthenia gravis are paraneoplastic syndromes in other species but have not been observed in rabbits.

Clinical signs are primarily dyspnea (76.9%) and exercise intolerance (53.9%) (Kunzel et al. 2012; Lewis 2016). Bilateral exophthalmos was observed in 46.2% of rabbits with thymomas resulting from compression of the cranial vena cava by the mass. The orbital venous sinus of rabbits drains into the cranial vena cava and the increased pressure causes exophthalmos and third eyelid prolapse which is intermittent (Vernau et al. 1995; Bennett 2009). Thymoma should be on the list of differentials in rabbits with exophthalmos and dyspnea. The heart and lung sounds are diminished in the cranial and ventral fields, and there is decreased compressibility of the cranioventral chest due to the mass. Hematologic and biochemistry values are often within normal limits.

Thoracic radiographs are strongly suggestive of thymoma demonstrating a large cranial mediastinal mass (Figure 17.17) (Bennett 2009). It is difficult to define the border between the mass and the heart, and a misdiagnosis of an enlarged cardiac silhouette can be made. The mass is often large enough to cause caudodorsal displacement of the heart and lungs and elevation of the trachea. Ultrasound is a very useful diagnostic tool. Thymomas tend to have mixed echogenicity and cavitations. Ultrasound can also direct a core needle biopsy instrument to obtain a sample avoiding fluid and major blood vessels. CT angiography can be useful to determine if the mass has invaded major vessels (Morrisey and McEntee 2005; de Mello Souza 2013) but cannot determine the extent of adhesions that makes excision difficult (Bennett 2009).

In a report of 13 rabbits with thymoma, 12 were diagnosed on cytology with 8 confirmed with histology with one sample having too few cells for evaluation (Kunzel et al. 2012). If the aspirate is primarily lymphocytes, cytokeratin stain will show the epithelial component confirming a diagnosis of thymoma (Bennett 2009; de Mello Souza 2013). In dogs and cats, the presence of eosinophils helps confirm the diagnosis of thymoma, but eosinophils have not been reported to be a feature of rabbit thymomas.

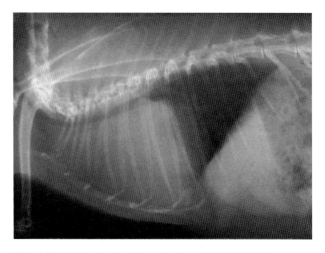

Figure 17.17 Lateral radiograph of a rabbit with a thymoma. The mass is displacing the trachea dorsally and the heart caudally. It is difficult to differentiate the heart from the mass because they are both soft tissue dense. Ultrasound or CT will be helpful to determine the extent of the mass.

In a prospective study, hypofractionated stereotactic volumetric modulated arc radiotherapy with adaptive planning was used to treat 15 rabbits with thymoma. In all 15 rabbits, contrast enhanced CT showed elimination of all enhancing tumor volume for 2 years after treatment. Ten still had no tumor recurrence at the time the study was published, two died of unrelated causes 618 and 718 days after treatment, and three were lost to follow up. No radiation side effects were observed. These results are very promising; however, this treatment option is not readily available. Megavoltage radiation therapy was not as promising and serious radiation side effects occurred (Andres et al. 2012).

The treatment of choice for thymomas has been surgical excision (Morrisey and McEntee 2005; Bennett 2009; Dirven et al. 2009; de Mello Souza 2013; Huston et al. 2012; Lewis 2016). Complete excision carries a good prognosis in most species; however, local recurrence has been reported in rabbits (Kunzel et al. 2012). In one study, three rabbits were treated with surgery alone and survived 8 months to 3 years (Huston et al. 2012). Lewis reported a 50% long-term survival rate with major complications most likely to occur during the first 10 days postoperative. The author has had an approximately 75% long-term survival with all fatal complications occurring during the first week after surgery (Bennett 2009).

In a retrospective study, 13 rabbits were diagnosed with thymoma in a 3 year period at a single institution supporting that it is a relatively common problem (Kunzel et al. 2012). Four rabbits were euthanized at the time of diagnosis and, in two, the mass was mainly fluid and fluid aspiration was the only treatment they received. Those two only survived 150 and 270 days. The mass was surgically removed in seven rabbits, but only two survived the perioperative period. In both survivors, a cranial mediastinal mass recurred at 6 and 34 months postoperative and euthanasia was elected. Recurrence is considered the result of incomplete excision (Lewis 2016).

A thymoma has been reported to be successfully removed using an intercostal approach (Kostolich and Panciera 1992); however, the recommended surgical approach is a ventral midline thoracotomy to allow access to both sides of the cranial thoracic cavity.

Lung Lobe Abscesses

Lung abscesses occur frequently in rabbits and may be underdiagnosed (Lewis 2016). In dogs and cats, medical management (long-term antibiotic therapy) and surgical treatment (lung lobectomy) have good success rates. While other organisms have been isolated from pulmonary abscesses in rabbits, *P. multocida* is the most common isolate (Lewis 2016). Its capsule is primarily made of hyaluronic acid which inhibits opsonization and phagocytosis resulting in the formation of caseous pus. Medical management is unlikely to resolve the infection, so it is logical to recommend lung lobectomy in rabbits (Bennett 2009) (Figure 17.18).

(a)

(b)

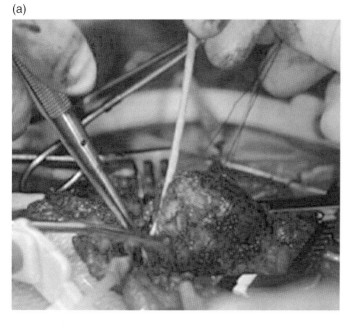 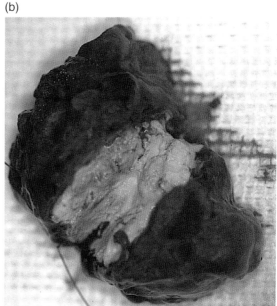

Figure 17.18 Intraoperative image of a lateral thoracotomy for a lung lobe abscess in a rabbit (a). The mass is being gently elevated with cotton-tipped applicators. After the lung lobe was removed, it was incised revealing the abscess for collection of culture samples (b).

Clinical signs include lethargy, depression, decreased appetite, weight loss, and other nonspecific signs of illness. Rabbits generally do not cough but sneezing may be part of the history. Affected rabbits may have a fever and increased white blood cell count. Thoracic auscultation reveals diminished sounds in the affected lung field.

Radiographs are generally consistent with a consolidated lobe. Ultrasound demonstrates a cavitated lesion in the affected lung and will allow collection of FNA samples for culture and cytology confirming the diagnosis. CT is also very useful especially with contrast. After contrast administration, the center of the abscessed lobe (pus) will not enhance because it does not have a blood supply while the area surrounding the pus is consistent with inflammation. CT can also be used to guide a needle into the lesion to obtain samples. It is best to get culture results and initiate antibiotic therapy prior to surgery so that an appropriate antibiotic will be circulating before manipulating the abscess. If the patient's condition indicates a more urgent need for surgical intervention, a Gram's stain may help direct preoperative antibiotic therapy. A variety of organisms have been isolated from abscesses in rabbits including anaerobic bacteria.

Ventral Thoracotomy

The first report of surgical excision of a thymoma in a rabbit used a lateral thoracotomy (Kostolich and Panciera 1992). That rabbit survived the surgery but died in the immediate postoperative period. The disadvantage of trying to remove a large cranial mediastinal mass through a lateral thoracotomy is the limited exposure. A ventral midline thoracotomy was used for the first reported successful excision of a thymoma where the rabbit survived long-term (Clippinger et al. 1998). It allows exposure to both sides of the chest and the important structures in the cranial mediastinum (Bennett 2009). The thoracotomy can be extended caudally as far as needed to achieve the necessary exposure. In most cases, the sternebrae of rabbits are too narrow to split longitudinally so the term "median sternotomy" is not applicable. A rotary woodworking tool has been recommended to cut sternebrae on midline (Lewis 2016; Szabo 2016). A sagittal saw is preferred because the blade oscillates rather than rotating so it is less likely to inadvertently cut through vital structures. It is difficult to determine if cutting sternebrae may be more painful than disarticulating ribs, but it is well recognized that many rabbits survive the surgical procedure only to succumb in the immediate postoperative period indicating the importance of providing intense postoperative monitoring and multimodal analgesia.

Place the rabbit in dorsal recumbency with the head pointing toward the surgeon and a towel under the neck to elevate it. Make a skin incision beginning mid-cervical (2–3 cm cranial to the manubrium) extending caudally along the manubrium to the xiphoid. A common error is not initiating the incision far enough cranially. There is a paired subcutaneous muscle (cutaneous muscle of the neck) on each side of midline (Popesko et al. 1992). Separate the sternohyoideus and sternocephalicus muscles in the cervical region on midline to the level of the manubrium using blunt dissection. Because the mass generally extends to the thoracic inlet, use a hemostat to bluntly dissect dorsal to (under) the manubrium into the cranial mediastinum to create a space between the sternebrae and the mass. Carefully, elevate the pectoralis muscles from the ventral aspect of the sternebrae. It is best to use electrosurgery for hemostasis. This will expose the articulations between the ribs and the sternebrae. Use fine scissors or a #11 scalpel blade to disarticulate the ribs along one side (Figure 17.19). Approximately, 44% of rabbits have 12 ribs and 56% have 13 ribs (Vella and Donnelly 2012). Only the first six are directly attached by the costal cartilage to the sternum and the last two usually have no attachment to the sternum. Continue this dissection to caudal to the mass undermining dorsal to (under), the sternebrae as the dissection progresses caudally to protect vital structures within the chest. Ideally, leave the xiphoid intact to provide more stability to the chest postoperatively, which is also believed to help with postoperative pain; however, it may not be possible to remove a large mass without completely separating the chest along midline.

Use a retractor, such as a Lone Star, to provide exposure to the mass (Figure 17.19). Be careful not to damage the intercostal muscles on the side where the ribs have been disarticulated by putting too much force to open the chest. To remove the mass, dissection must be meticulous and can be time-consuming. Cotton-tipped applicators are useful for lifting the mass away from important structures without damaging blood vessels. At the thoracic inlet, these masses generally wrap around the subclavian artery and vein as well as the jugular veins and carotid arteries. It is best to avoid ligating these vessels.

Once the mass has been removed, check for hemorrhage and air leaks prior to closing. Place an intercostal thoracostomy tube (5–10 fr) for control of the pleural space postoperatively. There is no need to reattach the ribs. Preplace figure-of-eight sutures through the intercostal muscles on the side where ribs were disarticulated, then around the sternebrae and contralateral rib (Figure 17.19). Once all sutures are placed, tie them from cranial to caudal. Appose the pectoralis muscles along the ventral midline with a slowly absorbed monofilament suture in a simple continuous pattern. This layer should create an air-tight seal. Use the thoracostomy tube to evacuate the chest cavity. Close

(a)   (b)   (c)

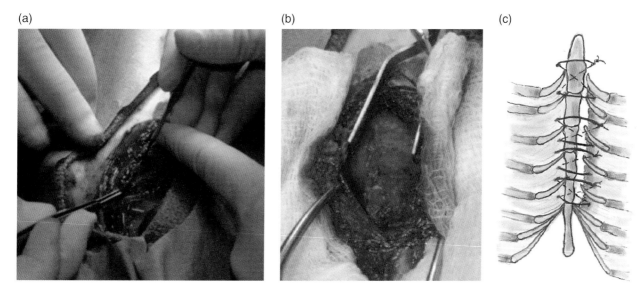

Figure 17.19 Intraoperative images of a ventral midline thoracotomy in a rabbit (a). Use a scalpel to disarticulate the ribs from the sternebrae. This rabbit has a thymoma (b) visible upon entry into the thoracic cavity obstructing the view of any normal structures. To close the chest wall, pass figure-of-eight sutures around the sternebrae and the intercostal muscles (c). Preplace all sutures and take large bites of the intercostal muscles. Once this layer has been closed, close the pectoralis muscles to prevent the legs from splaying and provide additional support to the sternebrae-intercostal closure.

the subcutaneous tissues and skin routinely. Submit the mass for culture (for abscesses) and histologic evaluation to direct long-term therapy. Kunzel et al. did not maintain the thoracostomy tube postoperatively and three of the five rabbits that died in the immediate postoperative period had a large amount of pleural effusion at necropsy (Kunzel et al. 2012). The author recommends leaving the thoracostomy tube in place for at least 24 hours, removing it only after a minimum of 24 hours with minimal fluid and air aspiration. Use the thoracostomy tube to provide intracavitary bupivacaine for postoperative analgesia as well.

The author has found intracavitary bupivacaine to be helpful in the postoperative period. The first dose can be given prior to closing the thoracotomy. The maximum dose of bupivacaine is 2 mg/kg q8h. During closure, this can be divided with some being used for an intercostal nerve block and the rest being placed into the chest cavity. For intracavitary analgesia, inject the bupivacaine through the chest tube. The volume is small and will need to be flushed into the chest with a small amount of air. Before putting the bupivacaine into the tube, determine the volume of air needed to completely fill the chest tube. After injecting the bupivacaine into the tube, flush it all into the chest with that volume of air.

Lateral Thoracotomy

The muscular anatomy of the lateral thorax of rabbits is similar to that of dogs (Bennett 2009). The latissimus dorsi lies under the skin and over the scalenus and serratus ventralis muscles. The scalenus extends caudally across the

fourth intercostal space as a fan-shaped muscle and the caudal end of the last belly inserts on the fifth rib. The serratus ventralis extends farther caudal to about the 10th rib, but its bellies are parallel to the ribs, so it is not necessary to transect them for an intercostal thoracotomy. The internal and external intercostal muscles are similar to those of dogs and cats, and the intercostal vessels and nerves are along the cranial aspect of the intercostal space.

Rabbits have only two lung lobes on the left: the left cranial and the left caudal lobes (Figure 17.20). The left cranial lobe has a small fissure that defines the cranial portion and the caudal portion. The division is incomplete, and both portions are supplied by a single bronchus. On the right side, there are four lobes: cranial, middle, caudal, and accessory. The right middle lobe is mainly ventral to the right cranial lobe. The accessory lobe is caudal to the middle lobe and ventral to the caudal lobe lying along the esophagus and caudal vena cava.

The location of the lateral thoracotomy will depend on the location of the lesion; however, for a lung lobectomy a fourth (cranial lobe) or fifth (caudal lobe) intercostal thoracotomy is generally used because it is the location of the hilum. As an external landmark, the caudodorsal border of the scapula is approximately at the level of the fourth intercostal space. Make an incision through the skin and subcutaneous tissues. Determine the location of the desired intercostal space and incise the latissimus dorsi from ventral to dorsal transecting the ventral 2/3 of the muscle. Bleeding from the vessels within the muscle can be

Figure 17.20 The anatomy of the lungs of a rabbit. (2) right cranial lobe; (3) right medial lobe; (4) right caudal lobe; (5) left caudal lobe; (6) cranial portion of left cranial lobe; (7) caudal portion of left cranial lobe. *Source:* Popesko et al. (1992). Reprinted with permission of Elsevier.

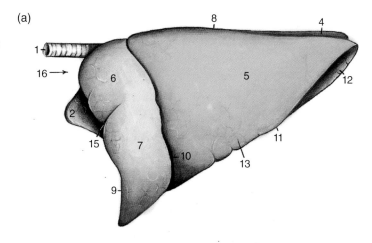

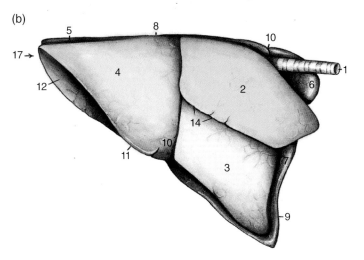

controlled with electrosurgery or hemostatic clips. Insert a hemostat under the latissimus cranially to identify the thoracic inlet, and then pull the hemostat caudally over each rib to count intercostal spaces confirming the location of the desired intercostal space. Separate the serratus ventralis at the appropriate intercostal space and transect the scalenus along the fifth rib (for a fourth intercostal thoracotomy). Incise the intercostal muscles being careful not to cut the internal thoracic vessels ventrally or the azygous vein dorsally. Once the chest is entered, assisted ventilation is required.

Identify the affected lung lobe and elevate it out of the chest cavity. Do not manipulate the affected lobe excessively to minimize the risk of pus going out the bronchus into other lobes. The bronchi and pulmonary artery and vein are small and can be ligated, clipped, or stapled, or sealed with a tissue sealing device. If a portion of the lobe is not affected, a partial lobectomy can be performed using a thoracoabdominal stapling device. The staples will seal the pulmonary parenchyma allowing a portion of the lung to be excised distal to the rows of staples. Carefully inspect

the stump for hemorrhage and air leaks prior to closure. Apply an intercostal nerve block for postoperative analgesia and an intercostal thoracostomy tube prior to closing the chest cavity.

Preplace sutures around the ribs cranial and caudal to the thoracotomy. There is normally a space between ribs, so they are not meant to be touching or overlapping. Once all sutures are placed, tie them from dorsal to ventral. Close the scalenus (if transected) and serratus ventralis, then the latissimus dorsi with a simple continuous pattern of a rapidly absorbable material. Submit the removed tissue for appropriate diagnostic testing.

Postoperative Care

Intracavitary bupivacaine can be repeated every 8 hours (Bennett 2009). Record the volume of both bupivacaine and air put into the chest so when fluid and air are evacuated via the tube, the volumes put into the chest are known and can be deducted from the totals. The chest tube should be aspirated for fluid and air (record amounts recovered)

(a)

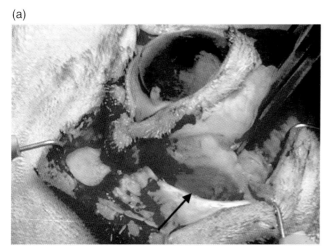

(b)

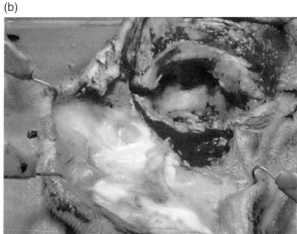

Figure 17.21 Intraoperative image of a rabbit undergoing exenteration for a retrobulbar abscess as a result of dental disease (a). Note the orbital sinus (arrow). All of the tissue has been removed from the orbit, but there is evidence of infection in the soft tissues nearby (b). If possible, remove all infected tissue prior to closing.

every hour or less initially. Extend the interval based on the amount of fluid and air recovered. The presence of a chest tube will induce an inflammatory reaction that will result in pleural effusion at a rate of approximately 1–2 ml/kg/d and evidence of infection (pyothorax) is observed 4–6 days after tube placement (Hung et al. 2016).

Enucleation and Exenteration

Enucleation refers to removing the globe, third eyelid, and the eyelid margins. Exenteration is the removal of all of the contents of the orbit. Rabbits have a large venous sinus surrounding the extraocular muscles and the Harderian gland extending caudal to the globe (Figure 17.21). If this sinus is damaged during surgery, substantial hemorrhage will occur. In rabbits, the two most common indications for enucleation are intraocular abscesses (Figure 17.22) and retrobulbar abscesses. For retrobulbar abscess, exenteration is recommended, and for intraocular abscesses, enucleation is preferred.

There are two types of enucleation commonly performed. For a transconjunctival enucleation, which is performed if there is no infection of the cornea or conjunctiva, make a circumferential incision in the bulbar conjunctiva at the limbus and remove the globe leaving as much soft tissue as possible in the orbit to minimize the sunken eye appearance postoperatively. After incising the bulbar conjunctiva, carefully dissect as close to the globe as possible. Transect the extraocular muscles at the globe as they are encountered. After removal of the globe, remove the third eyelid and Harderian gland as well as the eyelid margins prior to closing.

When performing a transpalpebral enucleation, suture the eyelids together 5 mm from the lid margins with a simple continuous suture of any material. This is typically indicated when there is an infection of the conjunctiva and/or cornea as it will contain the infection and minimize contamination of the soft tissues that will be exposed during the dissection. Incise the skin of the eyelids circumferentially down to the conjunctiva. Incise the medial and lateral canthal ligaments to free up the globe. Dissect soft tissues off the globe by transecting the extraocular muscles at their attachments to the globe as they are encountered. The eyelid margins, third eyelid, and Harderian gland will all be in the tissue excised.

Exenteration is indicated for management of retrobulbar abscesses as all of the soft tissues are removed making it

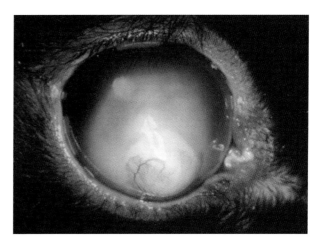

Figure 17.22 Image of an intraocular abscess caused by *Pasteurella multocida*. Since there is no corneal or conjunctival infection, a transconjunctival enucleation can be performed.

easier to control the infection postoperatively. Because the venous sinus extends around and caudal to the globe, it is likely there will be substantial hemorrhage. Control the hemorrhage by removing all of the soft tissues as quickly as possible, and then controlling hemorrhage with hemostatic aids and applying digital pressure.

With either enucleation or exenteration, consider making a prosthetic globe of polymethylmethacrylate (PMMA) if there is no evidence of infection. When infection is present such as with a retrobulbar abscess, make a prosthetic globe of PMMA impregnated with an appropriate antibiotic to provide a slow release of antibiotic over time (see under Section "Abscess Management").

Ear Surgery

Anatomy

As in other mammals, there are three components: external, middle, and inner ear (Capello 2004b; Chow 2011; Chow et al. 2011; Csomos et al. 2016). The external ear is comprised of the pinna and the tubular ear cartilage distal to the tympanum. The middle ear is contained within the tympanic bulla and houses the ossicles. The inner ear is encased in the temporal bone and contains the semicircular canals involved in balance and the cochlea and cochlear nerves involved in sound conduction. Animals with otitis interna typically have vestibular signs because of the intimate association of the vestibular and auditory systems. Many animals with only otitis media are asymptomatic because the disease is confined within the bulla. It is likely these animals experience pain but until they develop clinical signs related to otitis interna (head tilt) or otitis externa, otitis media goes undiagnosed. Primary bacterial or fungal otitis externa is uncommon in rabbits while primary otitis media is common.

In nature, rabbits have large upright pinnae used for sound amplification, thermoregulation, and communication with other rabbits. They are vertically oriented as is the bony acoustic meatus, the cartilaginous acoustic meatus (annular cartilage), the tragus, and auricular cartilage (Figure 17.23). The tympanic membrane is protected inside the bony acoustic meatus. The ear canal is formed by three interlocking cartilages: the cartilaginous acoustic meatus (annular cartilage) that wraps around the bony acoustic meatus (part of the tympanic bulla), the scutiform cartilage, and the auricular cartilage. The tragus is the proximal part of the auricular cartilage and interlocks with the cartilaginous acoustic meatus and scutiform cartilage to form the external ear canal.

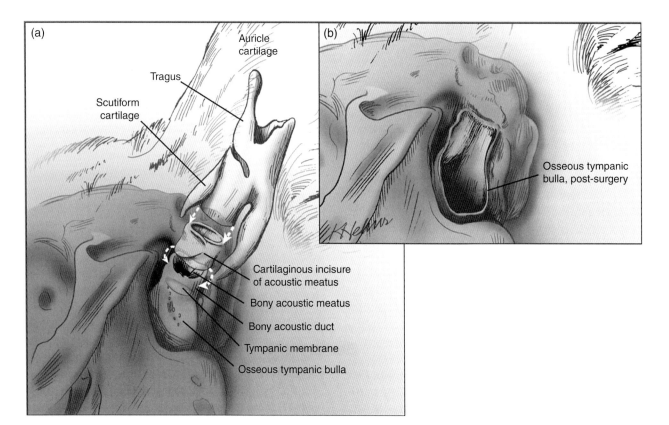

Figure 17.23 Image of the anatomy of the ear canal of a rabbit. *Source:* Chow (2011). Reprinted with permission of Elsevier.

Rabbits with upright ears have a relatively wide and rigid ear canal, and otitis externa is uncommon. Lop-eared rabbits have a narrow and weak ear canal predisposing them to accumulating cerumen. Additionally, lop-eared breeds have a 3–5 mm gap between the tragus and the cartilaginous acoustic meatus, which results in the ear bending over, typical for the breed. This potentially results in complete occlusion of the ear canal. If the external ear canal is occluded by this anatomy, normal ceruminous secretions cannot drain properly setting up an environment for bacterial and fungal growth. Over time, the accumulations can push out through the gap and create an outpouching full of cerumen, debris, and microorganisms resulting in formation of an abscess at the base of the ear.

The major vessels supplying the pinna are on the convex surface and include the rostral, intermedial, and caudal auricular arteries located more centrally and the rostral and caudal marginal veins around the perimeter.

The facial nerve (CN VII) exits the stylomastoid foramen just caudal to the tympanic membrane and courses craniolaterally around the tympanic bulla. Facial nerve paresis/paralysis can occur if a disease process expands into this area. It can also sustain damage during surgical manipulations. The most obvious clinical sign of facial nerve damage is an inability to blink (Figure 17.24). It also provides parasympathetic innervation to the salivary and lacrimal glands. Loss of the ability to blink and decreased tear production predisposes to exposure keratitis especially in rabbits with prominent globes. Facial nerve injury does not affect mastication; however, hypoglossal nerve damage (another reported complication of bulla osteotomy) can.

History and Clinical Signs

Otitis media is relatively common in rabbits and underdiagnosed because of the lack of clinical signs. Otitis media without otitis externa is generally the result of ascending infection from the nasopharynx via the auditory tube into the bulla. In one report, approximately 80% of rabbits with upper respiratory tract infections also had otitis media and in 70% of them, it was bilateral (Deeb et al. 1990). In apparently healthy rabbits, 11% had otitis media. In another study, 33% of rabbits had evidence of otitis media at necropsy, and it was an incidental finding on CT in 27% of rabbits (Snyder et al. 1973; Fox et al. 1971). Lop-eared rabbits are at an increased risk of developing otitis media (de Matos et al. 2016). Otitis media in humans is a painful condition, and it is likely painful for rabbits as well.

Clinical signs are vague and include anorexia, lethargy, behavioral changes, and discomfort. They are usually not noticed until otitis externa or an abscess and physical mass have developed, or vestibular signs related to otitis interna manifest. Once vestibular signs are present, it is unlikely they will resolve even after the infection has resolved. Once these signs develop, the disease has advanced significantly. For this reason and the frequency of dental disease in rabbits, five-view skull radiographs to evlaute the bullae and teeth should be recommended as part of an annual wellness exam in rabbits.

Diagnostic Evaluation

As part of a routine physical examination, palpate the base of the ear canal for evidence of swelling or pain. Assess for pain on opening the jaw. Because of the proximity of the mandible to the bulla, bulla osteitis can cause pain when opening the mouth.

Otoscopy is difficult in rabbits, especially lop-eared breeds because the canal is narrow and folded over. Heavy sedation or general anesthesia is required, and it is still very difficult to visualize the tympanum. Consider making skull radiographs under the same sedation/anesthesia. It is best not to instill any fluid into the ear if other diagnostics such as skull radiographs or CT are to be performed because if fluid gets into the bulla it will create a soft tissue dense artifact. Normal ceruminous secretions in rabbits are white and can look like pus; however, on cytology there will be no white blood cells. Evaluate the ear canal for signs of inflammation and any exudates cytologically. Collect samples for culture if cytology is consistent with infection. A Gram's stain can be helpful for deciding what antibiotic to use empirically. Biopsy any masses seen.

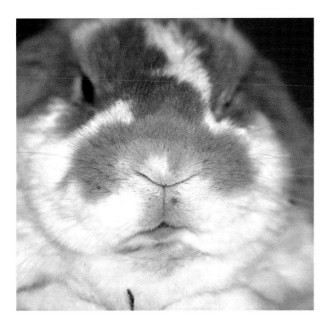

Figure 17.24 Facial nerve palsy in a rabbit with an abscess surrounding the external ear canal. Notice the right eye is not closed and the right upper lip is drooping.

Skull radiographs are useful for assessing the health of the tympanic bulla. Five views are recommended: VD or DV, lateral, right and left lateral oblique, and rostral-caudal, with the obliques and rostral–caudal being most helpful. The bone should be thin and smooth, and the bulla full of air. If the bulla is filled with soft tissue dense material, it may be pus or tissue. Changes in bone suggestive of otitis media include increased thickness, irregular surface, proliferation, and lysis. Also, compare sides for evidence of asymmetry.

CT is preferred because there is no superimposition, contrast allows differentiation between pus and tissue, and periotic soft tissues can be evaluated (abscess, mineralization) (de Matos et al. 2016) (Figure 17.25). In patients with vestibular signs and normal CT scan, an MRI is recommended to assess the brain.

Medical Management

Because of the anatomy and nature of rabbits, medical management is not usually successful at curing otitis media and externa causing clinical signs in rabbits (Meredith and Richardson 2015). Long-term (at least 6 weeks) antibiotic therapy has been suggested to be helpful but not curative. Many will experience temporary improvement while on antibiotics, but signs recur after they are discontinued. A variety of organisms have been isolated and antibiotic therapy (with or without surgical intervention) is best directed by results of culture and sensitivity testing.

Auricular Surgery

Partial Pinnectomy

Partial pinnectomy is mainly indicated for tumor excision but can be performed for lacerations that fail to heal primarily and for avascular necrosis of the pinna that can occur after venous or arterial catheterization. Epithelial tumors are most common in the pinna of rabbits. Shope fibromas, papillomas, trichoblastomas, and melanomas have been reported.

Mark appropriate margins around the mass and incise full thickness to excise the mass. Cut the cartilage 1–2 mm shorter than the skin so the skin can be opposed over the cut edge. One way to accomplish this is to pull the skin proximally while making the incision so it is retracted from the cut edge. When released, the skin on both sides will be slightly longer than the cartilage. Oppose the skin with fine monofilament suture in a simple interrupted or continuous pattern. Be careful to avoid damaging the caudal and rostral auricular vessels because their compromise can result in necrosis of the pinna distal to the site of damage.

If a complete pinnectomy is required, make a full thickness incision around the base of the ear from the intertragic incisure circumferentially. It will be necessary to isolate and ligate vessels at the base of the ear. Again, make the skin incision so the edges are 1–2 mm longer than the cut edge of the cartilage.

Auricular Hematomas

Auricular hematomas are the result of trauma, including self-trauma, to the pinna resulting in blood accumulating between the skin and cartilage on the concave side. It is vital to determine and treat the cause of trauma. Self-trauma is most common and often results from otitis. Left untreated the hematoma becomes organized and scar tissue contracts resulting in deformity. It is believed these are painful, but, in many respects, surgery is performed for cosmetic reasons.

In dogs, systemic and intralesional glucocorticoids have shown promise likely because they inhibit scar tissue contraction. Because rabbits are more sensitive to the negative effects of glucocorticoids and their use for treatment of auricular hematomas in rabbits has not been studied, surgery is generally recommended.

The surgical procedure recommended is analogous to that used in dogs. Make an S-shaped skin incision on the concave side of the pinna and remove the blood clot. Remove any fibrin debris and irrigate thoroughly. Place

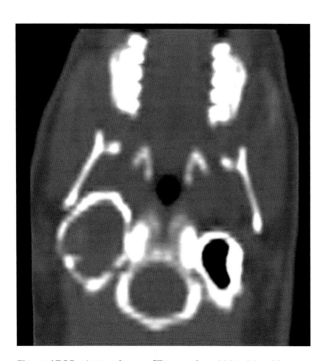

Figure 17.25 Image from a CT scan of a rabbit with otitis media on the right side. The bulla has enlarged, and the normally air-filled bulla is full of soft tissue dense material. Note the proximity of the mandible to the affected bulla which causes pain when opening the mouth.

partial or full thickness vertical mattress sutures as described for pinna lacerations to oppose the skin onto the cartilage. The goal is to get the skin to adhere to the cartilage again. Make a roll of gauze appropriate to the diameter of the curl of the pinna. Place a nonadherent pad on the incision, then place the roll of gauze on top of that. Place tape (Elastikon, Medline Industries, Inc. www.medline.dom) in strips around the outer pinna and the packing material. Leave the opening of external ear canal out of the bandage especially if topical otic treatments are indicated. In one week, cut the tape on the concave side and remove the packing. Do not remove the tape, as this will cause skin irritation. Gently clean the wound and replace the packing. Place another layer of tape on top of the original tape. At week two, remove the bandage completely. By this point, desquamation of cells allows the tape to be easily removed. Do not replace the bandage. A week later remove the sutures. The bandage will help keep the pinna flat during the healing process minimizing crinkling.

Ventral Bulla Osteotomy (VBO)

Ventral bulla osteotomy (VBO) has been described in rabbits (Chow et al. 2009; Chow 2011; Csomos et al. 2016). VBO is indicated for treatment of otitis media with or without otitis interna. The goal is to remove debris and purulent material from the bulla, collect diagnostic samples, and allow tissue ingrowth into the normally air-filled bulla allowing systemic antibiotics to penetrate. The approach is easier with fewer complications compared with ear canal ablation and lateral bulla osteotomy.

Position the patient in dorsal recumbency with a pillow under the neck to elevate the angle of the mandible. Make a 4–5 cm incision parallel and medial to the prominent mandibular angle and incise the platysma muscle medial to the mandibular salivary gland (Figure 17.26). Bluntly dissect the digastricus from the hyoglossus and styloglossus muscles being careful to avoid the hypoglossal nerve which is lateral to the hyoglossus muscle. Palpate the ventral aspect of the bulla and use a Gelpi retractor to maintain the separation. Use a periosteal elevator to remove soft tissue from the ventral surface of the bulla then a Steinmann pin to create an opening in the ventral aspect of the bulla. Use rongeurs to enlarge the opening enough to be able to remove any debris and the entire epithelial lining. Be careful at the dorsomedial aspect of the bulla which is the location of the oval and round windows. Aggressive dissection in this location will cause vestibular signs. Collect samples for culture and histopathology. Irrigate copiously to remove any pus. Place appropriate antibiotic impregnated beads into the site if there has been bone destruction resulting in infection of surrounding soft tissues and bone. Suture the digastricus back to the hyoglossus and styloglossus ventrally, and then appose the platysma.

Reported complications of VBO in other species include recurrence of infection, draining tract formation (due to not removing all of the epithelium lining the bulla), facial nerve damage (usually transient and more common with lateral bulla osteotomy), Horner's syndrome (usually transient), and hypoglossal nerve damage, which can affect tongue function but is rare. If dissection is extensive, swelling can

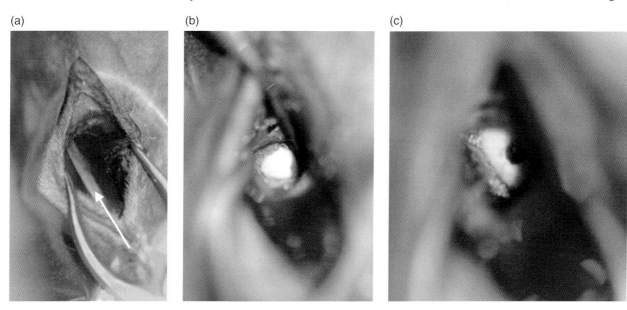

Figure 17.26 Intraoperative image of a rabbit undergoing a ventral bulla osteotomy for otitis media without otitis externa. Make a skin incision medial to the angle of the mandible (a) and dissect down to the tympanic bulla. Use a periosteal elevator to remove the soft tissue to expose the white bone of the tympanic bulla (b). Create a hole in the bulla with a Steinmann pin (c) and enlarge the opening. Collect samples, irrigate, and close. Consider placing antibiotic impregnated beads for topical antimicrobial therapy.

impinge on the oropharynx. Because of the difficulty intubating rabbits, it may be best not to do this procedure bilaterally under one anesthesia to minimize the risk of swelling causing airway obstruction, which is more likely to occur if there is bilateral swelling.

Ear Canal Ablation and Lateral Bulla Osteotomy

In dogs, total ear canal ablation is typically recommended because the underlying disease process affects the skin and cerumen glands of the entire external ear canal causing otitis externa and secondary otitis media (Chow 2011; Chow et al. 2011; Eatwell et al. 2013; Csomos et al. 2016). In rabbits, this is uncommon as most infections of the external ear canal occur secondary to otitis media breaking out the tympanum or from the folded cartilage causing partial or complete obstruction with resultant abscess formation at the base of the ear and secondary otitis media. Therefore, it is not necessary to remove all of the ear canal, only the segment proximal to the fold. It is vital to remove all of the ear canal predisposing to the accumulation of cerumen. When performing a partial or subtotal ear canal ablation a blind-ended ear canal is created (Figure 17.27).

Position the patient in lateral recumbency with a pillow under the neck to elevate the ear and bulla. Make a skin incision over the vertical ear canal proximal to the opening of the ear canal from about 1–2 cm from the intertragic incisure to 1–2 cm ventral to the tympanic bulla (Figure 17.28). Distally, dissect circumferentially around the ear canal isolating it from muscles and other soft tissues. Transect the ear canal at an appropriate level based on the underlying disease and continue dissection circumferentially proximally staying as close to the cartilage as possible to avoid injury to the facial nerve. Dissect down to the bony acoustic meatus which is part of the tympanic bulla and transect the cartilaginous acoustic meatus to remove the affected segment of external ear canal.

Use a periosteal elevator to dissect soft tissues from the lateral and ventral aspects of the bulla being careful to protect the facial nerve. Compared with dogs, the bulla of rabbits is more superficial and accessible. Place Gelpi retractors to maintain isolation of the bulla while using rongeurs to remove the lateral and ventral wall of the bulla starting with the bony acoustic meatus. Make the opening large enough to be able to clean out pus and debris and to be able to remove the entire lining of the bulla being gentle in the dorsomedial aspect. Collect samples and irrigate copiously. If the infection has caused bone destruction and has extended into the soft tissues place antibiotic impregnated beads into the site prior to closing. Close the distal ear canal with monofilament absorbable mattress sutures between the lateral and medial aspects of the ear canal. Place a few sutures in the deep tissues to eliminate dead

(a)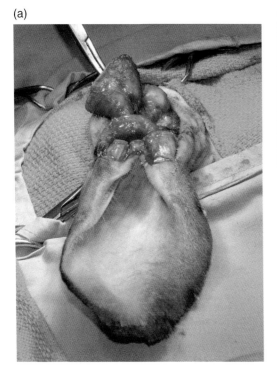

(b)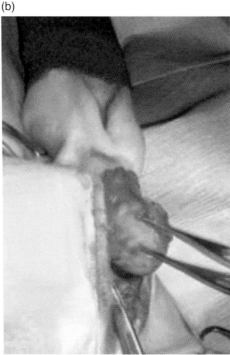

Figure 17.27 A partial or subtotal ear canal ablation with lateral bulla osteotomy is indicated in rabbits without otitis externa. (a) The affected segment of the external ear canal is excised, and the remaining ear canal is sutured closed. This leaves a blind end deep in the external ear canal. (b) Intraoperative image of an abscess at the base of the ear. *Source:* Images courtesy of Rebecca Csomos.

(a)

(b)

(c)

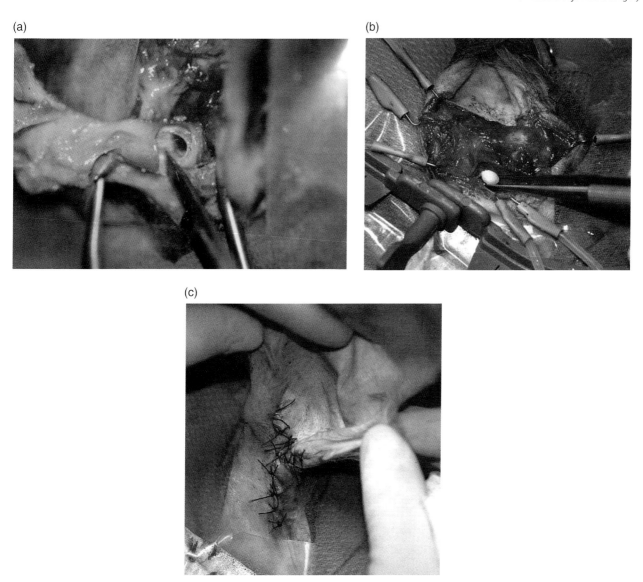

Figure 17.28 Rabbits do not have a horizontal ear canal and the tympanum is located inside the bony tube (bony acoustic duct – see Figure 17.23). Transect the external ear canal from the bony acoustic duct (a) to remove the external ear canal. Following the lateral bulla osteotomy, place antibiotic impregnated beads to provide topical antibiotic therapy (b). Close routinely (c).

space but be careful to avoid the facial nerve. Oppose the subcutaneous tissues and skin routinely. Marsupialization of the surgical site, drains, and postoperative flushing have not been shown to be beneficial compared to primary closure (Eatwell et al. 2013).

Abscess Management

As explained previously, rabbits tend to make caseous pus rather than the more liquid pus produced by dogs and cats. They also tend to produce a thick fibrous capsule around the abscess in an effort to wall it off. This capsule often contains pockets of pus that may contain bacteria. These

factors make it difficult to resolve abscesses in rabbits because they tend to quickly recur. The standard treatment for abscesses, lance, drain, irrigate, and place a drain generally results in recurrence. Even when left open to heal by second intention or marsupialized, typically the skin heals over the abscess before the infection has been controlled resulting in recurrence.

The author has had the best success in curing rabbit abscesses by approaching their resection as if they are a malignant tumor. Perform a marginal resection if possible, to excise the abscess intact without rupturing it (Figure 17.29). If this is possible, perform a routine closure. Often, the abscess will rupture or may contaminate the wound bed following excision which may lead to

(a)

(b)

(c)

(d)

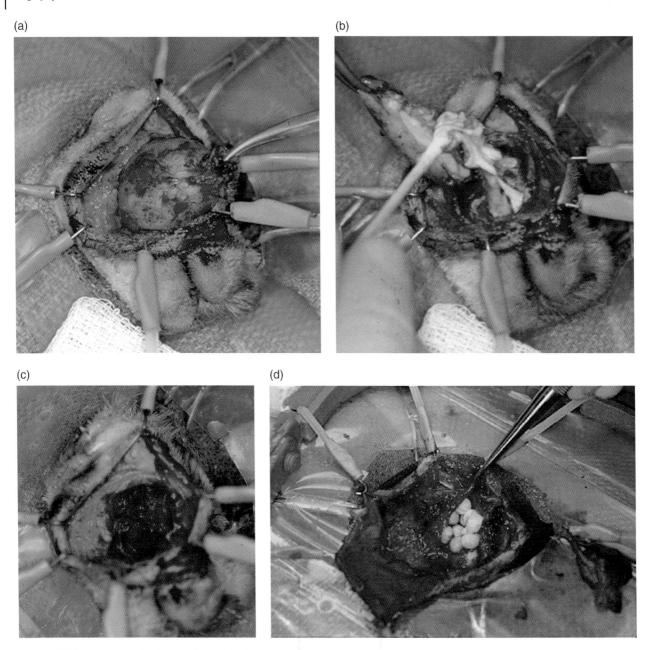

Figure 17.29 Intraoperative image of a rabbit with a maxillary abscess resulting from dental disease. Dissect the abscess from surrounding structures as if performing a tumor removal making every effort not to rupture the abscess (a). If the abscess ruptures (expected with dental abscesses because they arise through bone), clean the pus as quickly as possible (b). Irrigate the site copiously and remove any obviously infected tissue (c). Place antibiotic impregnated beads in the wound bed to fill the dead space created by the abscess excision (d). Then close routinely.

recurrence of the abscess. In order to reduce the risk of recurrence, place antibiotic impregnated beads into the wound bed to provide slow long-term release of antibiotic locally with minimal systemic absorption.

Historically antibiotic impregnated beads were primarily made with PMMA, and there are a number of studies evaluating the elution properties of various antibiotics from PMMA beads. The disadvantage of PMMA beads is that they are not absorbable so if the antibiotic chosen is not effective against the bacteria or the bacteria develop resistance, the beads become a nidus for infection. More recently, plaster of Paris (calcium sulfate hemihydrate) has been used to make beads (Kerrier™, info@kerrier.com). These beads are absorbable and provide a source of calcium when treating osteomyelitis such as with dental abscesses in rabbits. Elution studies are underway as of this writing.

Postoperative Care

Intensive postoperative care is essential in rabbits following surgery. Recover the patient in a warm, quiet environment, and continue IV fluid support as well as GI prokinetic therapy to reduce the risk of the patient developing postoperative ileus. Multimodal analgesia and antianxiety therapy are essential to reduce the risk of fatal complications resulting from pain, stress, and anxiety. Antibiotic therapy is indicated because of the potential for subclinical infection with *P. multocida*. Offer food as soon as the patient is awake, especially long fiber items such as fresh grasses. If the patient does not begin eating within three hours, begin syringe feeding a critical care diet. Continue these therapies until the rabbit is eating and drinking adequately on its own and is defecating normally.

References

Adin, C.A. and Nelson, R.W. (2018). Adrenal glands. In: *Veterinary Surgery: Small Animal*, 2e (eds. S.A. Johnston and K.M. Tobias), 6182–6183. St. Louis, MO: Elsevier.

Andres, K.M., Kent, M., Siedlecki, C.T. et al. (2012). The use of megavoltage radiation therapy in the treatment of thymomas in rabbits: 19 cases. *Veterinary and Comparative Oncology* 10: 82–90.

Bennett, R.A. (2009). Thoracic surgery in rabbits. *Proceedings of the First Southern European Veterinary Conference*, Barcelona, Spain.

Berent, A., Weisse, C., Bagley, D., et al. (2011). The use of subcutaneous ureteral bypass device for the treatment of feline ureteral obstructions. *Proceedings of the European College of Veterinary Internal Medicine*, Seville, Spain.

Bergdall, V. and Dysko, R.C. (1994). Metabolic, traumatic, mycotic, and miscellaneous diseases. In: *The Biology of the Laboratory Rabbit*, 2e (eds. P.J. Manning, D.H. Ringer and C.E. Newcomer), 336–355. San Diego, CA: Academic Press.

Bollinger, C., Walshaw, R., Kruger, J. et al. (2005). Evaluation of the effects of nephrotomy on renal function in clinically normal cats. *American Journal of Veterinary Research* 66: 1400–1407.

Capello, V. (2004a). Diagnosis and treatment of urolithiasis in pet rabbits. *Exotic DVM* 6 (2): 15–22.

Capello, V. (2004b). Surgical treatment of otitis externa and media in pet rabbits. *Exotic DVM* 6 (3): 15–21.

Capello, V. (2005). Surgical techniques for orchiectomy in the pet rabbit. *Exotic DVM* 7 (5): 23–32.

Chow, E.P. (2011). Surgical management of rabbit ear disease. *Journal of Exotic Pet Medicine* 20: 182–187.

Chow, E.P., Bennett, R.A., and Dustin, L. (2009). Ventral bulla osteotomy for treatment of otitis media in rabbits. *Journal of Exotic Pet Medicine* 18: 209–305.

Chow, E.P., Bennett, R.A., and Whittington, J.K. (2011). Total ear canal ablation and lateral bulla osteotomy for treatment of otitis externa and media in a rabbit. *Journal of the American Veterinary Medical Association* 239: 228–232.

Cikanek, S.J., Eshar, D., Nau, M. et al. (2018). Diagnosis and surgical treatment of a transitional cell carcinoma in the bladder apex of a pet rabbit. *Journal of Exotic Pet Medicine* 27: 113–117.

Clippinger, T.L., Bennett, R.A., Alleman, A.R. et al. (1998). Removal of a thymoma via median sternotomy in a rabbit with recurrent appendicular neurofibrosarcoma. *Journal of the American Veterinary Medical Association* 213: 1140–1143.

Csomos, R., Bosscher, G., Mans, C. et al. (2016). Surgical management of ear diseases in rabbits. *The Veterinary Clinics of North America. Exotic Animal Practice* 19: 189–204.

Deeb, B.J., DiGiancomo, R.F., Bernard, B.L. et al. (1990). *Pasteurella multocida* and *Bordatella bronchisepticum* infections in rabbits. *Journal of Clinical Microbiology* 28: 70–75.

Di Girolamo, N., Bongiovanni, L., Ferro, S. et al. (2017). Cystoscopic diagnosis of polypoid cystitis in two pet rabbits. *Journal of the American Veterinary Medical Association* 251: 84–89.

Dirven, M.J.M., Cornelissen, J.M.M., van den Ingh, T.S.G.A.M. et al. (2009). Malignant thymoma and uterine carcinoma in a rabbit. *Tijdschrift voor Diergeneeskunde* 134: 146–150.

Dolera, M., Malfassi, L., Mazza, G. et al. (2016). Feasibility for using hypofractionated stereotactic volumetric modulated ARC radiotherapy (VMAT) with adaptive planning for treatment of thymoma in rabbits: 15 cases. *Veterinary Radiology & Ultrasound* 57: 313–320.

Eatwell, K., Mancinelli, E., Hedley, J. et al. (2013). Partial ear canal ablation and lateral bulla osteotomy in rabbits. *Journal of Small Animal Practice* 54: 325–330.

Florizoone, K. (2005). Thymoma-associated exfoliative dermatitis in a rabbit. *Veterinary Dermatology* 16: 281–284.

Fox, R.R., Norberg, R.F., and Meyers, D.D. (1971). The relationship of *Pasteurella multocida* in otitis media in the domestic rabbit. *Laboratory Animal Science* 21: 45–48.

Gahring, D., Crowe, D., Powers, T. et al. (1977). Comparative renal function studies of nephrotomy closure with and without sutures in dogs. *Journal of the American Veterinary Medical Association* 171: 537–541.

Gleeson, M.D., Guzman, D.S., and Paul-Murphy, J. (2019). Clinical and pathological findings for rabbits with dystocia: 10 cases (1996–2016). *Journal of the American Veterinary Medical Association* 254: 953–959.

Gookin, J.L., Stone, E.A., Spaulding, K.A. et al. (1996). Unilateral nephrectomy in dogs with renal disease: 30 cases (1985–1994). *Journal of the American Veterinary Medical Association* 208: 2020–2026.

Graham, J. and Basseches, J. (2014). Liver lobe torsion in pet rabbits – clinical consequences, diagnosis, and treatment. *The Veterinary Clinics of North America. Exotic Animal Practice* 17: 195–202.

Graham, J., Orcutt, C.J., Casale, S.A. et al. (2014). Liver lobe torsion in rabbits: 16 cases (2007–2012). *Journal of Exotic Pet Medicine* 23: 258–265.

Greenacre, C.B., Allen, S.W., and Ritchie, B.W. (1999). Urinary bladder eversion in rabbit does. *Compendium on Continuing Education for the Practicing Veterinarian* 21: 524–528.

Greene, H.S.N. (1941). Uterine adenomata in the rabbit. *Journal of Experimental Medicine* 73: 273–292.

Griffiths, C.T., Craig, J.M., Krister, R.W. et al. (1975). Effect of castration, estrogen, and timed progestins on induced endometrial carcinoma in the rabbit. *Gynecologic Oncology* 3: 259–275.

Grunkemeyer, V.L., Sura, P.A., Baron, M. et al. (2010). Surgical repair of an inguinal herniation of the urinary bladder in an intact female domestic rabbit (*Oryctolagus cuniculus*). *Journal of Exotic Pet Medicine* 19: 249–254.

Harcourt-Brown, F. (2016a). Neutering. In: *BSAVA Manual of Rabbit Surgery, Dentistry, and Imaging* (eds. F. Harcourt-Brown and J. Chitty), 138–149. Gloucester, UK: British Small Animal Veterinary Association.

Harcourt-Brown, F. (2016b). Gastric dilation and intestinal obstruction. In: *BSAVA Manual of Rabbit Surgery, Dentistry, and Imaging* (eds. F. Harcourt-Brown and J. Chitty), 172–189. Gloucester, UK: British Small Animal Veterinary Association.

Hoyt, R.F. Jr. (1998). Abdominal surgery in pet rabbits. In: *Current Techniques in Small Animal Surgery*, 4e (ed. M.J. Bojrab), 777–790. Philadelphia, PA: Williams & Wilkins.

Hung, G.C., Gaunt, M.C., Rubin, J.E. et al. (2016). Quantification and characterization of pleural fluid in healthy dogs with thoracostomy tubes. *American Journal of Veterinary Research* 77: 1387–1391.

Huston, S.M., Lee, P.M.S., Quesenberry, K.E. et al. (2012). Cardiovascular disease, lymphoproliferative disorders, and thymomas. In: *Ferrets, Rabbits, and Rodents – Clinical Medicine and Surgery*, 3e (eds. K.E. Quesenberry and J.W. Carpenter), 263–268. St. Louis, MO: Elsevier.

Jenkins, J.R. (2012). Rabbits – soft tissue surgery. In: *Ferrets, Rabbits, and Rodents: Clinical Medicine and Surgery*, 3e (eds. K.Q. Quesenberry and J.W. Carpenter), 269–278. St. Louis, MO: Elsevier.

Keeble, E. and Benato, L. (2016). Urinary tract surgery. In: *BSAVA Manual of Rabbit Surgery, Dentistry, and Imaging* (eds. F. Harcourt-Brown and J. Chitty), 190–211. Gloucester, UK: British Small Animal Veterinary Association.

King, M., Waldron, D., Barber, D. et al. (2006). Effect of nephrotomy on renal function and morphology in normal cats. *Veterinary Surgery* 35: 749–758.

Klaphake, E. and Paul-Murphy, J. (2012). Rabbits – disorders of the reproductive and urinary systems. In: *Ferrets, Rabbits, and Rodents: Clinical Medicine and Surgery*, 3e (eds. K.E. Quesenberry and J.W. Carpenter), 223–231. St. Louis, MO: Elsevier.

Kostolich, M. and Panciera, R.J. (1992). Thymoma in a domestic rabbit. *The Cornell Veterinarian* 82: 125–129.

Kunzel, F., Hittmair, K.M., Hassan, J. et al. (2012). Thymomas in rabbits: clinical evaluation, diagnosis, and treatment. *Journal of the American Animal Hospital Association* 48: 97–104.

Kyles, A.E., Hardie, E.M., Wooden, B.G. et al. (2005). Management and outcome of cats with ureteral calculi: 153 cases (1984–2002). *Journal of the American Veterinary Medical Association* 226: 937.

Lewis, W. (2016). Mediastinal masses and other thoracic surgery. In: *BSAVA Manual of Rabbit Surgery, Dentistry, and Imaging* (eds. F. Harcourt-Brown and J. Chitty), 257–268. Gloucester, UK: British Small Animal Veterinary Association.

Maratea, K.A., Ramos-Vara, J.A., Corriveau, L.A. et al. (2007). Testicular interstitial cell tumor and gynecomastia in a rabbit. *Veterinary Pathology* 44: 513–517.

Markovich, J.E. and Labato, M.A. (2014). Medical management of nephroliths and ureteroliths. In: *Kirk's Current Veterinary Therapy XV* (eds. J.D. Bonagura and D.C. Twedt), 892–896. St. Louis, MO: Elsevier.

Martorell, J., Bailon, D., Majo, N. et al. (2012). Lateral approach to nephrotomy in the management of unilateral renal calculi in a rabbit. *Journal of the American Veterinary Medical Association* 240: 863–868.

de Matos, R., Ruby, J., Van Hatten, R.A. et al. (2016). Computed tomographic features of clinical and subclinical middle ear disease in domestic rabbits: 88 cases (2007–2014). *Journal of the American Veterinary Medical Association* 246: 336–343.

McLean, E.J., Woodward, A.P., and Ryan, S.D. (2020). Comparison of the use of a vessel-sealing device versus ligatures for occlusion of uterine tissue during ovariohysterectomy or ovariectomy in rabbits (*Oryctolagus cuniculus*). *American Journal of Veterinary Research* 81: 755–759.

de Mello Souza, C.H. (2013). Thymoma. In: *Withrow and MacEwan's Small Animal Clinical Oncology*, 5e (eds. S. Withrow, D. Vail and R. Page), 688–691. St. Louis, MO: Elsevier.

Meredith, A.L. and Richardson, J. (2015). Neurological diseases of rabbits and rodents. *Journal of Exotic Pet Medicine* 24: 21–33.

Milligan, M. and Berent, A.C. (2018). Medical and interventional management of upper urinary tract uroliths. *The Veterinary Clinics of North America. Small Animal Practice* 49: 157–174.

Morrisey, J.K. and McEntee, M. (2005). Therapeutic options for thymoma in the rabbit. *Seminars in Avian and Exotic Pet Medicine* 14: 175–181.

Pilney, A.A. and Reavill, D.R. (2008). Chlyothorax and thymic lymphoma in a pet rabbit (*Oryctolagus cuniculus*). *Journal of Exotic Pet Medicine* 17: 295–299.

Pompeu, E., Liberti, E.A., Di Loreto, C. et al. (1995). Eversao da vesicular urinaria no coelho. *Brazilian Journal of Veterinary Research and Animal Science* 32: 238.

Popesko, P., Rajtova, V., and Horak, J. (eds.) (1992). *A Colour Atlas of Anatomy of Small Laboratory Animals*, vol. 1. London: Wolfe (Mosby) Publishing Ltd.

Redrobe, S. (2000). Surgical procedures and dental disorders. In: *BSAVA Manual of Rabbit Medicine and Surgery* (ed. P. Flecknell), 117–134. Glouchester, UK: British Small Animal Veterinary Association Publications.

Rhody, J.L. (2006). Unilateral nephrectomy for hydronephrosis in a pet rabbit. *The Veterinary Clinics of North America. Exotic Animal Practice* 9: 633–641.

Richardson, C. and Flecknell, P. (2006). Routine neutering of rabbits and rodents. *Practice* 28: 70–79.

Rostaher Prelaud, A., Jassies-van der Lee, A., Mueller, R.S. et al. (2013). Presumptive paraneoplastic exfoliative dermatitis in four domestic rabbits. *Veterinary Record* 172: 155.

Sanders, R., Redrobe, S., Barr, F. et al. (2009). Letter to the editor – liver lobe torsion in rabbits. *Journal of Small Animal Practice* 50: 562.

Smeak, D.D. (2018). Abdominal wall reconstruction and hernias. In: *Veterinary Surgery: Small Animal*, 2e (eds. S.A. Johnston and K.M. Tobias), 4234–4305. St. Louis, MO: Elsevier.

Snyder, S.B., Fox, J.G., and Soave, O.A. (1973). Subclinical otitis media associated with *Pasteurella multocida* infections in New Zealand white rabbits. *Laboratory Animal Science* 23: 270–272.

Stanke, N.J., Graham, J.E., Orcutt, C.J. et al. (2011). Successful outcome of hepatectomy as treatment for liver lobe torsion in four domestic rabbits. *Journal of the American Veterinary Medical Association* 238: 1176–1183.

Steinleiter, A., Lambert, H., Kazensky, C. et al. (1990). Pentoxyfilline, a methylxanthine derivative, prevents postsurgical adhesion reformation in rabbits. *Obstetrics & Gynecology* 75: 926–928.

Stock, E., Vanderperren, K., Moeremans, I. et al. (2019). Use of contrast-enhanced ultrasonography in the diagnosis of a liver lobe torsion in a rabbit (*Oryctolagus cuniculus*). *Veterinary Radiology & Ultrasound* https://doi.org/10.1111/vru.12709. [Epub ahead of print].

Stone, E.A., Robertson, J.L., and Metcalf, M.R. (2002). The effect of nephrotomy on renal function and morphology in dogs. *Veterinary Surgery* 31: 391–397.

Szabo, Z. (2016). Rabbit soft tissue surgery. *The Veterinary Clinics of North America. Exotic Animal Practice* 19: 159–188.

Szabo, Z. (2017). Transurethral urinary bladder eversion and prolapse in a castrated male pet rabbit. *Acta Veterinaria Hungarica* 65: 556–564.

Tahas, S.A., Pope, J., Denk, D. et al. (2017). Diagnostic challenges and surgical treatment of hydroureteronephrosis in a rabbit (*Oryctolagus cuniculus*). *Veterinary Record Case Report* 5: e000379.

Taylor, H.R. and Staff, C.D. (2007). Clinical techniques: successful management of liver lobe torsion in a domestic rabbit (*Oryctolagus cuniculus*) by surgical lobectomy. *Journal of Exotic Pet Medicine* 16: 175–178.

Thas, I. and Harcourt-Brown, F. (2013). Six cases of inguinal urinary bladder herniation in entire male domestic rabbits. *Journal of Small Animal Practice* 54: 662–666.

Thode, H.P. and Johnston, M.S. (2009). Probably congenital uterine developmental abnormalities in two domestic rabbits. *Veterinary Record* 166: 242–244.

Vannevel, J. (2002). Formation of a urinary calculus in the urethra of a rabbit. *Exotic DVM* 4 (1): 6–7.

Varga, M. (2016). Basic principles of soft tissue surgery. In: *BSAVA Manual of Rabbit Surgery, Dentistry, and Imaging* (eds. F. Harcourt-Brown and J. Chitty), 123–137. Gloucester, UK: British Small Animal Veterinary Association.

Vella, D. and Donnelly, T.M. (2012). Basic anatomy, physiology, and husbandry. In: *Ferrets, Rabbits, and Rodents – Clinical Medicine and Surgery*, 3e (eds. K.E. Quesenberry and J.W. Carpenter), 157–173. St. Louis, MO: Elsevier.

Vernau, K.M., Grahn, B.H., Clarke-Scott, H.A. et al. (1995). Thymoma in a geriatric rabbit with hypercalcemia and periodic exophthalmos. *Journal of the American Veterinary Medical Association* 206: 820–822.

Wagner, F., Beinecke, A., Fehr, M. et al. (2005). Recurrent bilateral exophthalmos associated with metastatic thymic carcinoma in a pet rabbit. *Journal of Small Animal Practice* 46: 393–397.

Weber, W.J., Boothe, H.W., Brassard, J.A., and Hobson, H.P. (1985). Comparison of the healing of prescrotal urethrotomy incisions in the dog: sutured versus nonsutured. *American Journal of Veterinary Research*. 46 (6): 1309–1315.

Weisbroth, S.H. (1975). Torsion of the caudate lobe of the liver in the domestic rabbit (oryctolagus). *Journal of Veterinary Pathology.* 12: 13–15.

Weisbroth, S.H. (1994). Neoplastic diseases. In: *The Biology of the Laboratory Rabbit*, 2e (eds. P.J. Manning, D.H. Ringler and C.E. Newcomer), 259–292. San Diego, CA: Academic Press, Inc.

Wenger, S., Barrett, E.L., Pearson, G.R. et al. (2009). Liver lobe torsion in three adult rabbits. *Journal of Small Animal Practice* 50: 301–305.

Whitfield, R.R., Stills, H.F., Huls, H.R. et al. (2007). Effects of peritoneal closure and suture material on adhesion formation in a rabbit model. *American Journal of Obstetrics and Gynecology* 197: 644.e1–644.e5. E645.

Zimmerman-Pope, N., Waldron, D.R., and Barber, D.L. (2003). Effect of fenoldopam on renal function after nephrotomy in normal dogs. *Veterinary Surgery* 32: 566–573.

18

Ferret Soft Tissue Surgery

Catriona MacPhail

Many soft tissue surgical procedures performed in dogs and cats can be adapted to domestic ferrets with notable differences in suture material choices and hemostasis. It is paramount for veterinarians undertaking surgical procedures in ferrets to have an understanding of several fundamental principles: anatomic differences from dogs, cats, and other small mammals; anesthetic and analgesic techniques; and clinical presentations associated with certain conditions requiring surgery. Abdominal surgery in ferrets is performed commonly for various diagnostic and therapeutic reasons. Typical abdominal surgical procedures of ferrets include abdominal organ biopsy, removal of gastrointestinal foreign bodies, adrenalectomy, partial pancreatectomy, splenectomy, and cystic calculi removal. Other soft tissue surgical procedures performed in ferrets include cutaneous and oral mass resection, anal sacculectomy, tail amputation, and salivary gland removal.

Surgical Abdominal Anatomy

The abdominal anatomy of the domesticated ferret is similar to that of the dog and cat with some notable differences.

Hepatobiliary System

The liver is relatively large with an estimated 4.3% liver:body weight ratio compared to 3.1% in dogs (Evans and Quoc 2014; Mayer et al. 2015). There are six lobes: left lateral, left medial, quadrate, right medial, right lateral, and caudate. The left lateral lobe is the largest, followed by the right medial. The caudate lobe has both caudate and papillary processes. The gallbladder is pear-shaped and sits in a fossa between the quadrate and right medial liver lobes. Multiple minor hepatic ducts form three major

hepatic ducts: right, central, and left (Poddar 1977). These ducts join the short cystic duct from the gallbladder to form the common bile duct. The bile duct opens into the duodenum at the major duodenal papilla. Blood supply to the liver is from the portal vein and hepatic artery, and drains from the liver to the caudal vena cava through hepatic veins.

Gastrointestinal Tract

Ferrets are carnivores with a short, simple digestive system. The stomach is roughly J-shaped and similar in conformation to dogs with a cardia, fundus, body, antrum, and pylorus. The size of the stomach varies with the amount of food contained within it and can hold 50–100 ml (Powers and Brown 2012). Overall, gastrointestinal transit time is relatively short (approximately four hours) (Bleavins and Aulerich 1981; Schwarz et al. 2003). Notably, there is a prominent normal lymph node in the lesser curvature near the pylorus (Figure 18.1) (Johnson-Delaney 2006).

The small intestine consists of duodenum, jejunum, and ileum. The duodenum is approximately 10 cm in length in adult ferrets and is divided into three segments: cranial, descending, and ascending. There is no gross anatomic distinction between the jejunum and ileum; therefore, it often referred to as the jejunoileum. In normal ferrets, the jejunoileum measures approximately 140 cm in length. Ferrets do not have a cecum or an ileocolic junction, making the transition to the large intestine indistinct. This junction is identified by the anastomosis between jejunal and ileocolic arteries. Intraluminally, there is a change from a smooth mucosal layer in the small intestine to one with longitudinal folds in the large intestine.

The large intestine measures approximately 10 cm in length and consists of the colon, rectum, and anus. The colon has ascending, transverse, and descending sections.

Surgery of Exotic Animals, First Edition. Edited by R. Avery Bennett and Geoffrey W. Pye.
© 2022 John Wiley & Sons, Inc. Published 2022 by John Wiley & Sons, Inc.

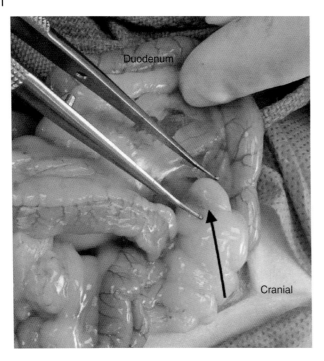

Figure 18.1 The gastric lymph node, normally prominent in ferrets (arrow).

Pancreas

The ferret pancreas is V-shaped with characteristic right and left lobes. The left lobe runs caudal and dorsal to the greater curvature of the stomach and medial to the spleen. The right lobe is larger and runs the length of the mesoduodenum. Ducts from the left and right lobes join to form a common pancreatic duct that enters the duodenum at the major duodenal papilla approximately 3 cm aborad to the pylorus. An accessory pancreatic duct entering the duodenum at minor duodenal papilla is absent in most ferrets (Powers and Brown 2012).

Spleen

The crescent-shaped spleen can be quite large in normal adult ferrets (Figure 18.2). During histologic examination of the spleen, diffuse extramedullary hematopoiesis is commonly found (Mayer et al. 2014). Care must be taken to differentiate between normal splenomegaly and pathologic splenic enlargement, for example, from primary or metastatic neoplasia.

Adrenal Glands

The left and right adrenal glands lie cranial and medial to the respective kidney. The left adrenal gland is easily located by following the prominent adrenolumbar vessels (equivalent to the phrenicoabdominal vessels) a short distance away from the vena cava crossing over the center of the gland. The right adrenolumbar vessels are difficult to visualize at the

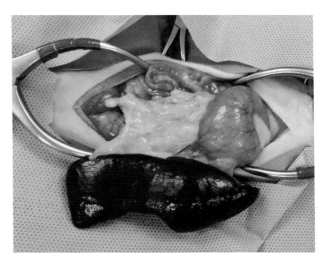

Figure 18.2 The appearance of a normal ferret spleen.

cranial aspect of the right gland. The right adrenal gland is dorsal to the caudate lobe of the liver and adhered to the right lateral and dorsal aspects of the caudal vena cava.

Urogenital System

Bean-shaped kidneys are present in the retroperitoneal space. In adult ferrets, normal kidneys measure 2.5–3.0 cm in length. The ureters run caudally and enter the urinary bladder on the dorsolateral aspect of the trigone. The urinary bladder is small and can hold up to 10 ml of urine.

The male reproductive tract is similar to that of a male dog. There is a palpable and radiographically apparent os penis; however, its tip is J-shaped with the tip curved dorsally distal to the urethral opening making urethral catheterization challenging (Figure 18.3). Male ferrets have a prostate

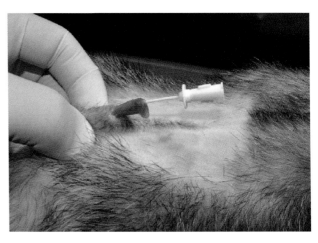

Figure 18.3 The urethral opening is located ventrally on the terminal curve of the J-shaped os penis (See Figure 18.19). A catheter has been placed in the urethra. *Source:* Reprinted with permission from Jekl and Hauptman (2017).

gland at the base of the bladder completely encompassing the urethra, potentially resulting in urinary obstruction with any condition causing hyperplasia or inflammation.

Female ferrets have a bicornuate uterus with two long tapering uterine horns ending in a short uterine body, and then a single cervix. The left and right ovaries lie caudal to the respective kidney and are attached to the abdominal wall by the suspensory ligaments. Visualization of the entire ovary may be obscured by fat, potentially predisposing ferrets to ovarian remnant syndrome following incomplete ovariohysterectomy.

Celiotomy and Closure

The small size of the ferret poses unique technical challenges to surgical procedures. Some advocate the use of clear adhesive drapes to allow improved visualization for the anesthetist and better thermoregulation; however, these drapes should be used with caution because they have been associated with an increased rate of surgical site infection in smaller patients (Webster and Alghamdi 2015). The author prefers straight and curved ring-tipped microsurgical forceps, in addition to Castroviejo needle holders for suturing delicate tissues.

A standard midline celiotomy in ferrets differs from other species. The skin is thin and there is little subcutaneous tissue. In male ferrets, the prepuce lies directly on midline just caudal to the umbilicus. Drape the prepuce out of the field to avoid iatrogenic damage.

Due to the long and narrow conformation of ferrets, the diaphragmatic reflection is more caudal than in other species. Start entry into the abdominal cavity approximately 1–2 cm caudal to the xiphoid to avoid entering the thoracic cavity. The linea alba is translucent and wide cranially (Figure 18.4). This allows controlled and careful entry into the abdominal cavity, as viscera beneath the abdominal

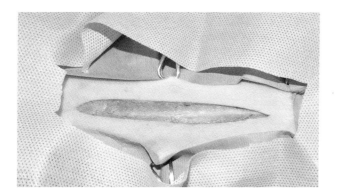

Figure 18.4 Ferrets have little subcutaneous tissue and a wide linea alba as shown.

wall can be visualized; however, due to the large size of the spleen, iatrogenic splenic laceration is possible. Tent the linea alba and make a stab incision with a #15 scalpel blade. Extend the incision caudally using the same scalpel blade or Metzenbaum scissors.

Once the abdominal cavity is open, place a retractor to allow visualization and palpation of the entire abdominal cavity and its contents. Ring retractors are the most commonly used in ferrets (see Chapter 1). Alternative methods for abdominal retraction include a pediatric Balfour and small Gelpi retractors.

Complete abdominal exploratory is indicated whenever performing abdominal surgery in ferrets. Perform a systemic or regional approach to evaluate for incidental findings such as gastrointestinal foreign material, adrenal gland disease, lymph node enlargement, and pancreatic nodules.

Close the abdomen in two layers: abdominal wall and skin. If there is enough subcutaneous tissue, this layer can be closed as a third layer. To minimize the amount of suture material, close the abdominal wall in a simple continuous pattern using 4-0 absorbable suture, such as polyglyconate or polydioxanone. Intradermal closure is not recommended in ferrets as it is technically challenging and often results in significant bruising. Close the skin using a simple or cruciate interrupted pattern, or a simple continuous or Ford interlocking pattern using 4-0 nylon or polypropylene.

Surgical Procedures

Adrenalectomy

Surgical excision of adrenal glands for adrenal gland disease is a reasonable and often preferred option particularly early in the course of disease; however, palliative medical options exist that provide good long-term survival without surgery through control of clinical signs. It must be noted that these medical therapies do not treat the adrenal tumor itself. As in other species, adrenalectomy offers the chance to cure the disease, whereas medical management does not.

Adrenal gland disease is the most familiar endocrinopathy in ferrets, with identifiable clinical signs of such as symmetric alopecia, pruritus, and vulvar swelling in females, and urinary obstruction due to prostatomegaly in males. Adrenal tumors were identified in 10.6% of ferrets in the United States and 21.9% of ferrets in Japan (Li et al. 1998; Miwa et al. 2009). Medical management addresses the clinical signs associated with increase in sex hormones produced by the diseased adrenal gland, but does not affect the progressive growth of abnormal adrenal tissue.

The most commonly used drugs for adrenal gland disease are gonadotropin-releasing hormone (GnRH) agonists. These drugs ultimately cause decreased production of sex hormones by suppressing luteinizing hormone and follicle-stimulating hormone from negative feedback to the pituitary gland. Monthly injections of leuprolide acetate have been shown to markedly improve clinical signs, although the effects are transient as resistance appears to develop over time resulting in the return of clinical signs (Wagner et al. 2001). Deslorelin acetate subcutaneous implants are currently considered the medical treatment of choice for adrenal gland disease in ferrets. Similar to leuprolide acetate, deslorelin implants effects are temporary. But in contrast, beneficial effects are much longer lasting for deslorelin implants with a mean time to return of clinical signs of 17.6 months (Wagner et al. 2009).

Surgical resection of affected adrenal glands is the preferred treatment option for many veterinarians, or it may be indicated in ferrets that are only partially responsive to medical management or become refractory to treatment. It should be noted that surgical excision is easier early in the course of the disease when the gland is smaller. In addition, it has been shown that ferrets that had undergone left adrenalectomy and then received deslorelin subcutaneous implants had a statistically significant longer time to recurrence of clinical signs than ferrets receiving implants with both adrenal glands left in situ (16.3 vs. 12.4 months) (Wagner et al. 2005).

Surgical resection of the left adrenal gland is straightforward. The gland is located in the retroperitoneal space cranial to the left kidney a few millimeters lateral to the caudal vena cava (Figure 18.5). Retract the descending colon ventrally and medially to allow the mesocolon to retract the spleen and small intestine to improve visualization. Bluntly dissect using mosquito hemostats or small right-angled forceps to isolate the gland from the surrounding tissue.

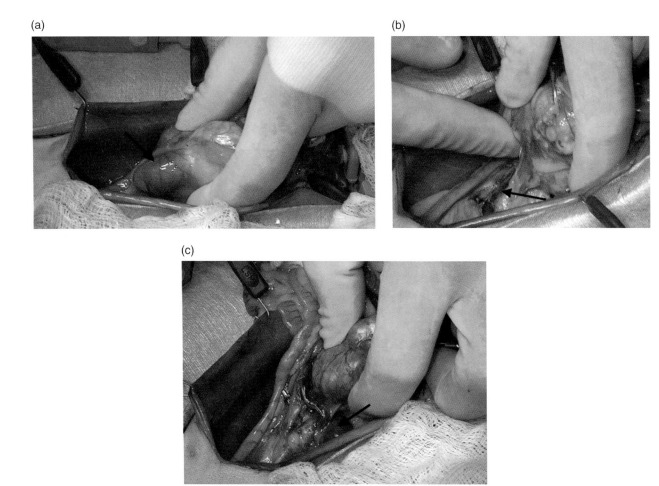

Figure 18.5 This ferret had a very large left adrenal mass that appeared to invade the capsule of the left kidney (a) Arrow is pointing at the left kidney. With careful dissection the kidney was separated from the mass (b) Arrow is pointing at the left renal vein. Dissection was continued. The left kidney (arrow) and left renal veins are free from the tumor (c). Ultimately, the entire left adrenal mass was removed, and it did not invade the vena cava or other surrounding tissues. *Source:* Images courtesy of R. Avery Bennett.

Identify the adrenolumbar vessels medial and lateral to the gland. Place encircling ligatures or hemostatic clips, or use a vessel-sealing device or bipolar electrosurgery across the vessels as they enter and exit the gland, and then transect them to remove the gland. Although uncommon, adrenal tumors involving the left gland can also invade into the neighboring cava.

Surgical resection of the right adrenal gland is technically more demanding. Diseased glands often wrap around the caudal vena cava dorsally and have been known to infiltrate the lumen of the vena cava (Figure 18.6). Retract the duodenum ventrally and medially allowing the mesoduodenum to retract the small intestines to visualize the caudal vena cava. Transect the hepatorenal ligament (from the caudate lobe to the cranial pole of the right kidney) to improve access to the right adrenal gland; alternatively, use the ligament to retract the caudate lobe by placing a mosquito hemostat on it or small stay suture (e.g. 4-0) through it. Begin dissection laterally to isolate the gland from the retroperitoneal space and locate the adrenolumbar vein exiting the cranial aspect of the adrenal. Ligate this vessel using suture ligatures, hemostatic clips, bipolar electrosurgery, or a vessel-sealing device. Continue isolating the gland with delicate sharp and blunt dissection using fine surgical instrumentation and cotton-tipped applicators. If possible, an encircling ligature or multiple hemostatic clips can be placed around the base of the gland to separate it from its relatively short and broad attachment to the caudal vena cava; however, this often results in incomplete removal of the gland. To isolate the gland away from the caudal vena cava, use a small tangential vascular clamp (e.g. neonatal Satinsky vena cava clamp or Cooley vascular clamp). Place the clamp proximal to the base of the adrenal gland with partial or complete occlusion of the caudal vena cava. Bluntly dissect the adrenal gland off the cava wall using cotton-tipped applicators. If there is tumor invasion, then resect the affected part of the wall of the vena cava. Manage any defect in or partial removal of the cava wall by suturing the wall with 5-0 to 7-0 suture in a simple interrupted or interrupted cruciate pattern. Release the clamp and observe the caudal vena cava for hemorrhage. Digital pressure for five minutes and topical hemostatic agents (e.g. Surgicel™ or Gelfoam ™. See Chapter 1) can be used to control minor hemorrhage.

If there is profound hemorrhage associated with removal of the right adrenal gland, or if the caudal vena cava has significant tumor invasion, resection of the right adrenal gland along with a section of the caudal vena cava between the liver and right renal vein can be performed if the resected area is small (<2 cm). Then perform an anastomosis of the caudal vena cava.

It has been shown that normal ferrets have naturally occurring collateral circulation in an acute temporary occlusion model (Figure 18.7) (Calicchio et al. 2016). Blood is rerouted through lumbar veins to vertebral venous sinuses to the azygous vein, and then to the cranial vena cava. Acute temporary caval occlusion for 20 minutes in eight normal ferrets resulted in no evidence of organ dysfunction. However, acute caval hypertension resulting in renal failure has been reported in approximately 30% of patients that have had acute caval ligation (Summa et al. 2015). Nonselective angiography was used to determine

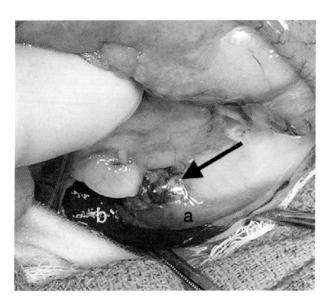

Figure 18.6 This invasive right adrenal mass is wrapping around dorsal to and left of the caudal vena cava in a six-year-old ferret (arrow). (a) Caudal vena cava. (b) Caudate process of the caudate lobe of the liver.

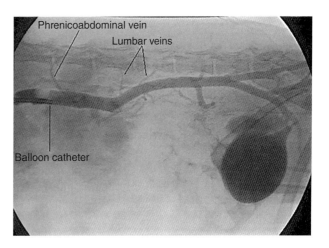

Figure 18.7 Temporary balloon occlusion of the caudal vena cava in ferrets consistently documented preexisting collateral circulation in all ferrets. Blood was rerouted through smaller veins such as the lumbar veins and phrenicoabdominal veins to the vertebral venous sinus, then the azygous vein and the cranial vena cava. *Source:* Reprinted with permission from Calicchio et al. (2016).

the degree of collateral circulation preoperatively (Summa et al. 2015). This technique could potentially be of use to predict the outcome in patients requiring caval ligation and resection for right adrenalectomy. An alternative two-stage technique using ameroid constrictors has also been described (Driggers 2008). Collateral circulation is induced by placing an ameroid constrictor on the caudal vena cava cranial to the renal veins, but caudal to the adrenolumbar veins. Several weeks later, a second surgery is performed to remove the right adrenal gland along with the affected segment of caudal vena cava; however, the casein in the ring stimulated formation of excessive granulation tissue that complicated the second surgery resulting in a mortality rate of 25%. Cryosurgery following partial debulking of right adrenal tumors has been associated with increased mortality and worse long-term outcome compared to other techniques and is no longer recommended (Swiderski et al. 2008).

Bilateral adrenal gland disease has been identified in up to 15% of ferrets (Weiss et al. 1999; Swiderski et al. 2008). The development of hypoadrenocorticism is of concern; however, only 4 of 28 (14.3%) ferrets undergoing bilateral adrenalectomy developed clinical signs of hypoadrenocorticism, all of which resolved following appropriate medical treatment. In a study of normal ferrets undergoing bilateral adrenalectomy, ferrets did clinically well receiving saline drinking water, although steroid and electrolyte levels were not evaluated (Filion and Hoar 1985).

Partial Pancreatectomy

The most common indication for partial pancreatectomy is hypoglycemia secondary to insulinoma. Insulinomas (functional pancreatic islet cell tumors) are the most common tumors diagnosed in ferrets (Li et al. 1998; Miwa et al. 2009). In a retrospective study of medical records of 574 ferrets, 39 (21.9%) were diagnosed with pancreatic islet cell tumor, the vast majority of which were functional (94.2%) (Li et al. 1998). In contrast to dogs, insulinomas in ferrets have a low incidence of metastasis (~7%) (Caplan et al. 1996); nonetheless, regional lymph nodes, liver, and spleen should be closely examined at surgery for pathologic enlargement or nodular changes. Diagnosis is usually presumptive based on clinical signs of lethargy and weakness with concurrent hypoglycemia (<60 mg/dl). Measurement of insulin levels or calculation of insulin:glucose ratios is generally unreliable and diagnostic imaging, such as abdominal ultrasound, is unrewarding due to the small size of the pancreatic nodules (Chen 2010). Medical management consists of diet modification and the use of oral corticosteroids (prednisone or prednisolone; 0.25–2.0 mg/kg BID); however,

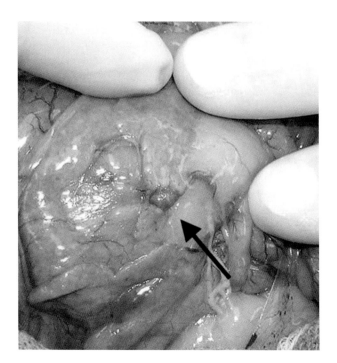

Figure 18.8 An insulinoma (arrow) in the right limb of the pancreas of a ferret.

this approach will only palliate clinical signs and not slow progression of disease. Surgical resection of the pancreatic nodule(s) with or without partial pancreatectomy is the treatment of choice.

Pancreatic nodulectomy is indicated for masses located in the right limb because the duodenum and pancreas share the same blood supply making partial pancreatectomy more difficult. Identify nodules as pale reddish tissue relative to surrounding pancreas and gentle palpation of a firm area. Often, there is an increase in vascularity to this region (Figure 18.8). For nodules located near the periphery of the right limb of the pancreas, use a suture fracture technique with small multifilament absorbable suture to resect the nodule. Incise the mesoduodenum, and encircle and tie a loop of suture around the base of the mass, crushing neighboring parenchyma, and ligating the local blood supply and small pancreatic ducts, which allow resection of the mass. For lesions within the right limb or near the pylorus, bluntly isolate the mass using mosquito hemostats, small right-angled forceps, gauze sponges, and cotton-tipped applicators, and resect taking care to avoid the pancreaticoduodenal vessels. Close defects in the body of the pancreas or mesoduodenum, while avoiding interference with the portal vein and the pancreaticoduodenal vessels. Avoid using electrosurgery and CO_2 laser in this procedure due to the potential to cause pancreatic inflammation and pancreatitis from collateral heat. Recently, the use of a bipolar vessel-sealing device (LigaSure™,

Medtronic, Minneapolis, MN) was described for insulinoma resection in dogs resulting in shorter surgical times and no postoperative pancreatitis (Wouters et al. 2011). Similar results would be expected in ferrets.

For lesions in the left limb or where a distinct nodule is not identified, perform a partial pancreatectomy. Locate the left limb in the omental bursa. Isolate the tip of the left limb from the surrounding mesentery using gentle sharp dissection. Continue this dissection toward the pylorus until just before the pancreas starts to turn into the mesoduodenum, just to the right of the pylorus, removing approximately 50% of pancreatic volume. Place an encircling ligature around the pancreas at this level and transect the limb distal to the ligature.

Major complications, such as diabetes mellitus or pancreatitis following pancreatic nodulectomy or partial pancreatectomy are uncommon. In a study of 66 ferrets with insulinoma(s), disease-free intervals were 22, 234, and 365 days with median survival times of 186, 456, and 668 days in ferrets receiving medical management, pancreatic nodulectomy, and nodulectomy with partial pancreatectomy, respectively (Weiss et al. 1998). In a separate study of 57 ferrets, persistent postoperative hypoglycemia was noted in 53% of ferrets following surgery. Recurrence of hypoglycemia was noted in 16 ferrets at a median of 10.6 months following surgery (Caplan et al. 1996). In another study of 20 ferrets with insulinomas, the disease-free interval following surgery was 240 days with a median survival of 483 days; however, 16 of 20 ferrets died or were euthanized for clinical signs consistent with insulinoma (Ehrhart et al. 1996). Necropsy of seven of the ferrets revealed recurrence of pancreatic tumors, but no evidence of distant metastasis. It is currently not known whether adjunctive chemotherapy or second resection of a recurrent pancreatic nodule further prolongs survival.

For long-term monitoring following pancreatic nodulectomy or partial pancreatectomy, evaluate fasting (one to three hours) blood glucose concentration two weeks postoperatively at the time of suture removal. If blood glucose concentration is normal, reevaluate this parameter every three to four months or if clinical signs develop.

Splenectomy

Indications for splenectomy in ferrets include neoplasia and trauma. Generalized splenomegaly is normal in most ferrets due to diffuse extramedullary hematopoiesis. Isoflurane anesthesia causes splenic sequestration of red blood cells contributing to splenic enlargement (Marini et al. 1994). The decision to perform a splenectomy should be based on cytology consistent with a neoplastic

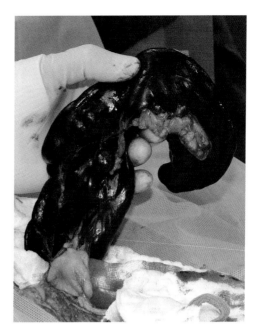

Figure 18.9 This enlarged spleen in a five-year-old ferret was histologically diagnosed as an acute splenic hematoma with severe red pulp congestion.

process and/or parenchymal irregularities observed on ultrasound or computed tomography (CT). In a study of 55 normal ferrets, the spleen was found to be hyperechoic to the liver with a mean thickness of $11.8 \pm 0.34\,mm$ (Suran et al. 2017).

The most common primary splenic neoplasia in ferrets is lymphoma, although hemangiosarcoma, mast cell disease, and liposarcoma have been infrequently observed (Dillberger and Altman 1989; Avallone et al. 2016) (Figure 18.9). A recent study described histiocytic sarcoma in four ferrets with extensive splenic involvement. Survival time following splenectomy was 9 days to 5 months (Thongtharb et al. 2016).

Total splenectomy can be performed in ferrets with relative ease. Ligate splenic vessels individually with absorbable suture (3-0 to 4-0) including the gastrosplenic vessels. Alternatively, hemostatic clips or vessel-sealing devices can be used to remove the spleen (Figure 18.10).

Gastrointestinal Surgery

The most common indication for gastrointestinal surgery in ferrets is removal of gastrointestinal foreign bodies (Mullen et al. 1992). As there are numerous intestinal diseases in ferrets, collecting gastrointestinal biopsies may be indicated. In addition, there have been isolated reports of pyloric adenocarcinoma and one recent description of gastric dilatation and volvulus syndrome (Rice et al. 1992; Sleeman et al. 1995; Geyer and Reichle 2012).

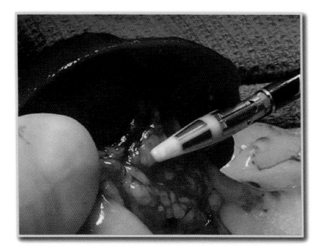

Figure 18.10 A vessel-sealing device being used for splenectomy in a ferret-making splenectomy very quick with minimal risk of hemorrhage.

Gastrointestinal Foreign Body Removal

Commonly ingested foreign bodies in young ferrets are often sponge, rubber, or foam objects taken from the environment. Trichobezoars are formed in the stomach of older ferrets due to excessive grooming. Clinical signs associated with gastrointestinal foreign material are variable and include lethargy, lack of appetite, and diarrhea, but vomiting may not occur or may not be observed in ferrets. Abdominal palpation is a key part of the physical examination as foreign material is often palpable and may elicit a pain response. Diagnostic imaging, such as abdominal radiographs, contrast radiography, and ultrasound can be helpful in definitively diagnosing gastrointestinal obstruction. Abnormalities observed on radiographs can include gaseous distension of the stomach, segmental intestinal dilation, and the presence of foreign material (Figure 18.11). Abdominal ultrasound has been shown to be of value in diagnosing gastrointestinal obstruction in dogs by providing greater accuracy, fewer equivocal results, and greater diagnostic confidence compared to plain radiographs (Sharma et al. 2011). Similar principles could be applied to

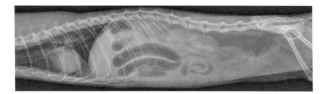

Figure 18.11 Lateral radiograph of a ferret with radiographic evidence of an intestinal obstruction with stacked pathologically dilated fluid and gas filled segments of intestine in the cranial abdomen.

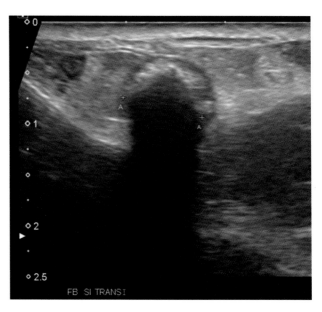

Figure 18.12 Ultrasound transverse image of a segment of small intestine in a two-year-old ferret demonstrating shadowing from a foreign body. The foreign object was determined to be a headphone ear bud at surgery.

ferrets when there is suspicion of gastrointestinal obstruction (Figure 18.12). Gastrointestinal foreign material is also often found incidentally during abdominal surgery underscoring the importance of complete abdominal exploration.

Gastrointestinal obstruction is a surgical emergency. Although there are several significant differences in the healing properties of the stomach, small intestine, and large intestine, the same suturing principles apply regardless of the location of the foreign body within the gastrointestinal tract. Ensure a secure closure with gentle tissue handling, adequate tissue purchase, appropriate suture material, and proper suture placement. Keep contamination of the peritoneal cavity to a minimum by isolating the section of intestine from the remainder of the abdominal contents.

Remove gastric foreign bodies through a routine gastrotomy. Place stay sutures at each end of the proposed incision to facilitate the procedure. Open the body of the stomach with a stab incision into the lumen in a relatively avascular area between the greater and lesser curvatures using a #11 or #15 scalpel blade. Continue the incision with Metzenbaum scissors to create an opening large enough to remove the foreign material.

Close the gastrotomy incision using a synthetic absorbable monofilament suture. There are various techniques to choose from when deciding how to close the stomach. Regardless of the suture pattern, the common theme for all gastrointestinal surgery is inclusion of the submucosal layer

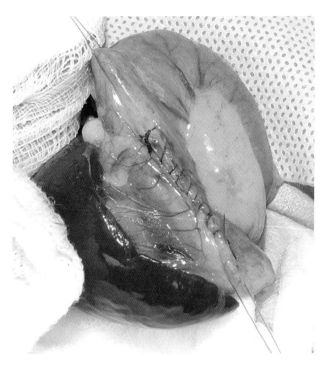

Figure 18.13 Single-layer simple continuous closure of a gastrotomy in a ferret with a gastric foreign body.

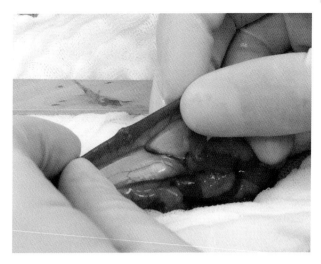

Figure 18.14 Transverse closure of an enterotomy following removal of a foreign body.

in the closure. Full-thickness purchase of the tissue ensures that this holding layer is incorporated in the suture line. Close the stomach in a single or double layer; however, there is increased concern for luminal compromise in ferrets and so a single-layer, full-thickness, simple continuous pattern is preferred due to increased efficiency and decreased amount of suture material used (Figure 18.13). A two-layer pattern may be more appropriate if performing a partial gastrectomy or if there is any concern about tissue viability. The second layer is typically done using an inverting pattern.

Approach foreign bodies located in the small intestine through a longitudinal incision aboral to the obstruction. Following removal of the foreign material, evaluate the intestine for viability. If there are any concerns about the viability of the small intestine, perform a resection and anastomosis. Otherwise, close the enterotomy incision with a single-layer appositional pattern using 4-0 to 5-0 monofilament absorbable suture. A single-layer appositional closure has been shown to be appropriate and preferred in dogs as double-layers caused marked reduction in lumen diameter, as well as increased intestinal wall thickness (Kirpensteijn et al. 2001). If there is any additional concern about luminal compromise with a longitudinal closure in ferrets, close small intestinal incisions transversely using simple interrupted sutures (Figure 18.14). Place sutures 2–3 mm from the incised edge and 2–3 mm apart. Begin and end continuous patterns beyond the edges of the enterotomy to ensure closure of the entire incision.

If there is a perforation or concern about intestinal viability, perform a resection and anastomosis. Assessing the tissue viability of the gastrointestinal tract can be challenging. Most often subjective parameters of viability are relied on to make the decision between enterotomy and resection. These parameters include color, peristalsis, arterial pulsation, capillary bleeding (cut-surface), and tissue thickness.

As with enterotomy closure, single-layer approximating patterns are preferred for intestinal anastomosis to avoid luminal compromise. Simple continuous patterns are more efficient and use less suture material, which is not only economical but also decreases the amount of foreign material in the abdominal cavity. A simple continuous pattern also creates a better seal minimizing the risk of leakage. The concern about creating a purse-string effect with a continuous pattern can be avoided if a modified simple continuous pattern is performed. In this technique, place two continuous suture lines, one originating at the mesenteric border and the other originating at the antimesenteric border. Good visualization of the mesenteric knot is imperative as this is the most common site of leakage. Place a single-layer full thickness continuous suture line from the mesenteric knot to a stay suture at the antimesenteric knot with tissue purchase 2–3 mm from the wound edge and 2–3 mm apart. Repeat this on the other side from the antimesenteric knot to the mesenteric knot. There is no difference in reported rates of dehiscence between animals with simple continuous anastomotic closures and animals with simple interrupted closures.

Following surgery, offer water and food once the ferret has fully recovered from anesthesia, within 2–4 hours. Outcome and prognosis following surgery for gastrointestinal obstruction is generally good to excellent as major complications are uncommon.

Pyloric Outflow Obstruction

Ferrets can occasionally present with acute gastric disten-sion due to obstruction of the pylorus (Figure 18.15). Causes of pyloric outflow obstruction include foreign material, pyloric hypertrophy, pyloric stenosis, and pyloric adenocarcinoma. Recently, two black-footed ferrets were reported to have acute gastric dilatation

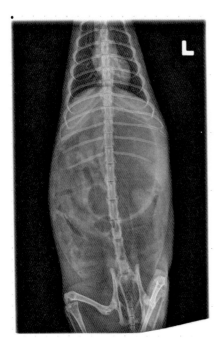

Figure 18.15 Ventrodorsal image of a ferret with gastric outflow obstruction.

resulting in death, but the cause could not be definitively determined (Hinton et al. 2016). Gastric dilatation and volvulus has only been reported in one ferret (Geyer and Reichle 2012). In the few reported cases of pyloric adenocarcinoma, there was concurrent infection with *Helicobacter mustelae* (Rice et al. 1992; Sleeman et al. 1995). Colonization of pyloric antrum and orad duo-denum with *H. mustelae* is common in domestic ferrets; however, clinical complications from infection such as gastritis or ulceration are infrequent.

Although it has not been reported, gastric surgical proce-dures should be feasible in ferrets for pyloric outflow obstruction. Removal of the pylorus and gastroduodenos-tomy (Billroth I) is indicated for pyloric masses (Figure 18.16). Identify the common bile duct entering the duodenum to avoid iatrogenic damage to this structure. Ligate the blood supply to the pyloric region, remove the omental and mesen-teric attachments, and excise the area of the pylorus to be removed. If possible, remove a margin of grossly normal tis-sue (0.5–1 cm) in addition to the pyloric mass. Anastomose the duodenum to the pyloric antrum. If the gastric and duo-denal lumens markedly differ in diameter, incise the duode-num at an angle and/or partly close the antrum. Close the far (dorsal) aspect of the incision first followed by the ventral aspect using 4-0 monofilament absorbable suture in a simple continuous or simple interrupted suture pattern.

Alternatively, close the pyloric antrum and create a gas-troduodenostomy on the dorsal aspect of the body of the stomach. This procedure has been used for palliative man-agement in a ferret with pyloric adenocarcinoma in which the resection of the mass was believed to be too difficult;

(a)

(b)

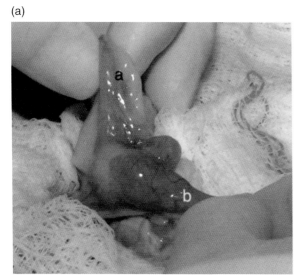 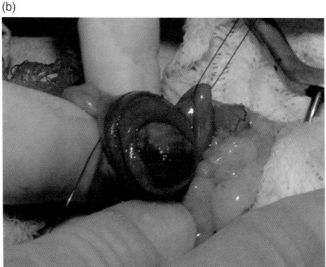

Figure 18.16 (a) A ferret with gastric outflow obstruction caused by a mass at the pylorus (a, stomach; b, duodenum). The mass was obstructing the pylorus and was confirmed to be a pyloric adenocarcinoma (b). A Billroth I was recommended, but the owner declined. *Source:* Images courtesy of R. Avery Bennett.

survival of this ferret following surgery was 80 days (Nankinishi et al. 2005).

Oral Cavity Disease

Other than dental disease, other oral conditions to take note of in ferrets include oral neoplasia and salivary mucoceles (salivary cysts). Squamous cell carcinoma is the most frequently reported oral neoplasm, although there are reports of osteosarcoma, osteoma, lymphoma, malignant melanoma, sarcoma, and fibromatous epulis (Johnson-Delaney 2016; d'Ovidio et al. 2016; Avallone et al. 2016). Advanced imaging and biopsy are required for definitive diagnosis and determination of the extent of disease. If possible, wide surgical excision including partial maxillectomy or mandibulectomy offers the best long-term yet limited prognosis. Rostral maxillectomy with adjuvant radiation therapy has been reported in one ferret with a disease-free interval of 5 months (Graham et al. 2006).

Like cats, ferrets have five pairs of salivary glands: parotid, molar, mandibular, sublingual, and the zygomatic glands. Unlike dogs, the mandibular salivary gland is not intimately associated with the monostomatic portion of the sublingual gland. Ferrets do not have a polystomatic portion of the sublingual salivary gland (Bennett 2009). Therefore, if indicated, the mandibular gland can be excised alone. The zygomatic gland has been most commonly implicated as the source of the mucoceles in ferrets, although a mandibular salivary mucocele has been reported (Thas 2014) (Figure 18.17). The etiology of salivary mucoceles is generally unknown, but trauma is most often implicated. Salivary mucoceles most often manifest as a subcutaneous swelling in the region of the affected salivary gland. Diagnosis is made by simple aspiration of the swelling revealing a viscous fluid with low cellularity. If indicated, periodic acid-Schiff stain can be used to confirm mucus in the sample. Surgical excision of the involved salivary glands leads to the quickest and most definitive resolution, although aspiration or marsupialization of the mucocele have been described. Advanced imaging or injection of contrast medium into the mucocele may be required to help identify the location of the affected salivary tissue, particularly for zygomatic mucoceles. In most cases, carefully dissect out the mucocele and then trace it back to the gland of origin. Once identified, remove the affected gland.

Abdominal Organ Biopsy

Diagnostic abdominal exploratory laparotomies and subsequent organ biopsy are common tools used in ferrets to assist in the diagnosis of chronic gastrointestinal disease. Abdominal surgery allows for complete exploratory

(a) (b)

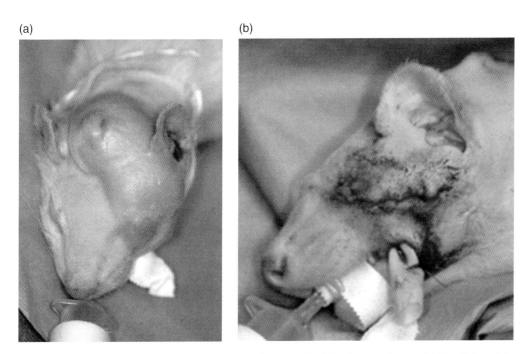

Figure 18.17 This ferret presented with a zygomatic mucocele following enucleation (a). The lining of the mucocele was carefully dissected out to the defect in the zygomatic gland. The affected gland was removed and a Penrose drain placed (b). The sialocele resolved with no recurrence. *Source:* Images courtesy of R. Avery Bennett.

examination of the entire length of the gastrointestinal tract. Full-thickness samples can be obtained from the stomach, duodenum, jejunum, and ileum.

To biopsy the intestine, make two 1 cm parallel, longitudinal, full-thickness incisions in the antimesenteric aspect of the bowel using a #11 scalpel blade. Excise the sample using Metzenbaum scissors. Close the defect with a simple continuous full-thickness pattern using 4-0 or 5-0 monofilament, absorbable suture material. An alternative to this technique is to use a 2–4 mm Baker's biopsy punch to take a full-thickness sample from the antimesenteric border. Close the defect longitudinally or transversely using a single-layer, full-thickness simple interrupted or interrupted cruciate pattern using 4-0 or 5-0 monofilament absorbable suture.

Liver biopsy is often indicated during abdominal exploratory as a screening for distant metastasis or to sample focal or diffuse hepatic abnormalities. There are multiple methods for sampling the liver. If there is a distinct lesion that needs to be biopsied, its size and location often dictate the biopsy method. For diffuse disease or routine sampling, biopsy the liver along the margin using a guillotine method or curved hemostats. Sample lesions away from the edge using Baker skin biopsy punch (2–4 mm).

To perform a guillotine biopsy, identify an accessible liver lobe with an easily sampled hepatic margin. Create a loop with a single throw out of a strand of 4-0 multifilament absorbable suture. Pass the loop around the tip of the isolated liver lobe and pull the suture snug to allow it to cut through the hepatic parenchyma. Small vessels and bile ducts will be bundled within the ligature. Secure the knot with three additional throws. Using Metzenbaum scissors, transect the hepatic tissue distal to the ligature. Control any bleeding from the cut surface using digital pressure, electrosurgery, or hemostatic agents such as Gelfoam™ or Surgicel™.

For partial or complete liver lobectomy, a variety of methods are available with use of encircling or overlapping mattress sutures being most common. An isolated report of successful complete liver lobectomy in a ferret using a self-ligating loop has been described (Goodman and Casale 2014) and this technique has been associated with minimal morbidity in other species, including rabbits.

Urogenital Surgery

Urethral obstruction is an emergency scenario encountered in ferrets. Obstruction most commonly occurs in male ferrets due to prostatic disease associated with adrenal gland disease and less commonly due to urolithiasis. Increased circulating sex hormone level from abnormal adrenal glands leads to squamous metaplasia of the prostatic epithelium resulting in prostatitis and cystic prostatic disease. Prostatic cysts can also become infected. Complete urethral obstruction can initially be managed with urethral catheterization, cystocentesis, or placement of a cystostomy tube.

Urethral catheterization can be challenging in male ferrets due to the small size and J-shaped os penis (Brown and Pollock 2011; Hoefer 2013) (Figure 18.3). A 24 ga catheter without the needle stylet can be used to dilate the urethral opening. Red rubber catheters (3.5 fr), jugular catheters (20–22 ga), tomcat catheters (3.5 fr), or specific 3.0 fr 11-in. urinary catheters (Slippery Sam™ Tomcat Urethral Catheters, Smiths Medical PM, Inc.) can be used for urethral catheterization. If catheterization cannot be achieved, cystocentesis can be performed to temporarily relieve the systemic complications associated with obstruction, as well as facilitating urethral catheter placement by decreasing backpressure. Decompressive cystocentesis followed by placement of an indwelling urethral catheter has been shown to be a safe procedure in cats with lower urinary obstruction (Hall et al. 2015).

If urethral catheterization is still unsuccessful, an alternative to cystocentesis for urinary drainage is placement of a cystostomy tube (Nolte et al. 2002). This short surgical procedure provides a route for urine diversion allowing stabilization of the ferret and providing access for contrast imaging studies of the urinary tract if indicated. Make a small caudal ventral abdominal midline approach over the distended urinary bladder. Place a small purse-string suture in a relatively avascular area of the ventral bladder. Pass a balloon-tipped catheter (5–8 fr) through a stab incision in the body wall just lateral to the main incision. Place the catheter into the urinary bladder through a small stab incision in the middle of the preplaced purse-string suture and inflate the balloon. Tie the purse-string suture and suture the bladder to the body wall using several tacking sutures. Secure the catheter on the outside of the abdomen using a finger trap suture.

Surgical or medical management of adrenal gland disease will often allow prostatic hypertrophy to subside, usually within a few days to a few weeks (Ludwig and Aiken 2004). With complete urethral obstruction due to large prostatic cysts or prostatic abscessation, adrenalectomy can be performed in addition to prostatic drainage, cyst resection, and/or omentalization. Complete resection of prostatic cysts is often not possible due to extensive adhesions to regional anatomy which puts the ferret at risk for urinary incontinence or vascular injury to the trigone and urethra. Omentalization is the preferred technique in dogs and has

(a)

(b)

(c)

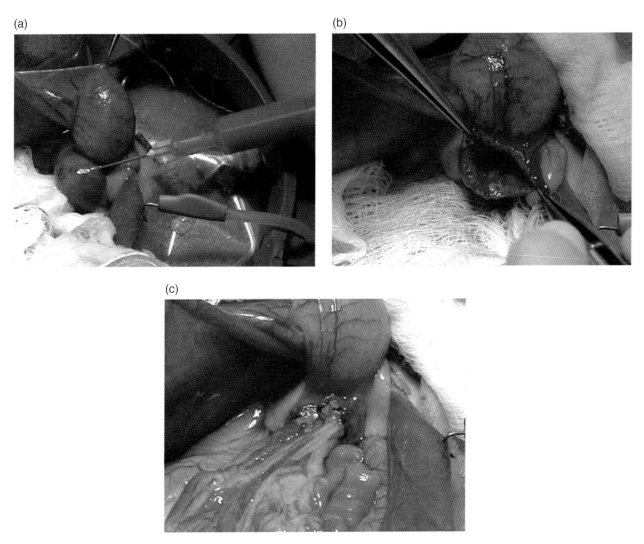

Figure 18.18 A male ferret with a prostatic cyst filled with green odiferous fluid which is typical (a). The cyst was opened and samples were collected. The cyst was then partially resected and irrigated (b), and then omentalized (c). *Source:* Images courtesy of R. Avery Bennett.

been performed with success in ferrets (Figure 18.18). Placement of a urethral catheter is ideal to avoid damage to the urethral wall. Incise into the capsule of the cyst or abscess and retrieve samples for bacterial culture, antimicrobial susceptibility testing, and histopathology. Excise as much of the capsule as possible while avoiding the dorsal aspect of the urinary bladder and prostate. If communication to the urethra lumen is identified, maintain the urethral catheter for 3–4 days to allow the urethral wall to heal. Insert the omentum deep into the remaining capsule and suture it in place using several simple interrupted monofilament absorbable sutures. Marsupialization of prostatic cysts is no longer recommended due to risk of major complications such as reabscessation and septic peritonitis (Powers et al. 2007).

Urolithiasis

Cystic calculi can occur in ferrets, but it is not as common as in dogs and cats or other small mammals. It was previously more common before commercial ferret diets became available and was shown to be caused by feeding cat foods with a plant protein base. Homemade diets and vegetable treats should be voided in ferrets. In a study of urolith composition in ferrets over a 25 year period, 67% were sterile struvite, 15% were cysteine, and 11% were calcium oxalate (Nwaokorie et al. 2011). Both struvite and cysteine uroliths were found predominantly in older, neutered male ferrets (Nwaokorie et al. 2011, 2013). It has been suggested, but not proven, that cysteine urolithiasis may have a familial predisposition (Nwaokorie et al. 2013).

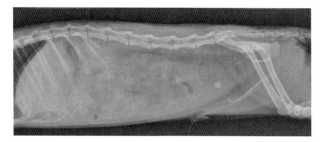

Figure 18.19 Lateral abdominal radiograph of a ferret with a cystic calculus. Note the J-shaped os penis and the urethral catheter placed along the ventral aspect of the tip of the penis.

Surgical removal of uroliths is the treatment of choice as success with diet-based medical dissolution for struvite stones has not been demonstrated. Perform a cystotomy using a routine caudal abdominal approach. Place stay sutures in the apex and near the trigone, and then make a ventral incision into the bladder in a relatively avascular area. Remove calculi from the bladder using forceps, a spoon, or other smooth instrument. Pass and flush a small urethral catheter several times antegrade and retrograde to make sure that no stones remain in the bladder neck or urethra (Figure 18.19).

The urinary bladder is unique in that it regains nearly 100% of its original tensile strength by 14 days following cystotomy. Synthetic absorbable suture material is most suitable for cystotomy closure. Monofilament suture is preferred as there is some concern that contact between urine and multifilament suture may lead to an increased rate of absorption or may promote urolith formation. Nonabsorbable suture and staples are contraindicated in urinary bladder closure as they are associated with the formation of urinary calculi. There are a number of suture patterns that can be used to close the urinary bladder. The surgical goals are to minimize tissue trauma, create a watertight seal, and avoid promotion of calculi formation.

It has been shown that there is no difference in circular bursting wall tension of urinary bladders closed with single-layer simple interrupted appositional pattern versus a two-layer continuous inverting closure and clinical outcomes are similar (Radasch et al. 1990; Thieman-Mankin et al. 2012). Luminal compromise may occur if two-layer inverting patterns are used in urinary bladders, particularly with severely thickened tissue. Most surgical texts state that the lumen of the bladder should not be entered with suture material and partial-thickness closure is recommended. Urinary calculi formation has been associated with multifilament absorbable suture, nonabsorbable suture, and metal staples; however, there have been no studies assessing the lithogenic potential of the newer monofilament rapidly absorbable sutures. Full-thickness

purchase of the bladder wall guarantees incorporation of the submucosal holding layer. Single-layer partial-thickness closures of the urinary bladder that miss the submucosa may be inadequate for preventing urine leakage. Therefore, it is optimal to close the urinary bladder in a ferret with 4-0 to 5-0 rapidly absorbable monofilament suture (e.g. glycomer 631). Postoperative radiographs provide documentation of complete stone removal.

For ferrets with distal urethral obstruction that cannot be unobstructed and ferrets suffering from recurrent urethral obstruction, urethrostomy is indicated. Urethrostomy is also considered in ferrets with distal urethral trauma, stricture, or neoplasia. Perform the urethrostomy approximately 1 cm ventral to the anus. At this location, the urethra is wide and superficial. Urethral catheterization facilitates palpation of the urethra. Make a 1 cm vertical incision on midline into the urethral lumen. Incisions straying off midline will encounter cavernous tissue that will result in persistent postoperative bleeding for as long as – 2–4 weeks. Place simple interrupted sutures from the urethral mucosa to the skin circumferentially with 5-0 or 6-0 monofilament rapidly absorbable suture. Complications associated with urethrostomy include hemorrhage, stricture, urine scald, urinary tract infection, and urine extravasation into the subcutaneous tissues.

Preputial Masses

Cystic preputial masses can develop secondary to increased circulating sex hormone levels from adrenal gland disease (Protain et al. 2009). However, other tumors can occur in this area as well, with preputial adenocarcinomas being most common (van Zeeland et al. 2014). Preputial adenomas and adenocarcinomas are apocrine scent gland in origin (Figure 18.17). Up to 75% of apocrine preputial tumors are malignant and exhibit aggressive local invasion of surrounding tissues and metastasis to regional lymph nodes (Antinoff and Williams 2012) (Figure 18.20). Wide surgical excision is the treatment of choice and may necessitate preputial and partial penile amputation with urethrostomy (Fisher 2002; van Zeeland et al. 2014). Dissect the diseased prepuce away from the surrounding tissue with 0.5–1 cm lateral margins and deep to the caudal abdominal fascia. Create a new preputial orifice by suturing the mucosal surface of the remaining prepuce to the skin using 4-0 or 5-0 monofilament absorbable suture in a simple interrupted pattern. If the penis is exposed, the skin of the penis undergoes keratinization and becomes tough resisting desiccation and environmental stress as occurs following circumcision (Figure 18.21). Alternatively, perform a partial penile amputation by excising the distal

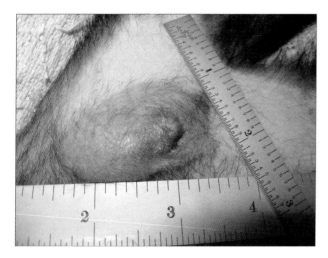

Figure 18.20 A large preputial adenocarcinoma. Resection required wide margins including body wall, perineal urethrostomy, and penile amputation. *Source:* Image courtesy of R. Avery Bennett.

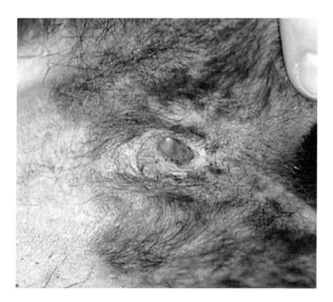

Figure 18.21 This ferret had a smaller preputial mass removed leaving the glans penis exposed. Through the process of keratinization (well studied in circumcised humans), the fragile skin on the penis becomes more keratinized so it is then less sensitive, but more resistant to desiccation and environmental trauma. *Source:* Image courtesy of R. Avery Bennett.

10–15 mm of the penis. Pass a 3-fr urethral catheter into the lumen to facilitate placement of simple interrupted mucosal sutures from the urethral mucosa to the outer surface of the penis. With large masses or if there is concern about the potential for local recurrence, consider complete penile amputation with perineal urethrostomy to achieve local tumor control (Jekl and Hauptman 2017). Survival following surgery has been estimated to be approximately 6 months; however, there is a report of a

ferret surviving 32 months following wide excision (1 cm histologic margins) using penile amputation and urethrostomy (van Zeeland et al. 2014).

Miscellaneous Procedures

Tail Amputation

A neoplasm overrepresented in ferrets is the chordoma, which is the fifth most common tumor in domestic ferrets and the most common musculoskeletal tumor. Chordomas originate from remnants of the notochord occurring near the tip of the tail or in the cervical or thoracic spine. Chordomas in ferrets are generally thought to be benign due to their slow growth, ease of excision (if on the tail), and low rate of documented metastasis. As the most common location is at the tip of the tail, tail amputation is considered curative. Incise the skin 0.5–1 cm distal to the area of the proposed amputation. Amputate the tail 2–3 coccygeal vertebral bodies proximal to the lesion following control of the ventral artery and vein. Due to the lack of subcutaneous tissues, close the incision using several simple interrupted nonabsorbable sutures (e.g. 4-0 nylon or polypropylene). Chordomas located in the cervical and thoracic region are impossible to completely resect; however, debulking may provide transient clinical relief (Pye et al. 2000; Frohlich and Donovan 2015). Isolated reports of distant metastasis have been noted (Williams et al. 1993; Munday et al. 2004; Frohlich and Donovan 2015).

Anal Sacculectomy

Removing the anal sacs (descending) is typically performed in ferrets at the time of early neutering to reduce the musky odor; however, the procedure can be performed at a later age if the sacs were not previously removed or incompletely removed. Disease (infection, neoplasia) of the anal sacs in ferrets is uncommon. The anal sac ducts open at the anocutaneous junction approximately at the 4 and 8 o'clock positions. Begin the anal sacculectomy by placing a mosquito hemostat across the opening of the duct (Figure 18.22). Using a #11 blade make a circumferential incision around the duct. Start dissecting from the incision around the duct working in a ventrolateral direction toward the apex of the sac using sharp and blunt dissection to free the glandular tissue from the surrounding soft tissues. The sac can be distinguished from the surrounding tissue by the unique yellowish color of the glandular lining. Once the sac is removed, lavage the surgical site and close with a single subcutaneous or dermal suture. Alternatively, leave the incision open to heal by second intention especially if the

(a)

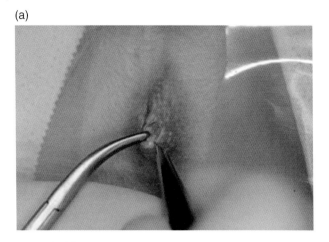

(b)

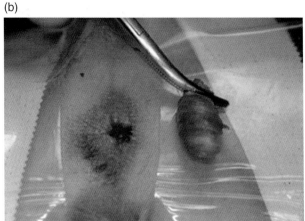

Figure 18.22 Because of the strong odor of the anal sac secretions, for dissecting, place a hemostat on the opening of the duct first to prevent secretions from coming out (a). Use a no. 11 blade or similar to carefully scrape the anal sphincter muscle off the sac working from the duct to the apex of the sac. Once removed (b) the defect can be closed or left open at the discretion of the surgeon. *Source:* Images courtesy of R. Avery Bennett.

defect is small (young animals) or contaminated. Complications are uncommon, but include fecal incontinence or rectal prolapse if the anal sphincter is severely damaged, or fistulous tracts if a remnant of the sac is left behind as this tissue is still secretory. Incomplete removal is recognized when draining tracts associated with a strong odor appear in the perianal region days to weeks after surgery. If there is evidence of infection, administer antimicrobials for 1–2 weeks prior to additional surgery in order to decrease inflammation and make identification of residual tissue easier. Place a 3 fr urethral catheter into the draining tract and follow the tract with meticulous sharp and blunt dissection, and then resect any yellow or gray tissue encountered. Close the area as described above and submit resected tissues for histopathology.

Cardiac Pacemaker

Second- and third-degree atrioventricular blocks are the most common conduction disturbances in ferrets. If there is a resulting bradycardia of less than 80 bpm, congestive heart failure develops with a subsequent poor prognosis without intervention. Significant bradycardia is treated with administration of isoproterenol or metaproterenol, or implantation of a permanent pacemaker (Sanchez-Migallon Guzman et al. 2006).

An epicardial pacemaker can be placed from an abdominal approach and incision through the ventral diaphragm (Figure 18.23). Make a transverse or longitudinal incision through the diaphragm and place stay sutures (3-0 monofilament suture) in the edges of the incised diaphragm to retract it out of the way. Incise the pericardium over the cardiac apex and implant a single-lead screw-in electrode or suture a single- or double-lead electrode directly to the epicardium using 4-0 nonabsorbable monofilament suture. Loosely close the pericardium with 4-0 monofilament absorbable suture with simple interrupted or interrupted cruciate sutures. Bring the lead wire through the diaphragmatic incision and connect it to the pulse generator. In contrast to dogs and cats where the generator is placed in a pocket created between the transversus abdominus and internal abdominal oblique muscles, leave the generator free in the abdominal cavity. Secure the lead to the dorsal diaphragm and the left abdominal wall using nonabsorbable simple interrupted sutures. Close the diaphragm in a simple continuous pattern and evacuate the thorax during diaphragmatic closure using a small red rubber tube to remove the air from the pleural cavity. Close the abdomen routinely. Previously reported pacemaker initial settings included activity-responsive variable heart rate from 140 to 180 bpm, ventricular refractory set at 200 ms, and ventricular pulse amplitude of 2.25 V (Sanchez-Migallon Guzman et al. 2006).

Vascular Access Port

The peripheral veins in ferrets are small and difficult to access. Repeated blood sampling or repeated intravenous injection (e.g. chemotherapeutics, antimicrobials) can be

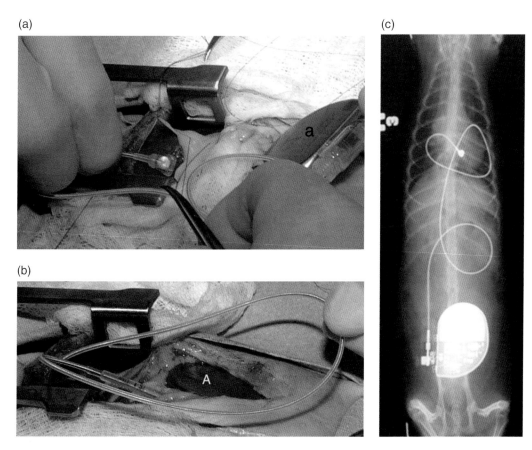

Figure 18.23 A ferret with third-degree heart block having a pacemaker placed. (a) The epicardial lead is being placed on the heart (a, pulse generator). (b) The pulse generator (A) is placed within the abdominal cavity and is not placed between muscles of the body wall which are too thin. (c) Postoperative radiograph showing placement of the epicardial lead on the heart and the pulse generator within the abdomen. *Source:* Images courtesy of R. Avery Bennett.

accomplished through the use of a vascular access port (VAP) (Harrison and Kitchell 2017). The most appropriate size for a ferret is a 4-fr catheter with the port the size of a United States dime (Le Petite™; Norfolk Veterinary Products). With the ferret in lateral recumbency, make a small incision over the jugular vein. Bluntly isolate a 1 cm segment of the jugular vein. Ligate the vein cranial to the level of proposed catheter insertion. Insert the catheter approximately to the level of where the cranial vena cava joins the right atrium. Tunnel dorsal from the skin incision for placement of the port. Advantages of the VAP is that it avoids the challenge of accessing a peripheral vein in a small mammal, reduces the stress of repeated injections to the animal, and minimizes the risk of extravasation. Small VAPs are prone to clotting, so it is crucial that the device is heparin-locked after each use.

References

Antinoff, N. and Williams, B. (2012). Neoplasia. In: *Ferrets, Rabbits, and Rodents: Clinical Medicine and Surgery*, 3e (eds. K.E. Quesenberry and J.W. Carpenter), 103–121. St. Louis, MO: Elsevier.

Avallone, G., Forlani, A., Tecilla, M. et al. (2016). Neoplastic diseases in the domestic ferret (*Mustela putorius furo*) in Italy: classification and tissue distribution of 856 cases (2000–2010). *BMC Veterinary Research* 12: 275.

Bennett, R.A. (2009). Nonabdominal surgeries in ferrets. *CVC in San Diego Conference Proceedings*. Baltimore, MD.

Bleavins, M. and Aulerich, R. (1981). Feed consumption and food passage with time in mink (Mustela vison) and European ferrets (*Mustela putorius furo*). *Laboratory Animal Science* 31: 268–269.

Brown, C. and Pollock, C. (2011). Urethral catheterization of the male ferret for treatment of urinary tract obstruction. *Laboratory Animals* 40: 19–20.

Calicchio, K., Bennett, R., Laraio, L. et al. (2016). Collateral circulation in ferrets (*Mustela putorius*) during temporary occlusion of the caudal vena cava. *American Journal of Veterinary Research* 77: 540–547.

Caplan, E., Peterson, M., Mullen, H. et al. (1996). Diagnosis and treatment of insulin-secreting pancreatic islet cell tumors in ferrets: 57 cases (1986–1994). *Journal of the American Veterinary Medical Association* 209: 1741–1745.

Chen, S. (2010). Advanced diagnostic approaches and current medical management of insulinomas and adrenocortical disease in ferrets (*Mustela putorius furo*). *Veterinary Clinics of North America: Exotic Animal Practice* 13: 439–452.

Dillberger, J. and Altman, N. (1989). Neoplasia in ferrets: eleven cases with a review. *Journal of Comparative Pathology* 100: 161–176.

d'Ovidio, D., Rossi, G., and Meomartino, L. (2016). Oral Malignant Melanoma in a Ferret (*Mustela putorius furo*). *Journal of Veterinary Dentistry* 33: 108–111.

Driggers, T. (2008). A novel surgery for right-sided adrenalectomies in ferrets (*Mustela putorius furo*). *Proceedings of the Association of Avian Veterinarians and the Association of Exotic Mammal Veterinarians*, pp.107–109.

Ehrhart, N., Withrow, S.J., Ehrhart, E.J. et al. (1996). Pancreatic beta cell tumor in ferrets: 20 cases (1986–1994). *Journal of the American Veterinary Medical Association* 209: 1737–1740.

Evans, H. and Quoc, N. (2014). Anatomy of the ferret. In: *Biology and Diseases of the Ferret*, 3e (eds. J.G. Fox and R.P. Marini), 23–67. Ames, IA: Wiley.

Filion, D. and Hoar, R. (1985). Adrenalectomy in the ferret. *Laboratory Animal Science* 35: 294–295.

Fisher, P. (2002). Urethrostomy and penile amputation to treat urethral obstruction and preputial masses in male ferrets. *Exotic DVM* 3: 21–23.

Frohlich, J. and Donovan, T. (2015). Cervical chordoma in a domestic ferret (*Mustela putorius furo*) with pulmonary metastasis. *Journal of Veterinary Diagnostic Investigation* 27: 656–659.

Geyer, N. and Reichle, J. (2012). What is your diagnosis? Gastric dilatation-volvulus (GDV) with secondary peritoneal effusion and splenic congestion or torsion. *Journal of the American Veterinary Medical Association* 241: 45–47.

Goodman, A. and Casale, S. (2014). Short-term outcome following partial or complete liver lobectomy with a commercially prepared self-ligating loop in companion animals: 29 cases (2009–2012). *Journal of the American Veterinary Medical Association* 244: 693–698.

Graham, J., Fidel, J., and Mison, M. (2006). Rostral maxillectomy and radiation therapy to manage squamous cell carcinoma in a ferret. *Veterinary Clinics of North America: Exotic Animal Practice* 9: 701–706.

Hall, J., Hall, K., Powell, L. et al. (2015). Outcome of male cats managed for urethral obstruction with decompressive cystocentesis and urinary catheterization: 47 cats (2009–2012). *Journal of Veterinary Emergency and Critical Care* 25: 256–262.

Harrison, T. and Kitchell, B. (2017). Principles and applications of medical oncology in exotic animal practice. *Veterinary Clinics of North America: Exotic Animal Practice* 20: 209–234.

Hinton, J., Aitken-Palmer, C., Joyner, P. et al. (2016). Fatal gastric dilation in two adult black-footed ferrets (Mustela Nigripes). *Journal of Zoo and Wildlife Medicine* 47: 367–369.

Hoefer, H. (2013). Excellence in exotics: practice tip: ferret urinary tract catheterization. *Compendium: Continuing Education For Veterinarians* 35: E6.

Jekl, V. and Hauptman, K. (2017). Reproductive disease of ferrets. *Veterinary Clinics of North America: Exotic Animal Practice* 20: 629–663.

Johnson-Delaney, C. (2006). Anatomy and physiology of the gastrointestinal system of the ferret and selected exotic carnivores. *Proceedings of the Annual Conference on Association of Exotic Mammal Veterinarians*, 29–38.

Johnson-Delaney, C. (2016). Anatomy and disorders of the oral cavity of ferrets and other exotic companion carnivores. *Veterinary Clinics of North America: Exotic Animal Practice* 19: 901–928.

Kirpensteijn, J., Maarschalkerweerd, R., van der Gaag, I. et al. (2001). Comparison of three closure methods and two absorbable suture materials for closure of jejunal enterotomy incisions in healthy dogs. *The Veterinary Quarterly* 23: 67–70.

Lennox, A. and Wagner, R. (2012). Comparison of 4.7-mg deslorelin implants and surgery for the treatment of adrenocortical disease in ferrets. *Journal of Exotic Pet Medicine* 21: 332–335.

Li, X., Fox, J., and Padrid, P.A. (1998). Neoplastic diseases in ferrets: 574 cases (1968–1997). *Journal of the American Veterinary Medical Association* 212: 1402–1406.

Ludwig, L. and Aiken, S. (2004). Soft tissue surgery of ferrets. In: *Ferrets, Rabbits, and Rodents*, 2e (eds. K.E. Quesenberry and J.W. Carpenter), 121–123. St. Louis, MO: Elsevier.

Marini, R., Jackson, L., Esteves, M. et al. (1994). Effect of isoflurane on hematologic variables in ferrets. *American Journal of Veterinary Research* 55: 1479–1483.

Mayer, J., Erdman, S.E., and Fox, J.G. (2014). Diseases of the hematopoietic system. In: *Biology and Diseases of the Ferret*, 3e (eds. J.G. Fox and R.P. Marini), 329–352. Ames, IA: Wiley.

Mayer, J., Marini, R.P., and Fox, J.G. (2015). Biology and diseases of ferrets. In: *Laboratory Animal Medicine*, 3e (eds. J.G. Fox, L.C.G.M. Anderson, K.R. Pritchett-Corning and M.T. Wary), 577–622. London: Elsevier.

Miwa, Y., Kurosawa, A., Ogawa, H. et al. (2009). Neoplastic diseases in ferrets in Japan: a questionnaire study for 2000 to 2005. *Journal of Veterinary Medical Science* 71: 397–402.

Mullen, H., Scavelli, T., Quesenberry, K. et al. (1992). Gastrointestinal foreign body in ferrets: 25 cases (1986–1990). *Journal of the American Animal Hospital Association* 28: 13–19.

Munday, J., Brown, C., and Richey, L. (2004). Suspected metastatic coccygeal chordoma in a ferret (*Mustela putorius furo*). *Journal of Veterinary Diagnostic Investigation* 16: 454–458.

Nankinishi, M., Kuwamura, M., Yamate, J. et al. (2005). Gastric adenocarcinoma with ossification in a ferret (*Mustela putorius furo*). *Journal of Veterinary Medical Science* 67: 939–941.

Nolte, D., Carberry, C., Gannon, K. et al. (2002). Temporary tube cystostomy as a treatment for urinary obstruction secondary to adrenal disease in four ferrets. *Journal of the American Animal Hospital Association* 38: 527–532.

Nwaokorie, E., Osborne, C., Lulich, J. et al. (2011). Epidemiology of struvite uroliths in ferrets: 272 cases (1981–2007). *Journal of the American Veterinary Medical Association* 239: 1319–1324.

Nwaokorie, E., Osborne, C., Lulich, J. et al. (2013). Epidemiological evaluation of cystine urolithiasis in domestic ferrets (*Mustela putorius furo*): 70 cases (1992–2009). *Journal of the American Veterinary Medical Association* 242: 1099–1103.

Poddar, S. (1977). Gross and microscopic anatomy of the biliary tract of the ferret. *Acta Anatomica (Basel)* 97: 121–131.

Powers, L. and Brown, S. (2001). Basic anatomy, physiology, and husbandry. In: *Ferrets, Rabbits, and Rodents: Clinical Medicine and Surgery*, 3e (eds. K.E. Quesenberry and J.W. Carpenter), 1–12. St. Louis, MO: Elsevier.

Powers, L., Winkler, K., Garner, M. et al. (2007). Omentalization of prostatic abscesses and large cysts in ferrets (*Mustela putorius furo*). *Exotic Pet Medicine* 16: 186–194.

Protain, H., Kutzler, M., and Valentine, B. (2009). Assessment of cytologic evaluation of preputial epithelial cells as a diagnostic test for detection of adrenocortical disease in castrated ferrets. *American Journal of Veterinary Research* 70: 619–623.

Pye, G., Bennett, R., Roberts, G. et al. (2000). Thoracic vertebral chordoma in a domestic ferret (*Mustela putorius furo*). *Journal of Zoo and Wildlife Medicine* 31: 107–111.

Radasch, R., Merkley, D., Wilson, J. et al. (1990). Cystotomy closure. A comparison of the strength of appositional and inverting suture patterns. *Veterinary Surgery* 19: 283–288.

Rice, L., Stahl, S., McLeod, C. et al. (1992). Pyloric adenocarcinoma in a ferret. *Journal of the American Veterinary Medical Association* 200: 1117–1118.

Sanchez-Migallon Guzman, D., Mayer, J., Melidone, R. et al. (2006). Pacemaker implantation in a ferret (*Mustela putorius furo*) with third-degree atrioventricular block. *Veterinary Clinics of North America: Exotic Animal Practice* 9: 677–687.

Schwarz, L., Solano, M., Manning, A. et al. (2003). The normal gastrointestinal examination in the ferret. *Veterinary Radiology & Ultrasound* 44: 165–172.

Sharma, A., Thompson, M., Scrivani, P. et al. (2011). Comparison of radiography and ultrasonography for diagnosing small-intestinal mechanical obstruction in vomiting dogs. *Veterinary Radiology & Ultrasound* 52: 248–255.

Sleeman, J., Clyde, V., Jones, M. et al. (1995). Two cases of pyloric adenocarcinoma in the ferret (*Mustela putorius furo*). *The Veterinary Record* 137: 272–273.

Summa, N., Eshar, D., Lee-Chow, B. et al. (2015). Clinical technique: imaging of the collateral caudal vena cava circulation using fluoroscopy guided non-selective contrast angiography in ferrets (*Mustela putorius furo*) with adrenocortical gland disorder for a presurgical evaluation. *Israel Journal of Veterinary Medical Science* 70: 31–35.

Suran, J., Latney, L., and Wyre, N. (2017). Radiographic and ultrasonographic findings of the spleen and abdominal lymph nodes in healthy domestic ferrets. *Journal of Small Animal Practice* https://doi.org/10.1111/jsap.12680.

Swiderski, J., Seim, H., MacPhail, C. et al. (2008). Long-term outcome of domestic ferrets treated surgically for hyperadrenocorticism: 130 cases (1995–2004). *Journal of the American Veterinary Medical Association* 232: 1338–1343.

Thas, I. (2014). Acquired salivary mucoceles in two domestic ferrets (*Mustela putorius furo*). *Veterinary Record Case Reports* 2: e000051. https://doi.org/10.1136/vetreccr-2014-000051.

Thieman-Mankin, K., Ellison, G., Jeyapaul, C. et al. (2012). Comparison of short-term complication rates between dogs and cats undergoing appositional single-layer or inverting double-layer cystotomy closure: 144 cases (1993–2010). *Journal of the American Veterinary Medical Association* 240: 65–68.

Thongtharb, A., Uchida, K., Chambers, J. et al. (2016). Histological and immunohistochemical features of histiocytic sarcoma in four domestic ferrets (*Mustela putorius furo*). *Journal of Veterinary Diagnostic Investigation* 28: 165–170.

Wagner, R., Bailey, E., Schneider, J. et al. (2001). Leuprolide acetate treatment of adrenocortical disease in ferrets. *Journal of the American Veterinary Medical Association* 218: 1272–1274.

Wagner, R., Piché, C., Jöchle, W. et al. (2005). Clinical and endocrine responses to treatment with deslorelin acetate implants in ferrets with adrenocortical disease. *American Journal of Veterinary Research* 66: 910–914.

Wagner, R., Finkler, M., Fecteau, K. et al. (2009). The treatment of adrenal cortical disease in ferrets with 4.7-mg deslorelin acetate implants. *Journal of Exotic Pet Medicine* 18: 146–152.

Webster, J. and Alghamdi, A. (2015). Use of plastic adhesive drapes during surgery for preventing surgical site infection. *Cochrane Database of Systematic Reviews* 4: CD006353.

Weiss, C., Williams, B., and Scott, M. (1998). Insulinoma in the ferret: clinical findings and treatment comparison of 66 cases. *Journal of the American Animal Hospital Association* 34: 471–475.

Weiss, C., Williams, B., Scott, J. et al. (1999). Surgical treatment and long-term outcome of ferrets with bilateral adrenal tumors or adrenal hyperplasia: 56 cases (1994–1997). *Journal of the American Veterinary Medical Association* 215: 820–823.

Williams, B., Eighmy, J., Berbert, M. et al. (1993). Cervical chordoma in two ferrets (*Mustela putorius furo*). *Veterinary Pathology* 30: 204–206.

Wouters, E., Buishand, F., Kik, M. et al. (2011). Use of a bipolar vessel-sealing device in resection of canine insulinoma. *Journal of Small Animal Practice* 52: 139–145.

van Zeeland, Y., Lennox, A., Quinton, J. et al. (2014). Prepuce and partial penile amputation for treatment of preputial gland neoplasia in two ferrets. *Journal of Small Animal Practice* 55: 593–596.

19

Rodent Soft Tissue Surgery

R. Avery Bennett

Introduction

There are five suborders within the order Rodentia, Anomaluromorpha (springhares), Castorimorpha (beavers, pocket gophers, kangaroo rats, and kangaroo mice), Hystricomorph (guinea pigs, chinchillas, degus, etc.), Myomorpha (mouse-like rodents including mice, rats, hamsters gerbils, etc.), and Sciuromorpha (squirrel-like rodents including squirrels, ground squirrels, prairie dogs, etc.). Hystrichomorph rodents have some unique reproductive characteristics including male genital anatomy.

Rodents are prey species and, when subjected to stress, pain, and fear, they seem to lose their will to live. They may die for no apparent medical reason. Sometimes they recover from surgery uneventfully and are discharged to their owner's care only to die a day or two later. In the author's experience, this occurs in hystrichomorph rodents more so than other suborders. It also seems that rodents that are more used to human contact are less susceptible to these stress related issues. Preemptive, multimodal analgesia combined with postoperative analgesic and anti-anxiety medications is very important.

Rodents ferment cellulose in the cecum and anorexia can have life-threatening consequences; therefore, a short preoperative fast is recommended to allow them to clear food material from their mouth since they are not able to vomit. After surgery, it is essential to ensure continued gastrointestinal function. Anorectic postoperative patients may need nutritional supplementation such as syringe feeding.

Rodents are prone to traumatizing their incision. Intradermal closure is recommended, but can be time-consuming. Steel skin staples are more difficult for them to remove. Midazolam is anxiolytic and can be helpful for preventing self-mutilation after surgery, particularly when paired with analgesic and anti-inflammatory drugs.

Reproductive Tract Surgery

Orchidectomy

Indications for orchidectomy in rodents include sterilization, treatment of testicular tumors, eliminating urethral and preputial plugs, and possibly to ameliorate aggressive behaviors. For population control, many feel it is easier to perform an orchidectomy than ovariectomy or ovariohysterectomy; however, female rodents are susceptible to various medical conditions, such as cystic ovaries, that can be prevented by ovariectomy. Urethral plugs have been reported in rats, mice, golden hamsters, and guinea pigs and can cause urethral obstruction, but after orchidectomy their size decreases by 99% (Lejnieks 2007). Preputial plugs occur as smegma accumulates within the prepuce, and they can become infected. Orchidectomy reduces the secretions from the preputial glands so plugs do not form. Testicular tumors, mainly Leydig cell tumors, occur in rodents, and orchidectomy is the recommended treatment. Testicular and prostatic tumors have been reported in gerbils (Toft 1992), and orchidectomy is indicated for their treatment or prevention. Orchidectomy has been shown to alter aggressive behavior as well.

Anatomy

The testes of rodents are relatively large for their body size and descend in the first one to two weeks (Harkness 1993). The inguinal canals are large, and a functional cremaster muscle allows the testes to move freely between the scrotum and abdomen. There is a large fat pad in the caudal abdomen on each side through which the spermatic cords pass blocking the viscera from migrating through the inguinal canal (Figure 19.1). There is also an epididymal fat pad within the vaginal tunic that blocks passage of viscera into the scrotum. It is attached to the head of the

Surgery of Exotic Animals, First Edition. Edited by R. Avery Bennett and Geoffrey W. Pye.
© 2022 John Wiley & Sons, Inc. Published 2022 by John Wiley & Sons, Inc.

(A)

(B)

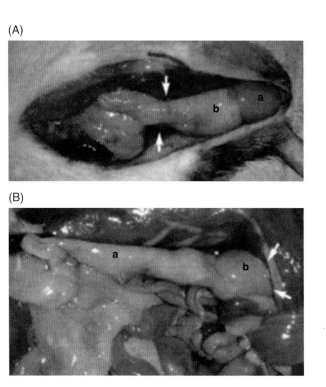

Figure 19.1 (A) The epididymal fat (b) is attached to the epididymis and extends cranially through the inguinal canal and into the abdomen to the caudal pole of the kidney, obstructing the inguinal canal and preventing inguinal hernia formation. Arrows indicate the location of the inguinal canal. The body wall, inguinal canal, scrotum, and vaginal tunic have been incised to show the normal location of the epididymal fat. Testis (a) (B) The epididymal fat (a) is being retracted cranially within the abdomen, pulling the testis (b) into the abdomen. In this image about half of the testicle is within the abdomen. *Source:* Bennett (2012b).

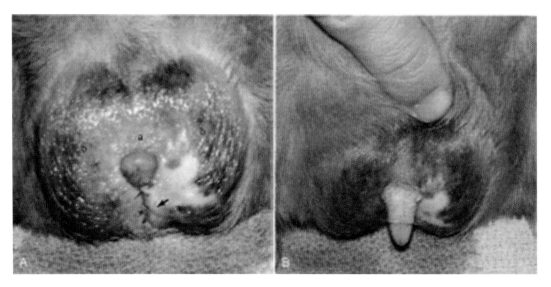

Figure 19.2 Histrichomorph rodents do not have a distinct scrotum and the testes are located on each side lateral to the penis. *Source*: Bennett (2012a).

epididymis and extends into the abdomen. Additionally, the coagulating glands and seminal vesicles partially obstruct the inguinal canal. Because of these anatomic features, despite having a wide inguinal canal, inguinal hernias are uncommon. The spermatic cord is comprised of the vaginal tunic with the cremaster muscle, and the ductus deferens and pampiniform plexus within. The vaginal tunic is an extension of the peritoneum that extends into the scrotum as the testes descend.

The large testes of most rodents are caudoventrally located under the tail and are quite prominent with little hair on the scrotum. Hystrichomorph rodents do not have a distinct scrotum, and the testes are located on each side lateral to the penis (Figure 19.2). The ligament of the tail of the epididymis (LTE) is a fibrous attachment between the vaginal tunic and the tail of the epididymis, and between the vaginal tunic and the inside of the scrotal skin.

Percutaneous Orchidectomy

The term "closed" indicates the vaginal tunic is not opened to remove the testis. Since the vaginal tunic is an extension of the peritoneum, if it is ligated at the external inguinal ring, it will reduce the risk of developing an inguinal hernia. Historically, many have recommended closing the external inguinal ring during orchidectomy to reduce the risk of developing an inguinal hernia; however, the caudal abdominal fat and epididymal fat block the inguinal canal preventing inguinal hernia. If the normal anatomy fails, an inguinal hernia can develop. The tunic must be dissected from tissues attached to it. This must be done carefully and can be time-consuming. The tissue to be ligated is thicker with a closed castration compared with the open technique.

For an open orchidectomy, incise the tunic and exteriorize the contents of the tunic effectively opening the peritoneal cavity. Detach the testis from the LTE, but there are no other attachments so once the ligament is broken the testis is easily be exteriorized. Place a ligature around only the pampiniform plexus and ductus deferens. Leave the tunic in place.

A modified open technique combines the advantages of both open and closed technique, making it easier to exteriorize the testis and occluding the external inguinal ring (Capello 2004). Open the vaginal tunic to make it easier to exteriorize the testis and detach it from the LTE. Then place the ligature proximal to the incision in the tunic to incorporate the entire spermatic cord, thus closing off the tunic at the external inguinal ring. Leave the tunic in place.

An intratesticular injection of 2% lidocaine at 1 mg/kg/ testis for intraoperative analgesia is recommended. The benefit is intraoperative to reduce the level of anesthesia needed to complete the procedure.

Hystrichomorph Rodents Position the patient in dorsal recumbency. Clip and prepare the skin around the penis and the inguinal area. Hold one testis between the thumb and first finger of the nondominant hand and make a skin incision over it parallel to, but lateral to, the penis. Be careful not to make the incision too close to the penis or it can be detached from the prepuce during dissection (Powers et al. 2008). Identify the spermatic cord and perform an open, closed, or modified closed orchidectomy. Be careful not to damage the epididymal fat and keep in mind that the goal is to remove the testis. Pulling the testis out far can damage the epididymal fat. Gently push the epididymal fat back into the inguinal canal and place the ligature at the junction of the epididymal fat and the head of the epididymis.

An alternative approach has been described where the skin incision is made over the ventral aspect of the tail of the epididymis (Nelson 2004). Be careful to not cut through the vaginal tunic. Clamp a hemostat onto the tail of the epididymis and apply caudal traction while pushing the skin proximally to break down the attachments allowing the testis to be exteriorized, and then perform either an open or closed orchidectomy.

Close the skin with an intradermal suture because these rodents are prone to developing scrotal abscesses. It is unknown why hystrichomorph rodents are predisposed, but it may be that the incision is close to the substrate and becomes contaminated with feces. Advise owners of this potential and stress the importance of keeping the substrate clean. Clean paper bedding should be changed twice daily for 7–10 days. Adhere to aseptic technique, use perioperative antibiotics, and handle tissues gently. Applying a thin layer of cyanoacrylate adhesive over the incision may provide a barrier to fecal contamination. If an abscess does occur open the incision, express the caseous pus from the abscess, obtain culture samples, irrigate the wound, and start systemic antibiotics. Consider implanting antibiotic impregnated plaster of Paris beads for patients with more aggressive infection. Most respond well and resolve with this therapy; however, a scrotal abscess increases the risk of developing an inguinal hernia due to tissue necrosis around the inguinal canal.

Non-Hystrichomorph Rodents There is little hair on the scrotum, but the surrounding hair can be clipped and prepared prior to surgery. Push the testes caudally and hold them out by placing the thumb and index finger at the base preventing them from moving into the abdomen. The author prefers to exteriorize both testes at the same time. Make an incision transversely being careful to only cut the scrotum and not into the tunic and testes for a closed orchidectomy (Figure 19.3). Alternatively, make two separate incisions from dorsal to ventral, one on each side over each testis. Incise as dorsal as possible to minimize the risk of the incisions being in contact with the substrate. Grasp one testis and retract it caudally only far enough to ligate proximal to the head of the epididymis preserving the epididymal fat. Place an encircling ligature between the epididymal fat and the head of the epididymis, and then transect distal to the ligature. The scrotal skin is too thin to suture so leave it open to heal by second intention or seal it with tissue adhesive.

Another modified open technique involves making two incisions, one on each side at the external inguinal ring cranial to the penis. The skin in this location is thicker and can be sutured closed with an intradermal pattern; however, the incisions are more likely to be in contact with

(a)

(b)

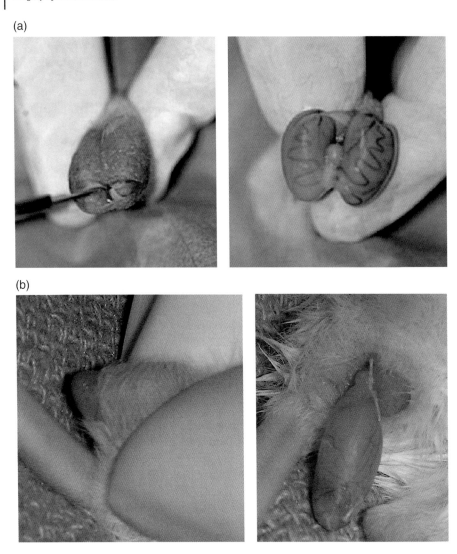

Figure 19.3 (a) When performing an orchidectomy in a murine rodent (mouse), make a transverse incision from one side to the other to allow both testes to be exteriorized. *Source:* Bennett and Mullen (2003a). (b) Alternatively, make two separate incisions, one over each testicle from dorsal to ventral.

the substrate. Identify the spermatic cord and preplace a suture circumferentially around it. Incise the tunic caudal to the ligature and exteriorize the testis. Ligate the vessels and ductus at the junction of the epididymal fat and head of the epididymis and transect distal to the ligature. Replace the fat into the inguinal canal, and then tie the preplaced ligature around the entire spermatic cord. Alternatively, detach the head of the epididymis from the testis and place the ligature to leave the head of the epididymis with the fat, and then replace the fat and head of the epididymis into the external inguinal ring to help block the inguinal canal (Capello 2003b). A closed technique can also be performed through this inguinal approach.

Postoperatively keep the substrate clean by changing it twice daily for a week. Following orchidectomy, rodents

may continue to display mounting and even intromission for several weeks, but activity decreases or is eliminated within one to two weeks (Harkness 1993). Do not put the patient with females for six to eight weeks because the ductus will still contain viable sperm. Complications include hematoma, self-trauma, inguinal hernia, and infection (Redrobe 2002).

Abdominal Approach for Orchidectomy

An abdominal approach for orchidectomy is possible in rodents as described in rabbits (see Chapter 17) because the inguinal canal is large enough for the testes to be pulled into the abdomen. The advantages of this technique are a single incision that is less likely to be contaminated by the substrate and the inguinal and epididymal fat are preserved (Bennett 2012b; Brown 2008). This approach is recommended in large rodents such as capybara (see Chapter 27).

Paraphimosis

Paraphimosis occurs most commonly in hystrichomorph rodents, especially chinchillas, and degus. It has been anecdotally not only reported following orchidectomy but also not associated with any procedure or known etiology. The penis is protected within the prepuce where it is kept moist and supple. If the penis is outside the prepuce for a prolonged period of time, the mucosa becomes more keratinized and thicker (called keratinization) to protect it from desiccation and environmental trauma. Because of this adaptation, it is unlikely paraphimosis would result in medical issues; however, most owners do not want to have their pet's penis exposed.

In a degu, paraphimosis was determined to be the result of preputial damage and lateral deviation of the penis into the subcutaneous tissues after orchidectomy (Powers et al. 2008). A phallopexy was performed by placing four polydioxanone sutures between the tip of the penis and the edge of the preputial orifice avoiding the urethral opening. They did not incise or scarify tissue, and the penis was still adhered to the prepuce two years later. The author recommends this procedure for rodents with paraphimosis.

Ovariectomy and Ovariohysterectomy

Indications for ovariectomy or ovariohysterectomy include cystic ovaries, ovarian tumors, sterilization, suppression of anxiety, and prevention of mammary and pituitary tumors in rats. Ovariectomy in most species prevents uterine diseases and may decrease the risk of developing mammary tumors. In a review comparing ovariectomy with ovariohysterectomy, nearly all complications with ovariohysterectomy were related to removing the uterus (van Goethem et al. 2006), and there was no need identified to remove the uterus. In rodents, when performing ovariohysterectomy through a ventral midline approach, the cecum and intestine must be manipulated, which can result in postoperative gastrointestinal ileus. Ovariectomy using a dorsolateral approach allows the surgeon to approach the ovaries directly without needing to manipulate other abdominal viscera. Unless there is uterine disease, ovariectomy is preferred over ovariohysterectomy.

Cystic Ovaries

Cystic ovaries have been reported in many species of rodents but are most common in guinea pigs and gerbils

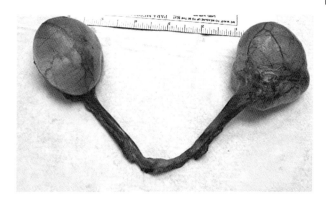

Figure 19.4 Bilateral cystic ovaries in a guinea pig. *Source:* Image courtesy Marc Silverman.

(Figure 19.4). Cystic ovaries are common in gerbils over two years age and may be unilateral or bilateral (Lewis 2003). In a study involving 43 guinea pigs from both pet owners and breeders, 53% had cystic ovaries and 36% of those were bilateral on ultrasound examination, and of the cavies over two years old 93% had cystic ovaries and 62% were affected bilaterally (Nielson et al. 2003). There was no difference in incidence between breeders and nonbreeding pet cavies. When there are multiple cysts, they are usually <5 mm, but when single they are larger and often multilobular (Quattropani 1977).

Histologically, the cysts are of the rete ovarii and do not produce hormones (Keller et al. 1987; Quattropani 1981, 1977; Rueløkke et al. 2003). Many guinea pigs are asymptomatic until the cysts become so large they compromise gastrointestinal and respiratory function. Some sows develop bilaterally symmetrical nonpruritic alopecia, become aggressive, and begin mounting others in the group (Mayer 2003). Many also have uterine disease and present for hemorrhagic discharge that the owner may perceive as hematuria (Eatwell 2003; Keller et al. 1987). Because cystic ovaries are so common in mature guinea pigs, consider recommending ovariectomy for young guinea pigs to prevent this condition and associated uterine disease.

Ovarian Tumors

Ovarian tumors including thecal cell, granulosa cell, and lutein cell tumors are common in gerbils (Bingel 1995; Greenacre 2004) with an incidence of 12.5% in one study (Benitz and Kramer 1965). In female gerbils with reproductive tumors, 29/37 had ovarian tumors and 8 had uterine tumors (Toft 1992). In hamsters, thecomas can become large enough to compromise gastrointestinal and respiratory function (Toft 1992). There are no reports of successful treatment of ovarian tumors in gerbils and hamsters.

Ovariectomy in four months old rats significantly reduced the incidence of both mammary and pituitary tumors, and prolonged survival; however, they were prone to developing osteopenia (Hotchkiss 1995). Ovariectomy in rats of any age resulted in significantly reduced anxiety behavior (de Chaves et al. 2009).

In guinea pigs, teratomas of the ovary occur commonly after age three and can be as large as 10 cm in diameter (Cooper 1994; Greenacre 2004; Toft 1992). They rarely metastasize and are typically unilateral. They are prone to rupture resulting in hemoabdomen and clinical signs of weakness, lethargy, collapse, and death.

Abdominal ultrasound is useful to determine the etiology of abdominal distention (ovary, uterus, or other organ), and is used to obtain samples for cytology. In animal with cystic ovaries, draining the fluid will help relieve any issues related to viscera compression; however, the fluid typically reforms quickly. Aspiration of fluid immediately prior to surgery makes ovariectomy easier to perform and, though malignant ovarian tumors occur in rodents, there are no reports of tumor seeding from draining the fluid. There may be adhesions between the diseased ovaries and uterus and other organs, so be cautious during the approach in animals with ovarian and/or uterine pathology.

Uterine diseases described in rodents include pyometra, mucometra, metritis, endometritis, tumors, and prolapse. Uterine tumors tend to be malignant in hamsters and gerbils and benign in rats occurring in over 65% of females over 21 months old (Greenacre 2004; Toft 1992). Hemorrhagic vaginal discharge often perceived as hematuria by the owner is a common presenting complaint. Metastasis and tumor seeding during surgery have been documents in hamsters with uterine adenocarcinomas (Toft 1992). Polyps, leiomyomas, leiomyosarcomas, carcinomas of the cervix, and squamous papillomas have been documented in hamsters (Greenacre 2004). The most common reproductive tract tumor of guinea pigs is leiomyoma and is associated with cystic ovaries (Field et al. 1989; Greenacre 2004; Harkness et al. 2010).

Pyometra

Pyometra is uncommon in most rodents, but it is important to note hamsters normally have a mucoid odiferous discharge during estrus. Pyometra occurs more commonly in guinea pigs and chinchillas (Bodri and Walker 1993). Clinical signs include lethargy, anorexia, polydipsia, and vaginal discharge. Vascular access is vital for these patients as they are dehydrated and often have other metabolic abnormalities, and it allows for administration of intravenous antibiotics.

Because of the high incidence of ovarian and uterine disease in older rodents, consider recommending ovariectomy in young rodents for prevention. The surgery is easier to perform with less morbidity in young healthy animals.

Anatomy

The uterus is bicornuate with the two horns coming together to form the uterine body, which is divided internally by an intercornual ligament with a single cervix. The horns are linear and are not coiled. The ovaries are located caudolateral to the kidneys, and the oviducts are dorsal to the ovaries encircling it extending cranially (Popesko et al. 1992). Fat is stored in the mesovarium, mesometrium, and broad ligaments. A single ovarian artery and vein are branches from the renal vessels. They split into ovarian and uterine branches, then run medial to each ovary and to the uterine horn. The reproductive tract is dorsal to the gastrointestinal tract, which must be retracted to achieve access through a ventral approach. The ovaries may be difficult to exteriorize through a small ventral approach if the suspensory ligament is short, in which case it is necessary to make a larger approach.

Ovariectomy

Ovariectomy is best achieved using a dorsolateral approach (Jenkins 2000; Redrobe 2002), which does not usually involve manipulation of the gastrointestinal tract that can result in postoperative ileus. Additionally, the incisions are smaller and are not in contact with the substrate making it less likely to be contaminated and for the weight of the viscera to stress the closure.

Position the patient in ventral recumbency and clip and prepare the dorsal thoracolumbar region for aseptic surgery (Figure 19.5). Make an incision on each side at the level of the third lumbar vertebra ventral to the erector spinae muscle just caudal to the last rib. Alternatively, make a single incision on dorsal midline or transversely across the dorsal midline, and then shift the incision from side to side to access each ovary. Use a mosquito hemostat to bluntly penetrate the body wall just caudal to the last rib and ventral to the erector spinae muscles at the level of the dorsal process of the third lumbar vertebra, then spread the jaws to enlarge the opening to 0.5–1 cm. Apply pressure to the abdomen to extrude the ovary out of the opening created. In older females with more perirenal fat, it can be difficult to get the ovary out. Use a hemostat or thumb forceps to retrieve it from its location caudal to the kidney. This is done without being able to visualize the ovary so use caution. Once the ovary is exteriorized, place a ligature or hemostatic clip at the base of the ovary to prevent hemorrhage. Transect distal to the ligature to complete the ovariectomy. Make sure to remove the entire oviduct along with the ovary because oviduct remnants filling with fluid

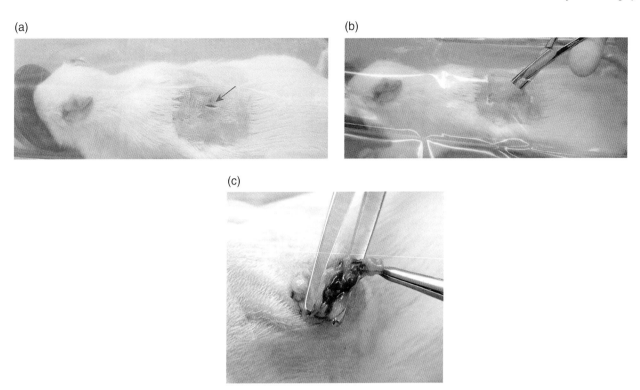

Figure 19.5 When performing an ovariectomy in a rodent (rat) make a skin incision on each side ventral to the epaxial muscles and just caudal to the last rib (a). Use a hemostat to puncture the body wall and spread the tips to enlarge the opening (b). Blindly use the hemostat to grasp the ovary and exteriorize it, and then place a hemostatic clip proximal to the ovary (c). Allowing it to be removed. Repeat the procedure on the contralateral side.

forming cysts has been reported (Jenkins 2000). Close the defect in the body wall with one or two sutures of an appropriately sized monofilament absorbable material, and then the skin with an intradermal suture or tissue adhesive.

Laparoscopic ovariectomy has been reported as a pilot study in three guinea pigs (McCready et al. 2020). A three-port technique with a 3.9 mm scope cannula and two 3.5 mm working ports with 3.5 mm cannulae with 3 mm instruments were used as well as a 3 mm vessel-sealing device were used. The abdomen was insufflated to a pressure of 6–8 mmHg. It was determined that it was critical to place the guinea pig in complete lateral recumbency to remove the ovary on each side with repositioning to remove the contralateral ovary.

Ovariohysterectomy

Ovariohysterectomy is indicated for patients with uterine disease that would not be expected to respond to ovariectomy alone. Nearly, all uterine diseases occur secondary to ovarian hormones (van Goethem et al. 2006).

Position the patient in dorsal recumbency, clip the fur, and prepare the skin for aseptic surgery. Center the incision midway between the umbilicus and pubis. Gerbils have a scent-marking gland on the ventral midline near the umbilicus, so in gerbils make the incision lateral to the scent gland and undermine the skin to expose the linea alba. In rodents, there is not usually much subcutaneous fat and the linea alba is easy to identify. The thin-walled cecum is just inside the body wall, so be careful entering the abdominal cavity. Iatrogenic damage to the cecum results in contamination and potentially life-threatening complications. It is recommended that a spay hook not be used. Using a finger or blunt instrument, retract the cecum and urinary bladder to one side to allow visualization of the contralateral uterine horn. Grasp the uterine horn, exteriorize it, and trace it cranially to locate the ovary. The mesovarium originates from the caudal pole of the kidney and is often short making it difficult to exteriorize the ovary compared with carnivores. Perform an ovariohysterectomy as in other species. It has been recommended that the ligature on the uterus be placed cranial to the cervix to prevent urine spilling into the abdomen (Jenkins 2000); however, a small amount of urine contamination would not be expected to cause clinical problems. Ligate the uterine body in a convenient location, as there is no concern for developing uterine disease if both ovaries are removed. Close the body wall with a simple continuous pattern of a slowly absorbed material such as polydioxanone or polyglycolic acid. Appose the subcutaneous tissues with a monofilament rapidly absorbed material, and then the skin with an intradermal suture or skin staples.

Ovariohysterectomy can be accomplished using the dorsolateral or flank approach described above for ovariectomy (Johnson-Delaney 2002; Rozanska et al. 2016). Make the dorsolateral approach on only one side, exteriorize the ipsilateral ovary, and ligate the ovarian pedicle. Exteriorize the ovary and ipsilateral uterine horn until uterine body and contralateral horn can be identified. Continue retraction until the contralateral ovary is exteriorized. Ligate the contralateral ovarian vessels and identify the uterine body, and then ligate the uterine body. Transect it distal to the ligature to complete the ovariohysterectomy. It can be technically challenging to remove the entire reproductive tract through this approach if there is uterine pathology and a lot of fat in the mesometrium.

Cesarean Section

Dystocia is relatively common in guinea pigs and chinchillas because the feti are precocious and large (Peters 1991) but is uncommon in other rodents. Degu feti are smaller and less well developed having sparse hair and closed eyes at birth (Johnson 2002). The pubic symphysis of guinea pigs may close at six to nine months age, and if this occurs prior to the first pregnancy, dystocia can occur (Peters 1991). If parturition occurs before fusion of the symphysis a cartilaginous union occurs and persists for life. Approximately 10 days prior to parturition, the symphysis begins to separate. When the gap is 1.5 cm parturition should occur within 48 hours and is about 2.2 cm during parturition. The gap is easy to palpate and clearly visible on radiographs (Figure 19.6). If the symphysis has spread and the sow has been in unproductive labor for 90 minutes administer oxytocin (0.5–1.0 IU IM). Offspring should be delivered within 15 minutes, and if they are not surgery is indicated (Peters 1991).

The pubic symphysis does not always fuse, and many primiparous older sows deliver normally. If the breeding date is known, teach the owner how to palpate the symphysis to determine if it is separating. If it has not separated at day 65 or if it has not separated and the patient is in labor, recommend surgery.

Position the patient in dorsal recumbency with the cranial half of the patient elevated so the abdominal contents fall caudally taking pressure off the lungs. Perform a caudal midline celiotomy being careful to avoid the mammary glands and their blood supply. Dystocia can be managed either by performing a Cesarean section or ovariohysterectomy. If it is not a breeding animal, ovariohysterectomy is recommended unless the uterine vessels are engorged and

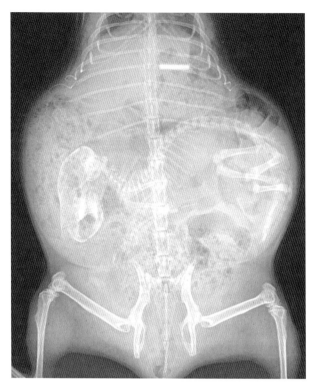

Figure 19.6 A dorsoventral radiograph of a gravid guinea pig about to farrow. Note the separation of the pubic symphysis (arrows). *Source:* Image courtesy of Kim Hester.

the patient is anemic. In these patients, it is best to perform a hysterotomy and quickly remove the feti, and then administer oxytocin to induce uterine involution to preserve the patient's blood.

Exteriorize the uterus completely and isolate it with moist sponges. Make a longitudinal incision in the uterine body either on the dorsal or ventral side. Deliver the feti and pass them to an assistant. Once all are removed, close with a simple continuous pattern of an absorbable monofilament suture, and then irrigate prior to routine closure. Salpingohysterectomy can be performed *en bloc* to deliver the feti and sterilize the patient. Ligate the ovarian vessels first because once the uterine vessels are ligated, there is no oxygen supply to the feti and time to revive them is limited. Clamp but do not ligate the uterine vessels and uterine body, and then transect distal to the clamp to remove the uterus. Pass it to an assistant to open the uterus and retrieve the babies while the surgeon ligates the vessels, irrigates, and closes.

While guinea pigs and chinchillas are precocious at birth and they even eat solid food, it has been shown that guinea pigs orphaned at less than one week of age have a high mortality rate indicating it is important for them to get colostrum from the mother (Harkness et al. 2010).

Uterine Prolapse

Prolapse is usually associated with parturition, and the patient may be stable to debilitated at the time of presentation. Prognosis is fair to good in patients that are stable. Stabilize debilitated patients prior to anesthesia and surgery. The exposed uterus is often contaminated and may be devitalized, so assess the tissue after cleaning. If it is edematous, apply 50% dextrose or other hypertonic solution to reduce the size. Replace the exposed uterus and, in most cases, perform an ovariohysterectomy. If it is important to preserve the patient's reproductive viability use a blunt probang to carefully push the horn back into the abdomen not just into the vagina. If the uterine tissue is replaced, but is only in the vagina, it can obstruct the urethra with potentially fatal consequences. If it will not stay in, consider an ovariohysterectomy or hysteropexy.

Cutaneous and Subcutaneous Masses

Mammary Tumors

Mammary tumors are the most common spontaneous neoplasm in rats and mice (Cooper 1994; Toft 1992). They appear to be uncommon in gerbils and hamsters with Russian hamsters more commonly affected. Mammary tumors are uncommon in guinea pigs (Peters 1991) and appear to be rare in chinchillas (Bennett 2012a) and have not been reported in degus. Approximately ⅓ of mammary tumors in guinea pigs are malignant, and they occur equally in males and females. Adenocarcinomas are locally invasive and rarely metastasize to the lungs (Cooper 1994; Eatwell 2003; Greenacre 2004; Harkness et al. 2010; Kitchen et al. 1975). There are no reports of

bilateral disease or development of a tumor in the contralateral side after excising one gland. Information regarding the effect of ovariectomy on the development or treatment of mammary tumors in guinea pigs is lacking.

Mammary fibroadenomas are benign and occur in 50–90% of female rats over one year of age and 16% of male rats (Hotchkiss 1995; Krohn and Barthold 1984; Vergneau-Grosset et al. 2016). These tumors are usually single, large, firm, not adhered, and do not cause systemic problems until they become so large they interfere with ambulation (Figure 19.7). Less than 10% of mammary tumors in rats are malignant (Greenacre 2004); however, presurgical cytology is recommended for appropriate surgical planning. It has been theorized that estrogen may stimulate the development of prolactin-secreting pituitary tumors that release large amounts of prolactin causing mammary fibroadenomas (Hotchkiss 1995). Exogenous estrogen does not increase the incidence of mammary tumor development. Ovariectomized Sprague–Dawley rats had a significantly lower incidence of mammary tumors compared to intact females (4% vs. 47%) and also had a lower incidence of pituitary tumors (4% vs. 66%). Ovariectomy also increased survival to 630 days (89% vs. 59%). In another study, ovariectomy in Sprague–Dawley rats at seven months age reduced the incidence of mammary tumor development by 95% (Planas-Silva et al. 2008). For these reasons, ovariectomy is recommended at four to seven months age. Estrogen antagonists have not been shown to prevent pituitary and mammary tumors (Greenacre 2004). Orchidectomy to alter the incidence in male rats has not been studied.

Mammary tumors in mice are associated with infection with mouse mammary tumor virus with an incidence of 30–70% (Collins 1988; Cooper 1994; Greenacre 2004).

(a)

(b)

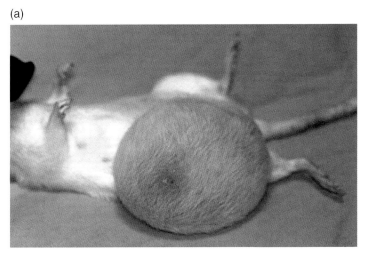
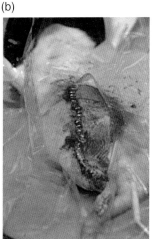

Figure 19.7 Rat mammary fibroadenomas can grow quite large (a). This tumor weighed more than the rat did after tumor removal. Because speed is important in removing large mammary tumors, a single-layer closure with skin staples is usually adequate (b). *Source:* Bennett and Mullen (2003b).

Ovariectomy has not been shown to have any effect and surgical excision does not prolong survival. Restricting the energy content of the diet has been shown to prolong survival. Preoperative cytology is indicated to confirm the mass is malignant before planning surgery.

Anatomy

Mammary tissue extends from the neck to the inguinal region and laterally up to the shoulders and flanks in rats and mice, so tumors can develop in unusual locations (Popesko et al. 1992); however, is only on the ventral abdomen and chest of hamsters and gerbils. Chinchillas have two pair of glands and guinea pigs only have one inguinal pair. The left and right glands of guinea pigs do not share blood and lymphatic supply (Mullen 2000).

Mastectomy

Treatment of mammary tumors in rodents includes removing the mass and associated mammary gland. The benefit of ovariectomy is clear in rats, is not beneficial in mice, and has not been well studied in other rodents. Other than mice, most recommend ovariectomy as part of the treatment of mammary tumors. If the patient is stable, perform ovariectomy immediately after mastectomy. In some circumstances, perform the mastectomy, and then the ovariectomy at a later date. If the tumor is benign, marginal excision is indicated. Removing the entire gland including the areola is recommended though the benefit of complete excision vs. lumpectomy has not been studied. Incise the skin at the base of the mass far enough onto the base to provide enough skin for a tension free closure. Dissect the skin off the base of the tumor and mammary gland. Be careful not to penetrate the mass because they tend to be very vascular, and this can result in significant hemorrhage that is difficult to control. Dissect around the mass down to the body wall ligating any vessels supplying the mass. If the mass is very large, ligate the arteries before the veins allowing blood to drain from the mass into the systemic circulation. Submit the tissue for histologic evaluation. After the mass has been removed, drains and bandages can be used to manage dead space, but are difficult to maintain in rodents. It is better to close dead space with sutures tacking the subcutaneous tissue to the body wall and potentially walking the skin for tension-free closure. If dead space is left, seroma formation is likely to occur. Close in two layers, subcutaneous tissue and skin. If the patient is not stable under anesthesia, quickly close the skin with staples.

Wide excision with 0.5–1.0 cm (depending on the size of the patient) margins around the mass is recommended for malignant tumors. If the mass is malignant, staging is recommended to include three view thoracic radiographs and cytology of the regional lymph node as well as histologic evaluation of the excised tissue for completeness of the excision. In addition to removing normal appearing skin margins, dissect down to and remove the external rectus fascia deep to the mass. Make sure to plan carefully because tissue is limited in this area. Identify and excise the regional lymph node for histologic staging. Close the defect in rectus abdominis fascia with appropriately sized monofilament slowly absorbed material in a continuous pattern or, if there is tension, an interrupted pattern. Closing the rectus fascia will bring the skin edges closer together. Close subcutaneous tissues as described above for benign mass excision.

Other Cutaneous and Subcutaneous Masses

A variety of benign and malignant cutaneous and subcutaneous masses have been reported in rodents. Trichofolliculomas are common in guinea pigs. They are benign cystic tumors of the basal cells that are typically large at the time of presentation and occur in the lumbosacral area. They contain keratin debris, sebum, and hair and are easy to diagnose with cytology.

Many rodents have scent-marking glands in various locations. Syrian hamsters have an area of alopecia and pigmented skin near each hip, while Djungarian hamsters have a single midventral sebaceous gland. Gerbils have a single gland on the ventral abdomen. Melanomas involving the scent glands of Syrian hamsters occur more commonly in males which also have larger glands (Harkness et al. 2010; Lipman and Foltz 1995).

Zymbal's glands are sebaceous and located around the external ear canal. Squamous cell carcinoma of the Zymbal's glands are often large and invasive but slow to metastasize to the lymph nodes, and then the lungs (Figure 19.8). Wide excision including total ear canal ablation and lateral bulla osteotomy with reconstructive techniques can be curative if performed before metastasis.

Both male and female rats have specialized sebaceous glands on each side of the urethral papilla, preputial, and clitoral glands, respectively. While inflammation is the most common problem associated with these glands, adenocarcinomas are invasive and can metastasize. Often, these animals present late in the course of the disease making it difficult to effect a surgical cure; however, if diagnosed early and treated with an appropriate surgical dose they can be cured. Place a 24 or 26 ga catheter into the urethral papilla to help avoid damaging the urethral opening during the dissection.

Melanomas of the scent glands are common in hamsters. In gerbils, squamous cell carcinomas, adenomas, and adenocarcinomas of the scent glands have been reported (Greenacre 2004; Jackson et al. 1996). Auricular

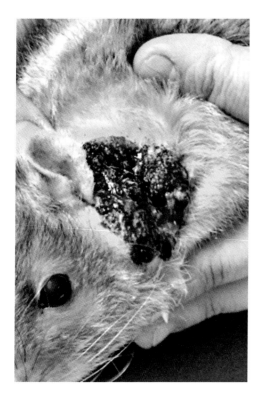

Figure 19.8 Histologically confirmed Zymbal's gland tumor in a rat. *Source:* Image courtesy of Christine Barber.

cholesteatomas have only been reported in humans, dogs, and gerbils (Greenacre 2004; Henry et al. 1983).

Obtaining a diagnosis of tumor type is essential for surgical planning. Marginal excision is expected to be curative for benign tumors; however, wide excision is recommended for malignant tumors. Most rodents have a moderate to extensive amount of loose skin. Excision of malignant tumors should include 0.5–1.0 cm of normal appearing tissue around the mass and one fascial plane deep.

Cervical Lymphadenitis in Guinea Pigs

In theory, cervical lymphadenitis (also known as "lumps") is caused by *Streptococcus* sp. bacteria that enter through traumatized oral mucosa resulting in abscessation of the draining lymph nodes (Peters 1991). This infection is highly contagious and infected individuals should be isolated until the infection is under control. Traditional abscess treatment of lancing, removing the pus, irrigating the abscess, allowing the wound to heal by second intention, and administering systemic antibiotic therapy does not usually resolve the infection due to the caseous nature of the pus of rodents. Excising the abscess *en bloc* has a better chance of resolving the infection, but contamination of the tissue bed can result in recurrence. It is important to submit samples for culture and sensitivity testing to determine what antibiotics to which the organism is sensitive.

Another treatment option for large abscess that cannot be easily excised is to lance, drain, and irrigate the abscess and then cauterize the inside of the abscess with silver nitrate (Mullen 2000). Silver nitrate not only is caustic and kills bacteria but also kills healthy tissue, so use it judiciously.

Placing antibiotic-impregnated polymethylmethacrylate (AIPMMA) or plaster of Paris (POP) beads into the wound bed after excision of the abscess will provide high concentration of antibiotic locally, and then they will continue to release antibiotic slowly for an extended period of time (Bennett 2012a). Excise the abscess as completely as possible, ideally without rupturing the abscess capsule so there is no gross infection remaining. Place the AIPPMA or POP beads into the defect loosely and close the subcutaneous tissue and skin over them. In most cases, the beads do not need to be removed.

Other Subcutaneous Abscesses

Abscesses in rodents are typically a result of dermal trauma, such as a cage-mate bite, allowing bacteria to enter. Some animals present ill while others are asymptomatic except for the mass. Take radiographs for abscesses of the head and feet to evaluate for bone and/or teeth involvement. Perform cytology to confirm that it is an abscess and determine if the bacteria are Gram positive or negative. Recurrence after treatment is common (Miwa and Sladky 2016). It is best to excise the abscess *en bloc* as for marginal resection of a tumor without rupturing the abscess capsule as described above. If the abscess ruptures, if it cannot be excised *en bloc* because of its location (e.g. dental abscesses), or if there is contamination of the wound bed from pus during excision, consider placing AIPMMA or POP beads. Select an antibiotic based on culture and sensitivity testing or Gram's stain characteristics. If there has been no contamination of tissue by pus, there is no need to place AIPMMA or POP beads. In severe cases of pododermatitis, amputation may be the best option. Most rodents adapt well after amputation; however, guinea pigs with forelimb amputation may have difficulty holding their body off the substrate (Miwa and Sladky 2016). They may traumatize the skin on their ventrum.

Gastrointestinal Surgery

Gastric Trichobezoars

Clinical illness caused by gastric trichobezoars has been described only in Peruvian long-haired guinea pigs (Figure 19.9) (Bennett and Russo 1985; Kuenzel and Hittmair 2002; Peters 1991). The proposed etiology is inadequate hay in the diet (Gerold et al. 1997). Feeding a

(a)

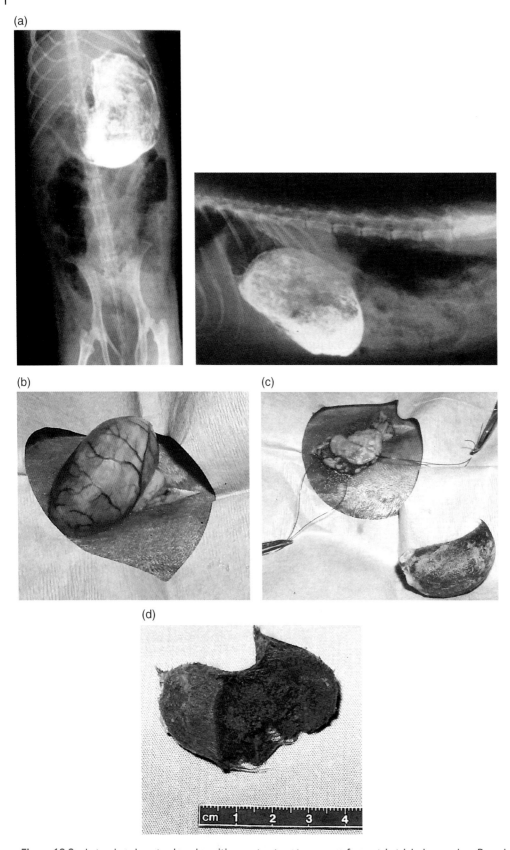

(b)

(c)

(d)

Figure 19.9 Lateral and ventrodorsal positive contrast gastrograms of a gastric trichobezoar in a Peruvian guinea pig (a). Intraoperative image of a firm mass in the stomach (b) that was removed via gastrotomy (c). After removal it was confirmed to be a firmly packed accumulation of hair (d). *Source*: Bennett and Russo (1985).

high-fiber pellet did not alter the development of alopecia indicating it is the length of the hay and not the fiber content. Without hay in the diet, the guinea pigs were eating the long hair and that, combined with inadequate exercise and possibly other stressors, results in the formation of hard trichobezoars (Theus et al. 2008).

These firmly compacted hair balls become very large (4–5 cm) and are unlikely to be broken down and passed with medical management, so surgical removal is recommended. Clinical signs may be acute from gastric outflow obstruction or more chronic and insidious, including hyporexia, weight loss, lethargy, and decreased production of feces. The trichobezoar is often palpable as a hard mass in the cranial abdomen. Radiographs with contrast (air or barium) or ultrasound are recommended for a definitive diagnosis.

Stabilize the patient prior to surgery including intravenous (IV) or intraosseous (IOs) fluid therapy. Perform a gastrotomy using a ventral midline celiotomy. Remove the hair ball and irrigate the stomach (Figure 19.9). Close the stomach with a simple continuous or simple interrupted pattern using a rapidly absorbed monofilament absorbable material on an atraumatic (taper) needle. Irrigate the abdomen with warm sterile saline and allow it to dwell to help increase body temperature prior to routine closure of the celiotomy.

Postoperatively provide multimodal analgesia, fluid therapy, nutritional support with syringe feeding as needed, and prokinetic medications. Provide free access to long hay, recommend frequent brushing to remove loose hair, encourage exercise, and minimize stresses. Some have recommended hair ball control medications for cats that contain petrolatum (Theus et al. 2008); however, this has not been studied in rodents and the effects of petrolatum on the cecal flora are unknown.

Cheek Pouch Eversion

Hamsters have well-developed bilateral cheek pouches for food storage that are lined with a thin epithelium. The pouches are very large and extend very caudal (Figure 19.10). Disorders of the cheek pouches include impaction, eversion or prolapse, abscessation, fistula formation, and neoplasia (Capello 2003a). Inappropriate material, such as cage bedding of paper or cotton, or large or small seeds may desiccate and adhere to the mucosa resulting in impaction. These animals present with a history of a mass effect on the lateral aspect of the head. Under sedation or anesthesia, moisten and lubricate the material, then manipulate the material carefully to free it from the mucosal lining of the cheek pouch. Educate the owner regarding cheek pouch impaction and how to reduce the risk of recurrence.

If there is impaction and the hamster tries to massage the material into its mouth, the pouch may evert. This can be unilateral or bilateral. These animals present with tissue protruding from the mouth. Sedate or anesthetize the animal and remove any material still adhered to the mucosa. Insert a small syringe case per os to replace the pouch into its normal position, and then place one or two sutures percutaneously to engage the cheek pouch, bouncing the needle off the syringe case, and then having it exit the skin near the point of entry. A cotton-tipped applicator can be used, but be careful not to suture into the cotton. Loosely tighten the sutures to hold the pouch in its normal position. Do not over tighten the sutures. Generally, after 10–14 days, the tissues will have adhered and the sutures can be removed.

In some cases, the impacted pouch will become infected resulting in an abscess or fistula or both. If the pouch is severely damaged or infected, it can be excised without clinical consequences since pet hamsters do not need to store food (Figure 19.10). If the pouch has everted, place a suture on one side of the exposed tissue proximal to the diseased pouch and excise it using a cut and sew technique. Cut a small section and place a simple continuous suture of a monofilament rapidly absorbable material, and then cut another section and suture that section. Continue until the entire base of the pouch has been transected and sutured. Withhold the normal diet for three to five days and provide a syringe fed soft diet so the tissues will start healing before allowing the hamster to try to pack food into the nonexistent pouch (Miwa and Sladky 2016). Also eliminate any bedding materials the hamster may attempt to push into the pouch.

If a fistula has formed so food and other material are exiting a hole in the skin, approach it from the external surface (Figure 19.10). Make a skin incision over the pouch, but not into it, and dissect the skin from the surface of the pouch. Excise the fistula opening as well. Clamp onto the pouch and apply traction while dissecting the skin off. Once it has been exteriorized enough remove the diseased tissue as described above. Irrigate the site and close the skin in two layers, subcutaneous tissue, and skin.

Neoplasia of the cheek pouch is often not noticed until the mass is large or causes eversion as the hamster tries to empty the pouch. Excise the pouch with the mass and submit it for histologic evaluation. The mass can be removed as described above for treatment of a fistula. Alternatively, it can be excised through an intraoral approach. Make an incision in the mucosa of the pouch and dissect an edge of the incision into the subcutaneous tissues. Grasp the edge of the incision and retract the pouch rostrally dissecting the attachments to the subcutaneous tissues off the pouch going through the incision,

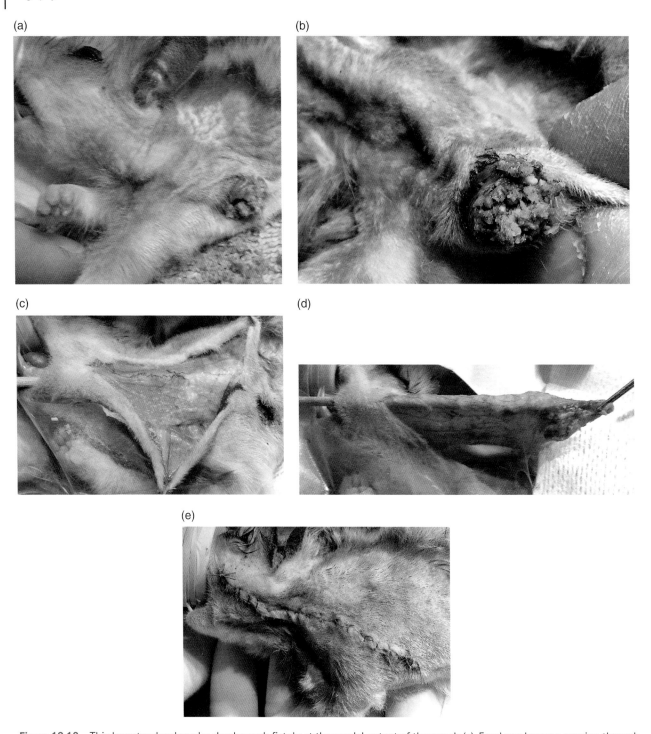

Figure 19.10 This hamster developed a cheek pouch fistula at the caudal extent of the pouch (a). Food can be seen passing through the fistula (b). To remove the pouch, a skin incision was made without incising the cheek pouch mucosa (c). The pouch was carefully dissected from the surrounding tissues from the caudal extent to the oral cavity (d). The oral mucosa was then closed with a simple continuous pattern. After copious irrigation of the remaining soft tissues, the skin was closed with a simple continuous pattern of polyglactin 910 (e). *Source:* Images courtesy of Suzanne Topor; Bennett (2012b).

essentially everting it. Once the mass and pouch have been exteriorized through the mouth, transect the mucosa to remove the pouch and mass, and then suture the mucosa closed with a simple interrupted pattern using a rapidly absorbed suture material.

Other Gastrointestinal Surgery

Rodents are physiologically unable to vomit, but typically do not eat indigestible items and gastrointestinal foreign bodies causing obstruction are rare. Gastrointestinal surgeries in rodents are performed as in other species except the size of suture and needles is small and delicate tissue handling is important.

Rodents are prone to developing adhesions following abdominal surgery, especially hamsters (Redrobe 2002). Reduce the risk of adhesions using gentle tissue handling, minimizing manipulation of the viscera, and avoiding the use of reactive suture materials such as chromic gut. In hamsters, verapamil at 200 μg/kg PO q8h for three days reduced the formation of adhesions (Dunn et al. 1991).

Surgical repair of unilateral perineal hernias has been reported in two chinchillas (Thole et al. 2018). Both presented with perineal swelling and the diagnosis was confirmed with ultrasound. In one chinchilla, the urinary bladder had herniated into the perineum. Both were treated with perineal herniorrhaphy using the internal obturator flap technique. One was orchidectomized and the other was not because of anesthesia concerns. Recurrence did not occur in either at 24 and 12 months postoperatively, respectively. Castration is strongly recommended in dogs with perineal hernias, but the effect of testicular hormones on the occurrence or recurrence of perineal hernias in chinchillas is unknown.

Urinary Tract Surgery

The urinary tract of rodents is similar to that of other mammals; however, the urethra in females does not open into the vagina. There is a separate urethral papilla ventral to the vaginal opening. The pelvic urethra of rodents is relatively large and stones often pass into the urethra and become lodged at the urethral papilla of females and penis of males.

Urolithiasis

Urolithiasis occurs commonly in guinea pigs and stones have been reported to be located in the ureter (Higbie et al. 2019), urinary bladder, and urethra; however, no reports of nephroliths were found. Cystic and urethral calculi were diagnosed in 15 chinchillas (Martel-Aroquette and Mans 2016). Cystic calculi have been diagnosed and surgically removed in hamsters (Bauck and Hagan 1984; Lidderdale and St Pierre 1990). In a laboratory setting, rats are commonly used as a model to study calcium oxalate urolithiasis (the most common type of uroliths diagnosed in humans) because there are stone-forming strains of rats and stone formation can be created using low doses of ethylene glycol; however, spontaneous urolithiasis has not been reported in pet rats or mice.

In guinea pigs, stones have historically been reported to be composed of calcium oxalates (Hoefer 2004); however, a study evaluating the composition of uroliths using infrared spectroscopy and X-ray diffractometry revealed 89% of 127 stones were composed of 100% calcium carbonate and suggests older reports of calcium oxalate uroliths were incorrectly diagnosed using old technology (Hawkins et al. 2015; Rogers et al. 2010; Jekl et al. 2017). Interestingly, chinchillas do not excrete excess dietary calcium in the urine, rather they excrete it into the colon (Martel-Aroquette and Mans 2016). Why they develop calcium carbonate urolithiasis is unknown.

The most common presenting complaint is hematuria (Harkness 1993). Other signs include anorexia, pollakiuria, dysuria, stranguria, incontinence, and pain on abdominal palpation. Partial or complete urinary obstruction can cause life-threatening consequence, so removal of uroliths is recommended. Consider surgical removal when the patient is a good candidate for surgery to determine the composition and prevent them from migrating causing obstruction.

A variety of factors have been proposed as predisposing to the development of urolithiasis in rodents; however, medical dissolution and prevention of urolithiasis in rodents have not been documented. Because of this, recurrence following removal of stones is common (Bennett 2009). A diet low in calcium and urine alkalinizers like potassium citrate may be beneficial; however, a low calcium diet has not been shown to be effective. The pH of rodent urine is normally alkaline. If the urine is acidic, urine alkalizing agents such as potassium citrate may be beneficial. Increasing water intake has been thought to help prevent recurrence. Compared to degus and guinea pigs, chinchillas drink more water when provided an open dish compared to a nipple drinker (Hagen et al. 2014). In one study, administration of hydrochlorothiazide 1 mg/kg once or twice daily was recommended to prevent recurrence (Becker and Schottstedt 2009). Stone analysis and culture of the stone and bladder mucosa provide information for determining a medical plan to try to prevent recurrence.

Radiolucent uroliths have not been documented in rodents. Some mineral dense objects observed on radiographs are actually not within the urinary system. Ultrasound is recommended for all patients with urolithiasis to determine the location of the stones and if they are causing obstruction, as well as to evaluate the kidneys and any secondary effects. Ureterolithiasis is rarely reported in rodents, but cystic and ureteral stones are relatively common.

In a chinchilla with a ureterolith causing complete obstruction resulting in hydroureter and hydronephrosis, nephroureterectomy was perform rather than ureterotomy or ureteral stenting for financial reasons (Higbie et al. 2019). Unfortunately, three months after nephroureterectomy the chinchilla presented with hydroureter and hydronephrosis caused by another stone in the contralateral ureter. Euthanasia was elected and semen-matrix calculi were diagnosed. It is likely that castration after the first obstruction would have prevented new stone formation.

Ureterotomy

While the ureters of rodents are small, microsurgical technique allows for successful removal of ureteral calculi. Ureteral stents are available in sizes as small as 0.7 mm, are hydrophilic, and allow urine to flow past ureteroliths. The ureteral artery and vein are branches of the renal artery and vein and must be preserved during ureteral surgery. Perform a standard ventral midline celiotomy from xiphoid to pubis to allow the body wall to be retracted enough to get exposure to the ureter. Retract the viscera to the contralateral side of the abdomen exposing the retroperitoneal space. Palpate the ureter along its length to identify the stone to minimize dissection. If the stone is in the distal ureter, it might be possible to massage it into the urinary bladder, and then perform a cystotomy.

Open the peritoneum at the stone location and isolate the segment of ureter being careful to preserve the ureteral artery and vein in the fat surrounding the ureter. It is generally recommended to incise the ureter distal to the stone in a normal segment; however, the stone is lodged because it cannot move more distally. Because the ureter cranial to the stone is dilated, it is easier to massage the stone toward the kidney and perform a ureterotomy in a dilated segment of the ureter. Once the obstruction is relieved, the dilated ureter recovers quickly. Use a #11 blade and make an incision as small as possible to allow retrieval of the stone. Irrigate the site and pass a small catheter (26 ga venous catheter) in both directions to flush out any debris. Pass a catheter or suture in both directions to assure the ureter is patent. This is especially important distal to the obstruction. With chronic ureteral obstruction, the lumen may be obliterated. It can be helpful to place a stent to prevent suturing the ureter closed inadvertently. Place a stent across the ureterotomy (use an appropriate size suture to function as the stent). Advance it proximally toward the kidney and distally into the urinary bladder across the incision. Consider closing a small ureterotomy transversely to widen the lumen and decrease the risk of stricture formation. Monitor the incision for leaks for several minute following closure. A simple continuous pattern of a very fine (8-0 or 10-0) monofilament absorbable material is recommended to create a better seal. If cystotomy is indicated to remove cystic calculi, remove the stent suture through the cystotomy. If cystotomy is not performed, use a rapidly absorbable suture for the stent or make a tiny stab incision into the bladder to retrieve the stenting suture, and then close the incision.

Antegrade hydropulsion was used to relieve a ureteral obstruction in a guinea pig (Eshar et al. 2013). Under general anesthesia with ultrasound guidance, pyelocentesis was performed using a 22 ga IV catheter to collect urine directly from the renal pelvis. A 5 ml syringe was connected and saline hydropulsion applied several times while monitoring with ultrasound. The stone did not pass into the bladder, but debris was visualized flowing through the ureter into the bladder past the stone. The owner declined any future evaluation; however, the cavy did well clinically until lost to follow up seven months later.

Cystotomy

Cystotomy can be performed using a caudal ⅓ ventral midline celiotomy if the status of the other abdominal viscera including the kidneys and ureters are known to be healthy based on ultrasound or other advanced imaging obviating a need for a complete exploratory. If possible, preplace a catheter retrograde to minimize the risk of stones migrating into the urethra. The ventral and lateral ligaments of the urinary bladder can be sacrificed if needed. Place stay sutures, retract the bladder cranially, and isolate it with saline moistened gauze. Make the incision on the ventral aspect of the bladder cranial to the trigone and use the stay sutures to open the incision allowing retrieval of stones. Trim a 1 mm piece of mucosa from the edge of the incision and submit it for culture and sensitivity testing. Use a bladder spoon or curette (be careful if the edge is sharp not to traumatize the mucosa) to carefully scoop out the calculi. Once bladder mucosa and stones have been collected, administer an appropriate IV antibiotic to be continued postoperatively. Withhold antibiotics until after samples have been collected in order to not affect the ability to culture organisms. Irrigate the bladder to flush any small stones out. Note that if stones escape into the abdominal cavity, it is not necessary to retrieve them as the minerals are quickly absorbed. If a retrograde catheter has been placed, once it appears all stones have been removed, slowly withdraw the catheter while injecting saline to flush any urethral stones into the bladder where they can be retrieved. Next, pass an appropriately sized catheter antegrade flushing with saline as the catheter is advanced through the urethra to clear any stones that may have passed into it. If possible, repeat this process both retrograde and antegrade to assure all stones have been removed. Close the bladder with a single layer of a rapidly absorbable material in a simple continuous or interrupted pattern. Instill warm saline into the abdomen and allow it to dwell for several minutes. Allow urine to accumulate in the bladder and apply pressure to check for leaks. Because of the small size and often-thin bladder wall, injecting saline into the bladder and expressing it to test for leaks may actually create leaks. Obtain postoperative radiographs to include the urethra to confirm that all stones have been removed. Diurese the patient after surgery for 36–48 hours.

Percutaneous cystolithotomy can be performed with minimal morbidity which may be important especially in patients with recurrent urolithiasis requiring multiple cystotomies. Euthanasia is a common cause of death in rodents with recurrent urolithiasis, often elected over treatment even the first episode (Martel-Arguette and Mans 2016). Place a catheter retrograde and instill enough saline to make the bladder easy to palpate. Make a 1–2 cm incision in the body wall over the midpoint of the bladder and enter the peritoneal cavity being careful not to incise the bladder. Being distended, it displaces other viscera and is easy to identify. Place sutures in the body wall and bladder wall circumferentially to create a seal so urine does not enter the peritoneal cavity. Incise the bladder wall and proceed as described above for cystotomy. The advantages of this procedure are that the incision is very small (1–2 cm), the entire peritoneal cavity is not opened reducing the risk of hypothermia, and the gastrointestinal tract is not manipulated. Once all stones have been removed, close the urinary bladder, replace it into the abdomen, close the body wall routinely, and then make radiographs to ensure all stones have been removed.

Because of the relatively large urethral diameter in rodents, cystic calculi up to 5 mm diameter can be removed from female guinea pigs using transurethral cystoscopy (Wenger and Hatt 2015; Pizzi 2009). This technique allows evaluation of the bladder and urethral mucosa as well.

Postoperatively, if the patient is not urinating after surgery, place a retrograde urethral catheter and leave it in place for 2–3 days, if possible, to allow the inflammation to subside. Administer nonsteroidal anti-inflammatory drugs (NSAIDs) to reduce inflammation, but be cautious if the patient has evidence of renal compromise.

Urethrotomy

Urethral obstruction with calculi seems to occur more commonly in female than male rodents. In most cases, urethral calculi can be retrohydropulsed into the bladder and removed by cystotomy. Many stones pass to the urethral papilla and become lodged. Often, these stones have been lodged for a long time. If stones are in the pelvic urethra, the best option is retrohyropulsion because the alternative is pubic symphysiotomy to access the pelvic urethra. For stones in the distal urethra perform a urethrotomy. Incise over the stone through the skin, subcutaneous tissues, and urethra to retrieve the stone(s). Close the urethrotomy primarily or allow healing by second intention. In a study in

dogs, there was no difference in healing between sutured and unsutured urethrotomies (Weber et al. 1985). Unsutured urethrotomies did bleed more after surgery, but it was not clinically significant.

For stones at the urethral papilla, incise over the stone and remove it (Figure 19.11). It is not necessary to suture the wound leaving it to heal by second intention. In one report, a urethral diverticulum was the reported location of a urethral calculus (Parkinson et al. 2017). The stone was removed and ablation of the diverticulum was attempted. Three months later two stones were within the diverticulum. This time the stones were removed, and a urethrostomy was created to include the diverticulum eliminating the location stones had accumulated and creating a large opening through which future stones might be able to pass and not obstruct the terminal urethra. In patients with recurrent urethroliths that lodge at the urethral papilla, this type of urethrostomy should be considered.

Intraabdominal Masses

Masses may arise in the abdomen associated with any visceral organ. Hamsters seem to be resistant to development of tumors, while older gerbils have a high incidence. Intraabdominal tumors reported in gerbils include tumors of the reproductive tract, spleen, liver, and pancreas; however, reports of successful surgical removal of these tumors are lacking (Toft 1992).

Polycystic disease involving the liver and kidneys are relatively common in hamsters (Capello 2003a). Surgery is not an option; however, if the disease is confined to one kidney or liver lobe surgical excision might be indicated. Lymphosarcoma is another common neoplasm affecting hamsters (Toft 1992). If there is a mass causing intestinal obstruction or a solitary mass, surgical excision may be indicated, but chemotherapy is recommended for diffuse disease. Rats are prone to developing renal neoplasia that may be bilateral. Unilateral nephrectomy can be performed, but surgery is not indicated for bilateral tumors (Cooper 1994; Greenacre 2004; Toft 1992).

Adrenal tumors have been reported in older rodents as an incidental finding at necropsy (Shumaker et al. 1974; Toft 1992). In older rats, adrenocortical tumors, malignant and benign, are common and pheochromocytomas have also been reported in rats. Metastasis has been reported (Toft 1992). Adrenal tumors in hamsters affect males more commonly than females and are usually benign cortical adenomas causing Cushing's syndrome with alopecia, hyperpigmentation, and behavioral changes (Toft 1992). The anatomic location of the adrenal glands is with the

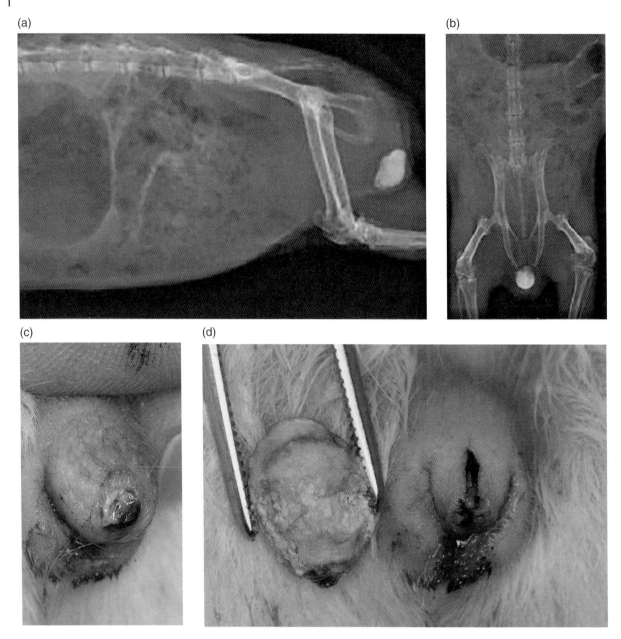

Figure 19.11 (a, b) A radiodense urethral calculus located at the urethral papilla in a guinea pig (arrow). (c) The stone can be seen at the urethral papilla. (d) Make an incision through the skin and urethra onto the stone to allow it to be removed. Allow the incision to heal by second intention. *Source:* Bennett (2012a).

right adhered to the caudal vena cava and the left a short distance away from it; however, there are no reports of successful removal of adrenal tumors in rodents.

Thoracic Surgery

The main indications for thoracic surgery in rodents are pulmonary tumors and lung lobe abscesses. Lung tumors are reported to be the most common neoplasm of guinea pigs representing 30–35% of tumors in guinea pigs over three years of age (Cooper 1994; Harkness et al. 2010). Bronchogenic carcinomas and alveolar carcinomas have

been reported, but the vast majority are benign bronchogenic pulmonary adenomas. Most are slow growing, and clinical signs are usually not recognized until late. In mice, lung tumors are the most common neoplasm with a reported incidence of 28% (Prejean et al. 1973). Lung tumors appear to be rare in other species of rodents (Greenacre 2004).

Another indication for thoracic surgery is lung lobe abscesses. These patients are typically more clinically ill than those with lung tumors. When the lung is manipulated, pus can go out the lobar bronchus into the mainstem and then into other lobes. It is essential to carefully lift the lung lobe out of the chest and immediately place a clamp at the hilum to stop any pus from exiting. Then place a ligature or hemostatic clip proximal to the clamp and transect between the ligature/clip and clamp to remove the lung lobe.

One of the big challenges with thoracic surgery in rodents is ventilating the patient when the chest is open. Techniques have been described for endotracheal intubation of guinea pigs (Kramer et al. 1998; Turner et al. 1992). It is feasible to intubate guinea pigs and chinchillas with a 2.0 mm endotracheal tube using a blind technique or using a rigid endoscope.

If an endotracheal tube cannot be placed per os, consider a temporary tracheostomy. Make a small (~1 cm) in the skin on the ventral midline of the neck. Identify and separate the sternocephalicus muscles to expose the trachea. Carefully dissect the areolar tissue from the trachea. Do not damage the recurrent laryngeal nerves on each side. Place a suture around a tracheal ring caudal to the proposed location of the tracheotomy and tie a large loop to be used to lift the trachea to the surface. Make a transverse incision between rings about ⅓ the diameter on the ventral aspect. Insert a mosquito hemostat into the incision and spread it to enlarge the opening without damaging the recurrent laryngeal nerves. Lift the suture to bring the incision into view and insert the tube. Once the procedure is complete and the patient well recovered, remove the tube and allow the incision to heal by second intention.

In rats, a technique for pulmonary lobectomy without endotracheal intubation has been reported with low mortality – 51 of 54 rats survived (Roman et al. 2002). The three fatalities occurred early in the study as a result of blood loss. Pulmonary lobectomy took <10 minutes total with the chest being open <3 minutes. Use a face mask that fits tightly around the muzzle to allow ventilation at 20 bpm during thoracotomy. Monitor lung inflation visually during the procedure. While the study was done in rats, it is likely this method would work well for other rodents needing a thoracotomy if endotracheal intubation is not feasible.

Lateral Intercostal Thoracotomy

For pulmonary lobectomy, under magnification perform a lateral intercostal thoracotomy at the fourth or fifth intercostal space to access the pulmonary hilum. After entering the thoracic cavity, place a Heiss retractor to maintain exposure. Identify and exteriorize the affected lung lobe. Because of the small size of most rodents, it is not feasible to isolate the pulmonary artery and vein to ligate or clip them individually. Rather, place a hemostatic clip or ligature at the hilum to ligate the artery, vein, and bronchus *en bloc*. Place a hemostat distal to the ligature and transect distal to the ligature to remove the lobe. Check the stump for hemorrhage, then fill the chest with warm saline to look for air leaks manifest as bubbles. Place a thoracostomy tube such as a 3.5 or 5 fr red rubber or commercially available thoracostomy tube at about the eighth intercostal space dorsally, then directed ventral and cranial. Place sutures circumferentially around the ribs adjacent to the thoracotomy to appose the ribs, but do not over tighten them causing the ribs to overlap. Close the muscles, subcutaneous tissues, and skin, and then evacuate the chest. Postoperatively, once there is minimal fluid and air for a two to three hours remove the tube. In a study in healthy dogs, a chest tube alone stimulated production of 1.43 ± 0.59 ml/kg/d pleural exudate that became septic in 4 days (Hung et al. 2016).

Ventral Midline Thoracotomy

For larger masses that cannot be remove through a lateral thoracotomy, perform a ventral midline thoracotomy analogous to a median sternotomy; however, the sternebrae are not divided. With the patient in dorsal recumbency, make a skin incision from the ventral thoracic inlet to the xiphoid. Dissect the pectoralis muscles off each side to expose the sternebrae. In rodents, the sternebrae are too small to split longitudinally as for a median sternotomy. Instead, disarticulate the ribs on one side at their attachment to the sternebrae from cranial (manubrium) to caudal or from caudal (xiphoid) to cranial. If possible, leave two to three ribs attached for stability after closure. After the lung lobectomy is complete, place a thoracostomy tube. To close, place figure of eight monofilament slowly absorbable suture around each sternebra and rib in the intercostal muscles to bring the ribs back into position (Figure 17.19c). Close the pectoralis muscles together along the midline which provides more stability. Finally, close the subcutaneous tissues and skin, and then evacuate the chest.

Enucleation and Exenteration

Proptosis is a common problem, primarily in hamsters. When exposed even for a short time the globe dries out and it is not possible to save, so enucleation or exenteration is recommended. Like rabbits, rodents have a large orbital venous sinus that surrounds the Harderian gland and extraocular muscles. Murid rodents do not have a third eyelid. These procedures in rodents are analogous to those in rabbits (see Chapter 17); however, there tends to be less hemorrhage and it is easier to control.

Ear Surgery

Otitis media is common in rodents. In a study of guinea pigs 13.4% of 426 animals had otitis media that was associated with respiratory disease (Boot and Walvoort 1986). The authors suggest otitis media is a "major disease problem" in guinea pigs. Access to the bulla of chinchillas is possible because it is large and easy to access through a dorsal approach (Meredith and Richardson 2015). Otitis media and interna in rats and mice are typically associated with infection with *Mycoplasma pulmonis* and *Streptococcus pneumonia* (Meredith and Richardson 2015).

Surgical management of otitis in rodents is rarely reported. In a rat with otitis media, a surgical approach was made to the acoustic meatus to allow irrigation of the bulla (Odberg 2001). Ear canal ablation with pinnectomy has been described for treating abscesses and neoplasia in hamsters (Capello 2011; Martorell et al. 2010).

Tail Degloving

Tail slip is the term used to refer to degloving of the skin off the tail and occurs most commonly in gerbils, chinchillas, and degus because their skin is more loosely attached, but it has been reported in other rodents (Miwa and Sladky 2016). Degloving of the tail occurs from holding the animal off the substrate by the distal ½ of the tail. Left untreated, the exposed denuded portion of the tail will desiccate and eventually slough. This condition may be painful or there may be denervation of the segment of tail resulting in self mutilation. While the risk of sepsis is remote, local infection is possible, so tail amputation is recommended.

This procedure can be accomplished under sedation with a local block using 0.01 ml of a 5% solution of bupivacaine injected proximal to the caudal edge of the skin. Use a tourniquet to control hemorrhage until the tail has been removed. Incise healthy skin proximal to the wound to provide a fresh incision for primary closure. Use a 25 ga needle to identify an intervertebral space proximal to the skin incision. Retract the skin proximally to expose the interspace and disarticulate the tail. When skin is released, it will cover the end of the exposed vertebra. Release the tourniquet and control any hemorrhage with electrocautery or electrosurgery. Ligatures are not usually needed as these vessels are small. Appose the skin in two layers over the vertebra, subcutaneous tissue and skin. With gentle tissue handling, self-mutilation postoperative is uncommon.

Pododermatitis

Pododermatitis in rodents is caused by inappropriate husbandry which may be due to not changing bedding frequently enough or the cage flooring is inappropriate with wire floors being especially problematic. In dealing with pododermatitis, the most important factor is correcting the underlying husbandry issues making the prognosis for complete recovery guarded. Much like elbow hygromas in dogs and other pressure/trauma-related wounds, surgery often makes the problem worse. It does not address the underlying husbandry problems and the wound often becomes larger after surgery.

Some success has been reported using aggressive surgical debridement with wound management daily to include debridement, wound irrigation, and bandaging to take pressure off the wound using donut-type padding around the wound. Obtain cultures and use appropriate systemic antibiotic therapy. Continue wound management until the wound has epithelialized. Scar tissue epithelium is fragile and the wound will open again if the husbandry is not corrected. Even then, it is helpful to continue to bandage and pad the area allowing time for the tissue to strengthen. Scar tissue will never be as strong as the original skin. Alternatively, apply a topical product such as New-Skin Liquid Bandage (Moberg Pharma, North America LLC, Cedar Knolls, NJ, USA) to help protect the new epithelium.

If it is possible to close the skin over the wound, the author has had success using aggressive surgical debridement, wound irrigation, implantation of small AIPMMA or POP beads, and closing the wound primarily. If the skin cannot be closed, place a simple continuous suture across the wound bed to hold the beads in place. It is vital to obtain cultures so appropriate antibiotics are used or the beads can become a nidus for bacteria.

Recovery

Pay attention to the patient's body temperature and provide thermal support as needed. Recovery should occur in a warm, quiet, well-ventilated area. Incubators are ideal because temperature and humidity can be controlled, and oxygen can be delivered if indicated. Alternatively, a small dark quiet cage with a circulating warm air or warm water blanket can be used. Be careful using supplemental heat sources where the temperature is unknown or cannot be controlled as these can cause serious thermal burns. If the patient remains recumbent, turn it from one side to the other every 60 minutes to minimize pulmonary atelectasis. Line the cage with clean paper towels until a scab has formed. Keep the patient isolated so other animals do not traumatize the wound or attack the patient perceiving it to be ill or injured. Continue to provide fluid therapy and nutritional support as needed until the patient is eating, drinking, urinating, and defecting well. Avoid using bandages because most rodents do not tolerate them. If a bandage is needed, try making a paste from metronidazole tablets and putting it on the bandage. It is bitter and discourages them from chewing the bandage. Antianxiety medications can also be very helpful for getting rodents used to having a bandage. A yoke can also be helpful to prevent self-trauma or chewing at bandages, and a technique for making them has been described (Figures 19.12 and 19.13) (Hoyt 1998). Make sure to observe the patient after applying a yoke to assure it adapts to the device and is able to eat and drink with it on.

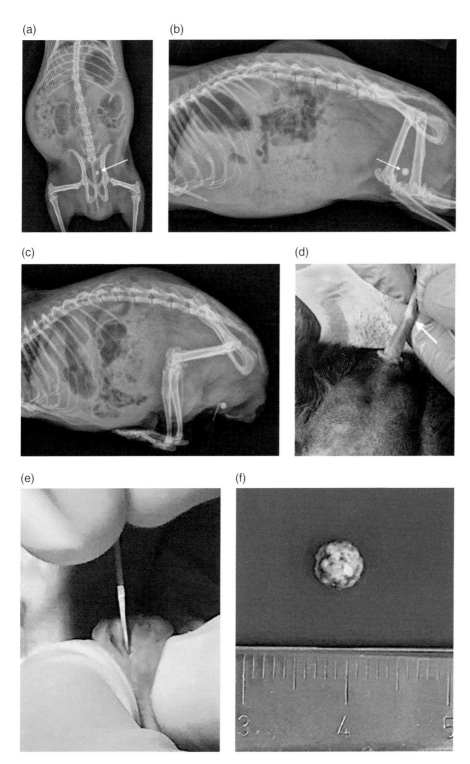

Figure 19.12 A male guinea pig presented for dysuria. Radiographs (a, b) show a urolith (arrow), but it is not possible to accurately determine the location: urethra or urinary bladder. With the legs pulled cranially (c), it is clear the stone is in the urethra. The guinea pig was sedated and the penis exteriorized exposing the stone (arrow) in the urethra (d). A urethrotomy was performed (e) and the stone removed (f). It is not necessary to suture the urethra. Allow it to heal by second intention.

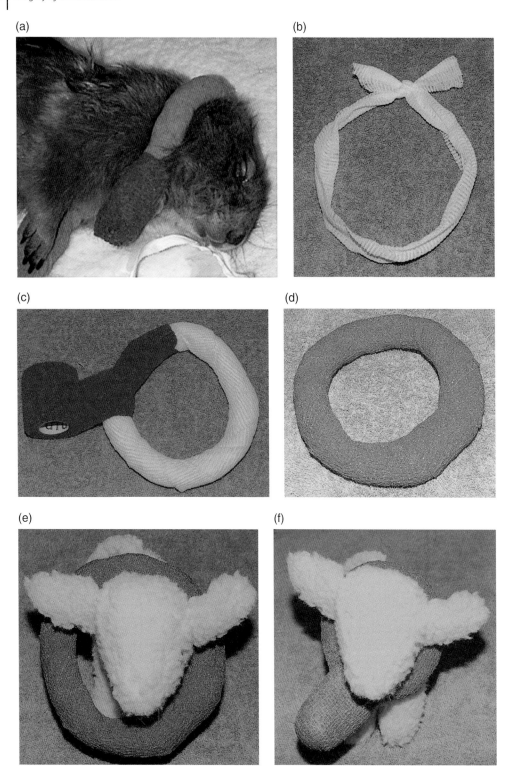

Figure 19.13 A yoke used to prevent self-mutilation in a prairie dog with a spinal cord injury (a). Make a yoke by creating a ring that will be large enough to pass over the head of the patient (b). Wrap cast padding and self-adhesive tape (c) to create a padded ring (d). Place the ring around the neck of the patient (e). Pinch one side of the ring until it is snug but not tight around the neck, and then wrap self-adhesive tape to hold it snug (f). *Source:* Images courtesy of Geoffrey Pye.

References

Bauck, L.A. and Hagan, R.J. (1984). Cystotomy for treatment of urolithiasis in a hamster. *Journal of the American Veterinary Medical Association* 184: 99–100.

Becker, W. and Schottstedt, T. (2009). Medical prophylaxis of calcium urolithiasis in two Guinea pigs. *Kleintierpraxis* 54: 389–392.

Benitz, K.F. and Kramer, A.W. (1965). Spontaneous tumors in the Mongolian gerbil. *Laboratory Animal Care* 15: 281–294.

Bennett, R.A. (2009). Rodents: soft tissue surgery. In: *BSAVA Manual of Rodents and Ferrets* (eds. E. Keeble and A. Meredith), 73–85. Gloucester: British Small Animal Veterinary Association.

Bennett, R.A. (2012a). Guinea pigs and chinchillas – soft tissue surgery. In: *Ferrets, Rabbits, and Rodents – Clinical Medicine and Surgery*, 3e (eds. K.Q. Quesenberry and J.W. Carpenter), 326–338. St. Louis, MO: Elsevier.

Bennett, R.A. (2012b). Small rodents – soft tissue surgery. In: *Ferrets, Rabbits, and Rodents – Clinical Medicine and Surgery*, 3e (eds. K.Q. Quesenberry and J.W. Carpenter), 373–392. St. Louis, MO: Elsevier.

Bennett, R.A. and Mullen, H.S. (2003a). Guinea pigs, chinchillas, and prairie dogs – soft tissue surgery. Guinea pigs and chinchillas – soft tissue surgery. In: *Ferrets, Rabbits, and Rodents – Clinical Medicine and Surgery: Includes Sugar Gliders and Hedgehogs*, 2e (eds. K.Q. Quesenberry and J.W. Carpenter), 274–284. St. Louis, MO: Elsevier.

Bennett, R.A. and Mullen, H.S. (2003b). Small rodents – soft tissue surgery. In: *Ferrets, Rabbits, and Rodents – Clinical Medicine and Surgery: Includes Sugar Gliders and Hedgehogs*, 2e (eds. K.Q. Quesenberry and J.W. Carpenter), 316–328. St. Louis, MO: Elsevier.

Bennett, R.A. and Russo, E.A. (1985). What is your diagnosis? Soft tissue density mass in the stomach consistent with a trichobezoar or phytobezoar. *Journal of the American Veterinary Medical Association* 186: 812–814.

Bingel, S.A. (1995). Pathologic findings in an aging Mongolian gerbil (*Meriones unguiculatus*) colony. *Laboratory Animal Science* 45: 597–600.

Bodri, M.S. and Walker, L.M. (1993). What is your diagnosis? Poor intra- and retroperitoneal contrast suggestive of emaciation and alimentary visceral displacement consistent with bladder and uterine mass. *Journal of the American Veterinary Medical Association* 202: 654–655.

Boot, R. and Walvoort, H.C. (1986). Otitis media in Guinea pigs: pathology and bacteriology. *Laboratory Animals* 20: 242–248.

Brown, C. (2008). Abdominal castration in the rat. *Laboratory Animals* 37: 36–37.

Capello, V. (2003a). Surgical techniques in pet hamsters. *Exotic DVM* 5 (3): 32–37.

Capello, V. (2003b). Techniques for neutering pet hamsters. *Exotic DVM* 5 (4): 21–26.

Capello, V. (2004). Prescrotal open technique for neutering a degu. *Exotic DVM* 6 (6): 29–31.

Capello, V. (2011). Common surgical procedures in pet rodents. *Journal of Exotic Pet Medicine* 20: 294–307.

de Chaves, G., Moretti, M., Castro, A.A. et al. (2009). Effects of long-term ovariectomy on anxiety and behavioral despair in rats. *Physiology & Behavior* 97: 420–425.

Collins, B.R. (1988). Common disease and medical management of rodents and lagomorphs. In: *Exotic Animals* (eds. E.R. Jacobson and G.V. Kollias), 261–316. New York: Churchill Livingstone.

Cooper, J.E. (1994). Tips on tumors. In: *Proceedings of the North American Veterinary Conference*, 897–898. Orlando, FL: NAVC.

Dunn, R.C., Steinleitner, A.J., and Lambert, H. (1991). Synergistic effect of intraperitoneally administered calcium channel blockade and recombinant tissue plasminogen activator to prevent adhesion formation in an animal model. *American Journal of Obstetrics and Gynecology* 164: 1327–1330.

Eatwell, K. (2003). Ovarian and uterine disease in Guinea pigs: a review of five cases. *Exotic DVM* 5 (5): 37–39.

Eshar, D., Lee-Chow, B., and Chalmers, H.J. (2013). Ultrasound-guided percutaneous antegrade hydropulsion to relieve ureteral obstruction in a pet Guinea pig (*Cavia procellus*). 54: 1142–1145.

Field, K.J., Griffith, J.W., and Lang, C.M. (1989). Spontaneous reproductive tract leiomyomas in aged Guinea pigs. *Journal of Comparative Pathology* 101: 287–294.

Gerold, S., Huisinga, E., Iglauer, F. et al. (1997). Influence of feeding hay on the alopecia of breeding Guinea pigs. *Zentralblatt für Veterinärmedizin. Reihe A* 44: 341–348.

van Goethem, B., Schaefers-Okkens, A., and Kirpensteijn, J. (2006). Making a rational choice between ovariectomy and ovariohysterectomy in the dog: a discussion of the benefits of either technique. *Veterinary Surgery* 35: 136–143.

Greenacre, C.B. (2004). Spontaneous tumors of small mammals. *Veterinary Clinics of North America: Exotic Animal Practice* 7: 627–651.

Hagen, K., Clauss, M., and Hatt, J.M. (2014). Drinking preference in chinchillas (*Chinchilla laniger*), degus (*Octodon degus*), and Guinea pigs (*Cavia porcellus*). *Journal of Animal Physiology and Animal Nutrition* 98: 942–927.

Harkness, J.E. (1993). *A Practitioner's Guide to Domestic Rodents*. Denver, CO: American Animal Hospital Association.

Harkness, J.E., Turner, P.V., Vande Woude, S. et al. (2010). *Harkness and Wagner's Biology and Medicine of Rabbits and Rodents*, 5e. Ames, IA: Wiley-Blackwell.

Hawkins, M.G., Ruby, A.L., Drazenovich, T.L. et al. (2015). Composition and characteristics of urinary calculi from Guinea pigs. *Journal of the American Veterinary Medical Association* 234: 214–220.

Henry, K.R., Chole, R.A., and McGinn, M.D. (1983). Age-related increase of spontaneous aural cholesteatoma in the Mongolian gerbil. *Archives of Otolaryngology* 109: 19–21.

Higbie, C.T., DiGeronimo, P.M., Bennett, R.A. et al. (2019). Semen matrix calculi in a juvenile chinchilla (*Chinchilla lanigera*). *Journal of Exotic Pet Medicine* 28: 69–75.

Hoefer, H.L. (2004). Guinea pig urolithiasis. *Exotic DVM* 6 (2): 23–25.

Hotchkiss, C.E. (1995). Effect of surgical removal of subcutaneous tumors on survival of rats. *Journal of the American Veterinary Medical Association* 206: 1575–1579.

Hoyt, R.F. Jr. (1998). Abdominal surgery of pet rabbits. In: *Current Techniques in Small Animal Surgery* (ed. M.J. Bojrab), 777–790. Baltimore, MD: Williams & Wilkins.

Hung, G.C., Gaunt, M.C., Rubin, J.E. et al. (2016). Quantification and characterization of pleural fluid in healthy dogs with thoracostomy tubes. *American Journal of Veterinary Research* 77: 1387–1391.

Jackson, T., Heath, L.A., Hulin, M.S. et al. (1996). Squamous cell carcinoma of the midventral abdominal pad in three gerbils. *Journal of the American Veterinary Medical Association* 209: 789–791.

Jekl, V., Hauptman, K., and Knotek, Z. (2017). Evidence-based advances in rodent medicine. *Veterinary Clinics: Exotic Animal Practice* 20: 805–816.

Jenkins, J.R. (2000). Surgical sterilization in small mammals. Spay and castration. *Veterinary Clinics of North America: Exotic Animal Practice* 3: 617–627.

Johnson, D. (2002). Exotic pet care: degus. *Exotic DVM* 4 (4): 39–42.

Johnson-Delaney, C. (2002). Ovariohysterectomy in a rat. *Exotic DVM* 4 (4): 17–21.

Keller, L.S., Griffith, J.W., and Lang, C.M. (1987). Reproductive failure associated with cystic rete ovarii in Guinea pigs. *Veterinary Pathology* 24: 335–339.

Kitchen, D.N., Carlton, W.W., and Bickford, A.A. (1975). A report of fourteen spontaneous tumors of the Guinea pig. *Laboratory Animal Science* 25: 92–102.

Kramer, K., Grimbergen, J.A., van Iperen, D.J. et al. (1998). Oral endotracheal intubation of Guinea pigs. *Laboratory Animals* 32: 162–164.

Krohn, D.E. and Barthold, S.W. (1984). Biology and diseases of rats. In: *Laboratory Animal Medicine* (eds. J.G. Fox, B.J. Cohen and F.M. Loew), 116–122. Orlando, FL: Academic Press.

Kuenzel, F. and Hittmair, K. (2002). Sonographische diagnosestrellung eines trichobezoars bei einem langhaarmeerschweinchen. *Wiener Tierärztliche Monatsschrift* 89: 66–69.

Lejnieks, D.V. (2007). Urethral plug in a rat (*Rattus norvegicus*). *Journal of Exotic Pet Medicine* 16: 183–2185.

Lewis, W. (2003). Cystic ovaries in gerbils. *Exotic DVM* 5 (1): 12–13.

Lidderdale, J.A. and St Pierre, S.J. (1990). Cystotomy for treatment of urolithiasis in a hamster. *The Veterinary Record* 127: 364.

Lipman, N.S. and Foltz, C. (1995). Hamsters. In: *Handbook for Rodent and Rabbit Medicine* (eds. K. Laber-Laid, M.M. Swindle and P. Flecknell), 65–82. New York: Pergamon.

Martel-Arquette, A. and Mans, C. (2016). Urolithiasis in chinchillas: 15 cases (2007–2011). *Journal of Small Animal Practice* 57: 260–264.

Martorell, J., Martinez, A., and Soto, S. (2010). Complete ablation of the vertical auditive conduct and ear pinna in a dwarf hamster with an aural spontaneous squamous cell carcinoma. *Journal of Exotic Pet Medicine* 19: 96–100.

Mayer, J. (2003). The use of GnRH to treat cystic ovaries in a Guinea pig. *Exotic DVM* 5 (5): 36.

McCready, J., Beaufrere, H., Singh, A. et al. (2020). Laparoscopic ovariectomy in guinea pigs: a pilot study. *Veterinary Surgery* 39: 131–137.

Meredith, A. and Richardson, J. (2015). Neurological disease of rabbits and rodents. *Journal of Exotic Pet Medicine* 24: 21–33.

Miwa, Y. and Sladky, K.K. (2016). Common surgical procedures of rodents, ferrets, hedgehogs, and sugar gliders. *Veterinary Clinics: Exotic Animal* 19: 205–244.

Mullen, H.S. (2000). Nonreproductive surgery in small mammals. *Veterinary Clinics of North America: Exotic Animal Practice* 3: 629–645.

Nelson, W.B. (2004). Technique for neutering pet chinchillas. *Exotic DVM* 6 (5): 27–30.

Nielsen, T.D., Holt, S., Rueløkke, M.L. et al. (2003). Ovarian cysts in Guinea pigs: influence of age and reproductive status on prevalence and size. *Journal of Small Animal Practice* 44: 257–260.

Odberg (2001). Treatment of middle ear infection in a rat. *Exotic DVM* 3: 8.

Parkinson, L.A.B., Hausmann, J.C., Hardie, R.J. et al. (2017). Urethral diverticulum and urolithiasis in a female Guinea pig (*Cavia porcellus*). *Journal of the American Veterinary Medical Association* 251: 1313–1317.

Peters, L.J. (1991). The Guinea pig: an overview. Part I and II. *Compendium on Continuing Education for the Practicing Veterinarian* 4: 15–27.

Pizzi, R. (2009). Cystoscopic removal of a uroliths from a pet Guinea pig. *The Veterinary Record* 165: 148–149.

Planas-Silva, M.D., Rutherford, T.M., and Stone, M.C. (2008). Prevention of age-related spontaneous mammary tumors in outbred rats by late ovariectomy. *Cancer Detection and Prevention* 32: 65–71.

Popesko, P., Rajtova, V., and Horak, J. (1992). *Atlas of the Anatomy of Small Laboratory Animals: Rabbit and Guinea Pig*, vol. 1, 148–240. London: Wolfe Publishing.

Powers, M.Y., Campbell, B.G., and Finch, N.P. (2008). Preputial damage and lateral penile displacement during castration in a degu. *Journal of the American Veterinary Medical Association* 232: 1013–1015.

Prejean, J.D., Peckham, J.C., Casey, A.E. et al. (1973). Spontaneous tumors in Sprague-Dawley rats and Swiss mice. *Cancer Research* 33: 2768–2773.

Quattropani, S.L. (1977). Serous cysts of the aging Guinea pig ovary. I. Light microscopy and origin. *The Anatomical Record* 188: 351–360.

Quattropani, S.L. (1981). Serous cystadenoma formation in Guinea pig ovaries. *Journal of Submicroscopic Cytology* 13: 337–345.

Redrobe, S. (2002). Soft tissue surgery in rabbits and rodents. *Seminars in Avian and Exotic Pet Medicine* 11: 231–245.

Rogers, K.D., Jones, B., Roberts, L. et al. (2010). Composition of uroliths in small domestic animals in the United Kingdom. *The Veterinary Journal* 188: 228–230.

Roman, C.D., Hanley, G.A., and Beauchamp, R.D. (2002). Operative technique for safe pulmonary lobectomy in Sprague-Dawley rats. *Contemporary Topics in Laboratory Animal Science* 41: 28–30.

Rozanska, D., Rozanska, P., Orzelski, M. et al. (2016). Unilateral flank ovariohysterectomy in Guinea pigs (*Cavia porcellus*). *New Zealand Veterinary Journal* 64: 360–363.

Rueløkke, M.L., McEvoy, F.J., Nielsen, T.D. et al. (2003). Cystic ovaries in Guinea pigs. *Exotic DVM* 5.5: 33–36.

Shumaker, R.C., Paik, S.K., and Houser, W.D. (1974). Tumors in Gerbillinae: a literature review and report of a case. *Laboratory Animal Science* 24: 688–690.

Theus, M., Bitterli, F., and Foldenauer, U. (2008). Successful treatment of a gastric trichobezoar in a Peruvian Guinea pig *(Cavia aperea porcellus)*. *Journal of Exotic Pet Medicine* 17: 148–151.

Thole, M., Schuhmann, B., Kostlinger, S. et al. (2018). Treatment of unilateral perineal hernias in two male chinchillas (*Chinchilla lanigera*). *Journal of Exotic Pet Medicine* 27: 43–49.

Toft, J.D. (1992). Commonly observed spontaneous neoplasms in rabbits, rats, Guinea pigs, hamsters, and gerbils. *Seminars in Avian and Exotic Pet Medicine* 1: 80–92.

Turner, M.A., Thomas, P., and Sheridan, D.J. (1992). An improved method for direct laryngeal intubation in the Guinea pig. *Laboratory Animals* 26: 25–28.

Vergneau-Grosset, C., Keel, M.K., Goldsmith, D. et al. (2016). Description of the prevalence, histologic characteristics, concomitant abnormalities, and outcome of mammary gland tumors in companion rats (*Rattus norvegicus*): 100 cases (1990–2015). *Journal of the American Veterinary Medical Association* 249: 1170–1179.

Weber, W.J., Boothe, H.W., Brassard, J.A. et al. (1985). Comparison of the healing of prescrotal urethrotomy incisions in the dog: sutured vs. nonsutured. *American Journal of Veterinary Research* 46: 1309–1315.

Wenger, S. and Hatt, J.M. (2015). Transurethral cystoscopy and endoscopic uroliths removal in female Guinea pigs (*Cavia porcellus*). *Veterinary Clinics of North America: Exotic Animal Practice* 18: 359–367.

20

Soft Tissue Surgery in Hedgehogs

Daniel J. Duffy and R. Avery Bennett

Hedgehogs are members of the family Erinaceidae in the order Insectivora. There are 16 species of hedgehogs with the African pygmy hedgehog (*Atelerix albiventris*) being the species most commonly kept as pets (Carpenter 2010). African hedgehogs have a simple stomach and are able to vomit. They have five toes on the front feet, but only four on the rear. They are also called four-toed hedgehogs and white-bellied hedgehogs (Carpenter 2010).

The tip of the prepuce is located on the caudal midline of the abdomen. It has been reported that the testicles of hedgehogs are intra-abdominal and orchiectomy must be performed through a celiotomy (Johnson-Delaney 2007); however, this does not appear to be the case. They do not have a defined scrotal sac, but each testicle is located lateral to the penis between the anus and the tip of the prepuce in para-anal recesses in the inguinal area (Ivey and Carpenter 2004).

The vulva is located immediately cranial to the anus. The uterus is bicornuate with a single cervix, but no uterine body (Figure 20.1). The horns are tightly curled, located in the caudal abdomen, and have been described as being similar to those of cows (Figure 20.2) (Johnson 2016). The vaginal vault is relatively long. It has been suggested that because the pubic symphysis does not fuse until 18 months of age, if a female hedgehog has not reproduced prior to that age it may be predisposed to dystocia (Ivey and Carpenter 2004); however, reports of dystocia in hedgehogs are rare (Vuolo and Whittington 2008).

There are two types of hair: the ventral aspect has more typical hair and the crown and dorsum have spines. The ventral haired skin contains numerous sweat and sebaceous glands while the spine covered skin does not have glands. The spiny skin has a thick dermis with a large amount of subcutaneous fat, but few blood vessels, while the epidermis is thin and fragile. The spines are composed of keratin with a complex internal structure making them strong and elastic but light weight. They are firmly attached to the follicle by a round bulb of basal cells. During anagen, they are very difficult to pull out. They are replaced every 18 months one by one, so there is no molting cycle. There are no spines on the midline of the crown, it is bald.

When preparing for surgery, cut the ventral haired skin as typical of other species. When preparing the spined skin, pull spines out as if plucking feathers (Miwa and Sladky 2016), though cutting them with a #10 clipper blade is easier. The teeth of a #40 blade, which is typically used in veterinary surgical preparation, are too close together and the spines will not fit between them. Like other types of hair, the spines and hair of hedgehogs regrow quickly after they have been cut. It does not take 18 months.

Hedgehogs have a unique defense mechanism whereby they roll into a ball so the soft ventral aspect is protected by tough spines. The panniculus muscle is thick around the edge forming the orbicularis muscle at the junction of the spiny and haired skin that functions as a purse-string pulling the spiny skin over the balled-up animal (Figure 20.3). If this orbicularis muscle is damaged, for example from a bite or during tumor resection, it should be repaired as a separate structure to maintain its integrity (Isenbugel and Baumgartner 1993).

Ovariohysterectomy and Mammary Tumor Removal

Uterine pathology is common (Raymond and White 1999; Raymond and Garner 2001a), and has been ranked the first (Miwa and Sladky 2016) or second most common (Reavill 2009) site for tumor development (Figure 20.4). It has been theorized that the influence of estrogen causes endometrial stromal hyperplasia that progresses to stromal polyp formation and then consequent endometrial stromal sarcoma development (Reavill 2009). Uterine tumors occur as early as two years of age (Miwa and Sladky 2016). Presenting complaints in hedgehogs with uterine disease

Surgery of Exotic Animals, First Edition. Edited by R. Avery Bennett and Geoffrey W. Pye.
© 2022 John Wiley & Sons, Inc. Published 2022 by John Wiley & Sons, Inc.

(a)

(b)

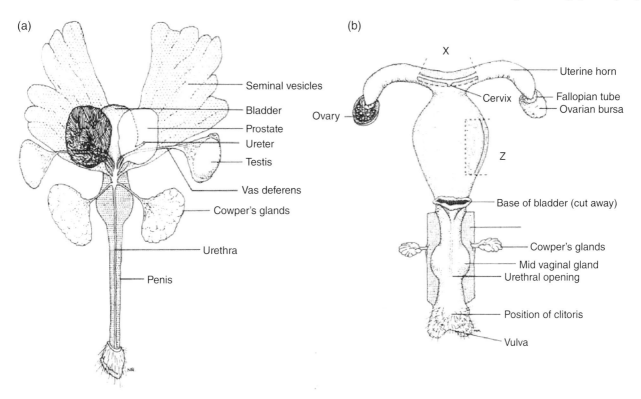

- Seminal vesicles
- Bladder
- Prostate
- Ureter
- Testis
- Vas deferens
- Cowper's glands
- Urethra
- Penis

X

- Uterine horn
- Cervix
- Fallopian tube
- Ovarian bursa

Ovary

Z

- Base of bladder (cut away)
- Cowper's glands
- Mid vaginal gland
- Urethral opening
- Position of clitoris
- Vulva

Figure 20.1 The uterus is bicornuate with a single cervix, but no uterine body (researchgate.net). Diagrammatic illustration of the reproductive organs of the male (a) and female (b) hedgehog in reproductive maturity. In the image the letter X shows a transverse section of the uterus demonstrating the lumen between the uterine horns. Z shows a transverse section through the vagina showing the relatively thin walled structure in this species. *Source:* Reeve (1994). Reprinted with permission of Dr. Nigel Reeve.

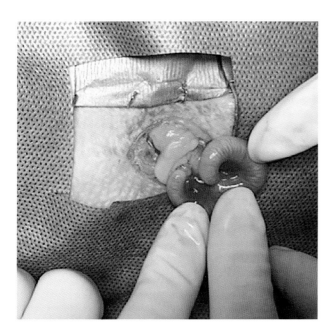

Figure 20.2 A female African hedgehog (*Atelerix albiventris*) undergoing a midline celiotomy for an elective ovariohysterectomy. The bicornuate uterus is being digitally examined for evidence of uterine pathology which is common in this species.

include weakness, hematuria, and hemorrhagic vaginal discharge (Figure 20.5). While surgery for uterine tumors is commonly performed, most veterinarians treating hedgehogs are not recommending prophylactic ovariectomy at the time of writing. If there is a connection between estrogen and the development of uterine tumors, it is likely that ovariectomy at a young age will prevent the development of uterine neoplasia obviating the need to perform an ovariohysterectomy on an unhealthy animal. Reavill suggests recommending early ovariectomy to prevent this common clinical problem as we would in other species (Reavill 2009).

Mammary tumors are also common in hedgehogs (Raymond and White 1999; Raymond and Garner 2000, 2001a; Reavill 2009). It has been reported that mammary gland adenocarcinoma is the single most common neoplasm of hedgehogs (Heatley et al. 2005). Mammary gland carcinoma and mammary papillary adenoma are also described (Raymond and Garner 2001a; Done 2002). Presenting signs include a singular or multiple subcutaneous masses along the ventral abdomen. Careful evaluation for concurrent neoplastic disease is recommended due to the high prevalence of additional neoplastic comorbidities

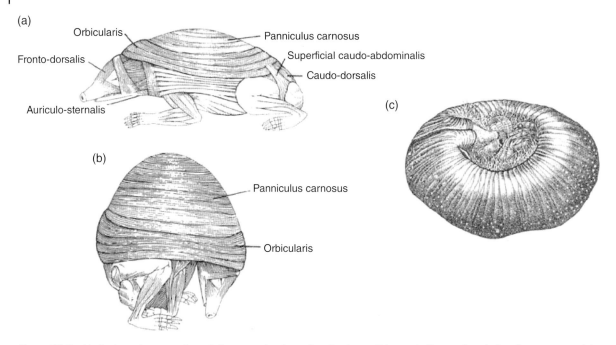

Figure 20.3 Hedgehogs have a unique defense mechanism whereby they roll into a ball exposing their spines to potential predators. The panniculus muscle is thick around the edge forming the orbicularis muscle at the junction of the spiny and haired skin that functions as a purse-string pulling the spiny skin over the balled-up animal. Diagrammatic illustration showing (a) the muscular anatomy of the hedgehog showing the main muscles involved in rolling to protect their ventral abdomen. (b) Hedgehog partly rolled up. Muscles can be seen to overlay the head, shoulders and tail of the animal. (c) In a hedgehog that is fully rolled into a ball neither the head nor feet are apparent to the external environment. *Source:* Reeve (1994). Reprinted with permission of Dr. Nigel Reeve.

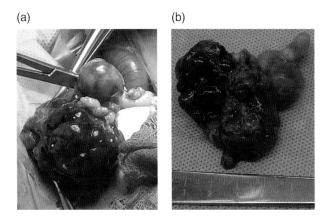

Figure 20.4 (a) Ventral midline celiotomy for removal of a granulosa thecal cell tumor in an adult female African hedgehog (*Atelerix albiventris*). The mass has been exteriorized from the abdomen and is being ligated at its base using circumferential and transfixing ligatures. (b) Insert shows excised mass (scale in millimetres).

in this species. Mammary tumors are usually malignant, characterized histopathologically as either solid or tubular. On histopathology there is evidence of epithelial cell proliferation with round to oval, anisokaryotic, and vesicular nuclei (Raymond and Garner 2001a). Fine needle aspirate cytology can be useful; however, if masses have outgrown their blood supply, central necrosis can lead to nondiagnostic samples being obtained. To date, there has been no correlation made between the influence of

estrogen and the development of mammary tumors in hedgehogs.

Excisional biopsy with wide margins (1 cm) and concurrent ovariohysterectomy through a midline ventral celiotomy are recommended for the treatment of mammary tumors in hedgehogs. Place the patient in dorsal recumbency. Clip widely to facilitate surgical resection and mobilization of tissues allowing skin closure without tension. Following surgical removal, submit masses for

(a)

(b)

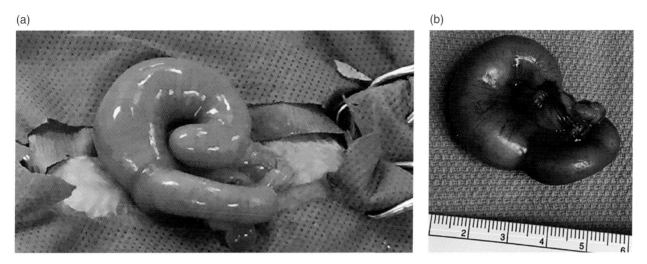

Figure 20.5 (a) An enlarged left uterine horn observed at the time of surgery. (b) The mass was histologically diagnosed as an adenosarcoma.

histopathologic assessment along with margin evaluation. In hedgehogs, the outcome of mammary tumor removal can be variable with some patients having no recurrence within a year of surgery (Wellehan et al. 2003), while in others, there has been reported early recurrence following surgical resection (Raymond and Garner 2001a; Ramos-Vara 2001). Early ovariectomy may reduce the incidence of mammary carcinoma, as in canine patients; however, further work is needed to confirm and elucidate this presumed association. Perform a standard caudal ventral midline approach to the reproductive tract similar to in canine and feline patients, with the important difference being the smaller and friable nature of hedgehogs' soft tissue. Use hemostatic clips or an electrothermal bipolar vessel sealing device as ligature placement may be challenging due to their small size. Gently manipulate each ovary and place a hemostat across the ovarian vessels. Apply hemostatic clips or suture ligatures to the ovarian pedicles and transect distally. Clamp and ligate the vaginal vault caudal to the cervix. Transect distal to the ligature and remove the uterus and ovaries. Perform a standard, three-layer closure of the abdomen.

Orchiectomy

Intact adult males are generally not overly aggressive. As such, elective orchiectomy is uncommonly performed; however, it may be requested by owners (Lightfoot 1997; Mikaelian and Reavill 2004; Greenacre 2004) to prevent or remove testicular pathology, to manage aggression, or prevent reproduction (Miwa and Sladky 2016; Lightfoot 1997). Gender determination in hedgehogs is not clinically challenging as males have a ventral prepuce located along the

abdominal midline. In similarity with some species, such as guinea pigs and chinchillas (Miwa and Sladky 2016), hedgehogs have a large inguinal canal allowing the testes to move freely into the abdominal cavity. Postulated reasons for this are hedgehogs' close proximity to the ground and relatively low core body temperature. Palpating the testes can be difficult in awakened males. Under sedation or general anesthesia, adult males have palpable testes, but do not have a defined scrotum (Lightfoot 1997). The testes are located subcutaneously within the para-anal recess (Bedford et al. 2000).

There are three different methods by which orchiectomy can be performed and the surgeon should be aware of the anatomy of the inguinal canal. The most commonly used approach is to make bilateral incisions over each individual testis and use an open or closed technique to remove the testes. Alternatively, make a single pre-scrotal incision and excise both testes using either an open or closed surgical technique (Miwa and Sladky 2016; Capello 2011). A third option is to perform a midline celiotomy and manipulate the testes into the caudal abdomen with gentle pressure or traction on the vasa deferentia. Take care to not damage the urethra because of the relative size and location of the prepuce and penis that are within the surgical field. There is no current literature to suggest that one technique is superior or associated with a higher degree of postoperative morbidity. The technique chosen is generally a matter of surgeon preference.

Once the patient is appropriately anesthetized and prepared using aseptic technique, infiltrate each testis with a local anesthetic (no greater than 2 mg/kg bupivacaine or 4 mg/kg lidocaine in total dose) for intraoperative analgesia. Due to the large inguinal canal, the authors prefer a closed technique to prevent possible herniation of abdominal contents. Place a single encircling or transfixation ligature around the tunic and its contents. Then place a second more proximal encircling ligature on the spermatic cord. If the tunic is inadvertently opened, suture across the external inguinal ring being careful not to compromise of the external pudendal vessels as they exit the inguinal canal prior to closing the subcutaneous tissues and skin in order to prevent herniation of abdominal contents. One of the authors (AB) ligates the vaginal tunic proximal to the defect or incision in the tunic to achieve functional closure of the inguinal canal as with the closed technique.

When performing a castration through a caudal ventral midline celiotomy, locate the vasa deferentia and gently retract them cranially. Simultaneously apply pressure externally to push the testes into the caudal abdomen through the inguinal canal. Identify the ductus deferens and pampiniform plexus. Due to the delicate nature of the male reproductive tract, these are frequently ligated together. Apply hemostatic clips or a vessel sealing device for ligating vessels to decrease surgical time. Alternatively, place two encircling ligatures using 4-0 absorbable suture. Detach the testis from the tunic by tearing the ligament of the tail of the epididymis allowing the testis to be removed. After removal of the testis, close the celiotomy in three-layers; body wall, subcutaneous tissues, and skin.

Posthitis and Paraphimosis

Inflammation of the prepuce and surrounding skin (posthitis) is a common presenting complaint in African pygmy hedgehogs caused by poor environmental hygiene and entrapment of bedding substrate within the preputial fossa (Ivey 2011). Patients can also present with paraphimosis. The skin surrounding the preputial orifice can invert causing constriction of the extruded penis impairing venous drainage from the highly vascular erectile tissues. Other causes of paraphimosis include abnormalities involving the preputial orifice, priapism, foreign bodies causing strangulation of the penis, trauma, or a constricting band of substrate, hair, or carpet fiber. Paraphimosis is easily differentiated from priapism, congenital deformities, penile neoplasia, or hematoma formation based on physical examination under anesthesia and concurrent palpation. The exposed penis quickly becomes edematous with associated swelling from the inciting cause or by trauma due to self-mutilation. After a period of time, the engorged penile skin might become dry and painful. Self-trauma and mutilation exacerbate the condition (Hernandez-Divers 2004).

If recognized early, paraphimosis can be treated with success. Treatment is initiated after assessment under general anesthesia with attempts to determine and address the underlying cause. Gently clean the penis by applying a copious amount of water soluble lubricant. Replace the penis inside the prepuce by first sliding the prepuce in a caudal direction, extruding the penis farther cranially. This everts the skin at the preputial orifice. Once the skin of the orifice is rolled out, replace the penis into the prepuce. Associated edema caused by the annular constriction and lack of drainage subsides rapidly after circulatory flow is reestablished. In cases where associated trauma or edema prevent reduction of the penis into the prepuce, apply hypertonic saline dressings, hyperosmolar solutions, or cold compresses to reduce the swelling. Once the penis has been replaced, place a temporary purse string suture circumferentially at the preputial orifice. If necessary, under magnification, incise the preputial skin to more thoroughly evaluate the preputial cavity and recess, remove any restrictive foreign material, and biopsy mass lesions. This will also often relieve the compromised venous flow; however, it is rarely necessary. Reconstruct the prepuce in three layers, internal mucosa, external skin, and subcutaneous tissue between them. If, after appropriate treatment, the penis will not stay within the prepuce, a phallopexy can be performed (see Chapter 19).

Neoplastic Disease in Hedgehogs

Numerous neoplastic diseases have been described in hedgehogs and individual treatments and management of such tumors is beyond the scope of this chapter; however, they have been described in detail elsewhere (Heatley et al. 2005). Cutaneous neoplasms reported in hedgehogs are common and include squamous cell carcinomas (Raymond and Garner 2001a; Rivera and Janovits 1992), mammary gland tumors (Raymond and Garner 2000, 2001a; Wellehan et al. 2003), and cutaneous mast cell tumors (Raymond and Garner 2001a; Raymond 1997). Mesenchymal tumors are reportedly less common in hedgehogs compared to epithelial and round cell tumors, with an incidence of 4% (Figure 20.6) (Raymond and Garner 2001a; Peauroi et al. 1994; Heatley et al. 2005). Tumors of the endocrine system comprise around 14% and include tumors of the thyroid, parathyroid, pituitary adenomas, and pancreatic and adrenocortical tumors (Raymond and Garner 2001a; Peauroi et al. 1994; Miller et al. 2002) accounting for 45% of endocrine diseases in hedgehogs (Done 2002; Raymond and Garner 2001a). A wide variety of tumors affecting the reproductive system have also been reported including uterine leiomyomas, leiomyosarcomas, and adenocarcinomas

(a)

(b)

(c)

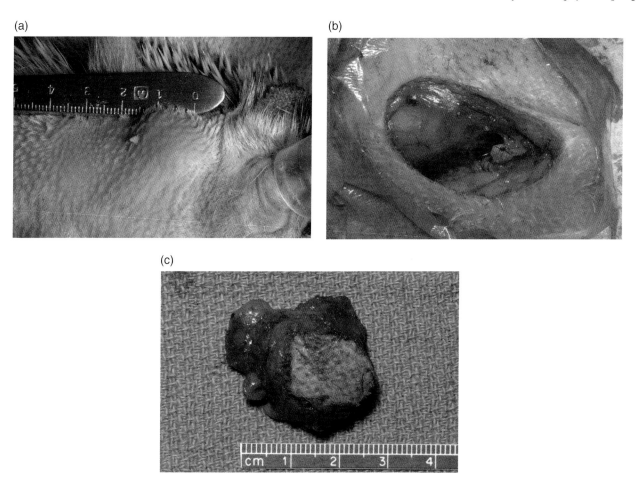

Figure 20.6 (a) Preparation of an adult female African hedgehog *(Atelerix albiventris)* for a subcutaneous adenocarcinoma diagnosed preoperatively with FNA cytology. (b) Intraoperative photo following mass removal and irrigation of the subcutaneous tissues. (c) The excised mass prior to submission for histopathologic analysis. *Source:* Images courtesy of Lorraine Corriveau, Purdue Veterinary Teaching Hospital.

with adenosarcomas being the most common malignant uterine neoplasms (Figure 20.5) (Raymond and Garner 2001a; Done et al. 1992). A retroviral origin for hedgehog lymphoma and multicentric skeletal sarcomas has been suggested (Heatley et al. 2005; Raymond et al. 1998; Peauroi et al. 1994). Lesions were similar to feline leukemia virus-induced osteochondromatosis (Peauroi et al. 1994).

Clinical signs of neoplastic disease, in addition to observation of masses, include weight loss, anorexia, lethargy, diarrhea, dyspnea, and ascites. Often signs are related to the body system affected and can rapidly progress. Early diagnosis is essential for developing targeted treatment plans and curative intent surgery. Because neoplasia is so common in hedgehogs, yearly examinations or even examinations every six months are recommended for hedgehogs beginning at a year of age including a through physical examination (ideally under sedation to facilitate a comprehensive assessment), abdominal palpation, and thoracic auscultation. Owners

should be advised to monitor for tumors as well. In patients with suspected neoplastic disease, diagnostic testing should include a minimum database: a complete blood count, serum biochemical profile, and urinalysis. Thoracic radiographs usually are indicated to evaluate for evidence of metastatic disease. Abdominal imaging allows for aspiration for cytology or biopsy, when indicated, as well as for surgical planning. Surgical treatment is recommended for most cases of local disease without metastasis. Surgical excision should be planned to achieve margins with submission of samples for histopathologic assessment that can be used to guide and facilitate treatment options (Figure 20.7).

Proptosis and Enucleation

Proptosis occurs when the eye is displaced rostrally and the palpebrae are trapped caudal to the globe prohibiting spontaneous repositioning of the globe within the orbit. Inciting

(a)

(b)

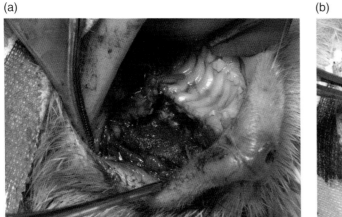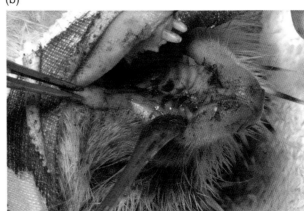

Figure 20.7 (a) Left partial maxillectomy for removal of an oral osteosarcoma. Gelatin sponge can be seen in the defect to aid in hemostasis. (b) A labial mucosal flap has been raised to close the defect using simple interrupted sutures.

etiologies in hedgehogs include trauma, acute orbital cellulitis with or without abscessation, neurologic disease, retrobulbar foreign bodies, and neoplastic disease (Wheler et al. 2001). The shallow orbits and relatively large palpebral fissures in hedgehogs may predispose them to proptosis in a similar manner to that of brachycephalic dogs. In a report of a hedgehog that underwent necropsy (Wheler et al. 2001), the orbital depth was only 1 mm deeper than the globe itself, which raises the question whether African pygmy hedgehogs are conformationally predisposed to proptosis. Inflammation, cellulitis, and fat accumulation within the retrobulbar space may also contribute to an effective reduction in orbital depth.

A complete ophthalmic examination under general anesthesia is recommended in all cases to thoroughly evaluate the globe and orbit. In five of eight hedgehogs presented for proptosis, the corneal damage was so severe that extrusion of the lens, uvea, vitreous, and retina were observed rendering the globe nonvisual and necessitating removal (Wheler et al. 2001). In patients with orbital cellulitis, cytology and culture and sensitivity testing with targeted antibiotic therapy should be initiated due to the fact that these clinical signs often progress to proptosis and further trauma.

Enucleation is usually reserved for cases in which previous attempts to treat the pathology involving the globe or orbit have failed and is the treatment of choice for a permanently blind, painful eye regardless of the cause. Other indications include perforating corneal and scleral injuries resulting in loss of ocular contents, intraocular or diffuse surface neoplasia, intractable intraocular inflammation (e.g. uveitis, panophthalmitis, or endophthalmitis), glaucoma not responsive to medical management, and chronic ocular pain (Cho 2008). An additional indication is

palliation for chronic exposure secondary to severe exophthalmos or proptosis (Holmberg 2007). Enucleation is not only for palliation of a painful eye, but is also an opportunity to address any concurrent orbital disease present (Holmberg 2007).

Enucleation involves the surgical removal of the globe along with a short segment of the optic nerve, the eyelid margins, third eyelid, conjunctiva, and lacrimal gland. The small size of the orbit in hedgehogs make ophthalmic surgery challenging. For enucleation, perform a lateral canthotomy with a scalpel blade or scissors. Gently grasp the conjunctiva with thumb forceps and make a radial perilimbal incision separating the conjunctiva, Tenon's capsule, and extraocular muscles from the sclera. Remove the lacrimal gland (beneath the orbital ligament) if it was not removed with the globe. Severe the optic nerve with curved scissors. Avoid excessive traction on the optic nerve to prevent injury to the optic chiasm and visual impairment in the remaining eye. Control hemorrhage with a hemostatic clip or gelatin sponge prior to closing. Close subcutaneous tissues with 4-0 or 5-0 absorbable appositional sutures and close the lid margins with 4-0 nonabsorbable appositional sutures. Due to the shallow conformation of the orbit, placement of a prosthesis is not a viable option. A prophylactic lateral tarsorrhaphy on the contralateral (unaffected) eye may be indicated for managing hedgehogs predisposed to proptosis.

Leg and Foot Injuries

Treatment of distal limb injuries in hedgehogs due to trauma from male–male interactions and aggression, pododermatitis, annular constriction of the limbs with

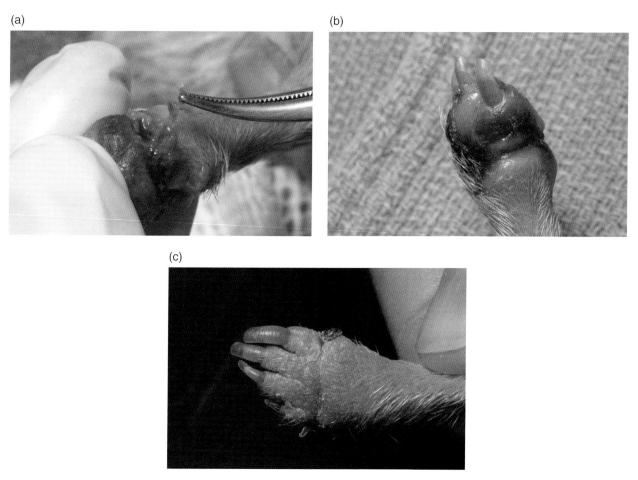

Figure 20.8 (a) A constricting string held in hemostats causing strangulation of the left hind limb of an adult female African hedgehog (*Atelerix albiventris*) that was carefully removed. The same limb 5 days (b) and 10 days (c) following removal of the string.

encircling fibers (Figure 20.8), neoplastic disease, abscessation, or fractures may require surgical intervention (Miwa and Sladky 2016; Smith 1992; Wroot 2001). Pododermatitis is occasionally observed in hedgehogs as in other small mammals (Miwa and Sladky 2016). Often specific surgical intervention is not required. Submerging the limb in an antiseptic solution (Smith 1992), topical application of antimicrobial ointments (triple antibiotic ointment or silver sulfadiazine), and protection from self-mutilation and contamination from the environment with regular bandage changes, appropriate antimicrobial administration, and analgesics are commonly implemented. The surgeon should ensure that the bedding is soft to prevent it from being a source of further abrasion and trauma. Surgical debridement may be indicated for treatment of severe wounds, osteomyelitis, or severe pododermatitis not responsive to conservative management. Although medical and surgical treatment of limb wounds parallels that used in dogs and cats, the intrinsic behaviors of hedgehogs and their evolution to protect against predation require modifications to postoperative management. Generally,

Elizabethan collars are not used as self-mutilation will ensue; however, bandaging and immobilizing the limb under general anesthesia is often well tolerated in this species (Smith 1992).

In some cases, limb amputation may be necessary. Remove the entire limb as proximal as possible. Remove the scapula when performing a forequarter amputation and perform a coxofemoral disarticulation for hind limb amputation (Miwa and Sladky 2016) to prevent self-mutilation and trauma to the remaining stump due to progressive muscle atrophy following the procedure. Limb amputation in small mammals is identical to procedures described in dogs with close attention to hemostasis, analgesic protocols, and thermoregulation under anesthesia. Hedgehogs adjust rapidly to amputation.

Intervertebral Disc Disease

Neurologic disease in hedgehogs is uncommon; however, reported etiologies include toxicosis, nutritional deficiencies, neoplastic disease, trauma, postparturient eclampsia, intervertebral disc disease (IVDD), polioencephalomalacia, otitis media, demyelination, wobbly hedgehog syndrome, rabies, parasite migration, and infarction (Díaz-Delgado et al. 2018; Johnson 2013; Ivey and Carpenter 2004, 2012; Lightfoot 2000; Larson 1999; Raymond 2009; Graesser et al. 2006; Garner and Graesser 2006; Palmer et al. 1998).

IVDD is a debilitating condition caused by progressive degeneration of one or more intervertebral discs resulting in compression of the spinal cord parenchyma. Signs reported with IVDD in hedgehogs are similar to those in chondrodystrophic dogs including lameness, proprioceptive ataxia, paresis, paralysis, and upper motor neuron signs affecting the urinary bladder (Raymond 2009). In a case series by Raymond et al., IVDD in hedgehogs that had

postmortem examinations had histologic features similar to those seen in chondrodystrophic breed-associated disc disease. In all hedgehogs, the nucleus pulposus had undergone a progressive decrease in proteoglycan content with subsequent dehydration and replacement of the mucoid nucleus with cartilage and eventual mineralization that was evident histologically (Raymond 2009). Degeneration of the disc leads to loss of the ability to withstand pressure leading to abnormal stress concentration and tearing of the annulus fibrosis, and eventual herniation into the spinal canal. To date, there are no reports of surgical intervention being utilized for the treatment of IVDD in hedgehogs; however, surgical decompression via hemilaminectomy and removal of inspissated disc material following appropriate imaging and lesion localization may allow alleviation of spinal cord compression and neuronal recovery.

References

Bedford, J., Mock, O., Nagdas, S. et al. (2000). Reproductive characteristics of the African pygmy hedgehog (*Atelerix albiventris*). *Journal of Reproduction and Fertility* 120: 143–150.

Capello, V. (2011). Common surgical procedures in pet rodents. *Journal of Exotic Pet Medicine* 20: 294–307.

Carpenter, J.W. (2010). Diseases and medicine of the African hedgehog. *Proceedings Western Veterinary Conference*, Las Vegas, NV.

Cho, J. (2008). Surgery of the globe and orbit. *Topics in Companion Animal Medicine* 23: 23–37.

Díaz-Delgado, J., Whitley, D.B., Storts, R.W. et al. (2018). The pathology of wobbly hedgehog syndrome. *Veterinary Pathology* 55: 711–718.

Done, L., Dietze, M., Cranfield, M. et al. (1992). Necropsy lesions by body systems in African hedgehogs (*Atelerix albiventris*): clues to clinical diagnosis. *Proceedings of the Joint Conference of the American Association of Zoo Veterinarians and the American Association of Wildlife Veterinarians*, Oakland, CA, pp. 110–112.

Garner, M.M. and Graesser, D. (2006). Wobbly hedgehog syndrome. *Exotic DVM* 8: 27–29.

Graesser, D., Spraker, T.R., Dressen, P. et al. (2006). Wobbly hedgehog syndrome in African pygmy hedgehogs (*Atelerix sp*). *Journal of Exotic Pet Medicine* 15: 59–65.

Greenacre, C.B. (2004). Spontaneous tumors of small mammals. *Veterinary Clinics of North America: Exotic Animal Practice* 7: 627–651.

Heatley, J.J., Mauldin, G.E., and Cho, D.Y. (2005). A review of neoplasia in the captive African hedgehog (*Atelerix albiventris*). *Seminars in Avian and Exotic Pet Medicine* 14: 182–192.

Hernandez-Divers, S.M. (2004). Principles of wound management of small mammals: hedgehogs, prairie dogs, and sugar gliders. *Veterinary Clinics of North America: Exotic Animal Practice* 7: 1–18.

Holmberg, B.J. (2007). Enucleation of exotic pets. *Journal of Exotic Pet Medicine* 16: 88–94.

Isenbugel, E. and Baumgartner, R.A. (1993). Diseases of the hedgehog. In: *Zoo and Wild Animal Medicine – Current Therapy*, vol. 3 (ed. M.E. Fowler), 294–303. Philadelphia, PA: W.B. Saunders.

Ivey, E. and Carpenter, J.W. (2004). Hedgehogs. In: *Ferrets, Rabbits, and Rodents: Clinical Medicine and Surgery*, 2e (eds. K. Quesenberry and J.W. Carpenter), 339–353. Philadelphia, PA: Elsevier.

Ivey, E. and Carpenter, J.W. (2012). Hedgehogs. In: *Ferrets, Rabbits, and Rodents: Clinical Medicine and Surgery*, 2e (eds. K. Quesenberry and J.W. Carpenter), 411–427. Philadelphia: Elsevier.

Johnson, D. (2013). Reproductive tract tumors and diseases in exotic companion mammals. *Proceedings ABVP Symposium*, Glendale, AZ.

Johnson-Delaney, C. (2007). What veterinarians need to know about hedgehogs. *Exotic DVM* 9: 38–44.

Lightfoot, T.L. (1997). Clinical techniques of selected exotic species: chinchilla, prairie dog, hedgehog, and chelonians. *Seminars in Avian and Exotic Pet Medicine* 6: 96–105.

Lightfoot, T.L. (2000). Therapeutics of African pygmy hedgehogs and prairie dogs. *Veterinary Clinics of North America: Exotic Animal Practice* 3: 155–172.

Mikaelian, I. and Reavill, D. (2004, 2, 2004). Spontaneous proliferative lesions and tumors of the uterus of captive

African hedgehogs (*Atelerix albiventris*). *Journal of Zoo and Wildlife Medicine* 35: 216–220.

Miller, D.L., Styer, E.L., Stobaeus, J.K. et al. (2002). Thyroid c-cell carcinoma in an African pygmy hedgehog (*Atelerix albiventris*). *Journal of Zoo and Wildlife Medicine* 33: 392–396.

Miwa, Y. and Sladky, K.K. (2016). Small mammals – common surgical procedures of rodents, ferrets, hedgehogs, and sugar gliders. *Veterinary Clinics: Exotic Animal Practice* 19: 205–244.

Palmer, A.C., Blakemore, W.F., Franklin, R.J.M. et al. (1998). Paralysis in hedgehogs (*Erinaceus europaeus*) associated with demyelination. *The Veterinary Record* 143: 550–552.

Peauroi, J.R., Lowenstein, L.J., Munn, R.J. et al. (1994). Multicentric skeletal sarcomas associated with probable retrovirus particles in two African hedgehogs (*Atelerix albiventris*). *Veterinary Pathology* 31: 481–484.

Ramos-Vara, J.A. (2001). Soft tissue sarcomas in the African hedgehog (*Atelerix albiventris*): microscopic and immunohistologic study of three cases. *Journal of Veterinary Diagnostic Investigation* 13: 442–445.

Raymond, J.T. and Garner, M.M. (2000). Mammary gland tumors in captive African hedgehogs. *Journal of Wildlife Diseases* 36: 405–408.

Raymond, J.T. and Garner, M.M. (2001a). Spontaneous tumors in captive African hedgehogs (*Atelerix albiventris*): a retrospective study. *Journal of Comparative Pathology* 124: 128–133.

Raymond, J.T. and Garner, M.M. (2001b). Spontaneous tumors in hedgehogs: a retrospective study of fifty cases. *Proceedings of the Joint Conference of the American Association of Zoo Veterinarians, American Association of Wildlife Veterinarians, Association of Reptilian and Amphibian Veterinarians, and the National Association of Zoo and Wildlife Veterinarians*, Orlando, FL, pp. 326–327.

Raymond, J.T. and White, M.R. (1999). Necropsy and histopathologic findings in 14 African hedgehogs (*Atelerix albiventris*); a retrospective study. *Journal of Zoo and Wildlife Medicine* 30: 273–277.

Raymond, J.T., Clarke, K.A., and Schafer, K.A. (1998). Intestinal lymphosarcoma in captive African hedgehogs. *Journal of Wildlife Diseases* 34: 801–806.

Reeve, N. (1994). *Hedgehogs*. London, UK: T & AD Poyser (Natural History).

Rivera, R.Y. and Janovits, E.B. (1992). Oronasal squamous cell carcinoma in an African hedgehog (*Erinaceidae albiventris*). *Journal of Wildlife Diseases* 28: 148–150.

Smith, A.J. (1992). Husbandry and medicine of African hedgehogs. *Journal of Small Exotic Animal Medicine* 2: 21–28.

Vuolo, S. and Whittington, J.K. (2008). Dystocia secondary to perineal fetal hernia in an African hedgehog. *Exotic DVM* 10: 10–12.

Wellehan, J.F., Southorn, E., Smith, D.A. et al. (2003). Surgical removal of a mammary adenocarcinoma and a granulosa cell tumor in an African pygmy hedgehog. *The Canadian Veterinary Journal* 44: 235–237.

Wheler, C.L., Grahn, B.H., and Pocknell, A.M. (2001). Unilateral proptosis and orbital cellulitis in eight African hedgehogs (*Atelerix albiventris*). *Journal of Zoo and Wildlife Medicine* 23: 236–241.

Wroot, A. (2001). Hedgehogs and moonrats: spines and curling in hedgehogs. In: *The Encyclopedia of Mammals* (ed. D. MacDonald). New York: Facts on File.

21

Surgery of the Sugar Glider
Geoffrey W. Pye

Introduction

Surgery of sugar gliders can be facilitated by the use of magnification, illumination, and microinstrumentation (see Chapter 3). Postsurgical self-mutilation is a common occurrence in sugar gliders. Factors that influence this self-mutilation include tissue irritation, tissue trauma, pain, and curiosity. When preparing sugar gliders for surgery, minimize tissue irritation by avoiding clipper trauma and clipper burn, and using less irritating solutions for aseptic preparation (see Chapter 2). Chlorhexidine scrub followed by rinsing with sterile saline are less irritating than using povidone-iodine and alcohol products. Rinsing well with saline also helps reduce residual scrub product that may attract attention to the surgical site postoperatively. Tissue trauma can be reduced by using magnification, illumination, microinstrumentation, lasers (both for incisions and phototherapy), and gentle tissue handling. Using preoperative multimodal analgesia and sedation can also reduce the incidence of self-mutilation. Buprenorphine (0.01 mg/kg), meloxicam (0.2 mg/kg), and midazolam (0.1 mg/kg) administered in combination intramuscularly and used in conjunction with a local anesthetic agent work well in sugar gliders. Curiosity in the surgical site can be displaced by feeding as soon as possible after surgery. Placing a piece of apple with the sugar glider in a cloth pouch works well to keep it from paying too much attention to the surgery site.

Orchiectomy

The most common surgical procedure performed in pet sugar gliders is orchiectomy (castration). Sugar gliders are a social species that are best kept in groups so permanent contraception of males is recommended unless breeding is wanted. Orchiectomy may also reduce the incidence of self-mutilation particularly due to overzealous masturbation,

in singly housed males. The testicles in sugar gliders sit in a scrotum that hangs from the body cranial to the penis. A number of methods for orchiectomy have been described (Pye and Carpenter 1999; Lightfoot and Bartlett 1999; Newbury et al. 2005; Morges et al. 2009; Ness and Johnson-Delaney 2011). While ages for orchiectomy have not been recommended, the procedure has been performed in a sugar glider as young as two months out-of-pouch (Morges et al. 2009). The simplest and quickest method is to use a CO_2 laser or radio frequency electrosurgery to perform scrotal ablation (Morges et al. 2009). Following anesthesia induction (typically isoflurane in oxygen supplied by a face mask) and analgesia administration, inject local anesthesia (lidocaine 1–2 mg/kg diluted as needed) into each testicle or into the scrotal stalk (Figure 21.1). After aseptic surgical preparation of the scrotal stalk, transect the scrotal stalk midway between the testicle and the attachment to the body wall using a CO_2 laser or radio frequency electrosurgical unit (Figure 21.2). Transecting the stalk distal to the body wall avoids the formation of a larger wound when the tension of the abdominal skin pulls on the wound edges. This method minimizes tissue irritation and trauma and, therefore, reduces the risk of postsurgical self-mutilation.

Scrotal ablation can also be performed using a scalpel. Careful dissection and ligation of the vessels is required (Figure 21.3). Use a small hemostatic clip (Weck Hemoclip® traditional, Teleflex Medical, NC, USA) or fine suture (6-0) to ligate the vessels (the vas deferens can be included) and then transect distal to the ligature. Close the surgical wound with an intradermal suture pattern. Tissue glue can be used to seal the skin over the surgical site, but this may attract the glider to mutilate the surgical site. Self-mutilation is more common with this method due to the increase in tissue trauma and irritation.

An open scrotal approach can also be used, similar to that used in domestic cats. Incise the skin overlying each testicle. Incise the tunic and expose the testicle (Figure 21.4).

Surgery of Exotic Animals, First Edition. Edited by R. Avery Bennett and Geoffrey W. Pye.
© 2022 John Wiley & Sons, Inc. Published 2022 by John Wiley & Sons, Inc.

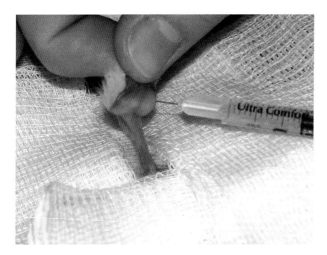

Figure 21.1 Intratesticular administration of lidocaine in a sugar glider, *Petaurus breviceps*. *Source:* Image courtesy of Matthew S. Johnston, VMD, DABVP – Avian, Colorado State University.

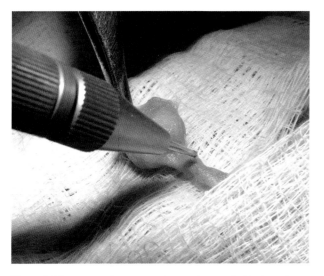

Figure 21.2 Laser-aided castration and scrotal ablation of a sugar glider, *Petaurus breviceps*. Transection is made away from the body wall. *Source:* Image courtesy of Matthew S. Johnston, VMD, DABVP – Avian, Colorado State University.

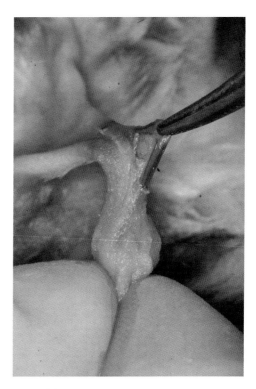

Figure 21.3 Scalpel-assisted castration and scrotal ablation of a sugar glider, *Petaurus breviceps*, with isolation and identification of the vascular cord and vas deferens for ligation.

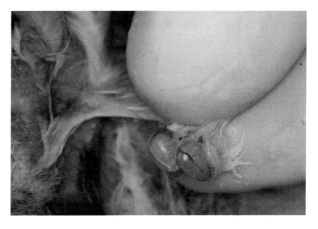

Figure 21.4 Castration of a sugar glider, *Petaurus breviceps*, using a scrotal approach.

Identify and ligate the vas deferens and vascular cord using either hemostatic clips or fine suture. Typically, the scrotum will reduce in size following castration using this method. Ablation of the scrotum avoids future trauma to the scrotum and also appears to reduce the risk of self-mutilation postsurgically.

Penectomy

Prolapse and trauma of the penis occurs in sugar gliders most commonly as a result of self-mutilation and overzealous masturbation in singly housed males. While replacement of the penis can be effective, recurrent prolapse, chronic prolapse, or necrosis of the penis may necessitate partial penectomy (penile amputation). The sugar glider penis is bifurcated, and the urethra exits at the point of bifurcation (Figure 21.5). In most circumstances, amputation of only a portion of the bifurcated part of the penis is required and does not impact the urethra. Catheterization using a 26 g intravenous catheter can help delineate the urethra to avoid inadvertent damage (Figure 21.6). Amputate the

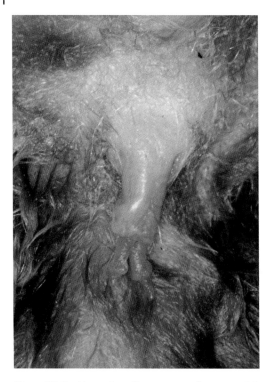

Figure 21.5 Normal penile anatomy of a sugar glider, *Petaurus breviceps*, showing the bifurcation of the distal penis.

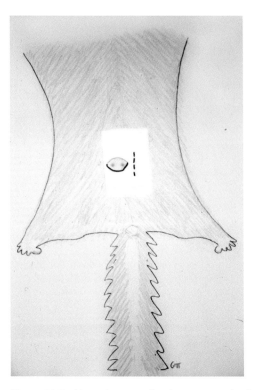

Figure 21.7 Ventral paramedian laparotomy site for a female sugar glider, *Petaurus breviceps*.

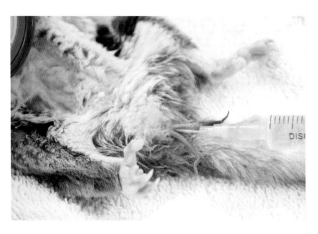

Figure 21.6 Catheterization of the urethra of a sugar glider, *Petaurus breviceps* using a 26 g IV catheter. *Source:* Image courtesy of Gina Geaudry DVM, photographer Sarah Gordon CVT, Packerland Veterinary Center, WI 54303, USA.

affected tissue using laser, radiosurgery, or cold steel and apply digital pressure for hemostasis if needed.

Abdominal Surgical Approach

After preparing the ventral abdomen for aseptic surgery, make a ventral midline incision. For female sugar gliders, either incise through the pouch or make a paramedian

incision (Figure 21.7), and then undermine and reflect the pouch and mammary tissues to expose the linea alba. Make an incision through the linea alba. Use a ring retractor (Lonestar Ring Retractors, Jorgensen Labs, Inc., Loveland, CO, USA) or a Heiss retractor to facilitate exposure of the abdominal contents. Close the abdominal cavity with a simple continuous suture pattern in the linea alba. If a paramedian incision was made, and tissue was undermined to reflect the pouch and mammary tissue, reduce dead space by apposing the subcutaneous tissues. Close the skin using a continuous intradermal suture pattern. Alternatively, place simple interrupted polyglactin 910 sutures using fine suture, trim the ends short, and glue the knots to prevent unraveling.

Ovariectomy and Ovariohysterectomy

After opening the abdomen with a ventral approach, elevate the bladder to expose the female reproductive tract. In nonreproductively active female sugar gliders, the ovaries are small (2–3 mm in length) and have a red granular appearance. Sugar gliders have two uteri that open into the vaginal cul-de-sac (Figure 21.8). The uteri can vary in appearance depending upon the reproductive status of the sugar glider with them being larger in gliders that have

Figure 21.8 Reproductive tract and lower urinary tract anatomy of a female sugar glider, *Petaurus breviceps.*

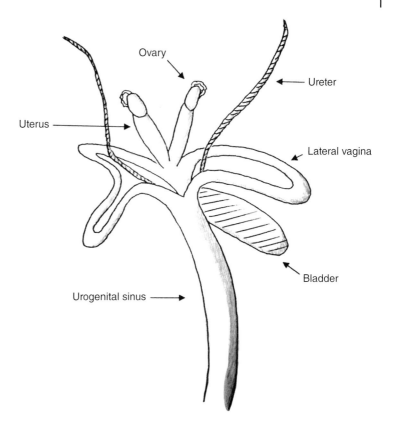

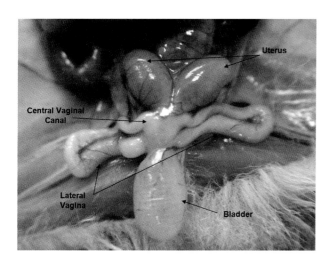

Figure 21.9 Reproductive tract and lower urinary tract anatomy of a multiparous female sugar glider, *Petaurus breviceps.* *Source:* Image courtesy of the Association of Sugar Glider Veterinarians.

been reproductively active (Figure 21.9). There are two lateral vaginae that are convoluted and come off each side of the vaginal cul-de-sac. Either an ovariectomy or an ovariohysterectomy can be performed, though there is no evidence to recommend removing the uteri and it makes the procedure more difficult. Identify and isolate the vessels

supplying the cranial portion of the ovary and ligate them with a small hemostatic clip or fine suture. For an ovariectomy, then isolate the ovary and place a hemostatic between the ovary and the uterus prior to transecting cranial to the clip. For an ovariohysterectomy, take care to identify and avoid the convoluted lateral vaginae and place a hemostatic clip at the junction of the uterus and vaginal cul-de-sac prior to transecting. Do not attempt to remove the lateral vaginae as they are intimately associated with the ureters and the risk of iatrogenic trauma is high.

Patagial Surgery

Patagial surgery may be required for traumatic injuries or mass removal (Ness and Johnson-Delaney 2011; Rivas et al. 2014). The patagium is formed by two opposing skin layers with little to no subcutaneous tissue and extends on each side of the body from the carpus to the tarsus (Figure 21.10). For closure, suture the skin of each side of the patagium separately (Figure 21.11). Using 6-0 absorbable suture, place a simple continuous suture from the subcutaneous side of the each skin layer, effectively burying the knots of the suture. Alternatively, place simple interrupted sutures using

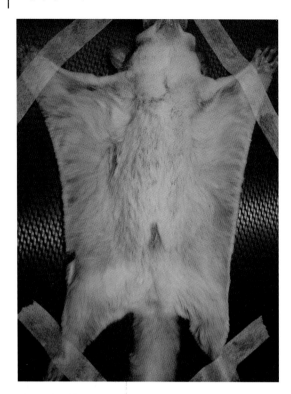

Figure 21.10 The patagium of the sugar glider, *Petaurus breviceps*, stretches from the carpus to the tarsus.

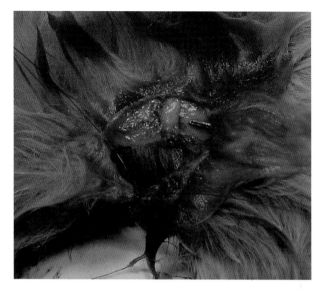

Figure 21.11 A dermal hemangiosarcoma from the patagium of a sugar glider, *Petaurus breviceps*, was removed and each side of the patagium was sutured separately with the knots tied internally. Minimal presurgical preparation was performed to minimize tissue trauma to avoid postsurgical self-mutilation.

fine suture, trim the ends short, and glue the knots to prevent unraveling.

Tail Amputation

Tail trauma can occur as a result of cage furniture (e.g. inappropriate exercise wheels), conspecific trauma, or self-mutilation. Partial tail amputation may be required. After aseptic surgically preparation of the tail (taking care to minimize tissue irritation), incise the skin on the dorsal surface and then ventral surface in a convex curved pattern. Gently pull the skin cranially to expose the underlying muscle, tendons, and bone. Using bone cutters, cut the bone and crush the tendons and muscle. Allow the skin to relax back to cover the stump. Ligation of the blood vessels is often not required and gentle digital pressure typically controls any hemorrhage. Place three or four simple interrupted skin sutures of fine material (5-0 or 6-0), cut the edges short, and glue the knots to prevent unraveling. Minimizing tissue trauma in this manner reduces the risk of further self-mutilation of the tail.

Removal of the Paracloacal Glands

On both sides of the cloaca the paracloacal glands that can get infected or impacted are located (Ness and Johnson-Delaney 2011). Secondary problems with constipation can occur as a result of swelling of the glands. With chronic infection or impaction of the paracloacal glands, surgical removal is recommended. Incise the skin directly over the gland taking care to keep the glandular wall intact. Bluntly dissect the subcutaneous tissues away from the gland to isolate the duct and blood vessels. Apply a single ligating clip or fine suture ligature and transect the duct and blood vessels. Close the skin with a single intradermal suture.

References

Lightfoot, T. and Bartlett, L. (1999). Sugar glider orchiectomy. *Exotic DVM* **1**: 11–13.

Morges, M.A., Grant, K.R., MacPhail, C.M. et al. (2009). A novel technique for orchiectomy and scrotal ablation in the sugar glider (*Petaurus breviceps*). *Journal of Zoo and Wildlife Medicine* 40: 204–206.

Ness, R.D. and Johnson-Delaney, C. (2011). Sugar gliders. In: *Ferrets, Rabbits, and Rodents: Clinical*

Medicine and Surgery, 3e (eds. K.E. Quesenberry and J.W. Carpenter), 393–410. St. Louis, MO: Elsevier, Saunders.

Newbury, S., Hanley, C.S., Paul-Murphy, J. et al. (2005). Sugar glider castration and scrotal ablation. *Exotic DVM* 7: 27–30.

Pye, G.W. and Carpenter, J.W. (1999). Clinical medicine and surgery of the sugar glider, *Petaurus breviceps. Veterinary Medicine* 10: 891–905.

Rivas, A.E., Pye, G.W., Papendick, R. et al. (2014). Dermal hemangiosarcoma in a sugar glider (*Petaurus breviceps*). *Journal of Exotic Pet Medicine* 23: 384–388.

22

Small Mammal Dental Surgery

Estella Böhmer

Incisor Extraction

Intraoral Approach

Indications for intraoral incisor extraction are congenital incisor malocclusion (superior brachygnathia), periodontal or apical tooth infection, and extremely thickened, longitudinally split, deformed, malpositioned, or structurally altered incisors.

In rabbits with superior brachygnathism, you can repeatedly trim the overgrown incisors using a diamond-coated cutting disc or extract them at about six months age. The latter helps preserve the initial normal occlusion of the cheek teeth long term and prevents dental-related compression of the nasolacrimal duct (NLD) caused by retrograde incisor elongation. Incisors that have stopped growing (missing pulp cavity on radiographs) do not need extraction unless they show signs of periodontal infection (Harcourt-Brown 2009a). For adequate assessment, intraoral radiographs are needed, including an isolated view of the maxilla or mandible in guinea pigs and chinchillas as described by Böhmer (2015).

To perform incisor extraction, use sterile gloves and instruments and prepare the oral cavity with 1% povidone-iodine- or 0.12% chlorhexidine gluconate solution immediately prior to surgery. If you have to extract all incisors, begin with the mandibular teeth. Use the tip of a scalpel (#15) to cut the gingival attachment from around the tooth. Starting mesially, introduce a blunt or sharp-edged arc-formed incisor luxator (iM3®, Vancouver, WA, USA) into the periodontal space on all four aspects of the incisor while applying gentle pressure at each side for approximately 20 seconds. This will cause the periodontal ligament fibers to tear (Figure 22.1) (Crossley 1994; Easson 2012). As soon as the incisor is sufficiently loose, grip the tooth with a smooth mosquito hemostat and gently rock and rotate the tooth while simultaneously applying gentle traction. Once it is completely free of attachments and very loose, pull it out with an arc movement that corresponds to the tooth curvature. Check the apex carefully

to assess if the "tooth sac" (germinal tissue) is adhered apically. If any pulp tissue is missing, destroy the intraalveolar remains by either curetting the apical tooth socket with a hypodermic needle (20 ga) bent into a shape based on the curvature of the extracted incisor or moisten the extracted tooth with iodine solution and reintroduce it into the tooth socket (Böhmer 2003). Pushing the incisor against the base of the alveolus (tooth intrusion) while gently rotating it will destroy the remaining germinal tissue with the sharp tooth edges (Steenkamp and Crossley 1999). Mobilize the relatively straight peg teeth using a fine hypodermic needle (21 ga) that you introduce deeply into the alveolus on all four sides of the tooth. Following incisor extraction, there is no need to suture the gingiva and it is not necessary to flush the wound postoperatively as there is no risk of "dry socket syndrome" (Mirdan 2012). Exceptions are severe intraalveolar infections that require postoperative wound irrigation and curettage.

Extraoral Approach (Osteotomy)

Indications for extraoral extraction are incisor-related rostral jaw abscesses, intraalveolar tooth fractures, intraalveolarly deformed incisors, elodontomas, very brittle teeth, or intradental tooth resorption.

Rostral mandibular abscesses are usually the consequence of infected incisors and tend to spread to the nearby premolar (P3) in rabbits or to the middle two cheek teeth in guinea pigs (M1-M2) (Figures 22.2 and 22.3). These infections do not usually resolve adequately if you merely extract the infected teeth and regularly flush the empty alveoli. By additionally performing an alveolar osteotomy access to the altered tooth socket and the infected peri-alveolar bone is improved. In guinea pigs, mandibular incisors often show a mid-body lysis (Böhmer 2003). In these cases, extract the coronal part of the tooth intraorally and remove the apical part safely using the osteotomy site (Figure 22.4).

Surgery of Exotic Animals, First Edition. Edited by R. Avery Bennett and Geoffrey W. Pye.
© 2022 John Wiley & Sons, Inc. Published 2022 by John Wiley & Sons, Inc.

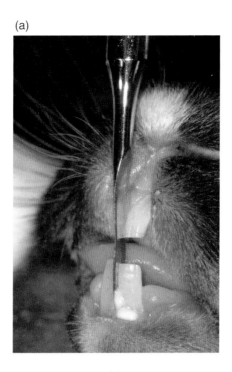

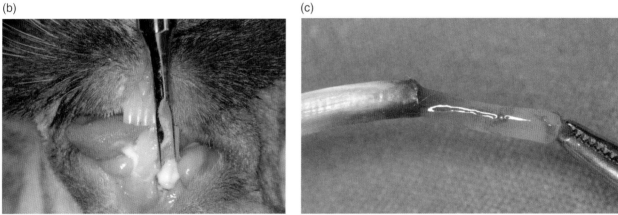

Figure 22.1 Apically infected left mandibular incisor in a rabbit: (a) luxator pushed into the medial part of the tooth socket, (b) luxator introduced into the rostral part of the tooth socket, (c) apical part of the extracted mandibular incisor showing the pulp being partially pulled out.

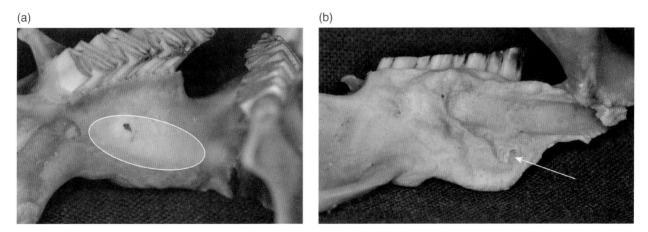

Figure 22.2 Mandibular abscess in two guinea pigs (mandible specimens, caudorostral view): (a) local osteomyelitis with fistula formation due to apical infection of the left incisor. The yellow area marks the osteotomy site. (b) After extraction of the left incisor via osteotomy with advanced inflammatory bone reaction and accidentally opened tooth socket of the first lower cheek tooth (P4) as an unwanted complication (yellow arrow).

(a)

(b)

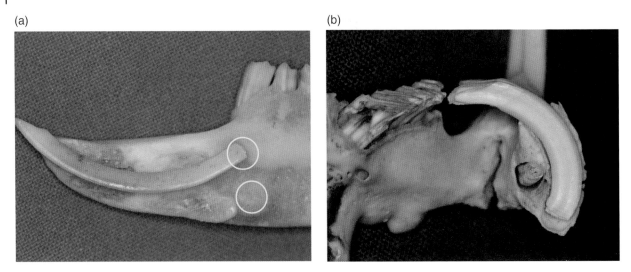

Figure 22.3 Anatomical relationship between the apices of the mandibular incisor and the first mandibular cheek tooth: (a) in a healthy rabbit specimen (medial view), (b) in a guinea pig with marked intraoral overgrowth of the premolar as a consequence of apical incisor infection; the so-called "bridge-formation" is a secondary finding due to local pain (caudorostral view).

(a)

(b)

(c)

(d)

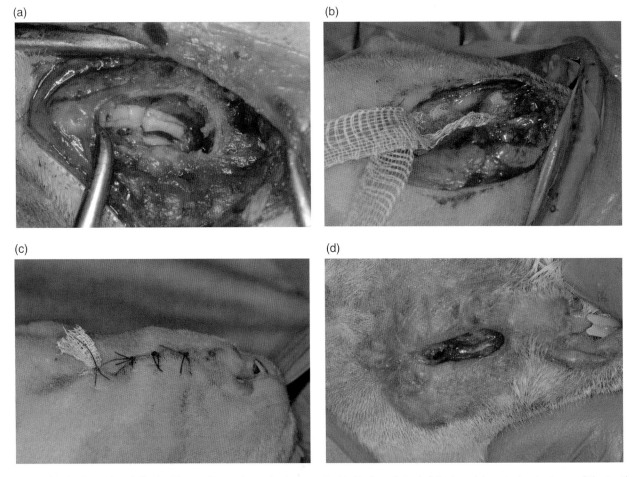

Figure 22.4 Rostral mandibular abscess in a guinea pig due to apical infection of the left incisor: (a) ventral osteotomy of the tooth socket to gain wide access to the infected site and the tooth fragments, (b) empty tooth socket packed with gauze, (c) temporary skin sutures, (d) three weeks postinitial surgery showing the healing osteotomy site (healthy granulation tissue).

To perform an osteotomy, use a suitably sized round burr on a high-speed compressed air drill to open the alveolus of the mandibular incisor at its deepest point (ventrolateral access in rabbits and ventromedial access in guinea pigs). Enlarge the initial fenestration by using a fine Luer bone rongeur, which facilitates the removal of any infected alveolar or dental tissue. Following radical debridement, thoroughly flush the empty alveolus and fill it through the osteotomy site with a gauze that has been coated with a mixture of granulated sugar and petroleum jelly or Furacin solution. Close the skin with simple interrupted sutures. Remove the sutures three days later and debride the wound again before placing another gauze. Repeat this procedure every two days until the wound has healed by secondary intention. Alternatively, gain access to the alveolus of the maxillary incisor by resecting the entire lateral wall of the tooth socket (Figure 22.5).

Even if the germinal tissue has been completely excised, an unstructured tooth may form (Steenkamp and Crossley 1999; Böhmer 2015). When this "dentinoid" shows no signs of infection (periodontal radiolucency) leave it in place (Figure 22.6); otherwise, extraction using an osteotomy is indicated. Complications following maxillary incisor extraction include postoperative epistaxis or purulent rhinitis; both can result from sharp instruments damaging the medial alveolar wall with penetration into the nasal cavity (Figure 22.5b). Iatrogenic symphysiolysis or mandibular fracture is an uncommon complication. More common is persistent infection that requires renewed radical wound debridement and management.

Prognosis for incisor extraction is very good as long as the cheek teeth are not involved secondarily. One remaining maxillary or mandibular incisor suffices to abrade both opposing incisors (Böhmer 2015).

The hypselodont mandibular incisors in omnivorous rodents are extremely long and their apices are located far caudal to the last molar (Figure 22.7). When extracting these teeth, take particular care to avoid iatrogenic jaw fracture or trauma to the molar apices, which lie in close proximity. Incisor extraction in these rodents is much easier if you perform a ventral osteotomy to section the tooth body there and extract it in two parts.

Elodontoma Treatment

Elodontoma is a benign and progressive tumor-like lesion of odontogenic origin that primarily affects the maxillary and mandibular incisors. It is common in captive black-tailed prairie dogs, degus, voles, squirrels, porcupines, and small laboratory rodents that tend to pull on cage bars repeatedly (Böhmer 2015). Apical dysplasia causes an extremely thickened and deformed apex of the incisor that is ankylosed in the surrounding bone. The space-occupying expansile growth of odontogenic tissue leads to severe dyspnea due to progressive obstruction of the nasal passages and/or causes severe deformation of the palatal bone (Phallen et al. 2000) (Figure 22.8). The primary therapeutic goal is to reestablish patent nasal airways or to improve air passage through the nasal cavity, which relieves the respiratory distress. Various palliative or surgical treatments have been used. At an early stage of disease, incisor extraction is indicated and is the easiest unless the apical dysplastic mass is too large. Remove the incisor and the elodontoma along with it by performing a dorsolateral osteotomy of the tooth socket. In more advanced cases, extract the incisor via a transpalatal or dorsal rhinotomy approach (Smith et al. 2013).

Extract apically altered maxillary incisors using a lateral osteotomy of the alveolus with opening the nasal cavity if needed. With the patient in lateral recumbency, make a

(a)

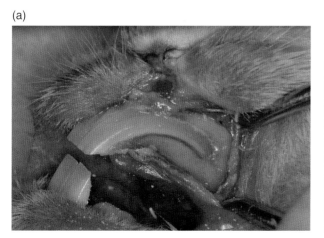

(b)

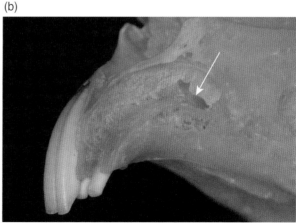

Figure 22.5 Lateral osteotomy of the left maxillary incisor tooth socket in a rabbit: (a) intraoperative view with exposed incisor, (b) specimen with extracted incisor showing an accidentally injured medial wall of the alveolus (exposed nasal cavity – yellow arrow).

(a)

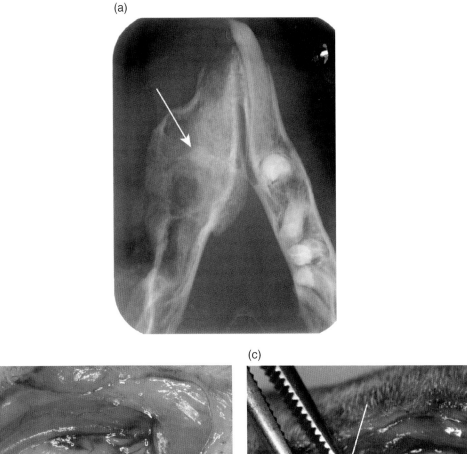

(b)   (c)

Figure 22.6 Dentinoid formation in two rabbits: (a) intraoral radiograph of the mandible showing a small dentinoid (white arrow) that can be left in place, (b) intraoperative view of the ventral mandibular cortex with a fistula (dental probe inserted) as a consequence of an infected dentinoid, (c) after osteotomy of the incisor alveolus and removal of the dentinoid (white arrow).

curved skin and subcutaneous tissue incision beginning dorsal to the infraorbital foramen and down to the naris. Retract the skin and elevate the periosteum overlying the lateral aspect of the maxillary bone with a periosteal elevator. Resect the lateral wall of the maxillary alveolus with a round burr on a high-speed hand piece as far as needed to be able to extract the incisor following its bisection (Figure 22.9).

To perform a unilateral dorsal rhinotomy, place the intubated animal in sternal recumbency. To expose the nasal bone, make a paramedian straight caudorostral incision through the skin and deeper soft tissue that reaches from the interocular region to the nares. Retract the skin and mobilize

the nasal bone by dissecting along its medial and lateral suture with the aid of an osteotome. Elevate the isolated bone and turn it up or remove it temporarily to gain adequate access to the nasal cavity and the alveolus of the apically malformed maxillary incisor (Figure 22.10). Perform a dorsal fenestration of the tooth socket and cut the maxillary incisor into two halves by using a cross-cut carbide fissure burr on a high-speed handpiece. Carefully elevate the thickened apical part of the incisor with the aid of a small osteotome and extract it via the rhinotomy. Do the same with the coronal part and remove it intraorally. Resect parts of the empty tooth socket to restore airway patency. Temporarily insert a soft red rubber catheter into the nasal passage

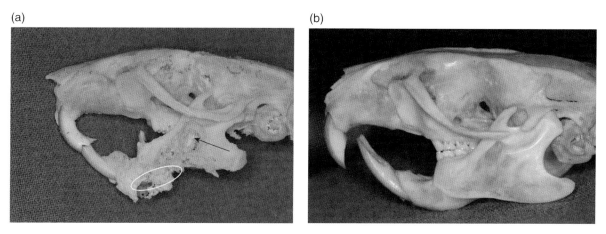

Figure 22.7 Two rat specimens: (a) incisor malocclusion and far advanced mandibular abscess due to apical infection of the left mandibular incisor whose apex perforates the mandible laterally (black arrow); the yellow oval marks the recommended osteotomy site for tooth extraction and abscess revision, (b) healthy rat for comparison.

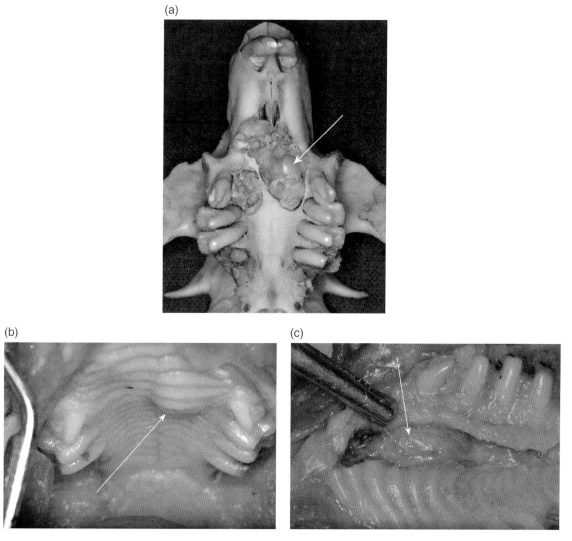

Figure 22.8 Prairie dog with elodontoma of both maxillary incisors and multiple carious lesions of the cheek teeth: (a) maxillary specimen (palatinal view) with bulbously deformed incisor apices, more pronounced on the left (yellow arrow), (b) intraoral view showing ventral bulging of the palatal bone due to expansile apical growth, (c) transpalatinal access to the left apex.

(a)

(b)

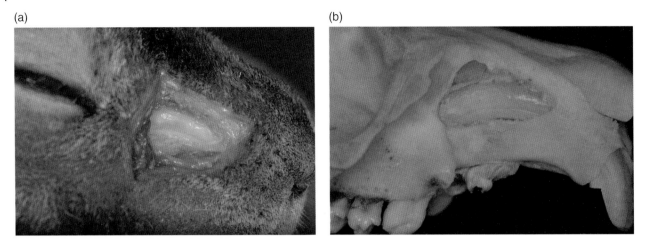

Figure 22.9 Lateral osteotomy of the right upper incisor alveolus in a prairie dog with elodontoma: (a) postmortem with partly exposed tooth, (b) the same animal with additional exposure of the nasal cavity.

(a)

(b)

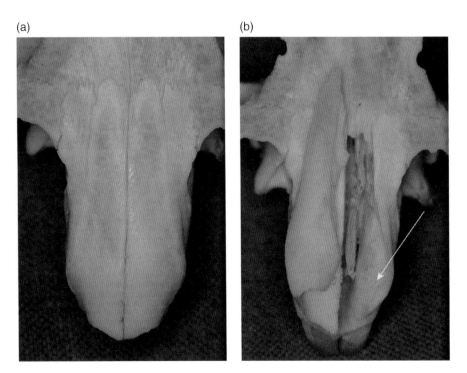

Figure 22.10 Maxillary specimen of a prairie dog: (a) dorsal aspect of the nose, (b) temporary resection of the left nasal bone to access the nasal cavity and the incisor tooth socket (yellow arrow).

sutured to the naris with a single simple interrupted suture to keep the airway open. Replace the nasal bone or remove it and close the skin incision with a simple interrupted pattern. Tension of the skin suture is sufficient to hold the repositioned bone in place, so there is no need for further stabilization. Place a temporary dorsal rhinostomy stent using a short red rubber catheter (Smith et al. 2013). Drill a hole into the caudal part of the nasal bone or cut out a suitable notch through which to place the tube. To perform a bilateral rhi-

notomy, make a dorsal midline skin incision, and mobilize and elevate or remove both nasal bones together.

To extract a severely malformed incisor apex an intraoral transpalatal approach can also be used. Place the patient in dorsal recumbency and open the mouth widely using an oral speculum. Incise the mucosa covering the hard palate and retract it carefully where the apex penetrates the palatine bone. Enlarge the approach as needed to be able to debulk the bulbous thickened incisor apex and remove it through the palatine osteotomy site, while extracting the remainder of the incisor crown intraorally (Wagner et al. 1999). Close the mucosa with a continuous suture.

As apical hyperplasia affects both dental and surrounding soft tissues, any surgical approach is challenging and carries a high risk of iatrogenic tooth fracture and turbinate damage resulting in serious hemorrhage. Common complications following a transpalatal approach are severe hemorrhage, hard palate fracture, and wound healing problems with formation of an oronasal fistula.

A purely palliative option to relieve respiratory distress caused by elodontomas is to insert a biologically inert plastic stent into the nasal cavity through a hole created on the flat dorsal part of the nose, immediately caudal to the altered incisor apices (Wagner and Johnson 2001). This temporary or permanent caudal stent rhinostomy does not include incisor extraction. It is indicated for end-stage disease, where the apical tooth malformations are associated with widespread inflammatory lesions of the intranasal structures causing severe dyspnea. Stent rhinostomy can be performed uni- or bilaterally and can rapidly establish airway patency, but requires regular stoma care and repeated stent replacement. The exact point of trephination into the nasal passages lies on a line connecting both facial surfaces of the lacrimal bone (Figure 22.11). Clip and prepare this area for aseptic surgery before performing a midline incision through the skin and periosteum. Open the nasal cavity by creating a dorsal fenestration using a 5 mm punch biopsy instrument, a 3 mm intramedullary pin, or a round burr on a high-speed dental handpiece. To keep stoma open, insert a suitable segment of an endotracheal tube or section of an 8 fr polypropylene urinary catheter and firmly lodge it in place. Fix the device in place with horizontal mattress sutures. Alternatively, create a permanent rhinostomy by inserting a human steel earlobe gauging device through the nasal bones (Bulliot and Mentre 2013).

The long-term prognosis is guarded to grave. Especially since, in most cases, the mandibular incisors show pathology as well, which tends to progressively affect the temporomandibular joint resulting in ankylosis. To help prevent this, extract the altered mandibular incisors as well.

Cheek Tooth Extraction

Intraoral Approach

Indications for intraoral cheek tooth extraction are individual teeth that are severely malpositioned, strongly curved, or markedly malformed that result in recurrent spur formation.

Since most premolars and molars that need to be removed are infected. It is rare to perform a purely intraoral extraction with subsequent closure of the gingival defect. If there is a periodontal infection, closing the gingival defect will increase the risk of spread of infection to the adjacent teeth.

Since tooth extractions always negatively influence the masticatory system, only remove teeth when there are strong indications to do so. This is particularly important with extraction of a single tooth from the center of an arcade as the adjacent teeth tend to tilt toward the extraction site over time. Therefore, in rabbits, it seems best to remove both the affected tooth and the teeth rostral or caudal to it, or even all teeth of the quadrant. This initially results in a delayed growth of the opposing teeth. Provided the remaining cheek teeth are no longer in occlusion (i.e. no axial load), they stop erupting about three to four months after extraction (Böhmer 2015). In parallel, the maxillary cheek teeth tend to tilt buccally while they progressively get covered with proliferative gingival tissue. This normally causes no further problems and repeated crown reduction is not needed. If a single cheek tooth is extracted in a rabbit, problems arise over time as most cheek teeth have two opposing teeth resulting in uneven wear.

In rabbits, cheek teeth even with severe pathologic changes due to advanced dental disease (e.g. marked malformation, abnormal tooth structure, and elongated and thickened apices) do not necessarily need to be removed as long as they do not show signs of periodontal infection. Those teeth or tooth remnants are ankylosed within the surrounding bone. They stop growing and are not painful as they lack a nerve supply if radiographically the pulp cavity is obliterated (Harcourt-Brown 2009a).

In guinea pigs, cheek tooth extraction without concomitant apical osteotomy is not recommended. Without retrograde access to the empty alveolus adequate aftercare is not feasible, especially since it is not possible to close the wide alveolus with gingival sutures. Extraction of two adjacent cheek teeth is not recommended as in rabbits because the opposing teeth do not stop growing in this species. If you remove only one cheek tooth, the opposing tooth will be ground down sufficiently over time due to their specific jaw movements (Böhmer 2015).

Prior to tooth extraction, prepare the oral mucosa with 1% povidone iodine or 0.12% chlorhexidine gluconate solution. Use the tip of a scalpel blade (#15) or a suitably sized hypodermic needle bent at a 90° angle (flat side facing the tooth) to cut the gingiva surrounding the tooth down to the alveolar bone on the buccal and lingual/palatinal aspect of the tooth. Then introduce a Crossley molar luxator (iM3) or a fine Heidemann spatula (ASA dental®, New York,

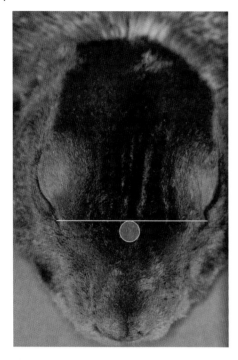

Figure 22.11 Site (yellow circle) just rostral to the eyes (yellow line) to perform a caudal stent rhinostomy in a prairie dog.

USA) into the periodontium to break down the periodontal ligaments. Since the closely contacting enamel ridges of both adjacent teeth impede axial insertion of the luxator, introduce the instrument into the interdental space from the lateral side (mandible) first and then rotate it coronally. Using gentle sliding movements, push the luxator deep into the alveolus on all four sides of the tooth. Repeat this procedure three to four times until the tooth is adequately mobilized. Grasp the tooth carefully and extract it with the aid of a special molar extraction forceps (iM3) or a smooth, curved mosquito hemostat. Tear the remaining intact ligament fibers by slightly rotating the tooth at the same time as pulling it along its long axis. If the germinal tissue is not observed, use a needle bent to conform to the extracted tooth body or repeatedly reinsert the tooth after coating the apex with iodine (Crossley and Aiken 2004; Böhmer 2015). Before suturing the gingiva, fill the empty tooth socket with a dental dressing (HemCon® Tricol Biomedical, Portland, OR, USA), a collagen sponge, or a synthetic bone graft (Vlaminck et al. 2007).

In rabbits, you can improve the access to all mandibular and some maxillary cheek teeth by performing a buccotomy. This approach is too traumatic to be used routinely. Incise the skin and the soft tissue from the labial commissure to the cranial border of the masseter muscle (Gorell and Verhaert 2006; Manso et al. 2011). This facilitates more complicated tooth extractions and enables resection of the lateral alveolar wall after making a vertical incision in the

lateral mucosa (Vlaminck et al. 2007). Incising the masseter is not recommended as it increases the risk of wound healing complications. To close, appose the oral mucosa with a continuous suture and close the subcutaneous tissue as well as the skin in two layers of simple interrupted sutures such as polyglactin 910.

Especially in rabbits, there is a relatively high incidence of dentinoid formation following any tooth extraction, even if the tooth has been extracted completely (i.e. apically attached germinal tissue). A few remaining germinal cells are sufficient to create unstructured odontogenic tissue (Böhmer 2015). Remove dentinoids that show signs of periodontal infection (e.g. radiolucent fringe), as they serve as a nidus for infection and cause recurring abscesses. Ankylosed dentinoids may be left in place.

A common complication of intraoral tooth extraction is fracture of the alveolar bone caused by the use of unsuitable instruments or impatience by the surgeon combined with inappropriate lever movements. If it happens, remove any bone fragments and sharp bone edges with small rongeurs before suturing the gingiva. Iatrogenic intraalveolar tooth fracture is another complication that usually occurs if a cheek tooth is brittle or has not been sufficiently loosened and is grasped with forceps. If it occurs with a mandibular cheek tooth, extract the apical part of the tooth using an apical osteotomy. For maxillary cheek teeth, a rostral (P2) or lateral (P3-M3) incision in the gingiva may improve access to the tooth socket (Figure 22.12). When extracting cheek teeth, always take care not to injure the alveolus or the germinal tissue of the adjacent teeth as this often results in spread of infection. Severe intraoperative bleeding is a rare complication that occurs primarily in rabbits because of trauma to a branch of the maxillary vein at the angle of the jaw. To stop bleeding apply pressure with a cotton-tipped applicator. Uncommon complications include postsurgical infection and iatrogenic fractures. In guinea pigs, the risk of fracture is higher when removing the last two molars as this part of the mandible is extremely thin.

Provided tooth extraction is indicated and correctly performed, the prognosis for uncomplicated healing is good.

Extraoral Approach (Apical Osteotomy)

Indications for extraoral cheek tooth extraction are apical or periodontal infections, longitudinally split teeth, splintered or transversely fractured teeth (apical remnant), apically thickened or severely malformed teeth due to the increased risk of iatrogenic fractures, and progressive carious defects or intradental resorptive lesions. In guinea pigs, any cheek tooth extraction should be performed with an osteotomy as the alveoli are very large and the gingiva cannot be sutured which leads to food impaction.

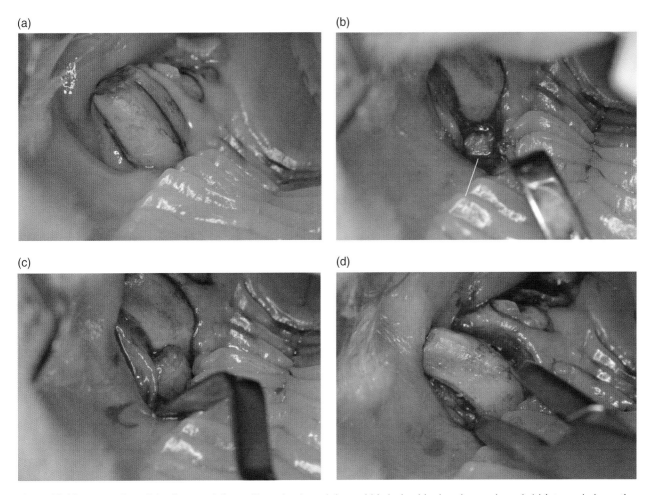

Figure 22.12 Extraction of the first two left maxillary cheek teeth in a rabbit (animal in dorsal recumbency): (a) intraoral elongation and buccal tilting of both teeth with secondary gingival hypertrophy, (b) iatrogenic horizontal fracture of the first premolar (P2); the yellow line marks the site for a gingival incision to enlarge the access to the alveolus, (c) tooth partially mobilized for extraction, (d) extraction of the adjacent premolar (P3).

Apical osteotomy is performed to gain access to an empty, infected alveolus allowing for repeated irrigation and debridement. Apical osteotomy is easy to perform on the mandible where it should be standard practice following any mandibular cheek tooth extraction. Access to the alveolus of maxillary cheek teeth is much more challenging and invasive due to species-specific anatomy (Böhmer 2015). Typically, less food becomes impacted into an empty maxillary tooth alveolus, so there is a reasonable chance for uncomplicated healing without an osteotomy. Apical access should be established in cases with widespread apical infection or if local infection persists. It should be part of the normal treatment for dental-related maxillary abscesses.

Mandibular Osteotomy (P3-M3 in Rabbits)

Apical osteotomy can be performed prior, during, or after, intraoral tooth extraction. The exact site of osteotomy depends on the specific pathology. After making a small skin incision and dissecting the subcutaneous tissue down to the bone, open the mandibular cortex overlying the apex using a suitably sized rose-headed bone burr on a high-speed compressed air drill (Figure 22.13). When performing an osteotomy following intraoral tooth extraction, insert a pointed explorer probe deep into the empty alveolus to perforate the apical bone plate prior to drilling. This helps avoid accidental injury to the adjacent apices from an incorrect trephination site.

Osteotomy can also help mobilize severely malformed, brittle, or fractured cheek teeth as it allows both ends of the tooth body to be adequately luxated prior to intraoral extraction or retropulsion (Figure 22.13). Perform any apical mobilization very gently using a dental probe and/or a Crossley molar luxator as the apical walls are extremely thin and friable in the area of the germinal tissue. Following tooth extraction, flush and gently debride the empty alveolus using a small bone curette to remove any loose bone, tooth fragments, and purulent debris. Save

(a)

(b)

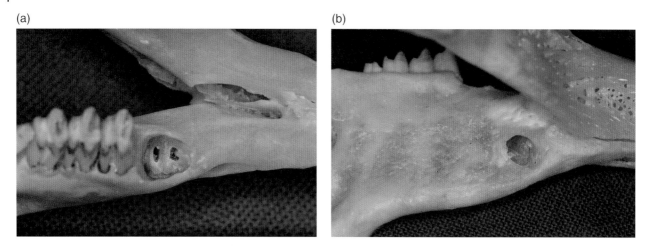

Figure 22.13 Mandible specimens of two rabbits: (a) horizontal intraalveolar fracture of the first mandibular cheek tooth being an indication to perform apical osteotomy for tooth extraction, (b) apical alveolar osteotomy of the first mandibular cheek tooth (P3).

healthy periodontal tissue as it may accelerate healing (Vlaminck et al. 2007). Remove any sharp bone edges using a small rongeur and pack the empty alveolus nearly up to the gingival margin with a gauze coated with a mix-ture of granulated sugar and petroleum jelly (Böhmer 2015) (Figure 22.14). Either suture the gingiva intraorally if possible (there is a high incidence of dehiscence) or leave it open to heal by second intention, which takes

(a)

(b)

(c)

(d)

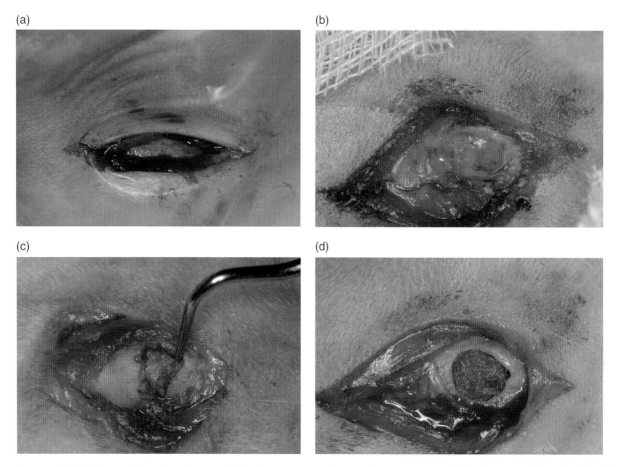

Figure 22.14 Intraoperative view of an apical alveolar osteotomy to gain retrograde access to the first mandibular cheek tooth (P3) in a rabbit: (a) ventral skin incision, (b) exposed bulb of the tooth apex, (c) retrograde tooth mobilization by means of a pointed probe, (d) empty alveolus packed in a retrograde manner with gauze.

about 7–10 days. Initially remove the packing, irrigate, debride, and pack the alveolus with new gauze every two to three days. Once there is healthy granulation tissue beginning to fill the alveolus, decrease the frequency to every week. Once the defect begins to fill with granulation tissue allow the wound to heal by second intention. In most patients, changing the packing can be done without sedation or anesthesia.

In guinea pigs, cheek tooth extraction is more challenging because they are more curved within the alveolus. Due to this curvature and the length of the tooth even an infected tooth will be firmly anchored within the alveolus. To mobilize the tooth adequately from both ends (coronally and apically), an alveolar osteotomy is always indicated (Böhmer 2015) (Figure 22.15). Whether the tooth is removed intraorally or apically depends on the situation. In contrast to rabbits, the gingiva generally cannot be sutured intraorally, so apical access is necessary and wound healing may take several months.

Maxillary Osteotomy (P2-P3 in Rabbits)

In rabbits, the apex of the second maxillary cheek tooth (P3) can be accessed relatively easily by performing an osteotomy at the zygomatic base (facial tuberosity) (Figure 22.16). Following a dorsal to ventral skin and subcutaneous tissue incision, visualize the facial tuberosity and make a hole in it using a burr to gain access to the apex of the premolar. Adequately treated (see packing protocol above), the osteotomy site usually heals without any complications.

Surgery is more challenging if an apical osteotomy of the first maxillary cheek tooth (P2) is necessary as its apex is in immediate proximity to the maxillary nerve (infraorbital foramen), the NLD, and the maxillary recess. It is vital to be familiar with the anatomy to not damage these structures while performing the osteotomy.

Maxillary Osteotomy (P4-M1 in Guinea Pigs)

In guinea pigs, the apices of the first two maxillary cheek teeth are very difficult to access as they are located far medial and rostral to the lacrimal bone. To access the apices of both teeth, resect the infraorbital part of the masseter muscle. Take care not to damage the nearby NLD, which courses rostrally between their apices (Figure 22.17).

If there are problems with wound healing or recurring local infection (pus accumulation) reassess the osteotomy site and the alveolus by obtaining intraoral radiographs in rabbits or using a special radiographic technique for an isolated view of the maxilla in guinea pigs (description in Böhmer 2015). Depending on the findings, a second surgical debridement may be required.

Surgery of Mandibular Abscesses

Tooth-related jaw abscesses generally do not heal after being lanced and drained, even if the local treatment is combined with systemic antibiotic treatment and frequent irrigation. Lancing an abscess will provide some temporary relief for the patient, but it will make any following surgical resection of the entire fibrous abscess capsule much more difficult (Crossley and Aiken 2004; Bennett 2008). Surgical intervention is the gold standard for jaw abscess treatment consisting of radical abscess resection, aggressive wound debridement, and extraction of all infected teeth (Harcourt-Brown 2009b). Performed at an early stage

(a)

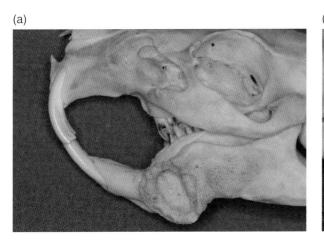

(b)

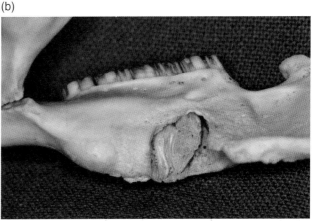

Figure 22.15 Specimens of two guinea pigs with mandibular abscesses: (a) after extraction of the first mandibular cheek tooth (P4) with the aid of a lateral alveolar osteotomy, (b) ventromedial alveolar osteotomy to gain retrograde access to the second mandibular molar (M2) (medial view).

(a)

(b)

(c)

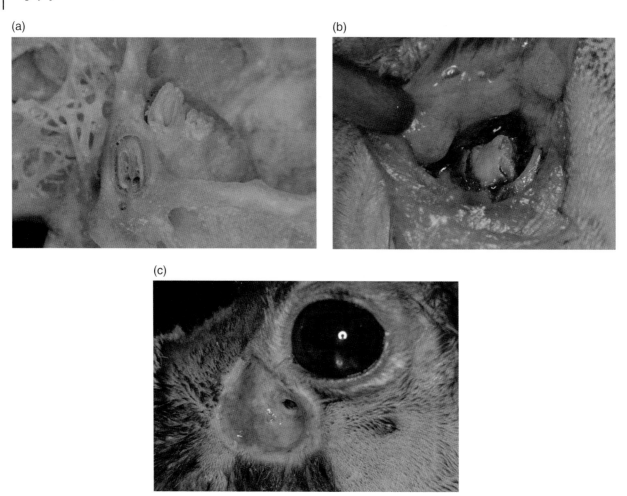

Figure 22.16 Anatomical sites of the facial tuberosity in rabbits: (a) maxillary specimen with perforation of the facial tuberosity due to retrograde cheek tooth elongation (P3), (b) intraoperative site with exposed tooth apex (P3), (c) two and a half weeks post tooth extraction with subsequent open wound healing.

of disease, it provides a relatively good chance of permanently resolving the abscess. Presurgical high-quality skull or dental radiographs (intraoral radiographs in rabbits and special views of the maxilla and mandible in guinea pigs) are essential for an accurate assessment of exactly how many teeth are involved and the extent of the infection (Böhmer 2015). While the initial surgery (tooth extraction and abscess resection) can be performed rather quickly, the aftercare is much more time consuming and involved. It often takes up to several weeks or months and the outcome is influenced much more by the follow-up treatments than the surgical technique. These re-examinations should include repeated radiographs, especially in cases with any wound healing problems or recurring local abscesses (Böhmer 2007).

Rostral mandibular abscesses mainly originate from infected incisors. In rabbits, the infection tends to spread to the first mandibular cheek tooth (P3), whereas in guinea pigs, the second (M1) or third molar (M2) are at risk, since

the apex of the mandibular incisor is adjacent to their apices (Böhmer 2015). Gain apical access to the primarily infected incisor through an osteotomy on the medial aspect of the mandible in guinea pigs. Open the infected alveolus ventrolaterally in rabbits (Figures 22.2 and 22.18).

Mandibular abscesses can also result from an apically infected (and, therefore, longitudinally split) cheek tooth. In rabbits, the first mandibular cheek tooth (P3) is most commonly affected. Since its elongated apex perforates the cortex of the mandible medially, access the apically infected tooth through a ventromedial approach (see osteotomy). If not treated at an early stage, the infection tends to spread laterally affecting both mandibular cortices and requiring lateral access for abscess management. The ipsilateral incisor and the adjacent premolar (P4) are usually involved as well and need extraction.

Caudal mandibular abscesses are initially confined to the medial aspect in most rabbits, as the apices of the last two molars (M2/M3) lie just adjacent to the inner mandibular cor-

(a)

(b)

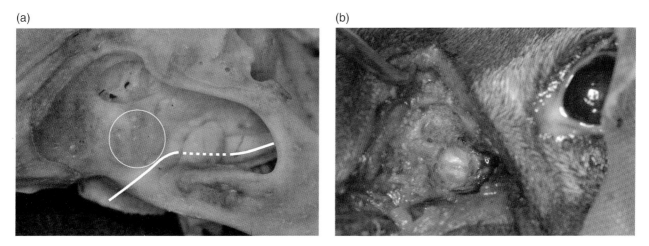

Figure 22.17   Anatomy of the area surrounding the first upper cheek tooth (P4) in a guinea pig: (a) maxillary specimen depicting the apical bulbs (yellow circle) of both first maxillary cheek teeth with the nearby nasolacrimal duct and maxillary nerve (white line) (lateral view), (b) intraoperative view after premolar apicoectomy (P4), the gauze is inserted near the nasolacrimal duct to stop local bleeding.

(a)

(b)

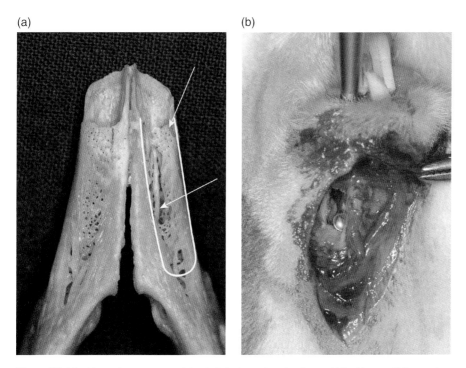

Figure 22.18   Ventral osteotomy of the left incisor alveolus in a rabbit: (a) mandible specimen with a small oblong incisor remnant (yellow arrow) being an indication for ventral alveolar osteotomy (yellow line), (b) intraoperative site of an alveolar osteotomy with a curette pushed into the empty alveolus.

tex. The infection can spread laterally, progressively involving the masseter muscle which undergoes liquefactive necrosis; an indication for its total resection. The ipsilateral temporomandibular joint is also at risk and infection there can result in temporomandibular joint ankylosis. Patients with temporomandibular joint ankylosis carry a poor prognosis and euthanasia is likely the most humane recommendation.

Although the mandibular cheek teeth in guinea pigs have a lingually concave curvature, their elongated apices tend

to perforate the jaw ventrally (P4/M1) or ventrolaterally (M2/M3). Cheek tooth-related mandibular infections are best managed using a ventrolateral approach. As in rabbits, caudal abscesses affecting both M2 and M3 often remain undetected well-hidden medial to the masseter muscle. The infection tends to spread medially and dorsally secondarily involving the temporomandibular joint and the masseter muscle which undergoes necrosis (Böhmer 2015). Due to extensive bone lysis, tooth extraction becomes very challenging with a high risk of iatrogenic mandibular fracture. In these cases, apicoectomy and packing the site with gauze as described previously may be a better option.

Unilocular mandibular abscesses are best excised "en bloc" (as if it were a tumor) as this minimizes risk of recurrence (Bennett 2009). With the patient in dorsal recumbency, resect a fusiform shaped area of the overlying skin and carefully dissect the entire tough and thick abscess capsule down to the bone using Metzenbaum scissors (Figure 22.19). Separate the abscess base from the underlying bone. A small depression will be visible in the bone corresponding to the apex of an infected tooth. Submit a tissue sample (abscess capsule and purulent material) for aerobic and anerobic bacterial culture and sensitivity testing. Following retrograde or intraoral tooth extraction and thorough excision of any necrotic tissue, irrigate the empty alveolus with a warm antiseptic fluid (e.g. 0.1% polyhexanide or 0.1% octenidine). Do not use povidone iodine as its effect may be decreased by purulent debris (Probst and Vasel-Biergans 2004). Use adequately sized strips of a suitable gauze coated with a 1:1 mixture of granulated sugar and petroleum jelly to pack the alveolus and surrounding wound (Böhmer 2015) (Figure 22.20). Close the skin with simple interrupted sutures leaving a small opening at the deepest point where the gauze exits. On the third postoperative day, remove all or some of the skin sutures and remove the wound dressing. Debride the wound thoroughly using curettage with resection of any necrotic tissue and irrigate both the soft tissue wound and the alveolus. Insert a new wound dressing as described above. Leave the wound open or close it temporarily with one or two interrupted sutures to prevent the gauze from falling out. Repeat wound care every two to three days until healthy granulation tissue begins to form and then weekly until the wound has closed (Figure 22.20). Healing time depends on the extent of infection, the number of extracted teeth, and any complications that may require additional surgery. Extensive abscesses may take up to 2 months to resolve using this technique.

Multilocular mandibular abscesses are firmly attached to the mandible making it difficult to perform an "en-bloc" excision. Dissect all of the individual abscesses down to the bone as radical as possible and resect any infected bone, ossified parts of the abscess capsule, spiculated periosteal proliferations, and bone sequestra with the aid of fine Luer bone rongeurs (Bennett 2009). To preserve jaw stability retain as much of the mandibular cortex as possible. This approach is vital for a positive outcome and the risk of recurrence increases if any necrotic bone is left (Bennett 1999; Böhmer 2015). Whether or not closing the intraoral defect is indicated following tooth extraction depends on the individual case and the size of the lesion. Small defects heal well by second intention. Large defects following removal of several teeth are best sutured closed if possible. This requires microsurgical instruments and fine suture on a small needle and is meticulous and tedious.

If wound healing complications or recurring local infections occur, radiographs should be made to evaluate the remaining teeth and surrounding bone. Depending on the findings (e.g. spread of infection), it may be necessary to open the apical access to the alveolus and the soft tissue defect again to excise any remaining necrotic bone or soft tissue and to extract any dentinoids or impacted food material. On a rare occasion, a fistula may develop between the oral cavity and the skin. Getting the fistula to close can be challenging. It will generally not close unless all of the infection is controlled. Once the tissues are healthy suture the oral mucosa, subcutaneous tissues, and skin in separate layers. Closure of the fistula may be challenging.

(a)

(b)

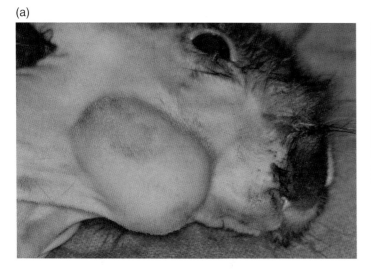
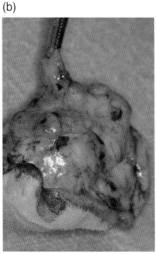

Figure 22.19 Unilocular mandibular abscess in a rabbit: (a) preoperative, (b) abscess capsule resected "en bloc."

(a) (b) (c)

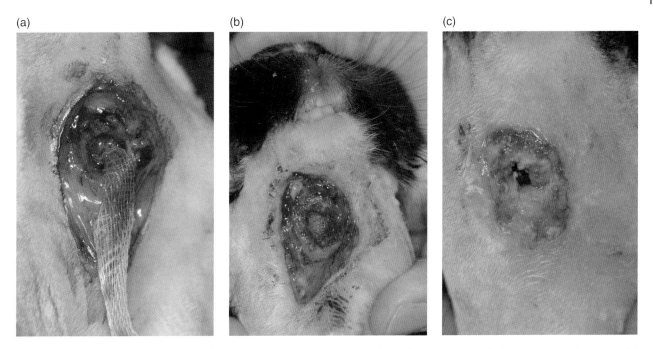

Figure 22.20 Open wound treatment following retrograde tooth extraction (mandibular P3) and radical abscess resection in a rabbit: (a) intraoperative view prior to temporary skin closure for about three days, (b) one week postsurgery with the empty alveolus packed with gauze, (c) two and a half weeks postsurgery.

Apicoectomy

Apicoectomy in combination with abscess management as described can be used to treat small, local abscesses due to apical infection of a single cheek tooth provided the tooth is not split longitudinally or loose. Following excision of the abscess, resect the apical dental tissue and the germinal tissue with a suitably sized burr (milling cutter) (Figure 22.21). Antibiotic-impregnated polymethylmethacrylate (AIPMMA) beads can be placed to provide local antibiotic therapy (see below). Apicoectomy prevents apical tooth growth, but the tooth continues to erupt (Massler and Schour 1941). In guinea pigs, the cheek tooth simply falls out some weeks later (Böhmer 2015). In rabbits, however, the tooth stops migrating out of the alveolus in most cases and remains ankylosed in place (Crossley and Aiken 2004).

Alternative Methods of Abscess-Treatment

As an alternative to packing the abscess site with medicated gauze, AIPMMA beads can be placed into the defect created by abscess excision. This technique has been used for many years to treat soft tissue and orthopedic infections in animals and humans (Tobias et al. 1996; Ethell et al. 2000; Weisman et al. 2000; Bennett 2009; Harcourt-Brown 2009b). This technique allows primary closure of

the abscess site and eliminates the need for open wound care. The beads elute antibiotic over a long period of time into the surrounding tissue at high local concentration while the systemic concentration remains low. This allows the use of antibiotics that are associated with ototoxicity, enterotoxicity, and renal toxicity when used systemically. The antibiotic used is best based on culture and sensitivity testing of the abscess. Antibiotic elution is bimodal with rapid release in the first few days and long-term release over several weeks to months (Bennett 2009). Heat-stable antibiotics such as clindamycin, gentamicin, amikacin, cefazolin, ceftiofur, ceftazidime, and tobramycin are best for incorporation in polymethylmethacrylate (PMMA) as an exothermic reaction occurs during curing (Bennett 2008). AIPMMA beads are commercially available from compounding pharmacies or you can make them yourself (described in Böhmer 2015). Mix the powdered copolymer and the antibiotic prior to the adding the liquid monomer. Put the semiliquid cement in a large syringe and squirt it out onto a sterile plastic sheet before cutting it with a scalpel blade into small fragments that can be molded into small beads. Polymerization is rapid so it can be helpful to have several people making beads from one package of cement. While a sphere has the most surface area and, thus, the most rapid elution of antibiotic, cylindrical implants are also useful as they can fit in small abscess niches. AIPMMA beads cannot be autoclaved, but can be gas sterilized and then stored for up to 12 months. The

(a)

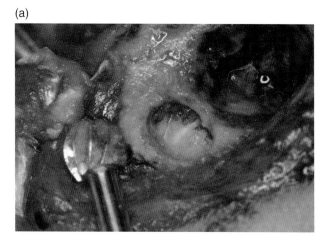

(b)

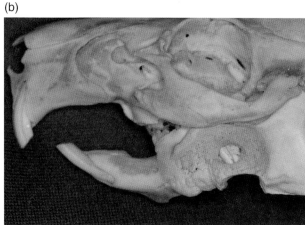

Figure 22.21 Apicoectomy in two different guinea pigs: (a) intraoperative view following exenterio bulbi and apicoectomy of the last maxillary cheek tooth (M3), (b) skull specimen with reactive proliferations of the mandibular bone and fistula formation due to periodontal infection of the last mandibular molar (M3) where apicoectomy has been performed.

package should be labeled with the antibiotic expiration date and the date of sterilization. Alternatively, the beads can be made in an aseptic environment and placed into sterile tubes for storage (Balsamo et al. 2007; Böhmer 2015).

AIPMMA beads are not absorbable but are biologically inert so they may remain within the tissues long term (Bennett 1999; Böhmer 2015) (Figure 22.22). It should be noted that if the bacteria in the wound are resistant to the antibiotic used, the beads can serve as a nidus for infection and will need to be removed.

As another treatment option is often referred to as marsupialization. Using this technique, suture the skin of the wound perimeter to the remainder of the abscess capsule with several simple interrupted sutures (Capello 2008; Harcourt-Brown 2009b). This will keep the abscess area open for a longer period of time allowing prolonged open wound management. With this technique, there is a risk of

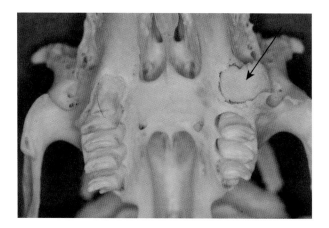

Figure 22.22 Maxillary specimen of a rabbit with implanted AIPMMA beads (black arrow) following extraction of both first upper cheek teeth (P2 + P3) two years before.

microabscesses within the abscess capsule developing into larger abscesses resulting in recurrence because the wound is infected when sutures are placed (Böhmer 2015).

Filling the abscess capsule with calcium hydroxide replaced weekly until the wound has healed has been reported to be effective in managing rabbit dental abscesses (Remeeus and Verbeek 1995). This method is not recommended based on clinical experience. The extremely alkaline calcium hydroxide not only is bactericidal but also causes severe necrosis of the soft tissues and bone (Eickhoff 2005; Gorell and Verhaert 2006; Harcourt-Brown 2009b).

Other biologically inert or biodegradable materials can be used as antibiotic carriers to fill an empty tooth socket or to provide local release of antibiotics. Some have angiogenic and osteoconductive properties including synthetic glass ceramics (e.g. PerioGlas, Block Drug Co., NJ, USA), calcium sulfate or phosphate pellets, and micro or macroporous hydroxyapatite granules (Yamamura et al. 1992; DeForge 1997; Kawanabe et al. 1998; Stoor et al. 1998; Bellantone et al. 2000; Liljensten et al. 2003; Stubbs et al. 2004; Richelsoph et al. 2007; Au et al. 2008; McConoughey et al. 2015). Most materials are available as dense blocks, porous solid pieces, granules, or even injectable solutions.

Another option for filling the defect and delivering local antibiotic is antibiotic-impregnated collagen sponges or fleeces (e.g. Septocoll®, Innocoll Inc., USA). However, the release time of antibiotics from different collagen implants was only four days (Wachol-Drewek et al. 1996). Similar problems with short duration of elution may arise if antimicrobial-impregnated gauzes are used (Taylor et al. 2010). There are many anecdotal reports of using various carriers without elution studies. It is best not to use carriers with unknown elution properties as they may elute antibiotic too rapidly and it may be absorbed in high enough concentrations to cause systemic toxicity.

Choosing a suitable wound dressing is not as critical as accurately identifying and eliminating the primary cause of infection (i.e. extraction of all infected teeth) and providing appropriate postoperative wound management either using repeated wound debridement over weeks to months or implanting an antibiotic carrier to provide long-term release of antibiotic locally (Böhmer 2015). For open wound management, some preparations have proven to be excellent topical dressings for infected wounds, such as sugar and honey. Both have rapid antimicrobial properties due to their hygroscopic activity (plasmolysis of bacterial cells), which also helps decrease inflammatory edema and draw lymph into the wound area. They keep the wound moist, attract macrophages, stimulate angiogenesis, accelerate sloughing of devitalized tissue, and promote formation of healthy granulation tissue without causing excessive granulation tissue formation or scarring (Chirife et al. 1982; Bergman et al. 1983; Topham 2002; Shi et al. 2007; Mphande et al. 2007; Bhat et al. 2014). Dry white sugar can cause a burning sensation when applied, mix it with an appropriate ointment (e.g. petroleum jelly). Alternatively, gauze soaked in 50% dextrose can be used (Gorell and Verhaert 2006).

The prognosis for healing in rabbits and rodents with mandibular abscesses depends on the extent of the infection, the site of the pathologic changes, the general condition of the patient, the experience of the practitioner, and the chosen method of treatment.

Focal abscesses of the mandible are rather rare in chinchillas and degus, except for rostral abscesses that originate primarily from infected incisors. If cheek tooth-related mandibular infections occur, surgical treatment is performed as described above.

Surgery of Rostral Maxillary Abscesses

Extraoral Tooth Extraction (P2, P3) and Sinusotomy in Rabbits

In rabbits, abscesses involving the cribriform plate and/or the facial tuberosity are relatively common. They may be tooth-related (maxillary incisors or both first maxillary cheek teeth) or caused by chronic NLD infections. In guinea pigs, rostral maxillary abscesses are rare, though the etiopathogenesis is similar. Abscess management and cheek tooth extraction using a maxillary osteotomy is challenging because the tooth apices are difficult to

access, especially in guinea pigs (see maxillary osteotomy). It is important to identify and remove infected teeth early to decrease the risk of the infection eroding into the nasal cavity due to the close anatomic relationship between the caudal aspect of the incisors, the premolars, and the nasal cavity.

In rabbits with an infection of the first maxillary cheek tooth (P2) that has spread into the maxillary sinus (unilateral purulent sinusitis), the premolar must be removed and the ventral aspect of the maxillary sinus must be opened at the most ventral point (Chitty and Raftery 2013). Use a lateral approach to gain access to the typically malformed and rostromedially displaced premolar and the infected maxillary sinus.

With the intubated rabbit in lateral recumbency, make a dorsoventral incision in the skin and subcutaneous tissue just rostral to the facial tuberosity. Use a self-retaining ring retractor (e.g. Lone Star retractor, Lone Star Medical Products, Stafford, USA) to facilitate access. Use a periosteal elevator to elevate the soft tissue caudally and rostrally to visualize the bony part of the NLD and the maxillary nerve where it exits the infraorbital foramen. The apex of the first maxillary premolar (P2) is located directly ventral to this foramen. Prior to or after intraoral tooth extraction, perform an alveolar osteotomy by resecting a part of the rostrolateral alveolar wall with a bone burr. Take care to not damage the maxillary nerve. The osteotomy provides access to the infected alveolus which lies on the ventral floor of the maxillary recess (Casteleyn et al. 2010). Using a high-speed air drill and a suitable round headed bone burr, drill a small hole into the maxillary bone just dorsal to P2 taking care to preserve the NLD (Figure 22.23). Access the conchomaxillary cavity by fenestrating the lamina cribrosa just dorsal to the NLD

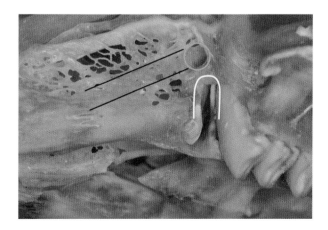

Figure 22.23 Maxillary specimen of a rabbit showing the osteotomy site (yellow line) for retrograde extraction of the first maxillary cheek tooth (P2). Note the immediate vicinity of the alveolus to the maxillary nerve (orange circle) (infraorbital foramen) and the nasolacrimal duct (black lines).

(Figure 22.24). Remove any purulent debris, infected tissue, and necrotic bone using a Volkmann curette, Lempert rongeurs, and cotton-tipped applicators soaked with sterile saline until the site is free of infected material. Pack both the thoroughly debrided sinus site and alveolus with sugar-impregnated gauze and close the overlying skin. Remove the sutures three days later and debride and repack the wound as previously described after irrigating the maxillary sinus (Chitty and Raftery 2013; Guevara et al. 2006).

Experimental studies have shown that long-term results are best if the surgical approach to the maxillary sinus is as small as possible (less mucosal damage) and if patency of the narrow, slit-like opening into the nasal cavity (ostium) can be preserved (Guevara et al. 2006; Harkema et al. 2006; Chitty and Raftery 2013). This ensures that the remaining sinus mucosa continues to produce adequate amounts of nitrous oxide, which enhances the local host defense mechanism through vasodilation and phagocytosis. It also stimulates the mucociliary activity, which is important as the ostium into the nasal cavity is not at the most ventral point of the conchomaxillary cavity, so active ciliary movement is necessary to remove normal secretions (Schlosser et al. 2000; Naraghi et al. 2007; Lundberg 2008).

In rabbits, an infection of the first maxillary premolar often spreads to the adjacent tooth (P3) whose tooth body is located deep within the facial tuberosity. Along with retrograde tooth elongation, this premolar becomes severely curved and its apex perforates the facial bone laterally (Böhmer and Crossley 2011). Where there is severe periodontal abscess, extract the affected tooth as well as a major part or even the entire facial tuberosity.

Lateral Fenestration of the Nasolacrimal Duct

Lateral fenestration of the NLD is indicated to treat a focal abscess of an obstructed and dilated NLD.

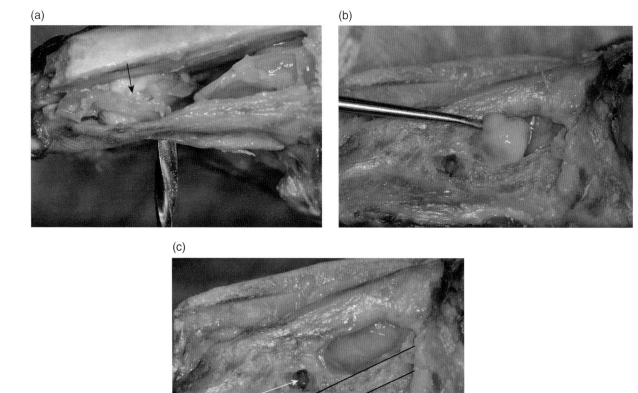

(a)

(b)

(c)

Figure 22.24 Postmortem specimen of a rabbit suffering from chronic rhinitis with purulent sinusitis and infected maxillary conchae: (a) opening of the conchomaxillary cavity at its deepest point just rostrodorsal to the nasolacrimal duct (black arrow) with the aid of a burr, (b) after sinusotomy to widely open the infected ventral recess of the maxillary sinus (curette filled with pus), (c) after sinusotomy showing entry point (yellow arrow) and the nasolacrimal duct (black lines).

Perform a dorsoventral incision in the skin and subcutaneous tissue rostral to the facial tuberosity to gain access to the lamina cribrosa with the bony part of the NLD. Fenestrate the lateral wall of the duct using a burr as wide as needed to access the infected area (Figure 22.25). Perform a thorough local debridement. Copiously irrigate the duct to relieve the obstruction and partially close the skin to form an adequate stoma for further flushing. Irrigate the duct twice daily until the infection improves and a small fistula develops. This fistula typically heals over with time. Recurring problems may not arise because in most cases, a connection develops between the NLD and the nasal cavity.

Dorsal Rhinostomy

Indication for a rhinostomy is widespread dental or NLD-related intranasal abscesses with accumulation of large amounts of caseous material within the dilated and mostly disintegrated maxillary sinus, combined with progressive necrosis of the turbinates.

Place the intubated rabbit in sternal recumbency and make a paramedian incision in the skin on the dorsal aspect of the nose. To obtain unilateral access to the nasal cavity, separate the nasal bone from the nasal process of the incisive bone laterally and from its counterpart medially with the aid of an osteotome or sharp scalpel along the bony suture. Carefully elevate the nasal bone and flip it caudally or temporarily remove it (Figure 22.26). Debride the nasal cavity as aggressively as needed to resect all necrotic bone and soft tissue using a Volkmann curette, bone ronguers, and cotton-tipped applicators. Irrigate the nasal cavity with warm sterile saline through the nares. Before replacing the nasal bone resect a small part its base. Insert a temporary drain into the nasal cavity through the hole created at the base of the nasal bone for twice daily postoperative irrigation. Close the skin with simple interrupted sutures. Administer a broad-spectrum antibiotic

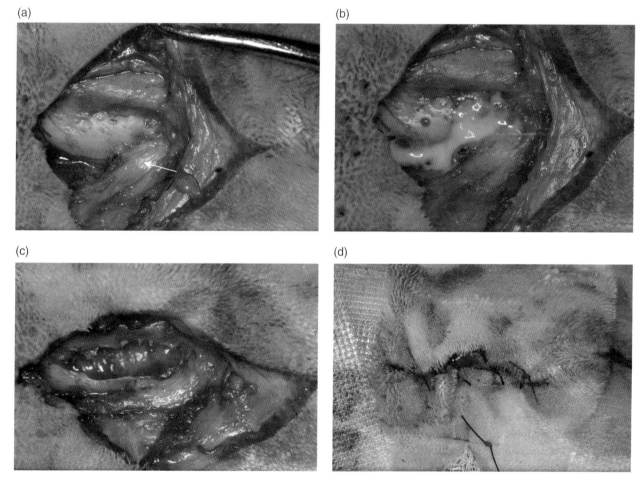

(a) (b) (c) (d)

Figure 22.25 Lateral fenestration of the nasolacrimal duct: (a) exposure of the nasolacrimal duct and the maxillary nerve (foramen infraorbitale) (white arrow), (b) pus oozing out of the nasolacrimal duct after drilling a hole in it, (c) widespread opening of the duct (fenestration), (d) skin sutures to form a persistent stoma.

(a)   (b)

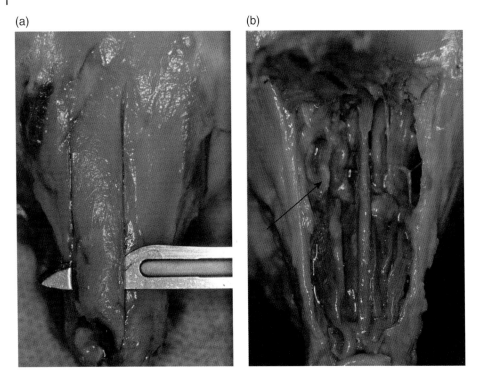

Figure 22.26 Dorsal rhinostomy in a postmortem rabbit specimen: (a) mobilization of the right nasal bone plate, (b) situation after removal of both nasal bone plates showing right-sided purulent rostral rhinitis and sinusitis (black arrow).

based on culture and sensitivity results for about 3 weeks (Chitty and Raftery 2013).

Surgery of Retrobulbar Abscesses

Extraoral Tooth Extraction Combined with Orbital Exenteration or Partial Resection of the Zygomatic Arch in Rabbits

In rabbits, retrobulbar abscesses are predominantly caused by periodontal infection of a single or the caudal four maxillary cheek teeth (P4-M3). Initial pathology is usually unrecognized because of the absence of clinical signs. The infection tends to spread to adjacent teeth, the retrobulbar soft tissue, and/or the intraorbital lacrimal glands until exophthalmos is noted, often combined with horizontal exposure keratitis. At the same time, the infected teeth become grotesquely deformed and elongated protruding far into the orbit. They are often obscured by a solid, fibrous capsule that tends to ossify forming a retrobulbar bullous bony structure (Böhmer 2015) (Figure 22.27).

In guinea pigs, retrograde elongation and apical infection of a single maxillary cheek tooth (M2/M3) is always accompanied by typical structural changes of its occlusal surface (e.g. abnormal enamel and dentin pattern) (Figure 22.28). Along with the retrobulbar tooth elonga-

tion, the eye becomes progressively more exophthalmic over a period of several months. If slight exophthalmos is present, skull or dental radiographs, including an isolated view of the maxillary molars as described by Böhmer (2015), are strongly recommended even if the patient is not showing any clinical signs.

To ensure a successful long-term outcome, extract all infected teeth and perform a radical abscess excision with removal of all necrotic or infected soft tissue and bone (Böhmer 2015). Equally important is the postoperative wound management (previously described) which may be challenging depending upon the number of extracted teeth that can cause a wide connection to the oral cavity. Intraoral tooth extraction and abscess management alone is not recommended (Martinez-Jimenez et al. 2007). Due to the poor exposure of the infected orbit with this method, parts of the abscess capsule or infected bone may not be excised, which increases risk of infection recurrence (Figure 22.29). Furthermore, it is difficult to perform adequate follow-up care with only intraoral access. This especially applies to guinea pigs with their strongly curved and long alveoli. Therefore, dental-related retrobulbar abscesses should be still combined with orbital exenteration. In rabbits, however, resection of the zygomatic arch may be a suitable alternative.

Orbital exenteration is a procedure to remove the globe along with all of the contents of the orbit. With the patient

(a)

(b)

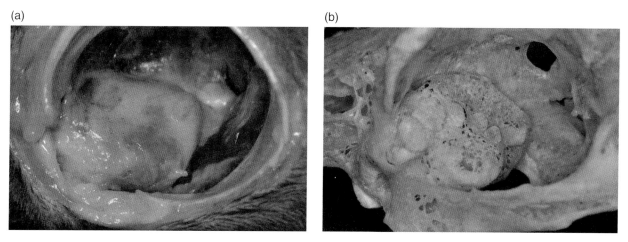

Figure 22.27 Rabbit with bulbous retrobulbar bone proliferation due to apical cheek tooth infection (P4-M3): (a) intraoperative view, (b) maxillary specimen of the same patient.

(a)

(b)

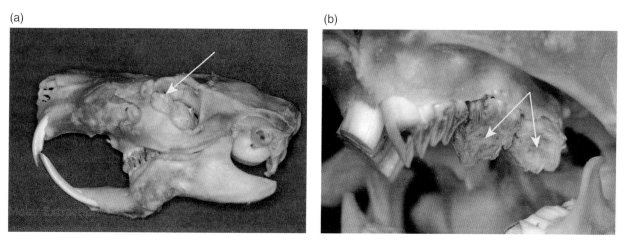

Figure 22.28 Specimen of a guinea pig with extreme retrograde elongation of both last two maxillary cheek teeth (M2 and M3): (a) malocclusion with secondary elongation of the incisors (yellow arrow), (b) intraoral view of the structurally changed occlusal plane of both caudal molars (M2+M3) (yellow arrows).

(a)

(b)

(c)

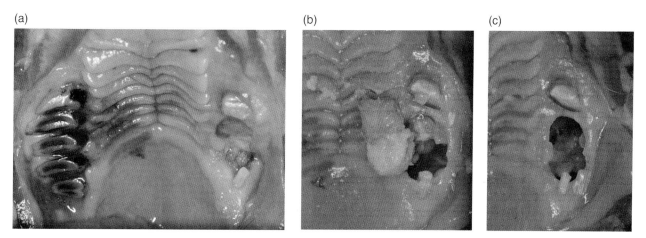

Figure 22.29 Rabbit with a dental-related retrobulbar abscess (P2-M3) (dorsal recumbency): (a) intraoral view, (b) postmortem with one molar being extracted (M2), (c) postmortem with two molars being extracted (note the poor view of the infected retrobulbar area).

in lateral recumbency, appose the eyelids with a curved arterial clamp. Make two curved skin incisions about 2 mm from and parallel to the upper and lower lid margins that meet nasally and temporally (Figure 22.30). Using small Metzenbaum scissors, transect all muscles and adnexas that are attached to the globe down to the orbital apex. Finally, transect the optic nerve, artery, and vein and remove the globe and resected intraorbital tissue including the intraorbital lacrimal glands. Use cotton-tipped applicators to apply pressure on the transected vessels to achieve hemostasis. To gain access to the infected teeth, penetrate the fibrous or ossified abscess capsule and enlarge the opening as needed. Extract all affected teeth and perform a radical abscess excision. This will result in a relatively large connection to the oral cavity which can be closed through the exenteration site with monofilament suture material. Alternatively, pack the empty tooth sockets and the abscess cavity with a gauze

coated with a mixture of granulated sugar and petroleum jelly (Figure 22.31). Close the wound for three days and then perform wound care as previously described.

In guinea pigs, retrobulbar abscess excision combined with extraction of one or both caudal maxillary molars always results in a wide connection to the oral cavity that cannot be closed surgically. Postoperative wound treatment is very challenging and time-consuming, and may result in fistula formation.

In rabbits, the apices of the caudal four maxillary cheek teeth (P4-M3) can be approached by partially removing the zygomatic arch (Figure 22.32). Make a skin incision along the zygomatic arch and isolate the underlying bone. Resect part of the arch by making two transverse osteotomies far enough apart to gain access to the tooth apices.

If the second maxillary cheek tooth (P3) is involved as well, resect the facial tuberosity as well. This affords lateral

(a)

(b)

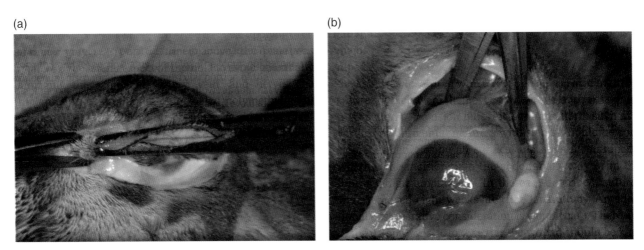

Figure 22.30 Exenteratio bulbi in a rabbit: (a) situation after skin incision and apposition of the eyelids with the aid of a arterial clamp, (b) transection of the retrobulbar soft tissue.

(a)

(b)

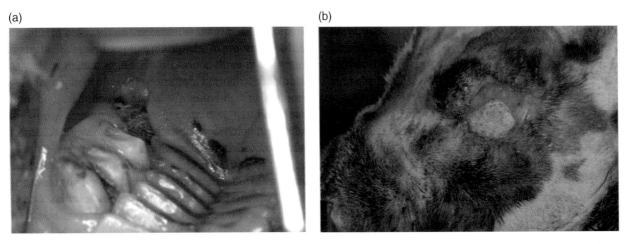

Figure 22.31 Post extraction of the last two maxillary molars (M2-M3) in a rabbit: (a) intraoral view with the alveolus packed with gauze, (b) orbit filled with gauze.

(a)

(b)

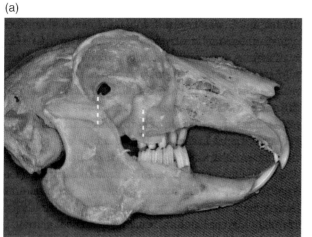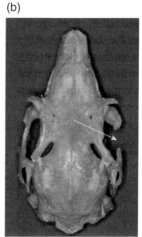

Figure 22.32 Skull specimen of a rabbit showing partial resection of the zygomatic arch: (a) lateral view (yellow dotted lines), (b) dorsal view (yellow arrow).

access to the tooth apices allowing radical abscess excision along with tooth extraction without needing to remove the eye. In guinea pigs, this approach is not feasible as the tooth apices are located too far medially.

Prognosis for cure depends on the extent of the retrobulbar bone damage and the number of infected and extracted cheek teeth. The outcome may be better if all maxillary cheek teeth are extracted because the intraoral defect is far easier to suture closed and the opposing teeth stop growing.

Treatment of Jaw Fractures

In rabbits and guinea pigs, mandibular fractures are more common than maxillary fractures. The choice of treatment depends on the location of the fracture and the species. A rapid return to normal function and normal tooth wear is the primary goal of surgical intervention (Villano and Cooper 2013). Precise surgical alignment and rigid stabilization of the fragments to reestablish normal occlusion allow rapid return to function. Conservative treatment will likely result in malunion causing secondary malocclusion. In rabbits, surgical intervention is indicated for rostral or mid-body mandibular fractures through the incisor or cheek teeth alveoli. Fractures caudal to the mandibular body can be treated conservatively since the mandibular angle is covered medially by the pterygoid muscles and laterally by the strong masseter muscle, both of which stabilize the fracture. However, comminuted fractures of the caudal mandible may heal in malunion causing severe malocclusion due to secondary skull deformity (Figure 22.33).

In rabbits, traumatic unilateral mandibular fractures can be stabilized by using an external fixator. Place at least two Kirschner wires or threaded pins for acrylic fixators (IMEX® Veterinary, Inc., Longview, TX) in each fragment that pass through one or, preferably both mandibles and then connect these with an acrylic connecting system. If a pathologic or iatrogenic fracture occurs due to osteomyelitis, make sure to place the pins only in healthy (noninfected) bone tissue and consider additionally placing AIPMMA beads in the abscess area. Alternatively, use a bone plate for fixation of a traumatic mandibular fracture (Guerrissi et al. 1994; El-Bialy et al. 2002; Campisi et al. 2003; Chen et al. 2012) (Figure 22.34). Mini 1.5 mm titanium plates (DePuySynthes®, West Chester, USA) (Bilgili and Orhun 2002; Horiguchi 2002; Erdogan et al. 2006; Uckan et al. 2009; Fernandez et al. 2012) or 1.5 mm absorbable miniplates (Lacto Sorb® system 1.5 mm, Marty Lemire and Associates, Royal Oak, USA) (Hochuli-Vieira et al. 2005) have been reportedly used with success. Most papers describing mandibular plating are experimental and published in human medicine. The techniques can be applied to pet rabbits as well when using an appropriately sized implant and the screws do not traumatize the reserve crowns of the teeth (Figure 22.35).

Another surgical option is interfragmentary wire stabilization which is best combined with an external fixation device (Bilgili and Orhun 2002; Enezei et al. 2014). Drill a small hole in each fragment, pass a suitably sized stainless steel wire (0.3–0.5 mm) through both holes and tighten it by twisting. Independent of the surgical approach, suture intraoral soft tissue defects meticulously as most jaw fractures are exposed to the oral cavity. In rabbits, fracture healing is characterized by relatively rapid callus formation. Jaw fractures heal by intramembranous ossification where the periosteum and endosteum grow across the fracture ends forming a callus that is later remodeled into bone

(a)

(b)

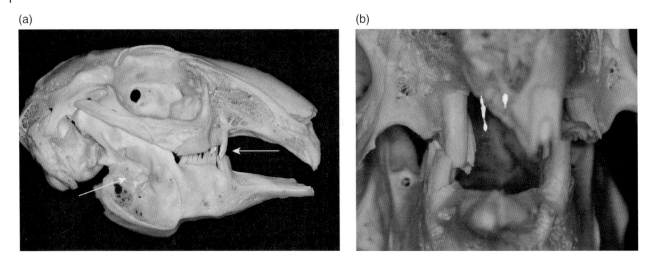

Figure 22.33 Rabbit specimen with a comminuted fracture of the caudal mandible healed in malalignment with secondary cheek tooth malocclusion: (a) note the pseudoarthrosis between the caudal mandible and the bony ear canal, (b) intraoral view with shift of the mandible to the right and secondary right-sided tooth elongation.

(a)

(b)

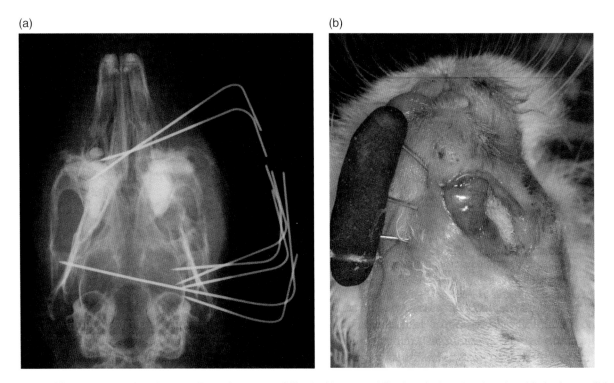

Figure 22.34 Two rabbits with mandibular fractures stabilized with external fixation devices: (a) pins placed in both mandibles, (b) Type I external skeletal fixator.

(Nalin 2013). Therefore, handle both structures very carefully in case of any surgical fixation.

Maxillary fractures are rare. They mostly affect the incisive bone immediately caudal to the incisors and can include trauma to the NLD and the nasal conchae, which can cause severe dyspnea. The best treatment is to perform a complete surgical resection of the isolated rostral part of the maxilla with closure of the soft tissue.

This helps avoid bacterial rhinitis or stenosis of the nasal cavity. Temporarily insert a small plastic tube into each naris. To stabilize a unilateral mid-incisive bone fracture, place threaded parapulpar pins into both maxillary incisors, and connect them with composite material (Figure 22.36).

Nonunion, malunions, and delayed union with secondary malocclusion, damage to tooth roots by implants, soft

(a)

(b)

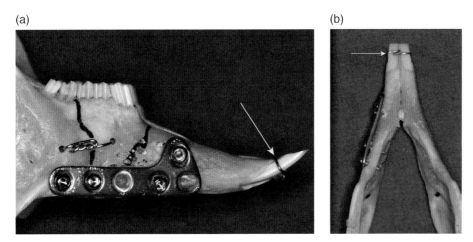

Figure 22.35 Mandibular specimen of a rabbit with an assumed mid-body fracture and symphysiolysis both stabilized with the aid of a mini bone plate and a cerclage wire fixation of the incisors (yellow arrow) without damage to the tooth apices: (a) lateral view, (b) ventral view.

(a)

(b)

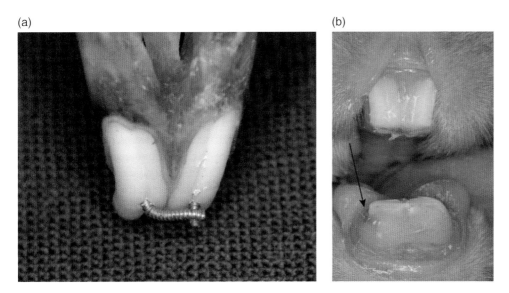

Figure 22.36 Fixation of jaw fracture-related incisor separations in two rabbits: (a) maxillary specimen with intradentally placed parapulpar pins that have to be covered additionally with a composite bridge, (b) situation after immobilization of a mandibular symphysiolysis with the aid of an incisor cerclage wire fixation (black arrow) and an additional composite bridge (shortened incisors reduce unwanted stress on the fracture site).

tissue infection, osteomyelitis, and bone necrosis are potential complications.

Prognosis for healing of jaw fractures depends on their location and the degree of accompanying soft tissue trauma. The most favorable prognosis is for fractures of the vertical ramus, whereas the prognosis for mid-body or rostral fractures depends on the individual situation. While most mandibular fractures treated conservatively tend to heal rather well in rabbits, complications are common in guinea pigs, in particular secondary abscess formation. In cases of iatrogenic jaw fractures following tooth extraction, the extent of the primary infection additionally influences the outcome.

Stabilization of a Mandibular Symphysiolysis

Trauma-related mandibular symphyseal separation is a common injury in rabbits and guinea pigs. Provided that the mandibular incisors have not been damaged, simply connect both incisors together with a composite to stabilize the symphysis allowing it to heal (Böhmer 2015). Prior to applying the composite, thoroughly clean and irrigate the site. Align both mandibles and stabilize with orthopedic wire placed around the incisors (Figure 22.36). Drilling a shallow notch into the lateral surface of each incisor will prevent the wire from slipping off the teeth when it is tightened. Clean the enamel with pumice powder and etch it with 40% phosphoric acid for about two minutes to improve the cohesive bond for the self- or light-cured composite material. Flush and dry the teeth. Apply the composite material in several thin layers over the cerclage wire (Figure 22.36). Due to tooth eruption, this dental bond progressively shifts coronally and will have to be replaced near the gingival margin about three weeks later. After six weeks, the symphysis should be healed and the device can be removed.

The prognosis for healing is good if the mandibles are adequately aligned and the incisors are not loose. It is guarded if it is severely contaminated due to the high risk of infection.

Condylectomy

Dysplasia, luxation, and anklyosis of the temporomandibular joint are very rare in rabbits and guinea pigs. More common are periarticular infections that arise from spread of a primary dental infection of the last mandibular or maxillary molar. Therapy depends on the individual situation and may be fatal if the jaw is ankylosed due to severe fibrosis. Experimental studies have shown that following condylectomy (gap of about 1 cm) rabbits can eat normally (Tuncel and Ozgenel 2011), however, expect secondary malocclusion to occur.

Alveolectomy and Mandibulectomy

Segmental, Partial, or Complete

Benign or malignant neoplasia affecting the jaw (odontogenic, osteogenic, or invasive soft tissue tumors) are relatively rare in small mammals, with the exception of elodontomas (Böhmer 2015). Resect locally limited soft tissue neoplasia by performing a fusiform excision with appropriate tissue margins as dictated by tumor type. Suture the mucosal defect in one or two layers using interrupted monofilament sutures. For larger defects, close the defect with a local buccal flap. If a more radical resection is indicated, a partial mandibulectomy may be necessary. This is also a therapeutic option for severely infected mandibular fractures, chronic mandibular abscesses with widespread bone loss, or temporomandibular joint ankylosis due to infection, muscle contracture, or tissue fibrosis. Following partial mandibulectomy, there often occurs a drift to the ipsilateral side (Figure 22.37). Malaligned cheek teeth and incisors will require repeated trimming at regular intervals.

Various techniques are used depending on how much tissue needs to be removed. For a segmental mandibulectomy, perform two osteotomies from the alveolar crest to the ventral border of the mandible. The resected section can encompass multiple cheek teeth and range from the area rostral to the first cheek tooth to the caudal aspect of the last molar. This technique offers an advantage to the partial mandibulectomy where the remaining caudal part of the mandible (caudal ramus with the condylar process of the temporomandibular joint) is resected as well. In the case of a complete hemimandibulectomy, remove the entire half of the mandible up to the symphysis.

Less aggressive procedures are the medial or lateral alveolectomy involving one or more alveoli or a horizontal bicortical full thickness resection of the alveolar ridge also referred to as nonsegmental partial mandibulectomy (Figure 22.38). Even if the entire medial or lateral wall of the mandible is resected continuity of the mandible is preserved as long as the ventral mandible remains intact. Some degree of mandibular bone regeneration may occur over time (Abrahamsson et al. 2010).

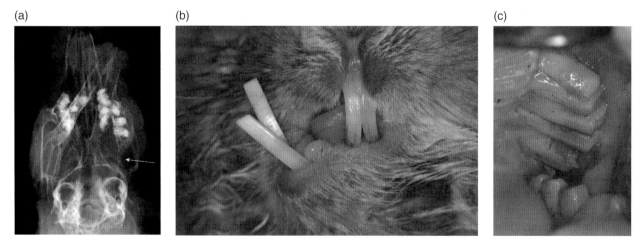

(a)   (b)   (c)

Figure 22.37 Long-term follow-up of a rabbit two years after partial (caudal) mandibulectomy: (a) radiograph of the partial mandibulectomy (yellow arrow) depicting marked lateral shift of the mandible (dorsoventral view), (b) front view with secondary lateral shift of the overgrown incisors, (c) intraoral view on the strongly tilted and overgrown left upper cheek teeth.

(a)

(b)

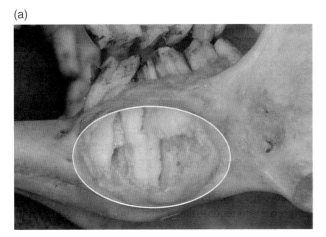 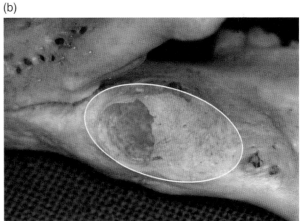

Figure 22.38 Mandibular specimen of two rabbits with a tooth-related mandibular abscesses: (a) the yellow area marks where a widespread lateral alveolectomy can be performed (P3-M1) (lateral view), (b) the yellow area depicts the site of an indicated medioventral alveolectomy (P3-P4) (medial view).

To perform a segmental mandibulectomy first rinse the oral cavity with a suitable antiseptic solution (0.12% chlorhexidine gluconate solution) and place the intubated rabbit in dorsal recumbency. In addition to general anesthesia, perform a caudal mandibular nerve block (Böhmer 2015). Make a skin incision along the ventral mandibular border that extends from the vertical ramus to the rostral part of the mandible. Extend the incision through the subdermal fascia. To gain access to the bone, reflect the rostral part of the masseter muscle as needed and elevate the medially located digastric muscle with a periosteal elevator. Following dissection of the pathologically changed tissue from the healthy bone perform a rostral and caudal osteotomy using an oscillating saw. To control hemorrhage, pack the medullary cavities of both mandibular ends with bone wax. Irrigate the wound to remove any bone dust and close oral mucosa, preserved muscle and fascial tissue, and skin in several layers.

To perform a complete hemimandibulectomy, make a skin incision from the mandibular symphysis to the temporomandibular joint. Transect all muscles and soft tissues from the mandible to the skull. Detach the masseter muscle from the lateral aspect of the mandible and transect the medially running digastric muscle. Transect the pterygoid and deep temporalis muscles to expose the medial surface of the mandible, which allows the oral mucosa to be elevated as well. Separate the symphysis with a periosteal elevator or a small osteotome and elevate the mandible. Retracting it dorsolaterally allows access to transect tissue up to the temporomandibular joint. Finally, disarticulate the condylar process. Control hemorrhage from larger blood vessels (e.g. mandibular alveolar artery) with electrosurgery, hemostatic clips, or suture ligation and stop diffuse capillary bleedings by applying pressure. Close the wound by apposing the different soft tissue layers using absorbable sutures. Close the oral mucosa with a continuous pattern and close the muscles to adjacent fascia and the skin with simple interrupted sutures. In case of a widespread abscess, coat the wound with sugar prior to closure and temporarily insert a gauze coated with a mixture of granulated sugar and petroleum jelly.

References

Abrahamsson, P., Isaksson, S., Gordh, M., and Andersson, G. (2010). Onlay bone grafting of the mandible after periosteal expansion with an osmotic tissue expander: an experimental study in rabbits. *Clinical Oral Implants Research* 21: 1404–1410.

Au, A.Y., Au, R.Y., Al-Talib, T.K. et al. (2008). Consil bioactive glass particles enhance osteoblast proliferation and maintain extracellular matrix production in vitro. *Journal of Biomedical Materials Research* A86: 678–684.

Balsamo, L.H., Whiddon, D.R., and Simpson, R.B. (2007). Does antibiotic elution from PMMA beads deteriorate after 1-year shelf storage? *Clinical Orthopaedics and Related Research* 462: 195–199.

Bellantone, M., Coleman, N.J., and Hench, L.L. (2000). Bacteriostatic action of a novel four-component bioactive glass. *Journal of Biomedical Materials Research* 51: 484–490.

Bennett, R.A. (1999). Management of abscesses of the head in rabbits. *Proceedings of the North American Veterinary Conference*, Orlando, Florida, pp. 821–823.

Bennett, R.A. (2008). Antibiotic-impregnated PMMA beads – use and misuse. *Proceeding of the Western Veterinary Conference*, Las Vegas, NV: Mandalay Bay Convention Center.

Bennett, R.A. (2009). Rabbit dental abscesses. *Proceeding of the Atlantic Coast Veterinary Conference*, Atlantic City, NJ

Bergman, A., Yanai, J., Weiss, J. et al. (1983). Acceleration of wound healing by topical application of honey. An animal model. *The American Journal of Surgery* 145: 374–376.

Bhat, R.R., Pai, M.V., Ram, S. et al. (2014). Comparison of sugar and honey dressings in healing of chronic wounds. *IOSR Journal of Dental and Medical Sciences* 13: 82–88.

Bilgili, H. and Orhun, S. (2002). Comparative study on the effects of wire, polydioxanone, and mini titanium plate osteosynthesis materials on the healing of mandibular fractures: an experimental study in rabbits. *Turkish Journal of Veterinary and Animal Sciences* 26: 1109–1116.

Böhmer, E. (2003). Extraktion von Schneidezähnen bei Kaninchen und Nagern – Indikationen und Technik. *Tierärztliche Praxis* 31: 309–320.

Böhmer, E. (2007). Intraoral radiographic technique in lagomorphs and rodents. *Exotic DVM* 9: 21–27.

Böhmer, E. (2015). *Dentistry in Rabbits and Rodents*. Oxford: Wiley Blackwell.

Böhmer, E. and Crossley, D. (2011). Objective interpretation of dental disease in rabbits, guinea pigs and chinchillas. Use of anatomical reference lines. *European Journal of Companion Animal Practice* 21: 47–56.

Bulliot, C. and Mentre, V. (2013). Original rhinostomy technique for the treatment of pseudo-odontoma in a prairie dog (*Cynomys ludovicianus*). *Journal of Exotic Pet Medicine* 22: 76–81.

Campisi, P., Hamdy, R.C., Lauzier, D. et al. (2003). Expression of bone morphogenetic proteins during mandibular distraction osteogenesis. *Plastic and Reconstructive Surgery* 111: 201–208.

Capello, V. (2008). Diagnosis and treatment of dental disease in pet rodents. *Journal of Exotic Pet Medicine* 17: 114–123.

Casteleyn, C., Cornillie, P., Hermens, A. et al. (2010). Topography of the rabbit paranasal sinuses as a prerequisite to model human sinusitis. *Rhinology* 48: 300–304.

Chen, T., Lai, R.F., Zhou, Z.Y., and Yin, Z.D. (2012). Application of ultrasonic inspection in monitoring dynamic healing of mandibular fracture in rabbit model. *Asian Pacific Journal of Tropical Medicine* 5: 406–409.

Chirife, J., Scarmato, G.A., and Herszage, L. (1982). Scientific basis for use of granulated sugar in treatment of infected wounds. *Lancet* 1: 560–561.

Chitty, J. and Raftery, A. (2013). Ear and sinus surgery. In: *BSAVA Manual of Rabbit Surgery, Dentistry and Imaging* (eds. F. Harcourt Brown and J. Chitty), 212–223. Gloucester, England: BSAVA.

Crossley, D.A. (1994). Extraction of rabbit incisor teeth. *Journal of the British Veterinary Dental Association* 2: 8.

Crossley, D.A. and Aiken, S. (2004). Small mammal dentistry. In: *Ferrets, Rabbits and Rodents – Clinical Medicine and Surgery* (eds. K.E. Quesenberry and J.W. Carpenter), 370–382. Philadelphia, PA: Saunders.

DeForge, D.H. (1997). Evaluation of bioglass/PerioGlas (Consil) synthetic bone graft particulate in the dog and cat. *Journal of Veterinary Dentistry* 14 (4): 141–145.

Easson, W. (2012). Tooth extraction. In: *BSAVA Manual of Rabbit Surgery, Dentistry and Imaging* (eds. F. Harcourt Brown and J. Chitty), 370–381. England: BSAVA Gloucester.

Eickhoff, M. (2005). *Zahn-, Mund- und Kieferheilkunde bei Klein- und Heimtieren*. Stuttgart: Enke.

El-Bialy, T.H., Royston, T.J., Magin, R.L. et al. (2002). The effect of pulsed ultrasound on mandibular distraction. *Annals of Biomedical Engineering* 30: 1251–1261.

Enezei, H.H., Azlina, A., and Igzeer, Y.K. (2014). The role of protein deficiency in the healing of mandibular fractures in rabbit model. *International Journal of Pharmacology and Pharmaceutical Sciences* 6: 351–357.

Erdogan, O., Esen, E., Ustün, Y. et al. (2006). Effects of low-intensity pulsed ultrasound on healing of mandibular fractures: an experimental study in rabbits. *Journal of Oral and Maxillofacial Surgery* 64: 180–188.

Ethell, M.T., Bennett, R.A., Brown, M.P. et al. (2000). *in vitro* elution of gentamycin, amikacin, and ceftiofur from polymethylmethacrylate and hydroxyapatite cement. *Veterinary Surgery* 29: 375–382.

Fernandez, H., Osorio, J., Russi, M.T. et al. (2012). Effects of internal rigid fixation on mandibular development in growing rabbits with mandibular fractures. *Journal of Oral and Maxillofacial Surgery* 70: 2368–2374.

Gorell, C. and Verhaert, L. (2006). Zahnerkrankungen bei Hasenartigen (Lagomorpha) und Nagetieren (Rodentia). In: *Zahmedizin bei Klein- und Heimtieren* (ed. C. Gorell), 189–212. Munich: Urban & Fischer.

Guerrissi, J., Ferrentino, G., Margulies, D., and Fiz, D. (1994). Lengthening of the mandible by distraction osteogenesis: experimental work in rabbits. *Journal of Craniofacial Surgery* 5: 313–317.

Guevara, N., Hofman, V., Hofman, P. et al. (2006). A comparison between functional and radical surgery in an experimental model of maxillary sinusitis. *Rhinology* 44: 255–258.

Harcourt-Brown, F. (2009a). Dental disease in pet rabbits 2. Diagnosis and treatment. *In Practice* 31: 432–445.

Harcourt-Brown, F. (2009b). Dental disease in pet rabbits. 3. Jaw abscesses. In: *Practice*, vol. 31, 496–505.

Harkema, J.R., Carey, S.A., and Wagner, J.G. (2006). The nose revisited: a brief review of the comparative structure, function, and toxicologic pathology of the nasal epithelium. *Toxicologic Pathology* 34: 252–269.

Hochuli-Vieira, E., Cabrini Gabrielli, M.A., Pereira-Filho, V.A. et al. (2005). Rigid internal fixation with titanium versus bioresorbable miniplates in the repair of mandibular fractures in rabbits. *International Journal of Oral and Maxillofacial Surgery* 34: 167–173.

Horiguchi, H. (2002). Bone mineral density and fracture healing of the mandible in rabbits receiving ovariectomy and a low-calcium diet. *Japanese Journal of Oral and Maxillofacial Surgery* 48: 145–153.

Kawanabe, K., Okada, Y., and Matsusue, Y. (1998). Treatment of osteomyelitis with antibiotic-soaked porous glass ceramic. *Journal of Bone and Joint Surgery. British Volume* 80: 527–530.

Liljensten, E., Adolfsson, E., Strid, K.G., and Thomsen, P. (2003). Resorbable and nonresorbable hydroxyapatite granules as bone graft substitutes in rabbit cortical defects. *Clinical Implant Dentistry and Related Research* 5: 95–101.

Lundberg, J.O. (2008). Nitric oxide and the paranasal sinuses. *The Anatomical Record* 291: 1479–1484.

Manso, J.E., Mourao, C.F., Pinheiro, F.A. et al. (2011). Molars extraction for bone graft study in rabbits. *Acta Cirurgica Brasileira* 26 (Suppl. 2): 66–69.

Martinez-Jimenez, D., Hernandez-Divers, S.J., Dietrich, U.M. et al. (2007). Endosurgical treatment of a retrobulbar abscess in a rabbit. *Journal of the American Veterinary Medical Association* 230: 868–872.

Massler, M. and Schour, I. (1941). Studies in tooth development: theories of eruption. *American Journal of Orthodontics and Oral Surgery* 27: 552–5576.

McConoughey, S.J., Howlin, R.P., Wiseman, J. et al. (2015). Comparing PMMA and calcium sulfate as carriers for the local delivery of antibiotics to infected surgical sites. *Journal of Biomedical Materials Research Part B: Applied Biomaterials* 103: 870–877.

Mirdan, B.M. (2012). A 980 nm diode laser clot formation of the rabbit's dental sockets after teeth extraction. *Iraqi Journal of Laser Part B* 11: 37–42.

Mphande, A.N., Killowe, C., Phalira, S. et al. (2007). Effects of honey and sugar dressings on wound healing. *Journal of Wound Care* 16: 317–319.

Nalin, L. (2013). The rabbit as an animal model in dental implant research – with special reference to bone augmenting materials. *Epsilon archive for student projects,* Uppsala ISSN: 1652-8697.

Naraghi, M., Deroee, A.F., Ebrahimkhani, M. et al. (2007). Nitric oxide: a new concept in chronic sinusitis pathogenesis. *American Journal of Otolaryngology* 28: 334–337.

Phallen, D.N., Antinoff, N., and Fricke, M.E. (2000). Obstructive respiratory disease in prairie dogs with odontomas. *Veterinary Clinics of North America: Exotic Animal Practice* 3: 513–517.

Probst, W. and Vasel-Biergans, A. (2004). Arzneimittel zur Schmerzreduktion. In: *Wundmanagement* (eds. W. Probst and A. Vasel-Biergans), 222–224. Stuttgart: Wissensch Verlagsgesellschaft.

Remeeus, P.G.K. and Verbeek, M. (1995). The use of calcium hydroxide in the treatment of abscesses in the cheek of the rabbit resulting from a dental periapical disorder. *Journal of Veterinary Dentistry* 12: 19–22.

Richelsoph, K.C., Webb, N.D., and Haggard, W.O. (2007). Elution behavior of daptomycin-loaded calcium sulfate pellets: a preliminary study. *Clinical Orthopaedics and Related Research* 461: 68–73.

Schlosser, R.J., Spotnitz, W.D., Peters, E.J. et al. (2000). Elevated nitric oxide metabolite levels in chronic sinusitis. *Otolaryngology–Head and Neck Surgery* 123: 357–362.

Shi, C.M., Nakao, H., Yamazaki, M. et al. (2007). Mixture of sugar and povidone-iodine stimulates healing of MRSA-infected skin ulcers on db/db mice. *Archives of Dermatological Research* 299: 449–456.

Smith, M., Dodd, J.R., Hobson, H.P., and Hoppes, S. (2013). Clinical techniques: surgical removal of elodontomas in the black-tailed prairie dog (*Cynomys ludovicianus*) and eastern fox squirrel (*Sciurus niger*). *Journal of Exotic Pet Medicine* 22: 258–264.

Steenkamp, G. and Crossley, D.A. (1999). Incisor tooth regrowth in a rabbit following complete extraction. *Veterinary Record* 145: 585–586.

Stoor, P., Soderling, E., and Salonen, J.L. (1998). Antibacterial effects of a bioactive glass paste on oral microorganisms. *Acta Odontologica Scandinavica* 56: 161–165.

Stubbs, D., Deakin, M., Chapman-Sheath, P. et al. (2004). in vivo evaluation or resorbable bone graft substitutes in a rabbit tibial defect model. *Biomaterials* 25: 5037–5044.

Taylor, W.M., Beaufrere, H., Mans, Chr., and Smith, D.A. (2010). Long-term, outcome of treatment of dental abscesses with a wound-packing technique in pet rabbits: 13 cases (1998–2007). *Journal of the American Veterinary Medical Association* 237: 1444–1449.

Tobias, K.M., Schneider, R.K., and Besser, T.E. (1996). Use of antimicrobial-impregnated polymethylmethacrylate. *Journal of the American Veterinary Medical Association* 208: 841–844.

Topham, J. (2002). Why do some cavity wounds treated with honey or sugar paste heal without scarring? *Journal of Wound Care* 11: 53–55.

Tuncel, U. and Ozgenel, G.Y. (2011). Use of human amniotic membrane as an interpositional material in treatment of temporomandibular joint ankyloses. *Journal of Oral and Maxillofacial Surgery* 69: e58–e66.

Uckan, S., Bayram, B., Kecik, D., and Araz, K. (2009). Effects of titanium plate fixation on mandibular growth in a rabbit model. *Journal of Oral and Maxillofacial Surgery* 67: 318–322.

Villano, J.S. and Cooper, T.K. (2013). Case report – mandibular fracture and necrotizing sialometaplasia in a rabbit. *Comparative Medicine* 63: 67–70.

Vlaminck, L., Verhaert, L., Steenhaut, M., and Gasthuys, F. (2007). Tooth extraction techniques in horses, pet animals and man. *Vlaams Diergeneeskundig Tijdschrift* 76: 249–261.

Wachol-Drewek, Z., Pfeiffer, M., and Scholl, E. (1996). Comparative investigation of drug delivery of collagen implants saturated in antibiotic solution and a sponge containing gentamycin. *Biomaterials* 17: 1733–1738.

Wagner, R. and Johnson, D. (2001). Rhinotomy for treatment of odontoma in prairie dogs. *Exotic DVM* 3: 29–34.

Wagner, A.R., Garman, R.H., and Collins, B.M. (1999). Diagnosing odontomas in prairie dogs. *Exotic DVM* 1: 7–10.

Weisman, D.L., Olmstead, M.L., and Kowalski, J.J. (2000). *in vitro* evaluation and antibiotic elution from polymethylmethacrylate (PMMA) and mechanical assessment of antibiotic-PMMA composites. *Veterinary Surgery* 29: 245–251.

Yamamura, K., Iwata, H., and Yotsuyanagi, T. (1992). Synthesis of antibiotic-loaded hydroxyapatite beads and in vitro drug release testing. *Journal of Biomedical Materials Research* 26: 1053–1064.

23

Large Mammal Dental Surgery

Allison D. Woody, David A. Fagan, and James E. Oosterhuis

Introduction

Dentistry and oral surgery are becoming more commonplace in the care of exotic animals. Just as we have learned the significance of oral health in humans (Li et al. 2000; Kim and Amar 2006) and companion animals (DeBowes 1998), we now realize that the oral health of even the largest of exotic mammals plays a role in their overall health. It stands to reason that oral pain and infection can significantly affect metabolic status, behavior, reproduction, and even social status of the exotic patient. The majority of treatments in large mammal dentistry and oral surgery are borrowed from either human or companion animal dentistry. Much of the time, procedures can be adapted with minimal changes from small animal, equine, and human dental text books according to the animal's closest domestic relative. Adequate knowledge of orofacial anatomy and basic dental and oral surgery principles is a must for proper treatment. Describing all dental and oral surgical procedures for the wide variety of large exotic mammals is beyond the scope of this chapter, and resources are already available for most species (Crossley et al. 2003; Wiggs and Lobprise 1997; Klugh 2010). This chapter will address surgical procedures that are unique in some way to the management of large mammal patients encountered in the authors' practice.

Preprocedure Considerations

Dental and oral surgery of large mammals requires an appreciation of the highly variable skeletal and soft tissue anatomy, and normal dentition of many genera. There is a considerable degree of variation from species to species, as well as from individual to individual within a species. For example, tooth eruption times and sequence can vary by as much as 6–18 months in some species. It is also a matter of importance that the patient's dental issue is not approached

as a solitary "tooth-problem." Each tooth is a necessary element associated with a masticatory apparatus. It matters not if a tooth is skillfully removed if the patient's temporomandibular joint is traumatized in the process. This same concept applies to all aspects of the patient's care surrounding any procedure. The oral procedure is not a success if the patient does not stand following recovery. Achieving an acceptable standard of care with large mammal dental cases is only possible by utilizing a team approach.

The management of each individual patient before and especially after surgery must be considered well in advance of every procedure. The ability to handle the patient awake may drastically change the treatment chosen from patient to patient. Detailed case-specific preparation is essential for each and every case. The patient's daily caretakers, trainers, nutritionist, etc., should be involved in the overall plan. A competent veterinary dentist with exotic animal experience can be a valuable resource as well.

The masticatory apparatus is one of the most efficiently vascularized portions of the mammalian body. Consequently, traumatic injury as well as postsurgical healing tends to favor the surgeon. Nearly all oral and maxillofacial surgery is considered contaminated and patient aftercare can be significantly more challenging in exotic patients. Aseptic practices should be followed, yet creating an aseptic environment for patients in the field can be nearly impossible. Antibiotic choice and regimens are ultimately decided on a case-by-case basis.

Anesthesia required to accomplish dental and oral surgical procedures is not discussed in this chapter, but requires extensive consideration. The authors strongly advise that a veterinarian who is educated in exotic animal anesthesia be responsible for the anesthesia and careful monitoring of the patient. The animal's well-being, as well as the safety of all individuals involved in the procedure, is vital. The task is far too big for the surgeon to reasonably undertake alone. In many cases (e.g. megavertebrates), it will take a team of

Surgery of Exotic Animals, First Edition. Edited by R. Avery Bennett and Geoffrey W. Pye.
© 2022 John Wiley & Sons, Inc. Published 2022 by John Wiley & Sons, Inc.

individuals for both the anesthesia and the surgery. The patient's metabolic health, joint health, muscular condition, positioning, and padding all play a role in anesthetic success. Detailed preoperative examination and laboratory work-up is essential and should be acquired routinely when circumstances allow. Assistance may be necessary following surgery to help the animal rise. This should be well thought out far in advance.

Terminology

Any discussion of injury to the mammalian dentition requires an understanding of the classification of tooth injury. Historically, there have been many such classifications based on a variety of factors, including etiology, anatomy, pathology, and/or therapy considerations. The American Veterinary Dental College (AVDC) currently uses an abbreviated classification similar to Andreason's modification of the World Health Organization system (Andreason 1981) used in human dentistry (http://AVDC.org 2012). A recent veterinary study has suggested that the AVDC classification system be expanded to include the remaining categories of tooth injury included in Andreason's classification system (Soukup et al. 2015). For the purposes of our chapter, we will remain consistent at this time with the current classification system (Box 23.1).

Elephants

Tusks have a wide, open apex and grow continuously at a rate of approximately 17 cm/year (Ungar 2010). They are often assumed to be equivalent to canine teeth, but are more technically maxillary incisors. A deciduous incisor, the "tush," never erupts but likely makes room for and guides the permanent successor (Raubenheimer 2000). The pulp of elephant tusks is vastly different from that of other mammals. It is highly vascular, resistant to trauma, and shows an exceptional ability to produce secondary dentin (Weissengruber et al. 2005). The pulp consists of densely packed collagen fibers with little nerve supply (Fagan et al. 1999; Weissengruber et al. 2005). The tusks are used for digging, carrying objects, and defense, but not for mastication.

The molars of the elephant are large and dense. They consist of multiple compressed laminae (enamel covered dentin) bound by cementum (Dumonceaux 2006). The number of laminae per molar increases with each successor, the largest containing 12+ laminae (Johnson and Buss 1965). They erupt caudally in the mouth and slowly move rostrally over the course of years. Once reaching the rostral mouth, the roots begin to resorb and the molar will gradually erode and exfoliate (Dumonceaux 2006). Elephants will have six sets of molars in their lifetime, but only one to two in each quadrant at any time (Johnson and Buss 1965). While many mammals exhibit continuously growing tusks, aside from the elephant, horizontal replacement of molars is found only in sirenia and macropods (Ungar 2010).

Common dental problems of the elephant include abraded, cracked, or broken tusks, impacted molars, and malocclusion due to improper exfoliation of molars. Problems of aged elephants arise as the last molars begin to break down. The final molar begins eruption around the age of 30 (Ungar 2010) and as early as 45 years of age, it will be the only molar left (Wiggs and Lobprise 1997). Elephants may live well into their 60s. As molar loss occurs, a softer diet with preground roughage must be formulated if the elephant is to maintain weight.

Tusks

Treatment of fractured tusks is determined following complete evaluation of the tusk. Visual inspection alone is often not enough to make a decision. For minor fractures,

---

Box 23.1 American Veterinary Dental College classification of tooth injury.

Enamel infraction (EI): an incomplete fracture of the enamel, no loss of tooth substance

Enamel fracture (EF): a fracture with loss of tooth substance, confined to the enamel

Uncomplicated crown fracture (UCF): a fracture of the crown, confined to the enamel and dentin and does not expose the pulp

Complicated crown fracture (CCF): a fracture of the crown that involves the enamel, dentin, and results in exposed pulp

Uncomplicated crown-root fracture (UCRF): a fracture of the crown and root involving enamel, dentin, and cementum (subgingival) that does not expose the pulp

Complicated crown-root fracture (CCRF): a fracture of the crown and root involving enamel, dentin, and cementum (subgingival) and results in exposed pulp

Root fracture (RF): a fracture of dentin-cementum-pulp, involving only the root

Source: AVDC Nomenclature Committee 2012.

(a)

(b)

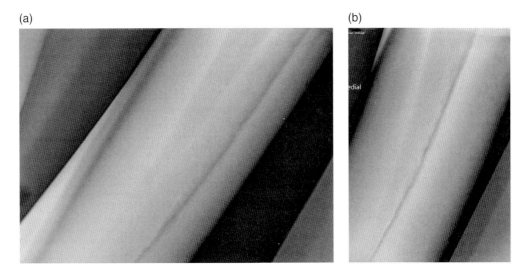

Figure 23.1 Two views of a newly fractured tusk in an African elephant (*Loxodonta africana*). Multiple views of the fracture are needed to evaluate if there is exposure of the pulp chamber. In the first view, the crack does not appear to communicate with the pulp chamber (a), but in the second view (b) it is apparent.

radiographs are essential in order to determine the fracture classification. Pulp may be involved if the fracture occurs approximately 15 cm or less beyond the gingival margin (Fowler 2006). Radiographs are also helpful in determining the extent of pulp damage and how far apically it may extend. Most elephants can be easily trained to allow radiographs to be obtained in a protected contact setting. A minimum of two views (dorsoventral and lateral) of the tusk are necessary (Figure 23.1), but a number of additional oblique views may be helpful. It is not possible to adequately evaluate the apex of the tusk radiographically due to the enormous density of the elephant skull. If it is determined that the tusk fracture is complicated (i.e. the pulp is exposed), surgical treatment of the tusk is indicated.

Severe complicated crown fractures resulting in pulp dangling from the tusk are the most challenging in deciding on treatment because the trauma not only removed a significant portion of the tusk exposing the pulp but also likely avulsed an undetermined length of pulp tissue away from the interior wall of the remaining tusk's pulp chamber. The pulp tissue near the fracture site stretches longitudinally and rips away from the tusk wall. The pulp then tears apart, the distal portion falls to the ground, and the proximal portion retracts back into the remaining pulp chamber. This action often pulls in an assortment of macro- and micro-contaminants. The injury to the cellular attachment of the pulp tissue to interior surface of the pulp chamber is particularly troubling as there is no way to determine the extent of the damage done or the degree of contamination. Sever the dangling pulp at the fractured

end of the tusk and immediately flush with 0.05% chlorhexidine solution. Use a zip tie to temporarily control bleeding if necessary. Elephants will tolerate this surprisingly well under sedation alone. Minimize additional contamination by covering the end of the tusk with acrylic until treatment decisions can be made. Multiple radiographic images and careful monitoring takes place over the next several weeks as an anesthetic procedure is planned. When the temporary cap is removed during the follow-up procedure, the appearance, or odor of the pulp tissue can help make decisions about the treatment plan.

Partial Pulpectomy

Fractured tusks with viable pulp tissue can be repaired by performing a partial pulpectomy under general anesthesia. The authors have found it beneficial to permanently restore the end of the tusk with a threaded pulp insert plug rather than dental acrylic alone. This technique does not require that the open end of the tusk be completely dry, allowing for a faster repair. It also provides an additional barrier should the acrylic be knocked off. The pulp insert plug can be made of polyether ether ketone (PEEK) for repairing pulp canals 5–15 mm in diameter. For larger canals, sterilized polyvinyl chloride (PVC) irrigation plugs can be used. These plugs will wear at a rate similar to that of the tusk as it is naturally worn down. Metal plugs have been successfully utilized as well.

Cut the distal end of the tusk at the length predetermined to successfully remove all nonvital pulp tissue.

Remove the nonviable pulp using a taxidermy blade, a large drill bit, and/or various custom-made sharp instruments. Remove the pulp a minimum of 10 cm proximal from the tusk end until viable tissue is identified (Figure 23.2). Prepare the end of the tusk for the pulp insert plug by drilling out the canal to a uniform diameter. Cut threads into the wall of the canal using an appropriately sized pipe thread tap. Before the pulp insert plug is screwed into the end of the tusk, fill the pulp canal with calcium hydroxide paste from the distal end of the pulp up to the proximal edge of the threads. Screw the plug into the end of the tusk, seating 2–3 cm proximal to the distal end (Figure 23.3). For the application of a final restoration, apply a seal of acrylic over the plug and the end of the tusk. Polymethylmethacrylate (PMMA) is generally the

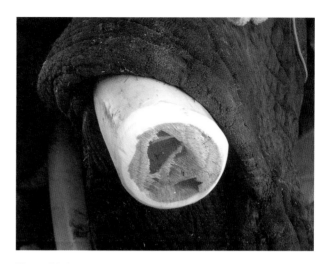

Figure 23.4 Final acrylic restoration following a partial pulpectomy on a vital tusk of an African elephant (*Loxodonta africana*). The restoration has been smoothed using a sander.

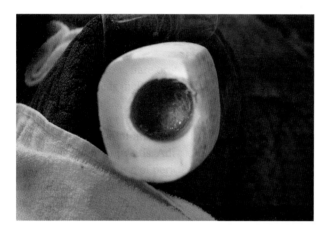

Figure 23.2 A partial pulpectomy of a vital tusk has been performed in an African elephant (*Loxodonta africana*). The pulp is removed a minimum of 10 cm proximal to the tusk and where viable tissue is identified.

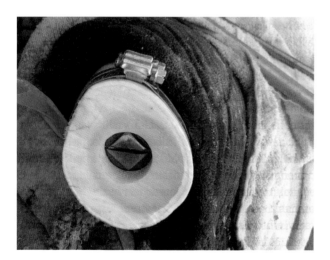

Figure 23.3 Following application of calcium hydroxide paste between the vital pulp tissue and the threads, a pulp insert plug is seated 3–4 cm beyond the end of the tusk in an African elephant (*Loxodonta africana*).

restorative of choice due to the large volume needed. Following restoration, sand the acrylic to form a smooth, uniform surface (Figure 23.4).

Aftercare following partial pulpectomy typically consists of standard nonsteroidal anti-inflammatory therapy for 3 days and antibiotic therapy for 10–14 days. Long-term radiographic monitoring in the postoperative period is essential. A minimum of two views (dorsoventral and lateral) of the tusk should be taken monthly for the first three months, then every three months for one year, and every six months in subsequent years. If the pulpectomy is successful, a transverse dentinal bridge will eventually form proximal to the pulp insert plug (Wiggs and Lobprise 1997) (Figure 23.5). Complications may arise following treatment when all of the necrotic or contaminated tissue was not removed. The authors have attempted to address this issue on several occasions with a repeat partial pulpectomy at a more proximal location with limited success. Clinical signs of pulpectomy failure include the patient chronically rubbing the face and the development of facial swelling and draining tracts. Radiographic signs of failure include gas pocketing and the development of longitudinal dentinal bridges, rather than horizontal, in an early effort to wall-off the infected pulp (Figure 23.6).

For animals that maintain a healthy tusk, but immediately return to behaviors that result in abnormal tusk wear, metal crowns can be fabricated (Figure 23.7). The crowns are most commonly made of cobalt steel for durability and cost. Cementation of the crown is accomplished using an industrial epoxy. Cementation typically will require a short second anesthetic procedure for a well-seated reliable crown.

(a)

(b)

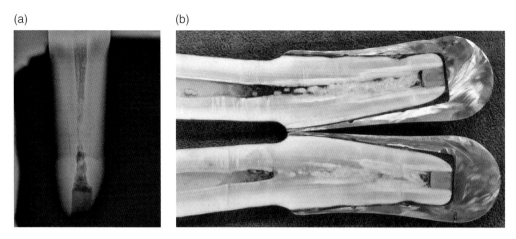

Figure 23.5 A radiograph (a) and a photograph (b) demonstrating normal dentinal bridge formation proximal to the plug insert following partial pulpectomy in an African elephant (*Loxodonta africana*).

(a)

(b)

(c)

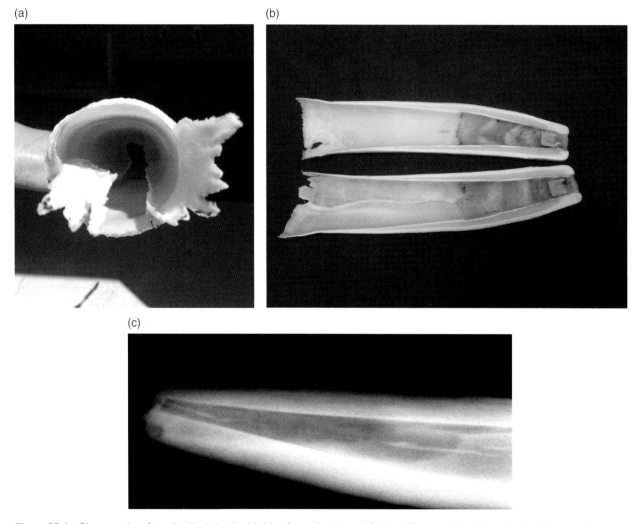

Figure 23.6 Photographs of longitudinal dentinal bridge formation in an infected African elephant (*Loxodonta africana*) tusk indicating treatment failure (a, b). Radiographic evidence of pulp necrosis can be seen here (c). The normally uniform, soft tissue density of the pulp chamber has developed more radiolucent areas where there is gas or air.

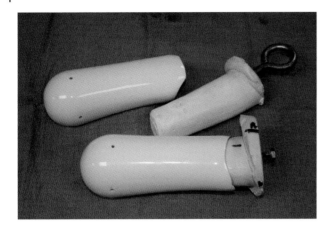

Figure 23.7 Stone models and metal crowns fabricated for the tusks of a juvenile African elephant (*Loxodonta africana*) who was a repeat offender for excessive wear.

Tusk Extraction

Fractured tusks with no remaining viable pulp, obvious infection from the fracture site, facial swelling, or mobility should be extracted. Previously published techniques for removing the tusks in pieces are both labor intensive and traumatic (Welsch et al. 1989; Kertesz 1990; Fowler 2006). Questions as to whether or not all pieces of the tusk are successfully removed with these techniques go unanswered by the inability to obtain apical radiographs. More recently, one case report describes removal of a traumatically intruded, partially mobile tusk by applying rubber elastics to the tusk at the gingival sulcus (Steiner et al. 2003).

A technique in which tusks can be completely removed is described here. Visualization of the feathered germinal edge is apparent following extraction reducing the opportunity for postoperative complications. Damage to the alveolar bone and apical tissues is minimized. Tusks (elephant and walrus) ranging in size from 5 to 15 cm in diameter have been successfully removed using this technique under general anesthesia.

Teeth, including tusks, are attached firmly in their alveolus, or sockets, by a network of tiny ligaments collectively known as the periodontal ligament. The periodontal ligament occupies a well defined, but relatively thin space surrounding the root. The goal of extraction, or exodontia, is to remove the tooth with minimal damage to the surrounding cortical bone of the alveolus. In small patients, this is accomplished by exhausting the periodontal ligament with prolonged applied pressure. This approach is nearly impossible with very large teeth, especially tusks. Tusk extraction is assisted by using periotomes, sharp knife-like instruments used to cut the periodontal ligament rather than fatiguing it. Hand-operated periotomes and, more recently, power versions are commercially available for human and small

veterinary patients. For megavertebrate patients, the authors use periotomes custom-made from stainless steel tubing the same diameter as the tusk (Figure 23.8). Drive the periotomes between the tusk and alveolar bone using one of three different methods: an air-driven palm nailer, a rotary hammer drill, or, for large tusks, a demolition hammer. Once the periodontal ligament is almost completely severed, apply torque with a standard plumber's chain wrench, and apply traction with custom-made external or internal extraction devices attached to an automotive slide hammer (Figure 23.8). When necessary, additional traction can be achieved using an electric winch attached to the slide hammer (Figure 23.9). For smaller tusks (juvenile elephants, walrus), use an electrician's wire mesh cable grip. Gentle debridement of the alveolus following extraction is essential and can be accomplished with a variety of stiff brushes or custom-made curettes. Control postoperative bleeding by tightly packing the alveolus with shaved ice.

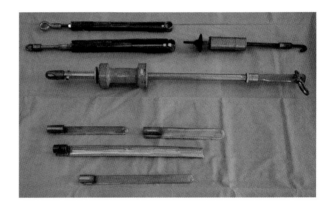

Figure 23.8 Custom-made internal extraction devices, automotive and custom slide hammer, and custom made periotomes.

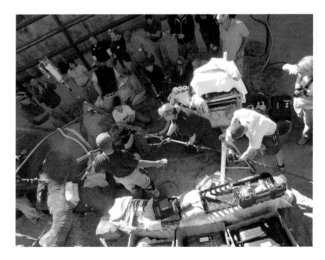

Figure 23.9 Automotive slide-hammer and wench-assisted extraction of a large African elephant (*Loxodonta africana*) tusk.

Challenges arise when there is significant curvature of roots or when ankylosis of part of the periodontal ligament occurs resulting in fusion of the bone and tooth. Removal of some alveolar bone may be necessary in these cases.

Molars

Odontoplasty

When the mandibular molars continue their normal movement rostrally in the jaw, but the process of exfoliation is interrupted, the molar may begin to turn upward and super-erupt at the mesial (rostral) margin. The portion of the molar that then exceeds the normal occlusal plane ("hooks" or "ramps") prevents the elephant from normal occlusion and normal mastication (Figure 23.10). The goal of therapy is to return the teeth to normal occlusion. Occasionally, this can be accomplished by offering the elephant larger diameter browse over a short period of time. This is more effective if the tooth is closer to exfoliation. More often, surgical correction is necessary.

Odontoplasty or surgical recontouring the tooth involves removal of the hooks or ramps of the molar. Use acrylic plastic paddles molded to fit around the molar to protect the tongue and buccal tissue. Transect the super-erupted portion of the molar with a reach die grinder fitted with a carbide-tipped circular saw blade (Figure 23.11). Round off the fresh edges of the tooth with an equine dental float.

Molar Extraction

In many cases, deformed or retained molars must be extracted in order to try to restore normal mastication. The usual case is that of a retained lower molar that is blocking

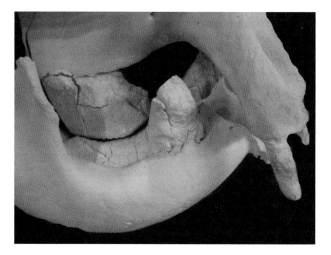

Figure 23.10 Elephant skull with mandibular molar ramps. Super-eruption of the mesial (rostral) aspect of the tooth results from delayed molar exfoliation and creates malocclusion.

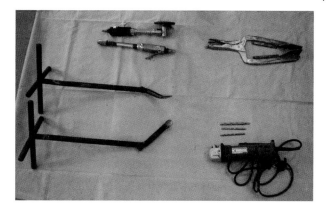

Figure 23.11 High-speed die grinders, custom-made molar extraction device, custom luxators, and right angle drill.

the normal progression of the incoming molar. Use acrylic plastic paddles (molded to fit around the molar in order to isolate it) to protect the tongue and buccal mucosa. Driving appropriately sized periotomes along the retained molar is nearly impossible due to the close quarters in the elephant's oral cavity. Sever the periodontal ligaments by using a drill bit in a right angle drill to cut a trench around the molar. Remove the retained molar by grasping it with a custom-made molar clamp (extraction forceps) (Figure 23.11) and twisting medially and laterally until the molar breaks loose. Debride the open socket to remove any retained molar shards, devitalized tissue, or impacted debris. Use a large ball-shaped carbide bur, driven by a high-speed die grinder to smooth rough edges of the alveolus (Figure 23.11). Lavage the socket with copious amounts of 0.05% chlorhexidine solution. Flush out the socket twice daily with warm water as the incoming molar moves rostrally (Figure 23.12). While dilute chlorhexidine solution may be ideal, it is difficult to achieve adequate volume and pressure to remove the accumulated debris, even using two garden sprayers simultaneously. A garden hose connected to a warm water source is readily available in most barns and will generally deliver the quantity and turbulence necessary to achieve a clean alveolus. Micro-contaminants are sufficiently diluted.

Extraction Site Maintenance

There is never enough gingival tissue to adequately provide primary closure of the site. Due to time constraints with anesthesia and challenges with postsurgical management, gingival flaps are not created. Elephants are very inquisitive and will often inspect their surgical sites immediately following recovery. Sutures, gauze packing, or even temporary crowns or other devices will often be removed in a matter of minutes to hours. Thus, extraction sites are typically left open to heal by second intention. Elephants are notorious for packing their sockets with food, debris, or

(a) (b)

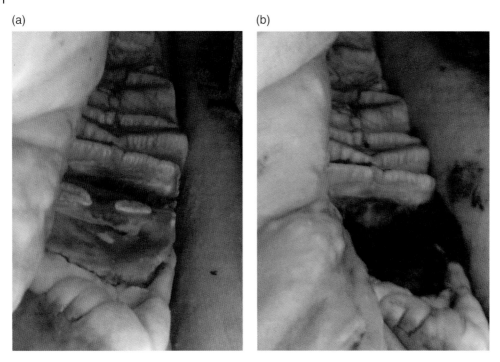

Figure 23.12 Impacted African elephant (*Loxodonta africana*) molar that resulted in a submandibular draining tract secondary to delayed molar exfoliation. The space between molars became impacted with food and debris resulting in infection (a). The remaining portion of the impacted molar was removed (b).

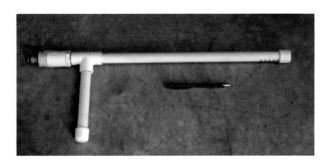

Figure 23.13 Custom-made elephant water flossing device. The device can be connected to a garden hose by quick connect for daily flushing.

even dung. The surgical area must be lavaged twice daily until healed, which can be six months to a year or more. Use 0.05% chlorhexidine solution in the first week of healing and gently administer using a garden sprayer. In subsequent weeks, connect a custom-made water flosser to a garden hose for daily flushing (Figure 23.13). Make the device using two ½″ PVC irrigation pipes connected and capped with a standard garden hose quick disconnect device on the handle end. Establish the working end with a series of five or six ¼″ holes drilled in line with the handle to be able to direct the flow of water. If at all possible, connect the hose to a warm water source rather than cold water to minimize the shock to exposed oral tissues.

Pain management following extractions should always be instituted for a minimum of five days. Antibiotic therapy is generally used for the first 10–14 days.

Chronic Alveolar Osteitis and Osteomyelitis

Chronic alveolar osteitis and osteomyelitis or "Lumpy Jaw" is a common problem in ungulates and macropods. It is often a chronic problem and is notoriously difficult to cure. The resultant bone infection may become life-threatening if not resolved. Once thought to be a manifestation of bacterial infection alone, the cause of lumpy jaw is now recognized as multifactorial. The primary underlying problem is tooth abscessation secondary to a periodontal and/or endodontic lesions. Opportunistic bacteria secondarily play a role (Wiggs and Lobprise 1994). Initial alveolitis may develop into osteomyelitis over time (Knightly and Emily 2003; Antiabong et al. 2013) and is often associated with overlying, diffuse, soft tissue cellulitis (Fagan et al. 2005). Lumpy jaw most commonly involves the premolars and molars of ungulates (Knightly and Emily 2003) and macropods (Butler and Burton 1980), and has been documented in the incisors of macropods (Kilgallon et al. 2010). Pulpitis or tooth fractures resulting from trauma or foreign body-induced periodontal lesions are common inciting insults (Wiggs and Lobprise 1994; Fagan et al. 2005).

A number of etiologic agents have been implicated in the development of lumpy jaw secondary to tooth injury (Antiabong et al. 2013). The most commonly isolated pathogens are anaerobic bacteria; *Fusobacterium* spp. in macropods and *Actinomyces* spp. in ruminants (Wiggs and Lobprise 1997; Sotohira et al. 2016). A mixed microbial population is often found. One recent study suggests that the pathogenic organisms may change as the condition progresses (Antiabong et al. 2013). There may be additional etiologic factors that are unidentified. Overcrowding, fecal contamination of food, dry feed stems, nutritional deficiencies, stress, and food impactions have all been investigated as playing a role (Wiggs and Lobprise 1994; Kilgallon et al. 2010). Application of a chlorhexidine varnish may help shorten the course of treatment and help prevent recurrence (Bakal-Weiss et al. 2010).

Animals affected with lumpy jaw will present with a large swelling of the cheek, often with a draining tract when the condition is advanced. Early detection is ideal and can occur with careful observation. Dropping food, hypersalivation, changes in prehension or mastication, and loss of body condition may be noted. The diagnosis is confirmed with a detailed intraoral examination including manual palpation and skull radiographs. Intraoral films may also be helpful. A recent study has shown that a hand-held portable test system to detect plasma endotoxin activity as a marker of systemic inflammation secondary to lumpy jaw disease may also be a useful diagnostic test (Sotohira et al. 2016).

Historically, treatment consisted of repeated episodes of opening the swelling, flushing, draining the debris, and closing the wound in combination with antibiotic therapy (Fagan et al. 2005). The effectiveness of this treatment was low and the high frequency of patient handling was difficult and stressful. Many species do not handle long-term hospitalization well. Once the dental origin of the problem was recognized, the treatment began to involve exodontia of the affected tooth/teeth (Wiggs and Lobprise 1994). Intraoral access is very limited in some species and postextraction healing can be challenging in that the sockets are typically not closed and may become impacted with food debris. Daily handling of these species for flushing is difficult and stressful for the animals. Permanent empty sockets have been reported following re-epithelialization of the extraction site trapping debris and requiring a second surgery with little intraoral access (Wiggs and Lobprise 1994). A buccotomy can be performed to improve access, but this is quite traumatic. Care

must be taken to preserve nerves and the vasculature in the cheek, and facial scarring will result. The most common down-side to this therapy is the development of postextraction malocclusion. As lumpy jaw is most frequently found in cheek teeth and most species depend on occlusive wear to maintain normal mastication, overgrowth of the opposing tooth or teeth develops. Thus, lifetime monitoring for malocclusion is needed. Routine dental examinations and intermittent rasping of overgrown opposing teeth becomes necessary and results in handling of the animal every 3–12 months, long-term.

We have developed a two-phase treatment protocol for ungulates that requires minimal intervention and handling, and has proven successful over the past decade. It is especially useful given the limitations commonly associated with the treatment of easily injured and stressed exotic species.

The first phase involves the trephination of the lateral alveolar wall followed by placement of an indwelling tomcat catheter to provide long-term access to the apical roots of the involved dentition. The clinical objective is to convert the chronic, invasive osteomyelitis into a contained, externally draining fistulous tract.

Trephination is the surgical perforation of the alveolar cortical bone to release the accumulated exudate from between the cortical plates (Wolcott et al. 2011). Historically, it was used in human dentistry as a means of relieving pain associated with periapical disease. Studies in the late 1990 and early 2000s showed that the resulting relief of pain in people was not significant and the therapy has primarily gone by the wayside (Moos et al. 1996; Nist et al. 2001; Wolcott et al. 2011). In exotic animals, the diagnosis of alveolitis is often made much later in the disease process and the objective is different. Trephination is not meant solely to eliminate pain, but to connect the apical abscess to the exterior surface allowing for direct drainage and flushing. The result over time is to eliminate surrounding cellulitis and distortion as well as preventing the spread of infection (Wolcott et al. 2011). The fistula phase is maintained for 6–8 weeks, a longer period of time than in human dentistry. For these reasons, the authors prefer the terminology "surgical fistulation" over trephination.

The second phase, periradicular surgery and endodontic treatment, is scheduled when the alveolar osteomyelitis has been contained. A compound apicoectomy is an advanced surgical and endodontic procedure that involves resection of the affected tooth root(s) apex(s) and periapical debris. All remaining pulp tissue is then removed, and the pulp canal system is sealed to block communication with the local tissues (Johnson and Fayad 2011). This phase eliminates the now more localized infection and restores the integrity of both the dentition and the alveolar bony defect. This requires familiarity with standard apicoectomy surgical access and procedure, including retrograde endodontic filling techniques. Consultation with a veterinary dentist is beneficial for completing this phase.

Diode laser-assisted decontamination and biostimulation are used throughout both phases. The diode laser energy interacts with soft tissues to decrease inflammation, increase tissue regeneration, and provide temporary analgesia (Carroll et al. 2014). Most diode lasers have a light wavelength within the 640–980 nm range, which is absorbed by the mitochondria of the target cells, leading to up-regulation of cellular adenosine triphosphate (ATP) production and modulation of cytokines, growth factors, and inflammatory mediators (Chung et al. 2012). Secretion of growth factors and activation of enzymes and other secondary messengers results in enhanced cell proliferation and differentiation (Chung et al. 2012). The effect has been shown to occur in hypoxic or stressed cells with little to no effect on healthy cells. Increased neovascularization and temporary vasodilation also result, enhancing neutrophil infiltration, and macrophage activity in the affected area (Carroll et al. 2014). Temporary inhibition of nerve conduction in small and medium diameter peripheral nerve fibers provides analgesia for approximately 48 hours (Carroll et al. 2014). Diode laser has also been shown to effectively seal dentinal tubules and eliminate bacteria (Gutknecht et al. 2004; Asnaashari and Safavi 2013).

Surgical Fistulation

With the patient under anesthesia, thoroughly assess the swelling. It may be localized or diffuse, firm or fluctuant. Obtain lateral and oblique skull radiographs. The location of the dental-related disease is usually obvious. The periapical region of one or more teeth may appear as a radiolucent, possibly cystic, zone (Figure 23.14). Use hypodermic needles in combination with radiographs to help establish the location externally. Conversely, if a draining tract is already present, insert radiopaque gutta percha points up the tract to help radiographically identify the tooth or teeth involved.

Make a stab incision over the tooth's apex or, most often, at the site of greatest fluctuation to establish drainage. Make an incision to widen the opening of the existing fistula. Carefully dissect through tissues to the level of bone overlying the offending tooth root. Reflect soft tissues using a molt periosteal elevator. Once the correct location

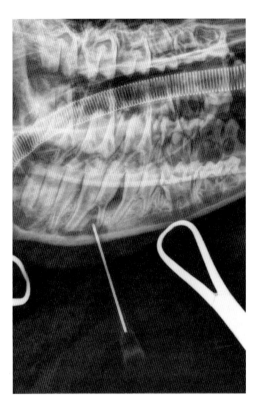

Figure 23.14 Radiograph of the right mandible of a southern steenbok (*Raphicerus campestris*) presenting with "lumpy jaw." Periapical lucency of both roots of the affected molar indicates the tooth is nonvital and has abscessed.

has been verified visually or radiographically, carefully remove approximately 0.5 cm diameter of the buccal cortical plate covering the tooth root apex using a water cooled high-speed dental handpiece and an appropriately sized round bur (#4, #6, #8, #10) until the apex and 1–2 mm ventral to the tooth is visualized. Collect and submit a swab for bacterial culture. Insert an open-ended tom-cat catheter into the apical area of the tooth. Flush the catheter initially with copious amounts of sterile saline solution to verify patency of the catheter and drainage of the periapical region. Using a second catheter, accomplish chemical debridement of the area by simultaneous flushing with a combination of hydrogen peroxide (H_2O_2) and sodium hypochlorite (NaOCl) from two separate syringe sources until no further debris is discharged (Visser 1988). Lavage the area thoroughly with sterile saline a second time. When available, perform direct diode laser decontamination of the periapical region. Finally, measure and cut to length a tom-cat catheter so that when the small open end is placed into the periapical region of the tooth, the syringe end remains on the external surface of the cheek. Secure the catheter in place and close the soft tissues around it using an appropriately sized nonabsorbable monofilament

(a)

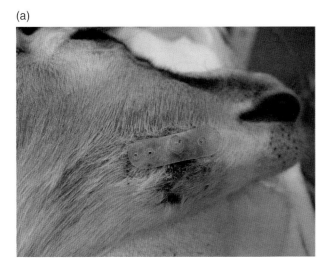

(b)

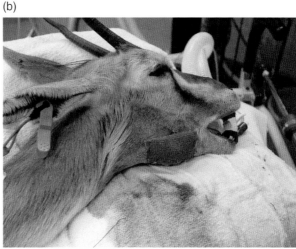

Figure 23.15 A southern steenbok (*Raphicerus campestris*) with alveolar osteitis. A tom-cat catheter is in place to maintain drainage for a period of six to eight weeks. (a) The catheter is secured with suture or staples and covered with a bandage to reduce the risk of ascending infection. (b) The patient is brought into the hospital for irrigation and diode laser biostimulation twice weekly.

suture (Figure 23.15). Perform a final catheter rinse with 2% povidone-iodine solution. In cases with profound soft tissue cellulitis where prolonged daily antibiotic therapy is not possible, consider direct injection of the 2% povidone-iodine solution into and around the infection site (Fagan et al. 2005). Though the solution has a temporary negative impact on healthy tissue in the area, it is not irreversibly damaged, yet the invasive microorganisms are killed and the host's ability to regenerate is ultimately improved (Fagan et al. 2005). Biostimulate the entire facial area using a low-level diode laser before the animal is recovered.

Prescribe analgesics and antibiotics when they can be used appropriately. Repeat flushing and diode laser biostimulation treatments once or twice weekly for six to eight weeks. These short immobilization (manual restraint or sedation) procedures enable the animal to remain with its group or with brief periods of separation.

Once the infection appears to be adequately contained (typically four to eight weeks), a second anesthetic procedure is performed to complete an apicoectomy and root canal procedure. A normograde root canal filling is desirable, but in most species, a retrograde filling is necessary due to limited intraoral access. In either case, removal of the diseased apical tissue is vital for a successful outcome.

For a retrograde filling, clip and clean the cheek area, and remove the tom-cat catheter. Make a 3-cm long and approximately 1.5 cm wide elliptical incision around the now fibrous tract, and bluntly dissect and remove the soft tissues to reveal the mandible (Figure 23.16). In addition to

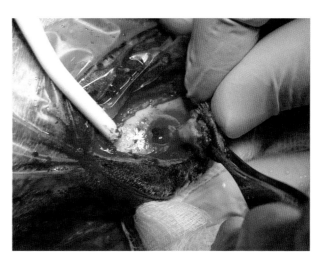

Figure 23.16 Photograph of the approach for an apicoectomy of a mandibular molar in a southern steenbok (*Raphicerus campestris*). Surgical fistulation has been accomplished and the fibrous tract that has developed around the tom-cat catheter is removed.

adequate exposure, consider the anatomic location of blood vessels and nerves. Extend the incision a minimum of 5 mm coronally and 5 mm apically to the point determined as the tooth apex. Use small Gelpi or Weitlaner retractors to establish good visualization, and then widen the opening of the alveolar cortex to approximately 1 cm diameter using a round bur. Perform an apical resection using a small tapered crosscut bur to remove diseased tissues and provide access for retrograde cleaning and filling. Incise the apex of the tooth at a 45° angle in an apical direction removing the apical-most 4–6 mm. Elevate and remove

(a)　　　(b)

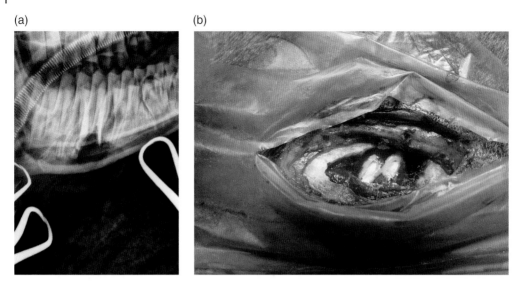

Figure 23.17 Radiograph (a) and photograph (b) of a mandibular molar of a southern steenbok (*Raphicerus campestris*) following apicoectomy and retrograde filling of a root canal.

the root-tip and debride the exposed socket thoroughly with a curette. Employ standard techniques for retrograde root canal preparation and filling. The complex anatomy of root structures in many species may prevent adequate instrumentation of the root canal. Anaerobic bacteria that persist in the dentinal tubules of the root canal walls may lead to treatment failure (Fagan et al. 2005). Chemical debridement and laser decontamination are relied on in these cases. Complete obturation can be quite challenging in teeth with complex anatomy as well. A good apical seal is vital in these cases. Confirm satisfactory endodontic obturation radiographically (Figure 23.17). Fill the remaining osseous defect with a bone graft product and complete the flap closure. If the soft tissue defect is large, horizontal mattress tension sutures can be helpful to oppose skin edges prior to a standard two-layer closure with a monofilament absorbable suture. Confirm adequate filling of the mandibular bony defect radiographically (Figure 23.18). Perform diode laser biostimulation of the area before the animal is recovered.

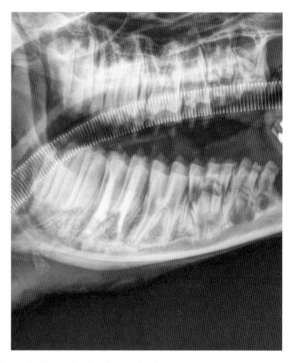

Figure 23.18 Final radiograph of a southern steenbok (*Raphicerus campestris*) following apicoectomy, retrograde root canal filling, and grafting of the bony defect.

References

Andreason, J.O. (1981). *Traumatic Injuries of the Teeth*, 2e, 19–24. Copenhagen: Munksguard.

Antiabong, J.F., Boardman, W., Moore, R.B. et al. (2013). The oral microbial community of gingivitis and lumpy jaw in captive macropods. *Research in Veterinary Science* 95: 996–1005.

Asnaashari, M. and Safavi, N. (2013). Disinfection of contaminated canals by different laser wavelengths, while performing root canal therapy. *Journal of Lasers in Medical Science* 4: 8–16.

AVDC Nomenclature Committee (2012). Dental fracture classification. http://www.avdc.org/nomenclature. html#toothfracture (accessed 28 November 2015).

Bakal-Weiss, M., Steinberg, D., Friedman, M. et al. (2010). Use of a sustained release chlorhexidine varnish as treatment of oral necrobacillosis in *Macropus* spp. *Journal of Zoo and Wildlife Medicine* 41: 371–373.

Butler, R. and Burton, J.D. (1980). Necrobacillosis of macropods-control and therapy. *Proceedings of the Conference of the American Association of Zoo Veterinarians*, pp. 137–140.

Carroll, J., Milward, M., Cooper, P. et al. (2014). Developments in low level light therapy (LLLT) for dentistry. *Dental Materials* 30: 465–475.

Chung, H., Dai, T., Sharma, S. et al. (2012). The nuts and bolts of low-level laser (light) therapy. *Annals of Biomedical Engineering* 40: 516–533.

Crossley, D.A. (2003). Oral biology, dental and beak disorders. *Veterinary Clinics of Exotic Animals* 6: 459–764.

DeBowes, L. (1998). The effects of dental disease on systemic disease. *Veterinary Clinics of North American Small Animal Practice* 28: 1057–1062.

Dumonceaux, G.A. (2006). Digestive system. In: *Biology, Medicine, and Surgery of Elephants* (eds. M.E. Fowler and S.K. Mikota), 299–307. Ames, IA: Blackwell Publishing.

Fagan, D.A., Benirschke, K., Simon, J. et al. (1999). Elephant dental pulp tissue: where are the nerves? *Journal of Veterinary Dentistry* 16: 169–172.

Fagan, D.A., Oosterhuis, J., Benirschke, K. et al. (2005). "Lumpy jaw" in exotic hoof stock: a histopathologic interpretation with a treatment proposal. *Journal of Zoo and Wildlife Medicine* 36: 36–43.

Fowler, M.E. (2006). Surgery and surgical conditions. In: *Biology, Medicine, and Surgery of Elephants* (eds. M.E. Fowler and S.K. Mikota), 119–130. Ames, IA: Blackwell Publishing.

Gutknecht, N., Franzen, R., Schippers, M. et al. (2004). Bactericidal effect of a 980-nm diode laser in the root canal wall dentin of bovine teeth. *Journal of Clinical Laser Medicine and Surgery* 22: 9–13.

Johnson, O. and Buss, I. (1965). Molariform teeth of male African elephants in relation to age, body dimensions, and growth. *Journal Of Mammology* 46: 373–384.

Johnson, B.R. and Fayad M.I. (2011). Periradicular surgery. In: *Cohen's Pathways of the Pulp*, 10e (eds. K.M. Hargreaves, S. Cohen and L.H. Berman), 738–768. St. Louis, MO: Mosby Elsevier.

Kertesz, P. (1990). The principles of elephant tusks and their extraction. *Proceedings of the 4th Elephant Keepers Workshop*, pp. 18–20.

Kilgallon, C.P., Bicknese, B., and Fagan, D. (2010). Successful treatment of chronic periapical osteomyelitis in a Parma wallaby (*Macropus parma*) using comprehensive endodontic therapy with apicoectomy. *Journal of Zoo and Wildlife Medicine* 41: 703–709.

Kim, J. and Amar, S. (2006). Periodontal disease and systemic conditions: a bidirectional relationship. *Odontology* 94: 10–21.

Klugh, D.O. (2010). *Principles of Equine Dentistry*. London: Mason Publishing Ltd.

Knightly, F. and Emily, P. (2003). Oral disorders of exotic ungulates. *Veterinary Clinics of Exotic Animals* 6: 565–570.

Li, X., Kolltveit, K., Tronstad, L. et al. (2000). Systemic diseases caused by oral infection. *Clinical Microbiology Review* 13: 547–558.

Moos, H.L., Bramwell, J.D., Roahen, J.O. et al. (1996). A comparison of pulpectomy alone versus pulpectomy with trephination for the relief of pain. *Journal of Endodontics* 22: 422–425.

Nist, E., Reader, A., Beck, M. et al. (2001). Effect of apical trephination on postoperative pain and swelling in symptomatic necrotic teeth. *Journal of Endodontics* 27: 415–420.

Oliphant, J.C., Parsons, R., Smith, G.R. et al. (1984). Aetiological agents of necrobacillosis in captive wallabies. *Research in Veterinary Science* 36: 382–384.

Raubenheimer, E. (2000). Early development of the tush and the tusk of the African elephant (*Loxodonta africana*). *Archives of Oral Biology* 45: 983–986.

Samuel, J. (1983). Jaw disease in macropod marsupials: bacterial flora isolated from lesions and from the mouths of affected animals. *Veterinary Microbiology* 8: 373–387.

Sotohira, Y. et al. (2016). Plasma endotoxin activity in kangaroos with oral necrobacillosis. *Journal of Veterinary Medical Science* 78: 971–976.

Soukup, J.W., Hetzel, S., Paul, A. et al. (2015). Classification and epidemiology of traumatic dentoalveolar injuries in dogs and cats: 959 injuries in 660 patient visits. *Journal of Veterinary Dentistry* 32: 6–14.

Steiner, M., Gould, A., Clark, T. et al. (2003). Induced elephant (*Loxodonta africana*) tusk removal. *Journal of Zoo and Wildlife Medicine* 34: 93–95.

Ungar, P. (2010). Xenarthra and afrotheria. In: *Mammal Teeth: Origin, Evolution, and Diversity*, 149–150. Baltimore, MD: The Johns Hopkins University Press.

Visser, C.J. (1988). The use of bleach and hydrogen peroxide in endodontics irrigation. *Journal of Veterinary Dentistry* 5: 3–4.

Weissengruber, G., Egerbacher, M., Forstenpointner, G. et al. (2005). Structure and innervation of the tusk pulp in the African elephant (*Loxodonta africana*). *Journal of Anatomy* 206: 387–393.

Welsch, B., Jacobson, E.R., Kollias, G.V. et al. (1989). Tusk extractions in the elephant (*Loxodonta africana*). *Journal of Zoo and Wildlife Medicine* 20: 446–453.

Wiggs, R.B. and Lobprise, H.B. (1994). Acute and chronic alveolitis/osteomyelitis ("lumpy jaw") in small exotic ruminants. *Journal of Veterinary Dentistry* 11: 106–109.

Wiggs, R.B. and Lobprise, H.B. (1997). *Veterinary Dentistry: Principles and Practice*, 343–347, 538–558, 559–579. Philadelphia, PA: Lippencott-Raven.

Wolcott, J., Rossman, L.E., and Hasselgren, G. (2011). Management of endodontic emergencies. In: *Cohen's Pathways of the Pulp*, 10e (eds. K.M. Hargreaves, S. Cohen and L.H. Berman), 42–45. St. Louis, MO: Mosby Elsevier.

24

Primate Surgery

Celia R. Valverde and Elizabeth Bicknese

Nonhuman primates (NHPs) are broadly divided into prosimians (lemurs, lorises, and tarsiers), monkeys (further separated into New World or Old World monkeys), lesser apes (gibbons), and great apes (chimpanzees, bonobos, orangutans, and gorillas). Having a general understanding of a primate's phylogeny, native diet, and habitat can aid medical and surgical care.

Personal Protective Equipment and Zoonotic Concerns During Surgery

Veterinarians who work with NHPs are at increased risk for acquiring zoonotic diseases (Burgos-Rodriguez 2011). NHP zoonotic diseases can vary from relatively mild ailments, such as dermatophytosis (Renquist and Whitney 1987), to potentially devastating diseases, such as macaque Herpes B virus causing fatal encephalomyelitis (CDC Center for Disease Control 2019). Additionally, human anthroponoses (reverse zoonoses) such as herpes simplex, measles, and chicken pox can potentially infect primates, sometimes with fatal outcomes (Schrenzel et al. 2003).

Veterinary standard precautions (VSP) should be followed (Table 24.1) to protect both the staff and the animal (National Association of Public Health Veterinarians 2010). VSPs and personal protective equipment (PPE) prevent exposure to bodily fluids and physical injury such as needle sticks and bites (Figures 24.1 and 24.2). One should refer to the Roberts (1995) publication for zoonotic and occupational safety recommendations. In surgery, it is especially important to not manipulate sharps by hand and only adjust sharps with instruments.

Integument and Appendages

NHPs have complex social structures and conspecific aggression is common. Injuries range from punctures and lacerations to crushing injuries. Clipping around wounds can help identify the extent of the injuries (Figure 24.3), though hidden soft tissue trauma can be surprisingly extensive. Male-induced injuries tend to be deep canine teeth lacerations and female-induced injuries are more muscle crushing. Crush injuries can induce distal extremity gangrene and severe rhabdomyolysis (Bicknese 1990).

Integument repair is similar to domestic animals (Figure 24.4). The decision to close traumatic wounds is multifactorial (e.g. size, depth, location, contamination, social ranking, and if repeat examinations are possible). Decontamination of the wounds by thoroughly irrigating and providing antibiotics (intravenous at examination, then oral), analgesics, and tetanus prophylaxis are important. Wounds can heal by second intention, but primary closure hastens resolution, especially in high motion areas. Partial closure can allow drainage as drains are not tolerated unless securely covered. Wet-to-dry debridement bandages are very effective but require frequent immobilizations. NHPs can remove sutures so intradermal or subcuticular sutures are preferred. Cyanoacrylate tissue adhesive can be used to secure knots or reinforce the primary closure, though overapplication causes stiffness which encourages picking.

During estrus some female NHPs, primarily Old World monkeys and great apes, have sexual swelling in the anovulvar region. Traumatized fully tumescent skin bleeds heavily and lacks tensile strength, so wound repair is best accomplished by horizontal mattress sutures with stents.

Table 24.1 Overview of common routes of NHP zoonotic exposure and partial list of personal protective equipment.

Exposure type	Prevention
Dermal exposure	Examination gloves. Double gloving if an Old World monkey, great ape, macaque, or very ill New world primate
	If handling NHP, long sleeves, consider disposable water-resistant gown and long pants
	Restraint gloves or restraint device based on animal demeanor and species
Punctures, bites, needle sticks	Double glove when appropriate for species and ailment
	Do not recap needles or use safe one-handed technique. Dispose sharps directly into an appropriate puncture resistant and leak proof sharps container. Readjust needles in surgery with thumb forceps and not by fingers
	Safety gear such as restraint gloves, gauntlets, and restraint cages as needed
Ocular or other mucus membrane exposure: potential of aerosolization or splash (i.e. with intubation and wound lavage)	Face shield or appropriate safety glasses
	Wash hands before eating, using the toilet or applying cosmetics, lip balm, handling contact lenses, or rubbing one's eyes
Inhalation	Appropriate face mask (sometimes more than a surgical mask, such as a NIOSH N95 mask, dust/mist respirator, Hepafilter, NIOSH-certified N95 duckbill masks)
	Robust suction if aerosolizing likely such as with dentals and some surgical events
Ingestion	No eating/drinking, handling contact lenses, or applying cosmetics (including lip balm) in a primate area
	Wash hands before eating

Source: Based on National Association of State Public Health Veterinarians (2010).

Old World monkeys have keratinized ischial callosities or "sit pads" covering their ischial tuberosities. Callosity wounds bleed heavily and suturing is challenging.

Sliding flaps and split/full thickness free skin grafts work well when protected with bandages. Bandaging NHPs can be challenging because of their strength and dexterity. It is best to incorporate hands and feet to prevent digit swelling

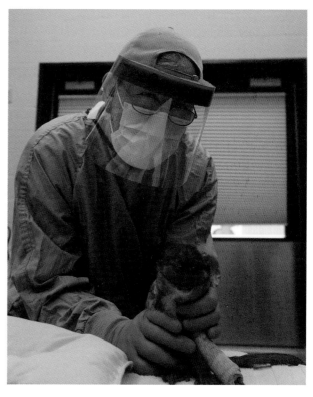

Figure 24.1 Personal protective equipment and veterinary standard precautions (VSP) are an essential part of providing veterinary care for nonhuman primates.

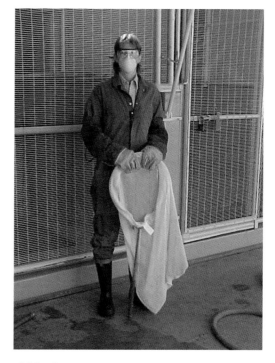

Figure 24.2 Personal protective gear used when netting a monkey to protect against physical injury and mucous membrane exposure.

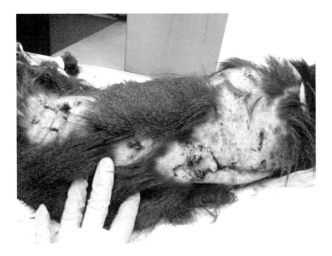

Figure 24.3 Clipping affected areas can reveal trauma that was not evident on the general exam as seen in this L'hoest guenon (*Cercopithecine lhoesti*).

and wrap dismantling. NHP digits are maceration prone, therefore, pad between the digits using conforming gauze or cotton, taking care not to apply excessive pressure to lateral digits. To prevent the bandage from slipping, use tape stirrups and bandage in flexion, minimizing extension. "Donuts" (round padding with a center hole) placed at elbows and heels help prevent pressure sores. Reinforce the proximal bandage end to protect the inner layers and the distal end with white tape or similar product to decrease moisture absorption. Alternatively, casts can be used due to their stiffness and difficulty in removing (Figure 24.5). It can be helpful to add a deterrent to wraps (e.g. Bitter apple or orange®, Tabasco® Hot Sauce, soap) or place "distractions" to encourage grooming on unaffected areas (e.g. tape loops, nontoxic children's paint, nail polish on nails) (Figure 24.4).

Digit and tail amputations are common surgical procedures, usually post-trauma. Digit and tail amputation is

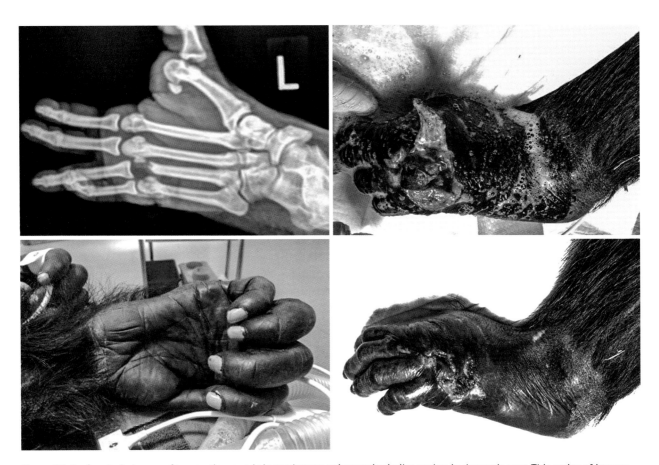

Figure 24.4 Surgical closure of traumatic wounds in nonhuman primates is similar to that in domestic pets. This series of images shows wound care in a chimpanzee (*Pan troglodytes*). A conspecific bite wound caused a fourth metatarsal avulsion fracture and a complex flap injury. Wound lavage and primary closure was successful. Nail panting on the unaffected limbs was used as a distractor from the suture line.

similar to domestic animal techniques (Figure 24.6). Utilize regional anesthesia and infuse a ring block proximally. Place a tourniquet before draping and maintain it less than 30 minutes to avoid vascular ischemia (Doyle 2010). Using a small hypodermic needle, locate the joint or intervertebral space. Incise the skin distal to the needle with a scalpel

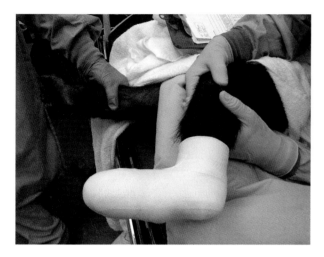

Figure 24.5 NHPs are often adept at removing bandages. Bandaging with joints in natural flexion and creating a stiffer bandage by reinforcing with casting material are techniques to retain bandages.

blade to create curved dorsal and ventral skin flaps. Transect the flexor and extensor tendons, ligaments, and joint capsule. Disarticulate the phalanx or vertebra with a scalpel blade. Release the tourniquet before suturing and provide hemostasis as needed. Appose subcutaneous tissues over the bone with interrupted absorbable sutures. Appose the skin with a subcuticular pattern or alternatively simple interrupted skin sutures. Exposed knots can be glued and the ends cut short to avoid unraveling and reduce picking by the NHP. Amputations can be bandaged until the skin begins adhering to the underlying tissues and starts healing across. Change the bandage within 24 hours to prevent moisture-induced skin maceration, then change as needed until healed.

Respiratory Tract

The NHP respiratory tract has differences compared to domestic animals: the right superior bronchus branches cranial to the main trachea bifurcation increasing the possibility of intubating a main stem bronchus, the mediastinum is complete, and lung lobe anatomy varies among NHP species with trends within taxa (Table 24.2). Unique to some NHPs are laryngeal air sacs; their function is unknown. Air sacs are present in most monkeys and all apes, except gibbons

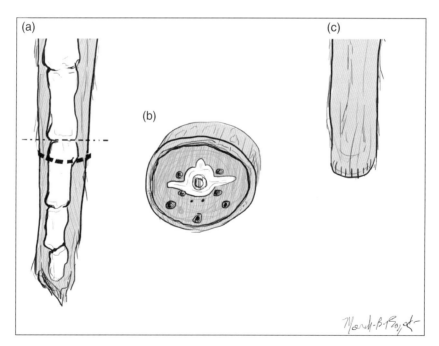

Figure 24.6 Amputation of distal tail. (a) Curved incisions are made to create dorsal and ventral skin flaps that should extend beyond the point of disarticulation of the coccygeal vertebrae. (b) Transverse view of the amputation site showing the locations of vessels that might need to be ligated are the paired: dorsal lateral coccygeal, ventral lateral coccygeal, superficial lateral coccygeal, and the smaller ventral coccygeal. The single large medial coccygeal vein is a large vessel ventral to the coccygeal vertebra. (c) The dorsal skin flap is extended over the stump and sutured to the ventral skin flap in two layers by either simple interrupted sutures in the subcutaneous or subcuticular layer and skin. Source: Medical illustration By Meriah Razak.

Table 24.2 Variations in number of upper and lower respiratory structures for different NHP taxa.

	Sinuses	Paranasal sinuses (laryngeal air sacs)	Right lung lobe	Left lung lobe
Prosimians		Most	4 (few species – 3)	2
New World primate		Most	4 (Cebidae – 3)	2
Old World primate	African monkeys – 4 (F, M, E, S)	Most	4	Small spp – 2
	Asian monkeys – 2 (M, S)	Baboons – moderate sized single central air sac		Larger spp – 3
Lesser apes		None in gibbons		
Great apes	Gorillas and chimpanzee – 4 (F,M, E, S)	Central air sac with bilateral cervical, pectoral, and axillary divisions	3	2
		Gorilla – Extensive – wraps around throat, across clavicle, and under axillary muscles		
Orangutan	2 (M, S)	2 (M,S)	1	1
		Extensive – wraps around throat, across clavicle, and under axillary muscles		

Sinuses: F, frontal; M, maxillary; E, ethmoid; S, sphenoid.
Source: Modified from Lowenstine and Osborn (2012).

(Lewis et al. 1975). Air sacs originate from paired ostia on the lateral larynx at the thyroarytenoid folds (Steinmetz and Zimmermann 2012). Smaller primates typically have a single, small, and minimally palpable air sac, baboons have a moderate-sized palpable single central air sac, and apes have a central air sac that leads into bilateral cervical, pectoral, and axillary divisions. Orangutans and gorillas have the most extensive air sacs that wrap around the throat, across the clavicles, and end under the axillary muscles.

Air sacculitis may occur as a sequel of sinusitis (Steinmetz and Zimmermann 2012). Sinusitis or air sacculitis symptoms are nonspecific including nasal discharge (intermittent, persistent), coughing, halitosis, and weight loss. Diagnosis may be made by palpation, ultrasonography showing fluid accumulation, horizontal beam radiographs showing a fluid line, or magnetic resonance imaging (MRI). Exudates vary from liquid to thick paste ("peanut butter" consistency), and when chronic, the air sac walls are thickened. Acute or chronic, it is usually a mixed culture of enteric bacteria along with *Pseudomonas spp*. Cases nonresponsive to conservative treatment or showing significant lesions on imaging are surgical candidates.

To avoid aspiration pneumonia during general anesthesia, great care must be taken to prevent the discharge from flowing out of the ostia into the larynx. If air sacculitis is suspected, NHPs should be held in a sitting upright position or partly inclined during anesthesia, especially great apes. Dorsal recumbence should be avoided until after intubation.

Air sac surgical drainage is critical for treatment success of air sacculitis (Hill et al. 2001). Open the air sac at the most dependent point through a horizontal skin incision (monkey 2 cm, chimpanzee 5 cm, orangutan 5–10 cm). Prior to incising the air sac, place stay sutures to prevent subcutaneous tissue contamination. Once open, flush the air sac carefully to avoid reflux through the ostia and risking aspiration pneumonia. Fibrotic bands forming pockets need to be broken down. In great apes, massage the entire air sac (including the axilla region) and rotate the animal to encourage drainage. Allow the incisions to heal by second intention over several weeks. To delay incision closure, marsupialize the stoma by suturing the air sac incision to the skin incision (Figure 24.7a–c). For cases requiring a permanent stoma, create a longer marsupialization or remove a triangular defect. Patients need multiple weeks on systemic antibiotics with selection based on culture results.

Surgical closure of the laryngeal ostia can prevent aspiration in chronic cases (McManamon et al. 1994). Using the air sac approach above, in the region of the larynx identify the ostia by digital palpation through the opened air sac. Place two ligatures around the stalk of each ostium or freshen and oversew tightly. The ostia may recanalize overtime.

Complete air sac resection has had excellent results with few complications in recurrent and refractile cases of air sacculitis (Lewis et al. 1975; Herrin et al. 2002). Incise the skin over the air sac, horizontally or vertically. Separate the skin from the air sac and dissect the air sac from the body

(a)

(b)

(c)

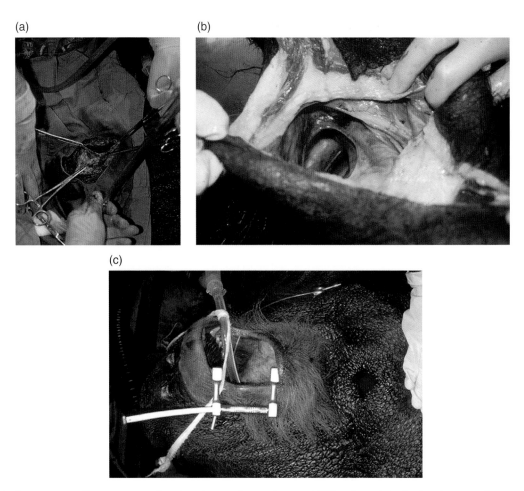

Figure 24.7 An orangutan (*Pongo pygmaeus*) undergoing an air sacculotomy. (a) The air sac is incised at the ventral aspect, using care not to contaminate the subcutaneous tissues. (b) Air sacs in great apes extend around the neck, to the axilla and under the pectoral and axillary muscles. This angle shows the depth and compartmentalization of the air sacs. (c) The finished marsupialization.

wall. Electrosurgery is useful for dissection and hemostasis. Ligate and resect the ostia close to the larynx. Tack the skin to the subcutaneous tissues to decrease dead space.

Orthopedics

Fracture management represents a great challenge with NHP's, primarily related to postoperative pain management, surgical site maintenance, external apparatus integrity, and self-trauma prevention. Orthopedic principals are the same for NHPs as for domestic animals. Due to logistical challenges, the capture, anesthesia, diagnostic, and surgical procedures are often performed in a single event which limits the ability for planning and procurement of proper implants (Figure 24.8a,b). Internal fixation is preferred as NHPs may dismantle external fixators. External fixators may be tolerated, but pins and clamps need to be protected from the animal's dexterous fingers with a padded wrap or light cast. Smaller primates may tolerate external coaptation; avoid heavy padding as this

encourages cast slippage (see Integument section for bandaging information). NHPs are extremely strong for their stature, so any form of fixation must stand up to extraordinary forces from manual challenges and high impact activities like jumping. Space confinement may be needed to allow healing before permitting increased activity, though social and enrichment needs must be met during this period (Figure 24.9).

Primary NHP musculoskeletal and connective tissue tumors are relatively rare. Surgical intervention is similar to domestic animals. Amputation is feasible as three-limbed primates can live quality lives, but an amputation decision should be assessed on a case-by-case basis.

Abdominal Surgery

NHP abdominal surgery uses the same principles as domestic animal surgery. The linea alba is more attenuated compared to domestic animals. The bladder is closer to the

(a)

(b)

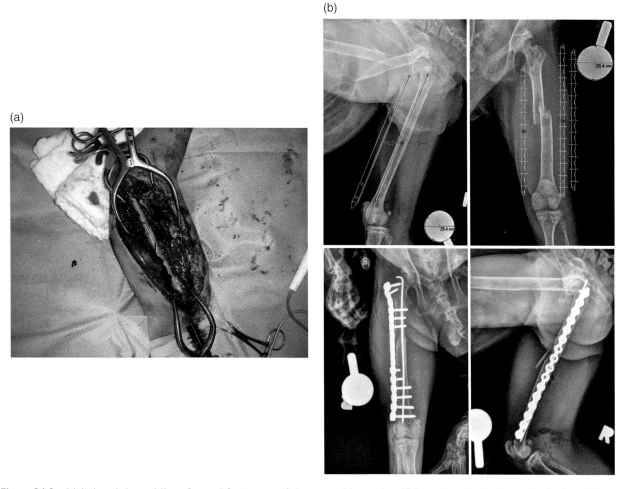

Figure 24.8 (a) A closed short oblique femoral fracture repair in a capuchin monkey (*Cebus sp*) repaired using a standard cranial lateral approach. (b) Procurement of proper implant size against radiographs is shown. The femoral fracture was stabilized with a locking SOP plate and an intramedullary pin construct. *Source:* Courtesy Dr. Seth Bleakley.

linea alba and is like a loose sac. When entering the caudal abdomen, take care to not puncture the urinary bladder. The omentum is more likely to migrate through small linea alba gaps; therefore, a well-sealed linea alba closure is critical. For animals with a sacculated stomach, such as langurs and great apes, it is challenging to work in the cranial abdomen so plan to use self-retaining abdominal retractors (e.g. Balfour) as surgical aids. A self-retaining elastic abdominal ring retractor, such as Lone Star or Alexis retractor, greatly enhances visualization, and is malleable and atraumatic, while keeping abdominal contents out of the operative field (Figures 24.10 and 24.11). NHPs are prone to developing adhesions, so using Halsted's principles is very important. Abdominal adhesions, prominent in gorillas, are sometimes encountered even in a surgically naive animal presumably secondary to prior trauma or inflammation.

Minimally invasive surgery (MIS) is beneficial in NHPs by allowing faster patient recovery, and reducing pain and analgesic requirements, and the risk of self-mutilation in the postoperative period. MIS has been mostly used for organ diagnostic sampling (spleen, kidneys, small intestine, lymph node, and liver) and surgical procedures and sampling of the reproductive tract (Bush et al. 1978; Wildt et al. 1982; Chai 2015; Newcomb et al. 2019; Pizarro et al. 2019).

Hernias

Diaphragmatic hernias have been reported in a variety of NHPs, including golden lion tamarins. Golden lion tamarins have a 9% incidence of heritable congenital Morgagni diaphragmatic hernia where abdominal viscera herniate through the foramen of Morgagni, the small triangular area of the diaphragm adjacent to the sternum (Figure 24.12) (Randolph et al. 1981). Surgical repair has been successful in the golden lion tamarin using a ventral midline abdominal approach and a primary repair by suturing the diaphragm to the xiphoid (Randolph et al. 1981).

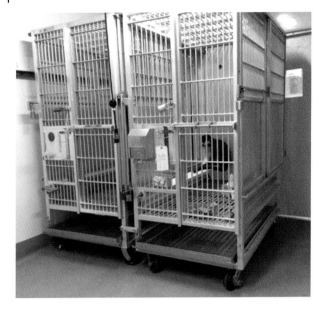

Figure 24.9 Fracture management requires limiting activity during fracture healing period. A lesser spot-nosed guenon (*Cercopithecine petaurista*) is on cage rest for a radius/ulna fracture stabilized with a bone plate. Note foraging puzzles in the cage for enrichment.

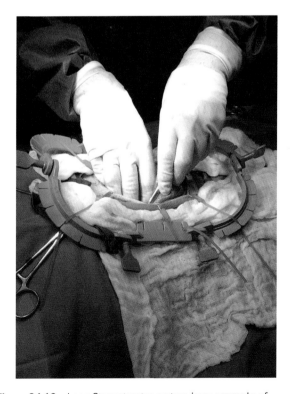

Figure 24.10 Lone Star retractor system is an example of self-retaining, atraumatic retractor that allow excellent visibility. Source: Photo by Catherine Wertis.

Inguinal hernias are relatively common in NHPs, especially in macaques, and are more prevalent in males, sometimes progressing to an inguinoscrotal hernia (Figure 24.13). Inguinal hernias occur when the inguinal canal becomes compromised and contents from the abdominal cavity and/or pelvic canal protrude into [called "indirect"; baboon, macaque, chimpanzee (Taylor et al. 1988)] or alongside [called "direct"; macaque (Carpenter and Riddle 1980)] the spermatic cord. Herniorrhaphy (either standard approach or MIS technique) is recommended to prevent abdominal organ incarceration and strangulation, or to maintain breeding capacity (Pizarro et al. 2019; Sadoughi et al. 2018). Intestinal involvement is more concerning and a combined inguinal and abdominal approach may be required.

For an indirect herniorrhaphy, incise the skin the over the hernia and open the hernial sac (Figure 24.14). Reduce the herniated tissues into the abdominal cavity through the internal inguinal ring. Incise the external abdominal oblique aponeurosis to enlarge the aperture if needed. Assess if the hernia sac needs to be ligated and removed. Displace the spermatic cord to allow suture placement through the muscular and fascial layers. Imbricate the deep inguinal ring by placing simple interrupted sutures that approximate the transversalis muscle fascia to the inguinal ligament. Use a synthetic, nonabsorbable suture with good tensile strength to provide wound support through the extended healing period. Reduce the inguinal ring adequately to prevent recurrence, but not excessively to constrict the femoral vessels leading to formation of a painful scrotal hydrocele. Next, appose the external oblique aponeurosis on each side of the inguinal ring with a simple interrupted pattern.

With direct herniorrhaphy (Figure 24.15), the internal inguinal ring is not affected; therefore, reinforce the transversalis fascia bulge using simple interrupted sutures, or by using a synthetic surgical mesh.

In macaques, chronic inguinal hernias may scar down and become irreducible. These cases should be evaluated to determine if surgery is required. If adipose or omentum has occluded and fibrosed in the hernia, herniorrhaphy is not needed. For each case, the risks and benefits of surgical intervention should be assessed.

Perineal hernias or incompetence of the pelvic support are almost invariably from tearing pelvic floor connective tissue during parturition followed by the additional loss of strength from gravitational forces and increased intra-abdominal pressure from any cause (Figure 24.16). An abdominal approach herniorrhaphy is described to pexy the vagina to the pelvic floor and attaching tissues surrounding the pelvic organs to the remaining pelvic inlet fascia with occasional success (Martin 1982). Until a better

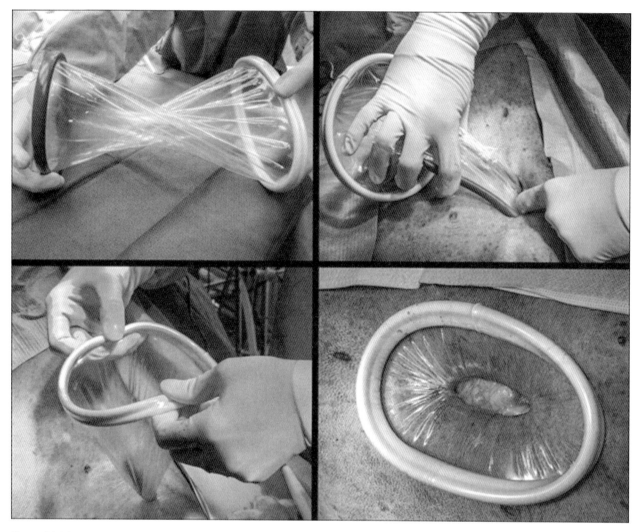

Figure 24.11 The self-retaining Alexis wound protector/retractors provide 360° of circumferential, atraumatic retraction.

surgical technique is developed, it might be advisable to remove the female from the breeding pool, minimizing the risk of morbidity associated with the herniation.

Retroperitoneal and Abdominal Abscesses

Retroperitoneal and abdominal abscesses have been reported in gorilla, orangutan, and chimpanzee (Mylniczenko 2003; Pollock et al. 2008; Hahn et al. 2014). Fistulae are common and often drain perirectally or perivaginally with older obese females overrepresented. Specific muscles such as the rectus abdominis, coccygeus, and iliopsoas muscles are occasionally associated with abscesses. Imaging techniques used include radiography (survey and contrast) (Figure 24.17), ultrasound, CT (Figure 24.18), and MRI (Hahn et al. 2014). Surgical abscess drainage is important for successful treatment. Minimally invasive techniques such as percutaneous ultrasound-guided peritoneal lavage and fluoroscope-guided

drainage catheter placement decrease overall surgical risks. Multiseptate lesions or the presence of thick purulent debris will require surgical intervention. Exploratory celiotomy for the management of abdominal abscesses usually reveals massive amounts of fibrous adhesions, while retroperitoneal abscesses may not have abdominal adhesions. Surgical resection of severely involved intestinal segments or reproductive tract and omentalization of the abscess cavity have been performed where complete abscess excision is not possible. Antibiotic-impregnated polymethylmethacrylate (PMMA) beads have been used; however, as PMMA is not biodegradable, if clinical failure occurs, removal surgery may be needed. Biodegradable antibiotic-impregnated beads may provide a better approach for the eradication of infection (Zilberman and Elsner 2008).

Treatment challenges with these abscesses are many. Medical challenges include mixed bacterial infections, multidrug-resistant isolates and evolving flora, frequent

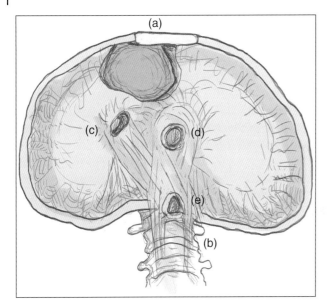

Figure 24.12 Morgagni hernia location shown on the diaphragm near the xyphoid in dark grey. The diaphragm and its associated normal structures are depicted: (a) xyphoid cartilage, (b) lumbar vertebra, (c) caval foramen, (d) esophageal hiatus (mid dorsally), and (e) aortic hiatus (dorsally). The Morgagni hernia is a congenital discontinuity on the muscular portion of the diaphragm adjacent to the sternum. It allows abdominal viscera to herniate into the thoracic cavity. Ultrasound evaluation is the simplest diagnostic method. Diagnostic imaging modalities include computerized tomography, plain or contrast radiographs (positive/negative contrast peritoneography and barium series). Source: Medical illustration By Meriah Razak.

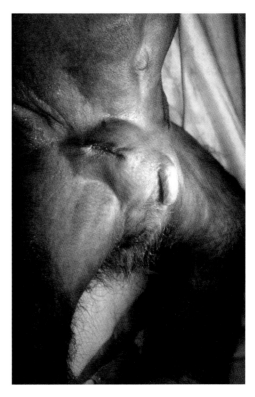

Figure 24.13 Inguinal hernia. Unilateral swelling at the region of the inguinal canal in an infant chimpanzee with an age-appropriate undescended testis. The skin incision depicts the location for the surgical approach. The surrounding scar tissue caused the rounded tissue mimicking a hernia despite surgical reduction.

recrudescence of disease, concurrent disease, misdiagnosis, and delayed diagnosis. Patient challenges include poor drug administration compliance and self-mutilation of surgical wounds postoperatively. Surgical challenges include severe adhesion formation impairing surgical access and identification of organs, incision dehiscence, recurrent abscess formation, repeated interventions required, intestinal torsion, peritonitis, and sepsis. Early diagnosis and aggressive intervention are more likely to result in a positive outcome (Mylniczenko 2003).

Intestinal *Acanthocephala* Infestation (Thorny-Headed Worms)

Acanthocephala infestations, an important disease of New World primates, are most frequently caused by *Prosthenorchis elegans* (inhabits the cecum and colon) and *P. spirula* (favors the terminal ileum; in heavy infestations the parasite is throughout the intestinal tract). Thorny headed worms are often a surgical or necropsy diagnosis. Surgery is required for nematode extirpation and a 10% postoperative mortality was reported in animals showing clinical signs and peritonitis at surgery (Wolff et al. 1990;

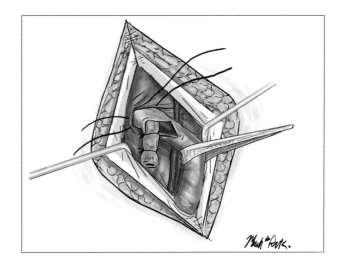

Figure 24.14 Demonstrating the surgical approach for a right indirect hernia. Note the hernial sac is abaxial to the spermatic cord and epigastric vessels. The hernial sac is resected in this image, and two simple interrupted sutures are in place to reduce the inguinal ring aperture to prevent recurrence. Source: Medical illustration By Meriah Razak.

Perez et al. 2008). Some animals require multiple surgeries. Perform a ventral midline approach to exteriorize the affected bowel and isolate it with moist laparotomy sponges. Free abdominal fluid, a modified transudate, is often found and the serosal surfaces of involved intestines and other organs might appear roughened. The parasites form small discrete raised white nodules on the serosal surface. To minimize intestinal spillage, isolate the affected segment using Doyen intestinal forceps or the fingers of an assistant. Make a 2 mm full-thickness incision on the anti-mesenteric border and use a mosquito forceps to grasp and remove the worms. A nodule can have several worms and removing all is difficult. Worms vary from 1–2 mm in diameter and

1–3 cm in length and can be numerous (Figure 24.19). Transilluminate the bowel to find remaining worms via recognizable shadows. At subsequent laparotomies, the serosal nodules of extirpated worms appear normal (Wolff et al. 1990). Most cases will test fecal negative by seven days. Fecal tests remain positive if all worms have not been removed.

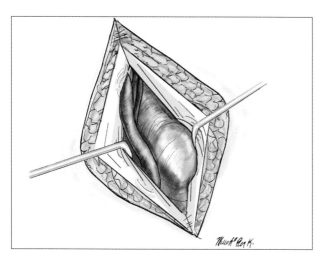

Figure 24.15 Demonstrating the surgical approach for a right direct hernia. Note the bulging muscle instead of a hernial sac, and the hernia being medial to the inguinal ring, epigastric vessels and spermatic cord. Source: Medical illustration By Meriah Razak.

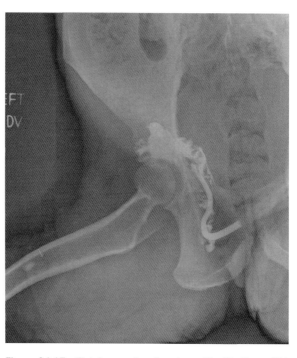

Figure 24.17 Fistulogram in a female gorilla (*Gorilla gorilla*) showing a retroperitoneal abscess tract exiting the perivulvar area, traveling between the retroabdominal muscles, and up and around the pelvis. At the time of the examination, a fistulous tract was evident and there was no defined abscess at its origin.

Figure 24.16 Perineal hernia in two female rhesus macaques (*Macaca mulatta*) with the animals in a sitting position. Images demonstrate a subcutaneous bulge at the two common locations, either next to the vulva (left image) or above the anus (right image). Entrapment of the intestines, urinary bladder, or uterus can occur and require surgical intervention via an exploratory celiotomy. During pregnancy, perineal hernias can preclude a vaginal delivery depending on the contents of the hernia, and may require a planned cesarean section.

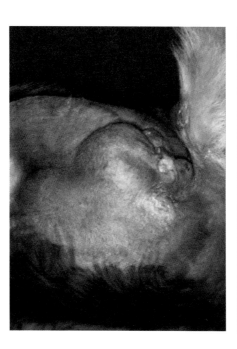 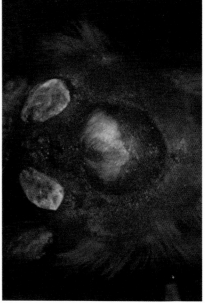

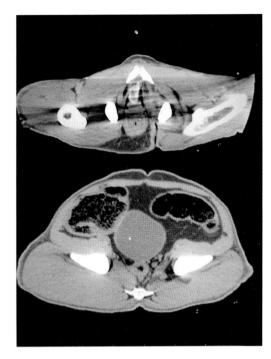

Figure 24.18 CT of a left-sided retroperitoneal abscess in a gorilla. Upper image shows a fistula coming from the retroabdominal area near the pelvis and exiting in the perianal area. Fistulas are common and tend to exit perirectally or perivaginally. The lower image shows the abscess within the muscles and tissues between the pelvis and the abdominal cavity.

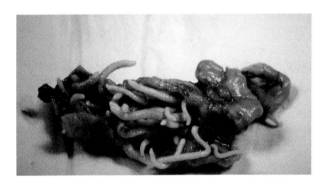

Figure 24.19 *Acanthocephala* parasites, aka thorny-headed worms, need to be removed surgically, often requiring multiple enterotomies. The ileum of a squirrel monkey (*Saimiri sciureus*) infested with *Prosthenorchis elegans* shows the typical presentation of multiple parasites attached at each reactive nodule (Formalin fixed specimen). Source: Courtesy of the Dr. Ming Wong, in memoriam.

Trichobezoar and Phytobezoar

Trichobezoars and phytobezoars have been reported in a variety of NHPs (Mook 2002). The folivorous colobine monkeys can retain indigestible fibers or stripped bark in their sacculated stomachs that can progress to phytobezoars (Calle et al. 1995). An exploratory laparotomy is both diagnostic and therapeutic (Figures 24.20 and 24.21).

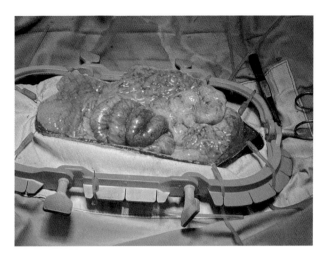

Figure 24.20 Bezoar surgery in an Angolan colobus (*Colobus angolensis*) showing roughened and hyperemic jejunal serosa. The intestines are starting to plicate or form "accordion pleats" as it tightens around the bezoar. *Source*: Image courtesy of Christine Miller.

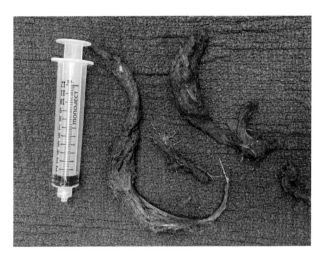

Figure 24.21 Phytobezoar removed from an Angolan colobus with intestinal blockage. Note how the long fibers had entwined together to form long rope-like structures that are strong and not prone to breaking apart. Bezoar was sectioned during removal. *Source*: Image courtesy of Christine Miller.

Surgical interventions might include gastrotomy, enterotomy, and enterectomy; apply the same techniques as used in small animal gastroenterotomies.

Cholecystectomy

Cholelithiasis has been described in several NHP species (Smith et al. 2006). Nonsurgical bile duct blockage (e.g. trematode *Platynosomum sp.*, nematode, *Trichuspirura leptostoma*) should be ruled-out before surgery is attempted (Sousa et al. 2008). Cholecystectomy, via an exploratory laparotomy or laparoscopy, is the surgery of choice for the management of cholelithiasis, cholecystitis (Figure 24.22), primary neoplasia, or gallbladder rupture. Expose the right medial and

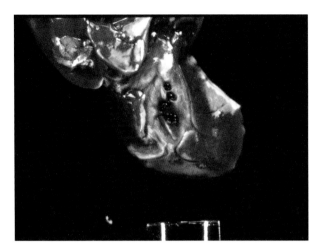

Figure 24.22 Cholelithiasis and cholecystitis in a rhesus macaque. A postmortem image showing a reactive gallbladder and surrounding liver parenchyma; surgical risks increase when this level of inflammation is present. Cholecystectomy, either surgical or laparoscopic, is the usual treatment in these cases. Gall bladder or bile duct surgeries via laparotomy should be performed with magnification. Source: Courtesy of the California National Primate Research Center image library.

quadrate lobes of the liver through a ventral midline abdominal approach. Using gentle caudal retraction, the gallbladder is dissected from the hepatic fossa. Ensure common bile duct patency by gentle manual expression or by catheterizing the duct, either normograde through the gallbladder or retrograde via the duodenal papilla. At the site of common bile duct confluence with the duodenum, make a small enterotomy to locate the duodenal papilla and place a small flexible catheter into the common bile duct to flush it. Elevate and remove the gallbladder, while identifying and ligating the common, cystic and hepatic ducts, and cystic and hepatic arteries to avoid life-threatening damage. Close the duodenal incision in a simple interrupted pattern with absorbable suture. Submit the gallbladder for histopathology and a portion of the wall and bile for aerobic and anaerobic culture. Choleliths should be submitted for chemical composition analysis since one of the most common, the cholesterol stone, might be managed with oral dissolution agents and prevented with a cholesterol restrict diet.

Choledochotomy, Choledochal Tube Stenting, and Cholecystoenterostomy

Choledochotomy, an incision in the bile duct, can be performed if a dilated duct cannot be relieved by flushing using a catheter (via a duodenotomy or a cholecystotomy). Choledochotomy has a high morbidity from dehiscence, bile leakage, and stricture formation. Magnification and illumination are required. An abdominal closed suction drain (e.g. Jackson–Pratt) might be used postoperatively to monitor for biliary leakage. A biliary diversion technique via a cholecystoenterostomy might be

preferable. Cholecystoenterostomy is indicated in cases where the bile duct is strictured or compromised and cannot be salvaged. Choledochotomy and choledochal tube stenting techniques are performed infrequently (Fossum 2013).

For cholecystoenterostomy, four suture lines will be needed. Dissect the gallbladder from the hepatic fossa and reflect it caudally. Bring the gallbladder into apposition on the antimesenteric border of the duodenum (cholecystoduodenostomy) or jejunum (cholecystojejunostomy) so that minimum anastomosis tension is present. Place stay sutures to stabilize the intestine and gallbladder. Create the back wall of the anastomosis with a 2–3 cm continuous suture line between the gallbladder serosa and the intestinal serosa near the mesentery border. Drain the gallbladder prior to making a longitudinal incision parallel to the back wall suture line, and incise the antimesenteric wall of the intestine similarly. The anastomosis is made by a full thickness continuous suture line from the gall bladder mucosa to the intestinal mucosa. Complete the stoma by suturing the serosal surfaces of the gallbladder and intestine over the near side of the stoma. Check the anastomosis patency by injecting saline into the intestine while occluding on each side of the anastomosis digitally.

Gastrointestinal Neoplasms

Intestinal neoplasms are likely to be malignant and when detected early are amenable to surgery with a low morbidity and prolonged survival. Intestinal resection and anastomosis with adequate margins and inclusion of adjacent enlarged lymph nodes is the cornerstone to therapy. In two studies of intestinal adenocarcinomas in geriatric macaques, metastases were evident in 34% and 42% of the cases (Valverde et al. 2000; Rodriguez et al. 2002) and involved mostly peripheral lymph nodes and liver. At the time of diagnosis or surgery, lymph node metastasis was not predictive for tumor recurrence or survival. Postoperative survival ranges from 1 month to 5.5 years (Valverde et al. 2000; Simmons and Mattison 2011).

Reproductive Surgery

It is important to be familiar with the normal anatomy and reproductive cycles for the different NHP taxa. Ovarian cycles vary by taxa relative to sexual swelling, visible menses, and seasonality (Hendrickx and Dukelow 1995a). NHP placentas are categorized in different ways, commonly by placental attachments and shape: prosimians have diffuse villous attachments; great apes and baboons have monodiscoid attachments (Figure 24.23); and most New World monkeys and Old World monkeys, including macaques have bidiscoid attachments (Benirschke 2012). Primates have two types of uterine shapes: bicornuate and unicornuate (Figure 24.24). *Tarsier*, *Callithrichinae*, and *Strepsirrhini* (lemuriformes) primates commonly birth twins and have a bicornuate uterus, while New World monkeys, Old World monkeys, and great apes have a unicornuate uterus (Hendrickx and Dukelow 1995b). Depending on the species, normal labor in NHPs generally occurs over five to seven hours, and the placenta

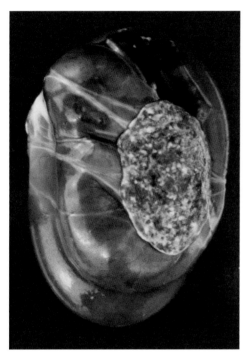

Figure 24.23 Stillbirth titi monkey fetus (*Callicebus sp*) depicting a monodiscoid placenta (this is an aberration as New World Monkeys usually have bidiscoid placentas). The placenta shows fibrin impregnation suggestive of placentitis. *Source:* Courtesy of the California National Primate Research Center image library.

is usually delivered within 15 minutes following parturition (Hendrickx and Dukelow 1995a).

Testes descend at puberty in New World monkeys, most Old World monkeys, and great apes. However, spider monkey (*Ateles spp.*) testes are scrotal at birth. Testes descend seasonally in some prosimians and most prosimians have seasonal testicular hypertrophy. Undescended testes are usually palpable between the deep inguinal ring and scrotum.

Cesarean section may be required due to dystocia, placenta previa or abruption (Figure 24.25), significant cervical prolapse, or intrauterine fetal death. The usual approach is to preserve the welfare of the dam at the expense of the fetus. During induction of anesthesia and surgical preparation, place the dam in left lateral recumbence to reduce fetal circulatory compromise from caudal vena cava compression. For surgery, place the NHP in dorsal recumbency and make a ventral midline abdominal approach by incising from the umbilicus to the cranial pubis. Take care to avoid the distended urinary bladder (due to protracted labor). Identify the gravid uterus and isolate it within the abdominal cavity with moist laparotomy sponges. Expediently perform a hysterotomy, taking care to avoid incising a placental disk, which causes profuse hemorrhage. Bidiscoidal placentas have a large intercommunicating plexus of vessels that should be avoided. Deliver the infant, clean the head, clamp and cut the umbilical cord, and hand the infant to the neonatal resuscitation team (Figure 24.26). Extract the placenta using gentle traction on the umbilical cord or blunt digital dissection. The best way to control uterine wall hemorrhage is to close the hysterotomy incision promptly rather than taking time to ligate or electrocoagulate vessels. We recommend closing the uterus using a two-layer continuous closure with an absorbable synthetic suture, although a single-layer closure technique is within acceptable standards of medical practice (Roberge et al. 2014).

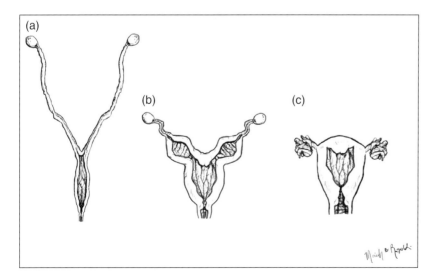

Figure 24.24 Comparing uterine types. (a) the bicornuate elongated carnivore uterus to (b) the bicornuate prosimian uterus and (c) the unicornuate uterus of Old World monkeys, New World monkeys, and great apes. *Source:* Medical illustration By Meriah Razak.

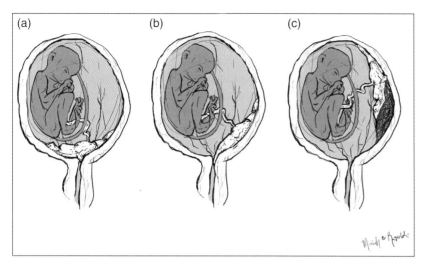

Figure 24.25 Abnormal placenta attachments which could precipitate a cesarean section surgery: (a) Complete placenta previa with placental implantation covering the internal cervical os, (b) Partial placenta previa with incomplete impingement onto the internal cervical os, (c) Partial placenta abruption with incomplete separation of the placenta with associated hemorrhage. *Source:* Medical illustration By Meriah Razak.

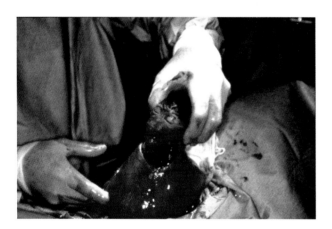

Figure 24.26 Cesarean section in a rhesus macaque showing the delivery of the infant. When incising the uterus, the implantation disks and any interconnecting plexus should be avoided. After delivery of the fetus and then the placenta, hemostasis is best accomplished by expedient closure of the uterus possibly followed by an oxytocin injection.

Good apposition without uterine leakage is required to prevent peritonitis and seeding endometriosis. If uterine hemorrhage is still significant, oxytocin can be administered systemically to enhance uterine contraction. Nursing postoperatively also will promote oxytocin release and further aid uterine involution. Lavage the abdominal cavity and close in a standard three-layer closure (Cline et al. 2012).

Ovariectomy and tubal ligations are commonly used for contraception in NHPs in lieu of ovariohysterectomy. Ovariectomy, performed by laparoscopy or laparotomy, is performed mostly for cessation of menstruation, management of endometriosis, or the excision of rare ovarian tumors. The technique is similar to that performed in domestic animals noting the ovaries are closer to the uterine body than the kidneys. For laparoscopic tubal ligation, place the primate in dorsal recumbency in a Trendelenburg (head down) position. Refer to Chapter 15 for MIS abdominal laparoscopic basic techniques. Place the camera cannula just caudal to the umbilicus, and two other ports for triangulation. Identify the uterus, fallopian tubes, and ovaries. Insert Babcock forceps through a cannula and isolate the fallopian tube by gently lifting the uterus. The salpinx is a delicate thin pink structure. Insert a vessel sealing and cutting device (e.g. LigaSure™, Covidien, Minneapolis, MN) or bipolar forceps. Hold the fallopian tube midsection with the grasping forceps and seal at both sides until the tissue turns white, indicating occlusion. Resect and remove the section through the cannula. Observe the surgical sites to ensure hemostasis. Deflate the abdomen. Appose the skin incisions using an intradermal absorbable suture (Chai 2015; Newcomb et al. 2019).

Postpartum cervical prolapse can be manually reduced after thorough cleaning as long as the cervical tissue is viable. Place a purse-string suture at the skin-mucosal junction to keep the cervix in place post-reduction for 3–7 days. If the tissue is severely compromised, a hysterectomy or ovariohysterectomy is indicated.

Ovariohysterectomy is primarily performed for medical and not contraceptive reasons including uterine rupture, placenta accreta or percreta, ectopic pregnancy, endometriosis, and uterine adenomyosis or neoplasia (Cline et al. 2012). Use a ventral midline approach being careful not to incise the urinary bladder. Given its relative cylindrical shape, the NHP uterus is deep in the pelvic inlet and usually cannot be exteriorized through the abdominal wall. With those anatomical considerations in mind, the remainder of the procedure is similar to a domestic animal

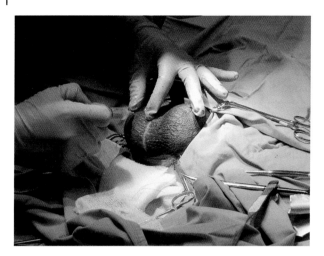

Figure 24.27 Lidocaine injected along but not into the vas deferens before starting the vasectomy will aid in intra- and postoperative pain management. For orchiectomy, it can also be injected intratesticular. The technique is shown in a bonobo (*Pan paniscus*).

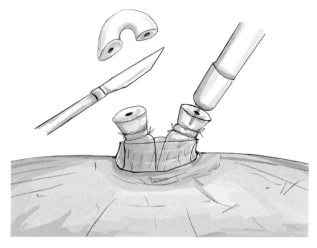

Figure 24.28 Vasectomy procedure showing the vas deferens protruding through the skin and vaginal tunic incision, double ligated and a section removed. It also shows fulgurating or electrosurgery applied to the vas deferens free ends to prevent recanalization. Source: Medical illustration By Meriah Razak.

Prostatic End   Testicular End

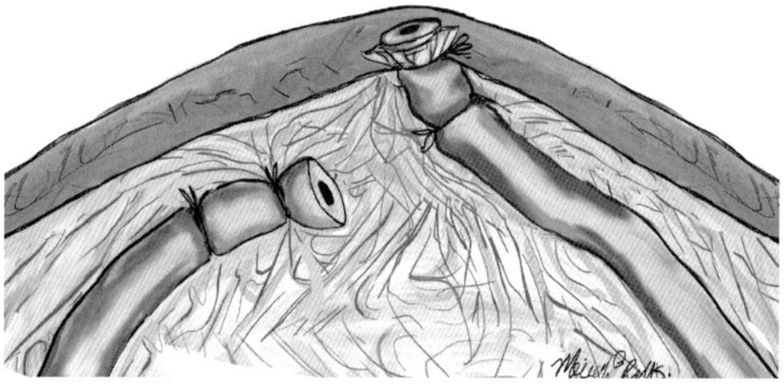

Figure 24.29 Vasectomy procedure showing interposing tunica vaginalis fascia between the two ends of the vas deferens as another technique that helps prevent vasectomy failure. Source: Medical illustration By Meriah Razak.

ovariohysterectomy. In contrast to domestic species, the ureteral location in primates is at the pelvic brim in close proximity to the suspensory ligament of the ovary. Prevention of ureteral injury occurs by direct visualization and palpation.

Endometriosis is an inflammatory, estrogen-dependent disease characterized by endometrial tissues outside the uterus occurring in Old World monkeys and great apes. Endometriosis, though benign, behaves like a malignancy invading the pelvic peritoneum, ovaries, rectocervical–vaginal areas, intestines, ureters, bladder, and other organs. Effective treatment involves ceasing further ovulation either chemically or surgically. Laparoscopy is important in diagnosing early lesions and can be used to perform bilateral ovariectomies, excision of endometriomas, and releasing adhesions. Laparotomy is required to manage moderate and advanced disease (Fanton et al. 1986).

Vasectomy and orchiectomy are recommended for permanent male contraception. Vasectomies are preferred as they are less invasive and normal species behaviors are retained. Vasectomy interrupts the vas deferens, and there are three general approaches. The first approach is used for small-to-medium sized monkeys. Palpate the spermatic cord between the penis and the inguinal ring; local anesthetic is applied along the sheath of the vas (but not into the vas) toward the inguinal ring. Additionally, local anesthetic can be placed intratesticular (Figure 24.27). Make a lateral prescrotal incision over each spermatic cord and the tunica vaginalis to expose the spermatic cord. Identify the vas deferens by white color, relative firmness, and lack of pulse. Isolate the vas deferens, double ligate, and transect between the ligatures. We favor excising 10–15 mm of the vas. Published lengths of vas deferens removed are drills 4 cm, man 1–5 cm, chimpanzees 3–5 cm. Confirmatory histology

on the tissues is recommended. In humans, fulgurating the vasa ends (Figure 24.28) using a battery-powered handheld cautery or electrocauterization is an important step as it decreases the incidence of sperm granulomas, recanalization, and postvasectomy pain syndrome (associated with chronic congestive epididymis from the continued accumulation of testicular fluid and sperm) (Viera 2015). The most effective method to prevent vasectomy failure, as reported in man, is a combined approach of cauterizing both ends of the vas and isolating each end by interposing it with a fascial layer (tunica vaginalis) (Figure 24.29) (Sokal et al. 2004). Appose the skin with subcuticular a suture, and the incision may be further sealed with a skin adhesive.

The second approach is similar except make a single prescrotal skin incision on the midline at the level of the pubic symphysis and isolate each cord through this incision (Morris and David 1992).

The third vasectomy approach is a scrotal incision caudal to the penis at the base of the scrotum like in man and is the preferred technique for larger NHP, especially chimpanzees and bonobos. It has been reported in drills (*Mandrillus leucophaeus*), chimpanzees, and bonobos (*Pan paniscus*) (Schexnider et al. 2007). Palpate the spermatic cord at the base of the scrotum just caudal to the penis. Administer local anesthetic near but not into the vas (Figure 24.27). Isolate the spermatic cord before incising the skin. Hold it by encircling it with a towel clamp, rather than grasping it with thumb forceps (Kumar and Raja 2012). Chimpanzees and bonobos have prominent cremaster muscles enveloping the vas deferens and vasculature, so identifying the vas deferens requires dissection. Use the fulguration and fascial interposition techniques as described above.

Reported vasectomy complications using only ligatures and length removal include recanalization of the vas deferens in common marmosets and chimpanzee, and sperm granulomas in rhesus macaques (Morris and David 1992; Peng et al. 2002). In chimpanzees there are concerns for vas deferens recanalization and the fulguration and fascial interposition technique above would decrease the likelihood (Viera 2015; WHO 2016). Vasectomy does not confer immediate sterility due to stored sperm, and it is unknown how long to separate breeding animals postvasectomy. In zoos, separation tends to be 4–6 weeks with the final decision based on risk tolerance.

Orchiectomy is not routinely performed for contraception; vasectomy is preferred. Historically, NHPs were neutered to alter behaviors, especially aggression, in pets or in the performing arts. This practice is not considered progressive and may not be effective as behaviors are complex and driven by more than hormones. Orchiectomy is usually performed for neoplastic processes. With testicular neoplasia, prosimians seem overrepresented and tend toward interstitial cell tumors (Remick et al. 2009). Orchiectomy is similar to domestic animals with preemptive local anesthesia (Figure 24.27), a prescrotal incision, and can be performed using an open or closed technique. NHP have more robust cremaster muscles than domestic animals. Perform bilateral orchiectomies through one prescrotal midline incision or two prescrotal incisions based on testicular mobility. Use a subcuticular skin closure.

Acknowledgment

We would like to thank Drs. Linda Lowenstine, Rita McManamon, Kirsten Gilardi, Terry Norton, Jan Ramer, and Mike Cranfield for sharing their expertise and knowledge on primate medicine, surgery, and pathology with us. We especially want to thank Orangutan Veterinary Advisory Group (OVAG) run by the Orangutan Conservancy and Dr. Steve Unwin of Chester Zoo and International Union for Conservation of Nature (IUCN) Wildlife Health Specialist for their generous sharing of knowledge about orangutan care. Thanks to Meriah Razak for her medical illustrations.

References

Benirschke, K. (2012). Comparative Placentation. http://placentation.ucsd.edu (accessed 07 November 2015).

Bicknese, E.J. (1990). Rhabdomyolysis in macaques. *Proceedings of American Association of Zoo Veterinarians Annual Conference*, South Padre Island, TX, pp. 316–318.

Burgos-Rodriguez, A. (2011). Zoonotic diseases of primates. *Veterinary Clinics of North America: Exotic Animal Practice* 14: 557–575.

Bush, M., Wildt, D.E., Kennedy, S. et al. (1978). Laparoscopy in zoological medicine. *Journal of the American Veterinary Medical Association* 173: 1081–1087.

Calle, P.P., Raphael, B.L., Stetter, M.D. et al. (1995). Gastrointestinal linear foreign bodies in *Trachypithecus cristatus ultimus*. *Journal of Zoo and Wildlife Medicine* 26: 87–97.

Carpenter, R.H. and Riddle, K.E. (1980). Direct inguinal hernia in the cynomolgus monkey (*Macaca fascicularis*). *Journal of Medical Primatology* 9: 194–199.

CDC Center for Disease Control (2019). B Virus (Herpes B). htpp://www.cdc.gov/herpesbvirus/ (accessed 13 October 2019).

Chai, N. (2015). Endoscopy and endosurgery in nonhuman primates. *Veterinary Clinics of North America: Exotic Animal Practice* 18: 447–461.

Cline, J.M., Brignolo, L., and Ford, E.W. (2012). Urogenital system. In: *Nonhuman Primates in Biomedical Research: Biology and Management*, 2e, vol. 1 (eds. C.R. Abee, K. Mansfield, S.D. Tardif and T. Morris), 482–562. San Diego, CA: Academic Press.

Doyle, G.S. (2010). Tourniquet first! *Journal of Emergency Medical Services*. http://www.jems.com/articles/2010/05/tourniquet-first.html.

Fanton, J.W., Yochmowitz, M.G., Wood, D.H. et al. (1986). Surgical treatment of endometriosis in 50 rhesus monkeys. *American Journal of Veterinary Research* 47: 1602–1604.

Fossum, T.W. (2013). *Small Animal Surgery Textbook*. Elsevier Health Sciences.

Hahn, A., D'Agostino, J., Cole, G.A., and Raines, J. (2014). Retroperitoneal abscesses in two western lowland gorillas (*Gorilla gorilla gorilla*). *Journal of Zoo and Wildlife Medicine* 45: 179–183.

Hendrickx, A.G. and Dukelow, W.R. (1995a). Breeding. In: *Nonhuman Primates in Biomedical Research: Diseases*, 2e (eds. T.B. Bennett, C.R. Abee and R. Henrickson), 335–374. San Diego, CA: Academic Press.

Hendrickx, A.G. and Dukelow, W.R. (1995b). Reproductive biology. In: *Nonhuman Primates in Biomedical Research: Diseases*, 2e (eds. T.B. Bennett, C.R. Abee and R. Henrickson), 147–191. San Diego, CA: Academic Press.

Herrin, K.A., Spelman, L.H., and Wack, R. (2002). Surgical air sac resection as a treatment for chronic air sacculitis in great apes. *Proceedings of American Association of Zoo Veterinarians Annual Conference,* Milwaukee, WI, pp. 369–371.

Hill, L.R., Lee, D.R., and Keeling, M.E. (2001). Surgical technique for ambulatory management of air sacculitis in a chimpanzee *(Pan troglodytes)*. *Journal of Medical Primatology* 51: 80–84.

Kumar, V. and Raja, A. (2012). No-scalpel vasectomy by electrocauterization in free range rhesus macaques (*Macaca mulatta*). *Open Veterinary Journal* 2: 6–9.

Lewis, J.C., Montgomery, C.A., and Hildebrandt, P.K. (1975). Air sacculitis in the baboon. *Journal of the American Veterinary Medical Association* 167: 662–664.

Lowenstine, L.J. and Osborn, K.G. (2012). Respiratory system diseases nonhuman primates. In: *Nonhuman Primates in Biomedical Research*, 2e (eds. C.R. Abee, K. Mansfield, S. Tardiff and T. Morris), 563–587. San Diego, CA: Academic Press.

Martin, D.P. (1982). Perineal cystocele in a cynomolgus monkey. *Journal of the American Veterinary Medical Association* 181: 1431–1432.

McManamon, R., Swenson, R.B., and Lowenstine, L.J. (1994). Update on diagnostic and therapeutic approaches to airsacculitis in orangutans. *Proceedings of American Association of Zoo Veterinarians Annual Conference,* Pittsburg, PA, pp. 219–220.

Mook, D.M. (2002). Gastric trichobezoars in a rhesus macaque (*Macaca mulatta*). *Comparative Medicine* 52: 560–562.

Morris, T.H. and David, C.L. (1992). Illustrated guide to surgical technique for vasectomy of the common marmoset. *Laboratory Animal* 27: 381–384.

Mylniczenko, N.D. (2003). A preliminary report on intra-abdominal abscesses in captive western lowland gorillas (*Gorilla gorilla gorilla*). *Proceedings of the American Association of Zoo Veterinarians Annual Conference*, Minneapolis, MN, pp. 62–66.

National Association of State Public Health Veterinarians (2010). Compendium of veterinary standard precautions for zoonotic disease prevention in veterinary personnel, National Association of State Public Health Veterinarians, Veterinary Infection Control Committee. *Journal of American Veterinary Medical Association* 237: 1403–1422.

Newcomb, L.K., Kruse, M.A., Minter, L.J., and Sobolewski, C.J. (2019). A modern approach to minimally invasive surgery and laparoscopic sterilization in chimpanzee. *Case Reports in Veterinary Medicine* 2019: Article ID 7492910. https://www.hindawi.com/journals/crivem/2019/7492910/abs/.

Peng, B., Zhang, R.D., Dai, X.S. et al. (2002). Quantitative (stereological) study of the effects of vasectomy on spermatogenesis in rhesus monkeys (*Macaca mulatta*). *Reproduction* 124: 847–856.

Pérez, J., Ramírez, M., and Hernández, C.A. (2008). Surgical intervention for removing intestinal *Prosthenorchis sp.* in a captive white-footed tamarin (*Saguinus leucopus*). *Revista Colombiana de Ciencias Pecuarias* 21: 608–613.

Pizarro, A., Amarasekaran, B., Brown, D., and Pizzi, R. (2019). Laparoscopic repair of an umbilical hernia in a Western chimpanzee (*Pan troglodytes verus*) rescued in Sierra Leone. *Journal of Medical Primatology* 48: 189–191. https://onlinelibrary.wiley.com/doi/abs/10.1111/jmp.12409.

Pollock, P.J., Doyle, R., Tobin, E. et al. (2008). Repeat laparotomy for the treatment of septic peritonitis in a Bornean orangutan (*Pongo pygmaeus pygmaeus*). *Journal of Zoo and Wildlife Medicine* 39: 476–479.

Randolph, J., Bush, M., Abramowitz, M. et al. (1981). Surgical correction of familial diaphragmatic hernia of Morgagni in the golden lion tamarin. *Journal of Pediatric Surgery* 16: 396–401.

Remick, A.K., Van Wettere, A.J., and Williams, C.V. (2009). Neoplasia in prosimians: case series from a captive prosimian population and literature review. *Veterinary Pathology Online* 46: 746–772.

Renquist, D.M. and Whitney, R.A. Jr. (1987). Zoonoses acquired from pet primates. *Veterinary Clinics of North America: Small Animal Practice* 17: 219–240.

Roberge, S., Demers, S., Berghella, V. et al. (2014). Impact of single-vs. double-layer closure on adverse outcomes and uterine scar defect: a systematic review and meta-analysis. *American Journal of Obstetrics and Gynecology* 211: 453–460.

Roberts, J.A. (1995). Occupational health concerns with nonhuman primates in zoological gardens. *Journal of Zoo and Wildlife Medicine* 26: 10–23.

Rodriguez, N.A., Garcia, K.D., Fortman, J.D. et al. (2002). Clinical and histopathological evaluation of 13 cases of adenocarcinoma in aged rhesus macaques (*Macaca mulatta*). *Journal of Medical Primatology* 31 (2): 74–83.

Sadoughi, B., Dirheimer, M., and Regnard et Fane`lie Wanert, P. (2018). Surgical management of a strangulated inguinal hernia in a cynomologus monkey (*Macaca fascicularis*): a case report with discussion, and review of literature. *Revue de Primatologie* (open edition) 9. https://journals. openedition.org/primatologie/3372.

Schexnider, J.M., Baker, D.G., and Hasselschwert, D.L. (2007). Semen evaluation for verification of azoospermia after vasectomy in chimpanzees (*Pan troglodytes*). *Journal of the American Association of Laboratory Animal Science* 46: 46–49.

Schrenzel, M.D., Osborn, K.G., Shima, A. et al. (2003). Naturally occurring fatal herpes simplex virus 1 infection in a family of white-faces saki monkeys (*Pithecia pithecia pithecia*). *Journal of Medical Primatology* 32: 7–14.

Simmons, H.A. and Mattison, J.A. (2011). The incidence of spontaneous neoplasia in two populations of captive rhesus macaques (*Macaca mulatta*). *Antioxidants & Redox Signaling* 14: 221–227.

Smith, K.M., Calle, P., Raphael, B.L. et al. (2006). Cholelithiasis in four callitrichid species (*Leontopithecus, Callithrix*). *Journal of Zoo and Wildlife Medicine* 37: 44–48.

Sokal, D., Irsula, B., Hays, M. et al. (2004). Vasectomy by ligation and excision, with or without fascial interposition: a randomized controlled trial. *BMC Medicine* 2 (1): 1. http://bmcmedicine.biomedcentral.com/artic les/10.1186/1741-7015-2-6.

Sousa, M.B.C., Leão, A.C., Coutinho, J.F.V. et al. (2008). Histopathology findings in common marmosets (*Callithrix jacchus* Linnaeus, 1758) with chronic weight loss associated with bile tract obstruction by infestation with *Platynosomum* (Loos, 1907). *Primates* 49: 283–287.

Steinmetz, H.W. and Zimmermann, N. (2012). Computed tomography for the diagnosis of sinusitis and air sacculitis in orangutan. In: *Fowler's Zoo and Wild Animal Medicine Current Therapy*, 7e (eds. R.E. Miller and M.E. Fowler), 422–430. St. Louis, MO: Elsevier Sanders.

Taylor, A.F., Smith, M., and Eichberg, J.W. (1988). Inguinal hernia surgery in an infant chimpanzee. *Journal of Medical Primatology* 18: 415–417.

Valverde, C.R., Tarara, R.P., Griffey, S.M. et al. (2000). Spontaneous intestinal adenocarcinoma in geriatric macaques (*Macaca sp.*). *Comparative Medicine* 50: 540–544.

Viera, A. (2015). Vasectomy and other vasal occlusion techniques for male contraception. http://www.uptodate. com/contents/vasectomy-and-other-vasal-occlusion- malecontraception?source=search_result&search=vasecto my&selectedTitle=2~28 (accessed 30 May16).

WHO World Health Organization Reproductive Health Library (2016). Vasectomy occlusion techniques for male sterilization: RHL summary (last revised 16 May 2016). http://apps.who. int/rhl/fertility/contraception/cd003991/en/.

Wildt, D.E., Chakraborty, P.K., Cambre, R.C. et al. (1982). Laparoscopic evaluation of the reproductive organs and abdominal cavity content of the lowland gorilla. *American Journal of Primatology* 2: 29–42.

Wolff, P., Pond, J., and Meehan, T. (1990). Surgical removal of *Prosthenorchis elegans* from six species of Callitrichidae. *Proceedings of the American Association of Zoo Veterinarians Annual Conference*, South Padre Island, TX, pp. 95–98.

Zilberman, M. and Elsner, J.J. (2008). Antibiotic-eluting medical devices for various applications. *Journal of Controlled Release* 130: 202–215.

25

Marine Mammal Surgery

Jennifer L. Higgins, Carmen M. H. Colitz, and Dean A. Hendrickson

Background

Marine mammals include pinnipeds (seals, sea lions, fur seals, and walruses), cetaceans (whales, dolphins, and porpoises), sirenians (manatees and dugongs), sea otters, and polar bears. This chapter will focus on surgical procedures performed in seals, sea lions, and dolphins as these are the most common marine mammals kept in captivity, as well as the species most likely to be taken in by rehabilitation centers. The number of surgeries performed in marine mammals remains limited as numerous challenges exist, including environmental constraints, anesthetic risks, anatomic challenges, incisional dehiscence, equipment limitations, and perceived risks. For these reasons, surgical procedures have been primarily limited to wound management, dentistry, ocular surgery, fracture repair, and upper gastrointestinal (GI) and respiratory endoscopy. There are many indications for abdominal surgery in marine mammals. Surgery is often the only treatment option for ureterolithiasis, severe enteritis, intestinal volvulus, and neoplasia. Both minimally invasive surgery (MIS) and laparotomy have been successfully performed in marine mammals. Lessons learned from these surgical procedures will improve treatment options for future patients.

Surgery of Pinnipeds

Ocular Surgery

Diseases of the cornea and lens are common in pinnipeds and can result in impaired vision and pain. Pathologic abnormalities frequently described include corneal ulcers, corneal edema, progressive keratopathy, cataracts, and lens luxation (Figures 25.1 and 25.2) (Miller et al. 2013; Kern and Colitz 2013). When the lens is involved, surgical treatment often becomes necessary to reduce pain, improve quality of

life in captive pinnipeds, improve sight, and allow release of stranded, wild pinnipeds. Cataract surgery is performed using similar techniques as in canine patients, depending on the situation, although a number of unique challenges are encountered in pinnipeds. Phacoemulsification, extracapsular lens extraction, and intracapsular lens extraction have all been successfully performed in pinnipeds (Dutton 1991; Barnes and Smith 2004; Colitz 2011; Esson et al. 2015).

After the patient is anesthetized and before surgery begins, evaluate the posterior segment using ultrasonography; electroretinography (ERG) is not routinely performed as it prolongs the anesthetic event and retinal degeneration has not been diagnosed in any pinniped to date. Ultrasound enables assessment of the posterior lens capsule, vitreous, and retina, and ERG evaluates photoreceptor function.

Position the pinniped either in sternal or lateral recumbency. Lateral recumbency may have negative effects on the lungs and respiration in larger patients; therefore, sternal recumbency is preferred.

Phacoemulsification

While phacoemulsification allows the use of the smallest surgical incision and diminishes risk of postoperative complications, this technique is impossible to apply in juvenile, subadult, and adult pinnipeds due to either lens instability or the presence of a dense cataract (Colitz 2011; Kern and Colitz 2013). Phacoemulsification can generally be utilized in pups or yearling animals (Esson et al. 2015; Kern and Colitz 2013; Colitz 2011). If phacoemulsification with a small incision single- or two-handed approach is chosen, use a #64 blade or keratome to create a deep partial thickness clear-corneal incision. Enter the anterior chamber with the keratome or #64 Beaver blade and inject approximately 0.2–0.3 ml 1:1000 preservative-free epinephrine (1 mg/ml) intracamerally to dilate the pupil (Barnes and Smith 2004; Esson et al. 2015; Kern and Colitz 2013). Topical 1:1000 epinephrine or 2.5% phenylephrine

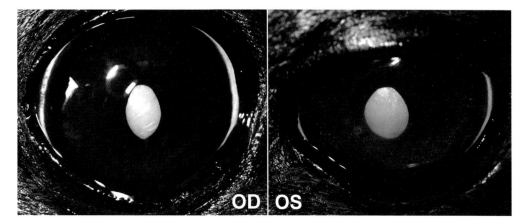

Figure 25.1 Both eyes of a harbor seal (*Phoca vitulina*). The right eye (OD) has a mature cataract and mild limbal hyperemia; there is also mild pigment crossing the limbus temporally. The left eye (OS) also has a mature cataract, as well as a gray-white round anterior stromal corneal opacity with a clear center and two other less dense superficial gray opacities.

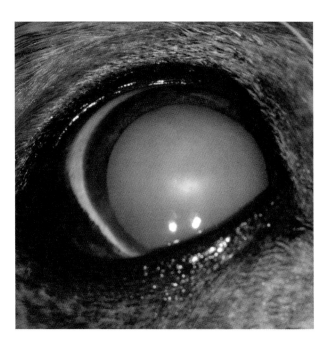

Figure 25.2 The right eye (OD) of a California sea lion (*Zalophus californianus*) with an anteriorly luxated cataractous lens. There is also faint diffuse gray opacity located ventrally and extending to the 7 o'clock position consistent with perilimbal edema. There is also mild limbal hyperemia.

administered three to four times over 20 minutes has also successfully dilated the pinniped pupil to approximately 4–5 mm. Dilation of the pupil is crucial to successful cataract extraction and is best attained with epinephrine as topical parasympatholytics (e.g. atropine and tropicamide) are ineffective. The pinniped pupil does not dilate as widely as the pupil of terrestrial mammals. This may be due to poor absorption across the thick fibrous tunic of the pinniped eye or too few cholinergic or adrenergic receptors in the iris (Miller et al. 2010). The anatomy of the dilator

muscle also differs from that of terrestrial animals, possibly affecting the efficacy of mydriatics.

After dilation of the pupil, maintain the anterior chamber shape with 1% or 2% sodium hyaluronate and perform a continuous curvilinear anterior capsulorhexis. The lens is large and globoid in pinnipeds and the choice of phacoemulsification needle length depends on the size of the animal and species. It is ideal to have the standard canine needle as well as the longer modified equine phacoemulsification needle available in order to reach the posterior aspect of the lens.

Perform phacoemulsification as standard for cataract surgery using high-frequency ultrasound waves, irrigation, and aspiration. Unlike the soft diabetic cataract in canine patients, most pinniped cataracts are very dense and unstable, making phacoemulsification challenging and lengthy. Pinnipeds over two years of age will have lenses that are denser than the phacoemulsification machines can emulsify and the chunky lens material will plug the aspiration tubing. In addition, the lengthy surgical time may damage the delicate corneal endothelial cells. Once the lens has been removed, extract the entire lens capsule, or as much of the lens capsule as possible, due to the 100% incidence of posterior capsular opacification (PCO) within one year in pinnipeds. PCO, also called lens capsule fibrosis, is severe and pinnipeds with lens capsules have become blind or impaired again. However, these fibrosed lens capsules have been removed successfully during a second surgery and sight restored. Suture the cornea with 8 or 9-0 polyglactin 910 and remove the sodium hyaluronate immediately prior to closure.

As intraocular lenses (IOLs) with the ideal dioptric strength have not been developed for any pinniped species, an IOL is not implanted in the pinniped capsule. However, IOLs would only potentially be necessary for pinnipeds returned to the wild who require the ability to focus at depths lower than most pools in captive facilities. Pinniped corneas have a flattened plateau through which they focus when in shallow water or on land (Hanke et al. 2009). Clinically, aphakic pinnipeds have not shown behavior consistent with having hyperopia, as they are able to catch fish from close and far away without issues and respond to visual cues. Stranded seal pups undergoing phacoemulsification procedures can regain sufficient vision for natural foraging behavior and are release candidates (Esson et al. 2015). Long-term survival of these animals, however, has not yet been established.

Due to the susceptibility of pinnipeds to corneal disease, extreme care must be taken when handling the cornea during surgery. Corneal endothelial cell loss can occur following exposure to the high-energy waves emitted by phacoemulsification. The success of the surgery also depends on management of uveitis, which is induced by exposure to the highly immunogenic lens proteins. Pinnipeds show very few clinical signs associated with uveitis compared to dogs and cats; they do not typically demonstrate aqueous flare or keratic precipitates. Signs of uveitis in pinnipeds include perilimbal edema, diffuse corneal edema, miosis, conjunctival hyperemia, and vision impairment. Preoperative, intraoperative, and postoperative administration of anti-inflammatory agents is crucial for management of uveitis. Administration of antibiotics is standard for prevention of perioperative infection. Options for medical management of pinnipeds postcataract surgery are detailed in Table 25.1. To minimize uveitis, pinnipeds are managed on a combination of a topical steroid (prednisolone acetate ophthalmic solution) and non-steroidal anti-inflammatory drugs (NSAID) (nepafenac or ketorolac). Either a systemic NSAID (carprofen or meloxicam) or corticosteroid (dexamethasone or prednisolone) are also prescribed. Neomycin-polymyxin-gramicidin and ofloxacin are utilized in combinations as topical antibiotics. Several treatment options exist for systemic antibiotics. Finally, either a topical or systemic carbonic anhydrase inhibitor is utilized to diminish risk of glaucoma. To allow the incision to heal, dry dock the animal for one week postoperatively.

Extracapsular Lens Extraction

In older pinnipeds without obvious lens instability, extracapsular lens extraction is often the best surgical approach (Figure 25.3). As with phacoemulsification, extract the anterior lens capsule, nucleus, and cortex, and remove the remaining lens capsule as it is not typically adhered to the zonules or ciliary processes after the age of 17 years. Make an approximate 160° partial thickness corneal incision using either a #64 Beaver blade or a keratome, then enter the anterior chamber using the keratome. Inject 0.2–0.3 ml 1:1000 epinephrine into the anterior chamber

and beneath the iris followed by a viscoelastic material (1.0%, 1.2%, or 2% sodium hyaluronate) to protect the corneal endothelium and maintain the anterior chamber vault. Using a Vannas scissor or a 22 g needle, start a curved incision in the anterior lens capsule and grasp the anterior lens capsule with Utrada lens capsule forceps. Perform a large continuous curvilinear anterior capsulotomy. Perform viscodissection to loosen the lens from its capsule. Gently insert a lens loupe beneath the lens to elevate it from the capsule and out of the eye. Once the lens has been removed from the eye, lactated Ringer's solution (LRS) is used to flush any remaining lens cortical material from the anterior and posterior chambers as well as from the lens capsule (Barnes and Smith 2004). Once the chambers are flushed, inject viscoelastic material again into the anterior chamber and behind the iris. Use Utrada forceps to gently tease the lens capsule from its position. In most cases, it will release from the vitreal attachment with patience. Close the incision with one simple interrupted suture at the 12 o'clock position and two separate simple saw tooth patterns (Nasisse 1997) on each side of the interrupted suture using 7-0 polyglactin 910. Perioperative and postoperative antibiotics and anti-inflammatory medications are as discussed in the phacoemulsification section.

Intracapsular Lens Extraction

Intracapsular lens extraction involves removal of the entire lens without opening of the lens capsule. This technique is best applied in pinnipeds with obvious lens luxation (Figure 25.2). Anterior lens luxation is more commonly observed than posterior luxation in seals, sea lions, and fur seals, and can lead to secondary uveitis, cataract, corneal edema, pain, and glaucoma (Colitz et al. 2010). Walrus have more commonly had posterior lens luxations than anterior lens luxations.

A few animals with cataract have had concurrent retinal detachment identified at the time of surgery with ultrasound. The choice was made to perform the lensectomy due to the sequelae likely if the lens was to be left in the eye. To date, only 2 out of 200 eyes, both from an elderly animal, have developed a retinal detachment following cataract surgery.

Some sea lions have had concurrent indolent ulcers at the time of lensectomy; therefore, debridement and burr keratotomy have been performed. In these patients, topical and oral corticosteroids are avoided and only NSAIDs are used along with appropriate antibiotics.

Conjunctival Graft

Corneal ulceration with stromal loss is not uncommon in pinnipeds. This can occur secondary to Otariid (or Pinniped) Keratopathy or from a chronic anterior lens

Table 25.1 Pharmaceutical options for management of pinnipeds post cataract surgery.

Drug	Dose	Route	Frequency	Duration	Comments
Antibiotics					
Cefazolin	10 mg/kg	IM, IV, SQ	Every 1.5 h	Intra-op	
Neomycin-polymyxin-gramicidin[a]		Topical	QID, then TID	4 wk	Use neomycin-polymyxin-gramicidin in combination with ofloxacin for 4 wk, then discontinue if no corneal ulcers present
Ofloxacin		Topical	QID, then TID	4 wk	
Enrofloxacin	3.5–5 mg/kg	PO	BID	3 wk	Either Enrofloxacin or Ciprofloxacin, not both
Ciprofloxacin	15 mg/kg	PO	SID	3 wk	Either Enrofloxacin or Ciprofloxacin, not both
Doxycycline	5 mg/kg	PO	BID	As long as needed	Indicated if corneal ulcer is present concurrently due to Pinniped Keratopathy
Convenia	4 mg/kg	SQ	Once	Unknown at this dose	At 8 mg/kg, lasts at least 53 d in sea lions
Excede	6.6 mg/kg	IM	Once	5 d	
Anti-inflammatories					
Carprofen	0.5–1.0 mg/kg	PO	BID	2–3 wk	Monitor for signs of GI ulceration; can use stomach protectants.
Meloxicam	0.05–0.1 mg/kg	PO	BID	2–3 wk	Monitor for signs of GI ulceration; can use stomach protectants
Dexamethasone	0.1 mg/kg	PO	SID	14 d, then taper	Steroids are used in place of NSAIDs in animals with renal or liver disease or if they are anorexic postoperatively
Prednisolone	1 mg/kg	PO	SID	Up to 3 mo, then taper	
Prednisolone acetate ophthalmic solution		Topical	QID	3–4 wk, then taper	Do not use if corneal ulcer is present
Nepafenac		Topical	TID	3–4 wk	Diclofenac and flurbiprofen are not typically used as they may sting and are not as potent
Ketorolac		Topical	TID	3–4 wk	
Carbonic anhydrase inhibitors					
Dorzolamide		Topical	TID, then BID	5–6 wk	Dorzolamide with Timolol combination also acceptable, same dose
Brinzolamide		Topical	TID, then BID	5–6 wk	
Dichlorphenamide	2 mg/kg	PO	BID		As an alternative to a topical carbonic anhydrase inhibitor
Methazolamide	2 mg/kg	PO	BID		
Gastroprotectants					
Sucralfate	10 mg/kg	PO	BID		Gastroprotectants may be indicated in animals on systemic NSAID therapy
Ranitidine	2.5 mg/kg	PO	SID		

[a] Always wait five minutes between administration of ophthalmic medications.

luxation causing the stroma to become malacic and thinned. Both situations have been surgically repaired successfully (Colitz et al. 2014). Use a BioSIS (Avalon Medical, Stillwater, MN) or A-Cell (ACell Inc., Columbia, MD) corneal graft to provide tectonic support and suture a conjunctival pedical flap over the initial graft (Figure 25.4). Conjunctival grafts provide fibrovascular tissue for the defect and provide a blood supply (Hakanson and Meredith 1987) as pinniped corneas do not readily vascularize or reestablish the stroma that has been degraded (Kern and Colitz 2013).

Create the conjunctival flap from the inferiotemporal conjunctiva extending to the dorsotemporal conjunctiva so that it will adequately cover the defect. Set aside the graft and address the corneal defect. Gently debride the ulcer

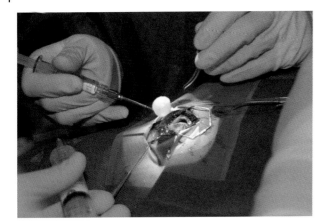

Figure 25.3 Intraoperative image of the cataractous lens being removed from the eye with a lens loupe cannula attached to viscoelastic syringe.

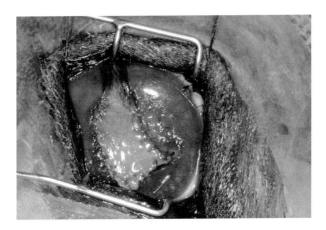

Figure 25.4 The right eye (OD) of a gray seal (*Halichoerus grypus*) that underwent a keratectomy and conjunctival graft as well as insertion of an episcleral cyclosporine implant.

and the adjacent epithelium. Suture a double layer of BioSIS graft using numerous simple interrupted sutures of 8-0 polyglactin 910. If there is a concurrent anterior lens luxation or cataract, remove this and close the incision as described above. Suture a conjunctival flap over the BioSIS with simple interrupted sutures; place two to three sutures as anchors at the dorsal aspect of the limbus. Administer topical and oral antibiotics as well as topical and oral NSAIDs, similar to management of cataract surgery patients. Tramadol (1–2 mg/kg PO BID) is often used for a few days to weeks.

Cyclosporine Implants for Keratopathy

Topical cyclosporine and tacrolimus have been utilized for over 11 years for management of Pinniped (including Otariid) Keratopathy. The positive response to these medications is not fully understood; however, both cyclosporine and tacrolimus are immunomodulatory agents that inhibit

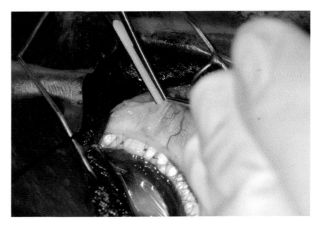

Figure 25.5 The left eye of a California sea lion (*Zalophus californianus*) immediately after having undergone lensectomy. Limbal sutures are in place in a simple saw tooth pattern with one simple interrupted suture at the 12 o'clock position. Approximately 5 mm dorsal to the limbus, a subconjunctival tunnel was made and a cyclosporine impregnated implant is being inserted into the tunnel, i.e. episcleral location.

calcineurin (Pflugfelder et al. 1986; Stern et al. 2004). Clinically, these medications also stimulate the lacrimal glands to secrete the aqueous portion of the tear film and improve mucin production. Keratopathy in pinnipeds is likely an immune-mediated disease; however, histopathology of corneal and globe samples has not shown excessive lymphocytes (R. Dubielzig, personal communication). Therefore, cyclosporine and tacrolimus may improve control of this disease by improving tear film quality and quantity and rebalancing the surface immunity of the eye. Cyclosporine implants have been used successfully in dogs for the control of keratoconjunctivitis sicca, and their use in pinnipeds over the past five years has been shown to be of benefit in diminishing flare ups of Otariid Keratopathy (Staggs et al. 2013).

Place cyclosporine implants in the episclera by making a small incision with Westcott scissors approximately 5 mm posterior to the dorsal limbus and bluntly dissecting a tunnel long enough for the implant (Figure 25.5). Use smooth forceps (e.g. tying forceps) to hold the implant and gently insert it into the tunnel. Close the incision with 7-0 polyglactin 910 in a cruciate or simple interrupted pattern.

Orthopedic Surgery

The most common indication for orthopedic surgery in pinnipeds is treatment of distal phalangeal fractures in the hind flippers of stranded animals. These fractures are often the result of bite wounds and contamination is a primary concern. Aggressively flushing the wound and administering systemic antibiotics is necessary for prevention or treatment of osteomyelitis. A high level of antimicrobial

(a)   (b)

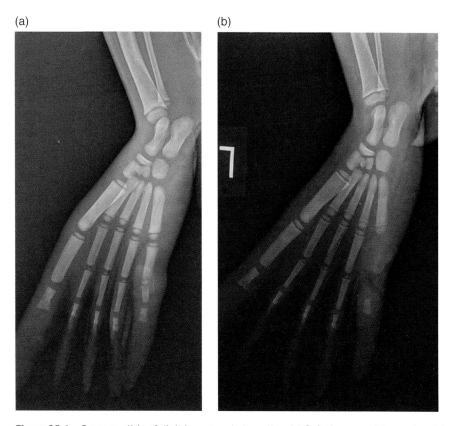

Figure 25.6 Osteomyelitis of digit in a stranded sea lion. (a) Soft tissue swelling and radiolucency of the proximal and middle phalanges of digit V is evident. (b) Postsurgical amputation of the affected bones. *Source:* Radiographs provided by C. Field, The Marine Mammal Center.

resistance has been found in bacteria isolated from stranded pinnipeds (Johnson et al. 1998). Thus, culture and antimicrobial susceptibility testing of penetrating wounds should routinely be performed in animals with flipper trauma. Surgery becomes necessary when medical management fails to treat the osteomyelitis. Amputation of the affected digits is the treatment of choice and the procedure is performed as in a canine patient (Figure 25.6). The primary surgical concern in pinnipeds is closure of the incision. An effort should be made to preserve as much soft tissue as possible by tunneling under the skin to the fracture site; however, if significant contaminated tissue is present, retaining sufficient tissue for closure can be challenging. To minimize wound dehiscence, use a horizontal mattress pattern or similar tension relieving pattern (Lucas et al. 1999).

The mandible is another common site for fractures in pinnipeds, although published reports of surgical repair are sparse. As with any animal, the choice of stabilization technique depends on the location and type of the fracture. A technique combining an acrylic intraoral splint and orthopedic wiring has been successfully utilized for treatment of a transverse mandibular fracture in a harbor seal (*Phoca vitulina*) (Lewer et al. 2007). This technique preserves the

tooth roots and neurovascular supply, provides adequate stabilization for fracture healing, and allows for immediate return to the animal's normal enclosure. Remove any loose or fractured teeth and place orthopedic wire circumferentially around the mandible. Position two to three wires both cranial and caudal to the fracture site. Place the wires interdentally with approximately 5 mm of space between the wire and gingiva. When positioning the wires, avoid the sublingual and mandibular salivary ducts. Once correct fracture alignment and proper occlusion are achieved, apply acrylic resin in layers to a thickness of approximately 8 mm. After the acrylic hardens, tighten the wires over the surface of the acrylic pulling the bone in tight apposition to the acrylic. Monitor bony union postoperatively to determine when sufficient healing has occurred to allow removal of the acrylic splint and wires. In one published report of a mandibular fracture repair in a harbor seal using this technique, evidence of sufficient bony union was not present radiographically until 12 months postoperatively (Lewer et al. 2007). A common complication of mandibular fracture in pinnipeds is osteomyelitis, evidence of which may be best appreciated on computerized tomography scans (Haulena et al. 1998).

Long bone fractures have only rarely been described in pinnipeds. A single published report describes the use of a string-of-pearls (SOP) locking plate for stabilization of a complete, transverse tibial fracture in a stranded gray seal (*Halichoerus grypus*) pup (Hespel et al. 2013). As is common with distal phalangeal fractures in pinnipeds, there was evidence of infection around the tibial fracture site in this animal. Even closed fractures with no evidence of penetrating wounds can have significant infection present. Thorough debridement and irrigation of the area is indicated before stabilization of the fracture. In young animals with distal diaphyseal fractures, the position of the growth plate must be taken into account when placing screws in a locking plate. Seals have a curved tibia with a concave medial surface. SOP and reconstruction plates can be bent from side to side as well as up and down. Locking plates are advantageous as they do not require perfect contouring to the bone surface. Since tight contact between plate and bone is unnecessary, use of locking plates also allows for better preservation of the periosteal blood supply. In the stranded gray seal pup described above, the plate was applied to the lateral aspect of the tibia to avoid potentially damaging the saphenous artery, vein, and nerve. The implantation of antibiotic-impregnated polymethylmethacrylate (PMMA) beads before closure may aid in the management of fractures with evidence of osteomyelitis or significant soft tissue infection, especially where blood supply is compromised. If culture and susceptibility testing are not able to be performed prior to surgery, gentamicin-impregnated PMMA beads are a good choice in stranded pinnipeds as approximately 75% of bacteria isolated have been reported to be Gram negative, most of which have been susceptible to gentamicin (Johnson et al. 1998).

Abdominal Surgery

Castration/Ovariectomy

Control of fertility is an important management concern in many facilities with captive pinnipeds. To prevent breeding as well as reduce aggressive behaviors, three main strategies are applied: physical separation, hormonal manipulation, and castration of males. While the first two options are most commonly utilized, castration has been performed in numerous California sea lions (*Zalophus californianus*). There are marked differences in the reproductive anatomy of otariids (sea lions and fur seals) and phocids (true seals) that must be taken into account during surgery. Otariid testicles are seasonally scrotal and surgery is typically performed during the breeding season to take advantage of the scrotal location of the testes. The procedure is similar to that in a canine patient with the testes removed through a prescrotal incision. In phocid species, the testes

are para-abdominal, positioned dorsal to the blubber layer in the inguinal region (Robeck et al. 2001).

Ovariectomy is rarely performed in pinnipeds. Abdominal surgery in these species is limited due to concerns of increased anesthetic risks associated with prolonged surgical procedures as well as challenges encountered during closure of the abdominal wall. The few reports of reproductive surgery in female pinnipeds have been for treatment of tumors of the reproductive tract, which are relatively common in California sea lions. These procedures are described in the MIS section of this chapter. There is a single historical report in the literature of ovariohysterectomy successfully performed by traditional laparotomy for treatment of vaginal prolapse in an Australian sea lion (*Neophoca cinerea*) (Read et al. 1982). While this procedure was performed over 30 years ago, several important lessons can be gained from the postoperative management. The surgery was performed using similar techniques as those used in a domestic dog. The main problem encountered was postoperative wound dehiscence, which is a major deterrent to performing abdominal surgery in pinnipeds. After initial breakdown of the subcuticular pattern, the skin was resutured with a row of deep vertical mattress sutures, which were then oversewn with a horizontal mattress pattern. A tension relieving suture pattern, such as a vertical or horizontal mattress with stents, should be considered when closing all surgical incisions in pinnipeds, whether the incision is in the abdominal cavity or in the limb for digit amputation. In the case described, sutures were removed eight weeks after the laparotomy. An additional postoperative consideration is wound care. There are differing opinions as to whether the wound should be kept clean and dry by maintaining the animal off exhibit and out of water or whether the animal can be returned to the water. In most circumstances, it is probably best to return the animal to the water, as this seems to minimize wound dehiscence and patient stress. Maintaining the animal in an aquatic environment eliminates strain that would be placed on ventral midline sutures if the animal were to move across the ground and likely aids in keeping the incision clean as well.

Telemetry Implantation

One recent application of laparotomy in pinnipeds is implantation of intraperitoneal telemetry devices. An intraperitoneally implanted satellite-linked life history transmitter (LHX tag) that allows for continuous recording of data throughout the life of an animal has recently been developed (Horning et al. 2008). Data is transmitted upon extrusion of the tag after the animal dies. The tags are 12 cm long and are implanted into the caudoventral abdominal cavity. While manipulation of the viscera is unnecessary, the challenges associated with closure of an incision in the abdominal wall still remain. To implant the LHX tags, make an 8.5–12 cm ventral midline incision. A six-layer closure with 1 or 0 polydioxanone sutures incorporating a tension-relieving suture pattern has been found to prevent incisional dehiscence. First, close the peritoneum with a simple continuous pattern. Second, close the linea alba with a simple interrupted or interrupted cruciate pattern. Third, close the subcutaneous fat with a simple continuous pattern. Fourth, close the intradermal fat (blubber) in a tension-relieving mattress pattern to reduce pressure on skin sutures. Fifth, use a subcuticular pattern to appose skin layers. Finally, place an interrupted cruciate pattern in the skin to provide additional support to the skin closure. Surgical glue or staples can also be utilized to further secure the skin. Closing in so many layers is advantageous as a single, strong holding layer is absent in the pinniped abdominal wall. Rather, it seems as if holding ability is more distributed throughout the body wall, unlike in land mammals. The success achieved with this method of closure in a large number of animals indicates that the abdominal wall can be reliably closed in pinniped species. Allowing animals with implanted LHX tags access to water after an initial recovery period from anesthesia may have also played a role in preventing wound dehiscence. It is believed that the salinity available in salt water improves wound healing.

MIS Procedures

Over the past decade, the application of MIS in pinniped species has expanded the number of abdominal surgeries performed. While recent experience with telemetry implantation has shown that a large abdominal wall incision can be successfully closed in pinnipeds without subsequent wound dehiscence, MIS further reduces the risk of dehiscence and decreases recovery time. Another advantage of MIS is improved visualization. The thick blubber wall of marine mammals is relatively inelastic, significantly restricting access to the abdominal cavity during open abdominal surgery. The amount of free space in the peritoneal cavity is also scant in comparison to the domestic animal, which further hinders manipulation of tissues. Thus, with a traditional open surgical approach a large incision is typically required. Imaging and study of pinniped landmarks is critical for any abdominal surgery in order to make the incision over the specific area of interest and minimize incision size. MIS offers more flexibility in incision location. An additional benefit of MIS that has not yet been explored in marine mammals is the potential to minimize the use of general anesthesia. MIS procedures are commonly performed in standing equine and bovine

patients with the use of sedation and a local anesthetic (Boure 2005; Hendrickson 2008).

The main indications for MIS in marine mammals are direct visual examination of abdominal organs, tissue biopsy, reproductive tract manipulations, and, in some cases, surgical treatment of gastrointestinal and urogenital diseases. To the authors' knowledge, there have been only five MIS procedures performed in pinnipeds that have been described in the literature (Fauquier et al. 2003; Dover et al. 2004; Roque et al. 2008; Lacave et al. 2009; Greene et al. 2015). These include three surgeries for removal of ovarian tumors or cysts, one exploratory surgery for visualization of the liver in a Northern elephant seal (*Mirounga angustirostris*) with hepatic disease diagnosed by serum chemistry values, and one gastropexy surgery in an elephant seal with a hiatal hernia. While the surgeries have had mixed success, important lessons have been learned. Factors critical to the success of MIS in all animals, but especially in marine mammals, are anesthetic time and patient condition. Anesthesia can be successfully performed in pinniped species; however, any underlying disease condition considerably increases anesthetic risk. The decision to go to surgery should be made before the patient's condition is severely compromised. Anesthetic morbidity and mortality in marine mammals is directly related to anesthetic duration. MIS procedures can be prolonged if the surgeon is not well trained in MIS or has a poor knowledge of marine mammal anatomy. Even experienced MIS surgeons may have to alter surgical treatments that are considered standard in domestic animals so as to minimize anesthetic time.

Ovariectomy performed for the purpose of removal of neoplastic or cystic tissue can be complicated by extensive vascularization or extensive connective tissue proliferation between organs. To excise the ovaries, identify the ovary and either remove with a vessel-sealing device or ultrasonic device. In the absence of an electrosurgical device, the ovaries are ligated using an absorbable suture tied with an endoscopic slip-knot, such as a 4S modified Roeder knot, and amputated with sharp dissection. One of the incisions for an instrument cannula may have to be enlarged to allow removal of the ovaries (Figure 25.7) (Dover et al. 2004).

There is a single report of surgical repair of a sliding hiatal hernia in a marine mammal (Greene et al. 2015), although this condition has been reported in a number of necropsies. The patient was a stranded Northern elephant seal pup suffering from regurgitation, poor weight gain, lethargy, and reduced lung sounds. A hiatal hernia was diagnosed by contrast radiography and GI endoscopy (Figure 25.8). Surgical repair using a MIS technique was successful, allowing the animal to be released into the

(a)

(b)

(c)

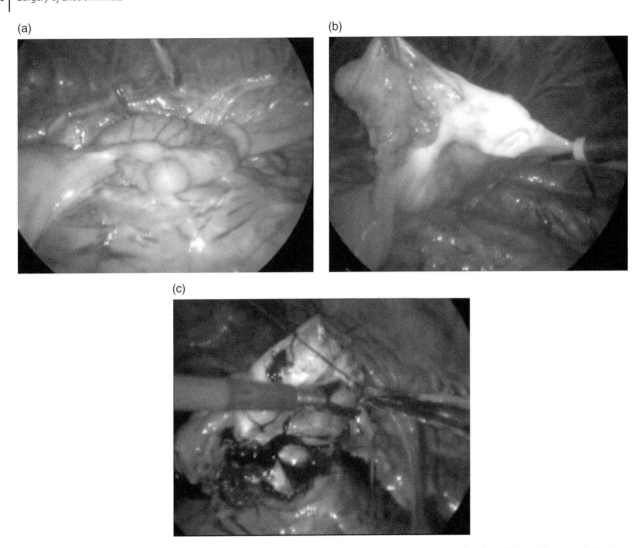

Figure 25.7 A three-port technique for laparoscopic ovariectomy in a gray seal. (a) Initial visualization of the right ovary following port placement. (b) Cauterization and transection of the suspensory ligament using a vessel-sealing device. The broad ligament, proper ligament, and uterine tube are similarly transected. (c) Three loop ligatures were placed around the ovarian artery and vein before transection. If available, electrosurgical devices can be used instead of ligatures. *Source*: Photographs provided by S. Dover, Channel Islands Marine & Wildlife Institute.

wild. While repair of hiatal hernias in dogs is typically by a combination of three procedures, diaphragmatic hiatal plication, esophagopexy, and left-sided gastropexy, the technique was modified in the elephant seal to reduce anesthesia time. The animal was placed in dorsal recumbency and an incision made just caudal to the umbilicus for insertion of a 10 mm rigid endoscope. An orogastric tube was placed, and the stomach was reduced into the abdominal cavity by placing the animal in a reverse Trendelenburg position and applying gentle traction with laparoscopic forceps. The hernia was left unrepaired and the stomach tacked to the left abdominal wall caudal to the last rib. To improve scar tissue formation, the serosal surfaces of the gastric fundus and body wall were scarified with electrosurgery. The gastropexy was performed with a

combination of extracorporeal and intracorporeal suture manipulation. The suture was started extracorporeally by passing suture material through the skin and body wall, then grasping the needle with laparoscopic forceps intracorporeally, passing it through the serosa, muscle, and submucosal layers of the prepared gastropexy site, and passing the needle back through the body wall. The sutures were tied extracorporeally to secure the gastropexy. It would be better to make a skin incision to bury the sutures and then close the skin incision.

Unlike the six-layer closure previously described, a two-layer closure is sufficient for portal sites made during MIS. The fascia and subcutaneous tissue can be closed with a single cruciate suture and the skin closed with another cruciate suture and sealed with surgical glue (Dover et al. 2004).

(a)

(b)

(c)

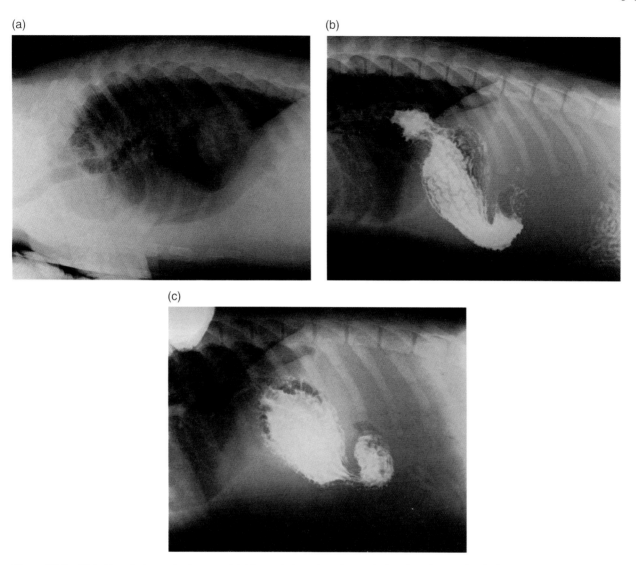

Figure 25.8 Hiatal hernia in an elephant seal. (a) Lateral thoracic radiograph showing abnormal soft tissue opacity within the thorax. (b) A positive contrast study shows herniation of the gastric cardia and fundus through the diaphragm into the caudal thorax. (c) Post-op lateral thoracic radiograph using contrast confirms position of the entire stomach within the abdominal cavity. *Source*: Radiographs provided by Greene et al. (2015), The Marine Mammal Center.

Surgery of Cetaceans

Oral Surgery

At the present time, surgery in cetaceans is primarily limited to treatment of oral and ocular disease. Although logistical and immobilization issues complicate treatment, tooth extraction is a relatively simple procedure owing to cetacean dental anatomy. Dolphins are homodont with shallow, single-rooted conical teeth. Fracture of teeth and exposure of the pulp cavity can occur subsequent to trauma, and extraction of the affected teeth is often necessary to prevent infection and development of periapical abscesses. Tooth extraction can be performed under sedation and

local anesthesia. Anesthesia of the mandible is achieved by infiltrating 2% lidocaine around the inferior alveolar nerve as it passes through the mandibular foramen. The mandibular foramen can be palpated intraorally lateral to the base of the tongue, and a 2 in. needle is typically required for the inferior alveolar nerve block in an adult bottlenose dolphin (*Tursiops truncates*) (Ridgway et al. 1975). Infraorbital nerve block has not been described in cetaceans. When extraction of a maxillary tooth is necessary in cetaceans, infiltrate the tissue surrounding the diseased tooth with 2% lidocaine. Once anesthesia has been achieved, extraction is a simple process requiring a dental elevator and extractor.

Mandible and maxilla fractures can occur subsequent to trauma in cetaceans. Marine mammals frequently strand with these traumatic lesions (Oremland et al. 2010). Unlike in pinnipeds, surgical stabilization of mandibular fractures has not been attempted in cetaceans. Instead, various splints have been fashioned out of Velcro® or neoprene material, which can easily be removed to allow for feeding. Following closed reduction, splint the maxilla to the mandible. Immobilization for three weeks has provided stabilization sufficient for fracture healing (Townsend and Sips 1996).

Another indication for oral surgery in dolphins is treatment of squamous cell carcinoma (SCC). In cetaceans, oral SCC typically presents as a nonhealing ulcerated lesion on the lips, hard palate, frenulum, or tongue. The tumors are locally aggressive, but seldom metastasize. Surgical excision is one method of treatment, but wide margins must be achieved to prevent recurrence (Renner et al. 1999; Doescher et al. 2007). These tumors often have an extensive vascular supply. Use a combination of ligatures and electrosurgery to control hemorrhage during surgery. As with tooth extraction, surgical removal of SCC is typically performed under sedation and local anesthesia. Either diazepam alone or a combination of an opioid and a benzodiazepine provide good sedation. Depending on the location of the lesion, local anesthesia is typically achieved with an inferior alveolar nerve block and infiltration of the mass with 2% lidocaine. After removal of the mass, close the submucosa in two layers, and finally the mucosa if sufficient tissue is available for apposition. Often, the size or location of the mass prevent complete excision. This is often the case with SCC in the intermandibular region. It is best to perform surgery before masses are greater than 1 cm in diameter. With these smaller masses, 5 mm surgical margins have successfully prevented local recurrence of the tumor (B. Doescher, personal communication). In cases when clean margins cannot be achieved, various treatments can be successfully applied to control tumor growth either alone or as an adjunct to surgery. Options include cryosurgery, intralesional chemotherapy, systemic chemotherapy, external beam photon radiation, brachytherapy, and laser ablation (Dover 1994; McKinnie et al. 2001, 2005; McKinnie and Dover 2003; Schmitt et al. 2010). With these approaches, repeated treatments are often necessary to control growth or prevent recurrence, but animals have been successfully managed for over 10 years on these treatments (B. Doescher, personal communication).

Ocular Surgery

Cetaceans develop degenerative changes of the lens less commonly than corneal changes, i.e. only 8.89% of eyes and 10.56% of animals were found to have lens lesions (Colitz et al. 2016). This number may be an underestimation

as it is difficult to examine cetaceans under dim or dark conditions and dilation is not easily attained. If a corneal ulcer is deep enough to threaten the integrity of the eye, surgical management with a conjunctival graft may be indicated, although dolphins have excellent healing abilities including intense vascular ingrowth to remodel the corneal defect. To date, aggressive medical management, if begun immediately following identification of the ulcer or trauma, has generally been successful in avoiding perforation and retaining sight. The suggested protocol for an acutely closed eye is oral doxycycline (4–5 mg/kg PO BID) until the eye has sufficiently healed and enrofloxacin (3.5–4 mg/kg PO BID) for five days. Doxycycline will protect the corneal stromal integrity, promote epithelialization, and provide some anti-inflammatory effects (Perry et al. 1986; Chandler et al. 2007). The enrofloxacin will protect against *Pseudomonas* sp., which are the most damaging of the bacterial flora present in most aquatic environments. Enrofloxacin is only administered for a short time at a low dose to minimize the risk of photosensitivity and horizontal keratopathy, which are associated with quinolone use in dolphins (Colitz et al. 2016). If the animal is well trained and allows manipulation of the eyelids, then topical medications can be given via a soft red rubber catheter gently inserted at the lateral aspect of the eyelids as often as possible, usually two to three times daily. Once the eyelids are beginning to open, topical antibiotics to cover the opportunistic flora should be initiated and doxycycline continued. Topical ophthalmic medications are often mixed with acetylcysteine at a final concentration of 3% or 3% acetylcysteine is given first, followed by the medication two minutes later. This has been used for approximately eight years and is believed to allow better penetration of the medications through the thick mucous tear film (Colitz et al. 2016). In addition to being a mucolytic, acetylcysteine is also a glutathione precursor as well as an antioxidant (Elbini Dhouib et al. 2016).

Abdominal Surgery

Abdominal surgery is rarely performed in cetaceans. The authors are aware of three such surgeries in the past 20 years. Despite the paucity of surgeries and the unfavorable results, important lessons have been learned. Experience suggests that both MIS procedures and traditional laparotomy are viable treatment options in cetaceans given sufficiently trained surgeons, a well-planned procedure to reduce the duration of anesthesia, and a patient that is not already in a considerably compromised state.

One major indication for abdominal surgery in the cetacean is for treatment of urinary calculi. Ammonium urate nephroliths are a common problem in captive bottlenose dolphins (Venn-Watson et al. 2010a,b). Ultrasonographic evidence of nephrolithiasis has been reported in over a third of captive dolphins, but is apparently rare in wild populations (Smith et al. 2013). Clinical disease characterized by azotemia, uremia, hematuria, ureteral or urethral obstruction, and decreased renal function often develops. Few treatment options exist. Medical management with oral fluid therapy is often attempted. Stones are dissolvable only by raising urine pH above 9.0, which is not feasible (Argade et al. 2013). Retrograde urethroscopy and ureteroscopy are extremely difficult in male dolphins due to challenges associated with passing the scope past the sigmoid flexure of the penis. Laparoscopic ureterotomy to remove ureteroliths has been attempted in one bottlenose dolphin (Meegan et al. 2012). This technique allows for either stone retrieval with instruments passed through a cannula or fragmentation of stones by laser lithotripsy. Stent placement is a potential treatment option but has not been attempted. Insertion of the laparoscope at the level of the umbilicus lateral to the rectus abdominis muscle provides access to the ureters. Ultrasound imaging prior to surgery allows for the locations of kidneys and ribs to be marked on the skin of the animal. Once the laparoscope is introduced into the abdomen and the kidney and ureter of interest are identified, make a small incision in the ureter and pass a guide wire. An ureteroscope is passed over the guide wire, through the laparoscopic cannula, into the abdominal cavity, and into the ureter to identify the stone(s). The stone is then destroyed with laser lithotripsy. The ureter is sutured using an intracorporeal technique. Although the dolphin on which this procedure was performed developed cardiac arrest and was ultimately euthanized, experience indicates that laparoscopic ureterotomy and closure of the ureterotomy can be successfully performed in a dolphin.

MIS techniques can be utilized to obtain a renal biopsy. This has successfully been performed in a bottlenose dolphin (Dover et al. 1999). Once the laparoscope is advanced into the abdomen and instrument ports made, incise the renal capsule. Pinnipeds and cetaceans have reniculate or multilobed kidneys. To obtain a renal biopsy, bluntly dissect a single reniculus from the remaining renal parenchyma, place a ligature at the base for hemostasis, and excise the tissue distal to the ligature to obtain the sample (Figure 25.9).

The second major indication for abdominal surgery in cetaceans is treatment of gastrointestinal disease. The gastrointestinal tract of cetaceans is characterized by a three-chambered stomach and a long intestinal tract. The first gastric compartment, the forestomach, can be visualized with flexible endoscopy. Regular endoscopic examination of the stomach is routine at many facilities as a result of some animals' propensity for ingesting foreign bodies. The anatomy of the cetacean three-chamber stomach reduces the risk of gastric or intestinal impaction secondary to foreign body ingestion; however, foreign bodies can cause heavy metal toxicosis, erosion, ulceration, gastritis, and occasionally peritonitis. Foreign bodies can be removed from the cetacean forestomach using gastroscopy.

Gastroscopy is not useful for visualization of structures aborad to the forestomach, and diagnosis and treatment of intestinal disease is limited in cetaceans. Intestinal volvulus has been reported in both captive and wild dolphins (Briggs and Murnane 1995; Anderson and Rawson 1997;

(a)

(b)

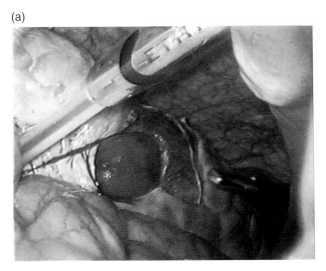
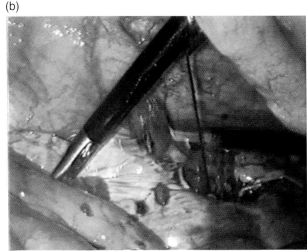

Figure 25.9 Laparoscopic renal biopsy in a bottlenose dolphin. (a) After incision of the renal capsule, a loop ligature is placed at the base of a single reniculus. (b) The reniculus is then dissected free of the surrounding parenchyma and removed through the portal incision. *Source*: Photographs provided by S. Dover, Channel Islands Marine & Wildlife Institute.

Manire 2003; Haulena et al. 2010). In captivity, animals with severe enteritis or intestinal volvulus will present with an acute onset of anorexia, abdominal pain, and vomiting. Ultrasound examination often reveals fluid-filled loops of bowel and peritoneal effusion. The condition of these animals rapidly deteriorates and euthanasia is the typical outcome. Surgical treatment is possible in some cases if the volvulus or enteritis is diagnosed early in the course of disease. To the authors' knowledge, there has been only a single attempt at surgical resection of diseased bowel in a cetacean. The animal, a Pacific white-sided dolphin (*Lagenorhynchus obliquidens*), presented with acute abdominal pain, anorexia, and lethargy, and had ultrasonographic signs of enteritis or an intestinal volvulus. The patient's condition continued to deteriorate over the course of four days at which time an open laparotomy was performed. This approach was chosen over a MIS procedure due to the degree of fluid distension of the bowel appreciated on ultrasound. The abdomen in patients with distended loops of bowel does not distend sufficiently to create a working space and the risk of bowel puncture during trocar placement is high. A ventrolateral approach was employed using ultrasound to determine the location of the incision site. While the linea alba provides the best holding layer, a lateral approach may be more appropriate if it provides better access to the distended loops of bowel in the tightly packed cetacean abdominal cavity. The incision has to be relatively large to provide adequate exposure. In the surgery performed, an 18 cm incision allowed exteriorization of most of the small intestines and access to the mesenteric root. Several important lessons were learned from the procedure. Anesthesia can be successfully performed in severely compromised animals if anesthetic time is limited (surgical time was one hour in this procedure) and an abdominal incision that is of adequate size for visualization and manipulation of tissues can be adequately closed without significant dehiscence. The dolphin was ultimately euthanized several days after surgery. While no intestinal volvulus was found during surgery, over half of the small intestine was diseased and considerable protein- and cell-rich free fluid was present in the abdomen. The devitalized sections of bowel could not be surgically removed due to the amount of tissue that would have required resection and the extension of the damage as far orad as the pylorus. The bowel was decompressed and the surgery completed with the hope that continued supportive care would allow the bowel to heal. While the animal recovered well from anesthesia and initially showed improvement of clinical signs, the condition of the bowel continued to deteriorate and euthanasia was performed.

Closure of Surgical Incisions

Closure of surgical incisions is a considerable challenge in cetaceans as with pinnipeds. Concerns over the ability to achieve a watertight closure, wound dehiscence, and potential evisceration are among the factors explaining the paucity of surgical procedures performed in cetaceans. The challenges associated with closure of the surgical incision are due to a thick, poorly vascularized blubber layer. This tissue heals slowly and excessive tension placed on the sutures can lead to underlying necrosis. If the abdominal cavity is entered, additional challenges exist. A strong holding layer for placement of sutures is absent within the abdominal wall of cetaceans, rather it seems that the holding layers are more distributed throughout the body wall. This can be a considerable obstacle for the surgeon as the tightly packed abdominal contents of cetaceans and the strong muscular activity of the rectus abdominis muscle during normal swimming place a tremendous amount of strain on an abdominal incision. There is much research that needs to be done to determine the best way to close the body wall of cetaceans.

The use of MIS techniques minimizes the risk of incision site dehiscence. Closure of cannula sites in two layers has yielded good results. For larger cannula incisions, such as those extended to remove tissue, the peritoneum, fascia, and subcutaneous tissue are closed together, followed by closure of the skin (Dover et al. 1999). For 5 mm cannula incisions, closing the peritoneum and fascia seems unnecessary, whereas 10 mm and larger incisions should include the peritoneum. The subcutaneous tissue and skin are simply closed in two separate layers.

Closing larger incisions is more challenging, but recent experience indicates that methods can be successfully applied to reduce the risk of dehiscence. Two concepts are key to preventing dehiscence – using tension-relieving patterns and closing in many layers to improve overall holding strength. These are similar concepts to those previously discussed with pinniped surgery. There have been two surgeries recently performed in cetaceans in which these techniques were successfully applied for closure of large incisions. In the Pacific white-sided dolphin undergoing laparotomy for treatment of enteritis, the transverse abdominis, internal abdominal oblique, and external abdominal oblique muscles were closed in separate layers, followed by closure of the hypodermis and the skin. The position of the diseased bowel required that an 18 cm incision be made in the location of the natural pivot point in swimming motion. Despite this additional stress, the technique for closure seemed to result in good healing up until the time of euthanasia. In a surgery performed to remove a large, multilobulated abscess in the ventral cervical region of a dolphin, a tension relieving near-far-far-near suture pattern was used to close the hypodermis (Meegan et al. 2015). Necrosis of the skin was generally averted by use of a horizontal mattress pattern with incorporated stents. Thus, recent experiences demonstrate that laparotomy or excision of large subcutaneous masses can be considered feasible techniques in cetaceans and should not be disregarded due to fear of unmanageable surgical site dehiscence.

References

Anderson, H.F. and Rawson, A.J. (1997). Volvulus with necrosis of intestine in *Stenella attenuata*. *Marine Mammal Science* 13: 147–149.

Argade, S., Smith, C.R., Shaw, T. et al. (2013). Solubility of ammonium acid urate nephroliths from bottlenose dolphins (*Tursiops truncatus*). *Journal of Zoo and Wildlife Medicine* 44: 853–858.

Barnes, J.A. and Smith, J.S. (2004). Bilateral phacofragmentation in a New Zealand fur seal (*Arctocephalus forsteri*). *Journal of Zoo and Wildlife Medicine* 35: 110–112.

Boure, L. (2005). General principles of laparoscopy. *Veterinary Clinics of North America: Food Animal Practice* 21: 227–249.

Briggs, M. and Murnane, R. (1995). Jejunal herniation and volvulus in an adult bottlenose dolphin (*Tursiops truncatus*). *Proceedings of the Internationlal Association of Aquatic Animal Medicine* 26. https://www.vin.com/apputil/content/defaultadv1.aspx?pId=11114&meta=Generic&id=3981303

Chandler, H.L., Colitz, C.M., Lu, P. et al. (2007). The role of the slug transcription factor in cell migration during corneal re-epithelialization in the dog. *Experimental Eye Research* 84: 400–411.

Colitz, C.M. (2011). When should your seal or sea lion have cataract surgery? *Proceedings of the International Marine Mammals Trainers Association* 39: 35.

Colitz, C.M., Saville, W.J., Renner, M.S. et al. (2010). Risk factors associated with cataracts and lens luxations in captive pinnipeds in the United States and the Bahamas. *Journal of the American Veterinary Medical Association* 237: 429–436.

Colitz, C.M., Bowman, M., Cole, G. et al. (2014). Surgical repair of a corneal perforation or descemetocele with concurrent lensectomy in three pinnipeds. *Proceedings of the Internationlal Association of Aquatic Animal Medicine* 45. https://www.vin.com/apputil/content/defaultadv1.aspx?pId=11397&meta=Generic&id=6251890

Colitz, C.M., Walsh, M.T., and Mcculloch, S.D. (2016). Characterization of anterior segment ophthalmologic lesions identified in free-ranging dolphins and those under human care. *Journal of Zoo and Wildlife Medicine* 47: 56–75.

Doescher, B., Sanchez, R., Lopez, A. et al. (2007). Radical surgical excision of an oral squamous cell carcinoma lesion in an Atlantic bottlenose dolphin (*Tursiops truncatus*).

Proceedings of the Internationlal Association of Aquatic Animal Medicine 38: 210–211.

Dover, S. (1994). Laser as a treatment for squamous cell carcinoma in a Pacific white sided dolphin. *Proceedings of the Internationlal Association of Aquatic Animal Medicine* 25: 145.

Dover, S., Beusse, D., Walsh, M. et al. (1999). Laparoscopic techniques for the bottlenose dolphin (*Tursiops truncatus*). *Proceedings of the Internationlal Association of Aquatic Animal Medicine* 29: 5.

Dover, S.R., Lacave, G., Salbany, A., and Roque, L. (2004). Laparoscopic ovariectomy in a grey seal (*Halichoerus grypus*) for treatment of hyperestrogenism. *Proceedings of the Internationlal Association of Aquatic Animal Medicine* 35: 51–52.

Dutton, A.G. (1991). Cataract extraction in a fur seal. *Journal of the American Veterinary Medical Association* 198: 309–311.

Elbini Dhouib, I., Jallouli, M., Annabi, A. et al. (2016). A minireview on *N*-acetylcysteine: an old drug with new approaches. *Life Sciences* 151: 359–363.

Esson, D.W., Nollens, H.H., Schmitt, T.L. et al. (2015). Aphakic phacoemulsification and automated anterior vitrectomy, and postreturn monitoring of a rehabilitated harbor seal (*Phoca vitulina richardsi*) pup. *Journal of Zoo and Wildlife Medicine* 46: 647–651.

Fauquier, D., Gulland, F., Haulena, M., and Spraker, T. (2003). Biliary adenocarcinoma in a stranded northern elephant seal (*Mirounga angustirostris*). *Journal of Wildlife Diseases* 39: 723–726.

Greene, R., Van Bonn, W.G., Dennison, S.E. et al. (2015). Laparoscopic gastropexy for correction of a hiatal hernia in a northern elephant seal (*Mirounga angustirostris*). *Journal of Zoo and Wildlife Medicine* 46: 414–416.

Hakanson, N. and Meredith, R. (1987). Conjunctival pedicle grafting in the treatment of corneal ulcers in the dog and cat. *Journal of the American Animal Hospital Association* 23: 641–648.

Hanke, F.D., Hanke, W., Scholtyssek, C., and Dehnhardt, G. (2009). Basic mechanisms in pinniped vision. *Experimental Brain Research* 199: 299–311.

Haulena, M., Gulland, F., De Cock, H., and Harman, J. (1998). The use of computerized tomography for diagnosis of osteomyelitis in pinnipeds. *Proceedings of the International Association of the Aquatic Animal Medicine* 29. https://vspn.vin.com/apputil/content/defaultadv1.aspx?pId=11119&id=3980402

Haulena, M., Huff, D., Ivancic, M. et al. (2010). Intestinal torsion secondary to chronic candidiasis caused by *Candida krusei* in a Pacific white-sided dolphin (*Lagenorhynchus obliquidens*). *Proceedings of the International Association of Aquatic Animal Medicine* 41. https://www.vin.com/apputil/content/defaultadv1.aspx?pId=11307&meta=VIN&id=4473866

Hendrickson, D.A. (2008). Complications of laparoscopic surgery. *Veterinary Clinics of North America Equine Practice* 24: 557–571, viii.

Hespel, A.M., Bernard, F., Davies, N.J. et al. (2013). Surgical repair of a tibial fracture in a two-week-old grey seal (*Halichoerus grypus*). *Veterinary and Comparative Orthopaedics and Traumatology* 26: 82–87.

Horning, M., Haulena, M., Tuomi, P.A., and Mellish, J.A. (2008). Intraperitoneal implantation of life-long telemetry transmitters in otariids. *BMC Veterinary Research* 4: 51.

Johnson, S.P., Nolan, S., and Gulland, F.M. (1998). Antimicrobial susceptibility of bacteria isolated from pinnipeds stranded in central and northern California. *Journal of Zoo and Wildlife Medicine* 29: 288–294.

Kern, T.J. and Colitz, C.M. (2013). Exotic animal ophthalmology. In: *Veterinary Ophthalmology* (eds. K.N. Gelatt, B.C. Gilger and T.J. Kern), 1782–1819. Oxford: Wiley.

Lacave, G., Maillot, A., Alerte, V., and Sampayo, J. (2009). Ultrasonic identification and laparoscopic approach of an abdominal mass in a Patagonian Sea lion (*Otaria flavescens*). *Proceedings of the International Association of Aquatic Animal Medicine* 40: 154.

Lewer, D., Gustafson, S.B., Rist, P.M., and Brown, S. (2007). Mandibular fracture repair in a harbor seal. *Journal of Veterinary Dentistry* 24: 95–98.

Lucas, R.J., Barnett, J., and Riley, P. (1999). Treatment of lesions of osteomyelitis in the hind flippers of six grey seals (*Halichoerus grypus*). *Veterinary Record* 145: 547–550.

Manire, C.A. (2003). Intestinal volvulus in two pygmy sperm whales, *Kogia breviceps*, undergoing rehabilitation. *Proceedings of the International Association of Aquatic Animal Medicine* 34. https://alpha.vin.com/apputil/content/defaultadv1.aspx?pId=11159&meta=generic&catId=29712&id=3980561

Mckinnie, C. and Dover, S. (2003). Diagnosis and treatment of lingual carcinoma in an Atlantic bottlenose dolphin (*Turisops truncatus*). *Proceedings of the International Association of Aquatic Animal Medicine* 34: 164–165.

Mckinnie, C., Dover, S., Ogilvie, G., and Bossart, G. (2001). Treatment of oral squamous cell carcinoma in an Atlantic bottlenose dolphin (*Tursiops truncatus*). *Proceedings of the International Association of Aquatic Animal Medicine* 32: 37–38.

Mckinnie, C., Dube, S., Fitzgerald, R. et al. (2005). Permanent I-125 seed implant in the treatment of squamous cell carcincoma in an Atlantic bottlenose dolphin, *Tursiops truncatus*. *Proceedings of the International Association of Aquatic Animal Medicine* 36: 71–72.

Meegan, J., Smith, C., Johnson, S. et al. (2012). Medical and surgical management of a male bottlenose dolphin (*Tursiops truncatus*) with chronic severe bilateral renal nephrolithiasis. *Proceedings of the International Association of Aquatic Animal Medicine* 43: 222–223. https://beta.vin.com/apputil/content/defaultadv1.aspx?pId=11354&catId=34822&id=5378002&ind=140&objTypeID=17

Meegan, J., Cotte, L., Ivancic, M. et al. (2015). Medical and surgical management of a chronic cervical abscess in a bottlenose dolphin (*Tursiops truncatus*). *Proceedings of the International Association of Aquatic Animal Medicine* 46.

Miller, S.N., Colitz, C.M., and Dubielzig, R.R. (2010). Anatomy of the California Sea lion globe. *Veterinary Ophthalmology* 13 (Suppl 1): 63–71.

Miller, S., Colitz, C.M., St Leger, J., and Dubielzig, R. (2013). A retrospective survey of the ocular histopathology of the pinniped eye with emphasis on corneal disease. *Veterinary Ophthalmology* 16: 119–129.

Nasisse, M.P. (1997). Principles of microsurgery. *Veterinary Clinics of North America: Small Animal Practice* 27: 987–1010.

Oremland, M.S., Allen, B.M., Clapham, P.J. et al. (2010). Mandibular fractures in short-finned pilot whales, *Globicephala macrorhynchus*. *Marine Mammal Science* 26: 1–16.

Perry, H.D., Kenyon, K.R., Lamberts, D.W. et al. (1986). Systemic tetracycline hydrochloride as adjunctive therapy in the treatment of persistent epithelial defects. *Ophthalmology* 93: 1320–1322.

Pflugfelder, S.C., Wilhelmus, K.R., Osato, M.S. et al. (1986). The autoimmune nature of aqueous tear deficiency. *Ophthalmology* 93: 1513–1517.

Read, R.A., Reynolds, W.T., Griffiths, D.J., and Reilly, J.S. (1982). Vaginal prolapse in a south australian sea lion (*Neophoca nove hollandia*). *Australian Veterinary Journal* 58: 269–271.

Renner, M.S., Ewing, R., Bossart, G.D., and Harris, D. (1999). Sublingual squamous cell carcinoma in an Atlantic bottlenose dolphin (*Tursiops truncatus*). *Journal of Zoo and Wildlife Medicine* 30: 573–576.

Ridgway, S.H., Green, R.F., and Sweeney, J.C. (1975). Mandibular anesthesia and tooth extraction in the bottlenosed dolphin. *Journal of Wildlife Diseases* 11: 415–418.

Robeck, T.R., Atkinson, S., and Brook, F. (2001). Reproduction. In: *CRC Handbook of Marine Mammal Medicine*, 2e (eds. L.A. Dierauf and F. Gulland), 193–236. Boca Raton, FL: CRC Press.

Roque, L., Salbany, A., Flanagan, C. et al. (2008). A novel approach to hypernatremia and hyperprogesteronemia through laparoscopy in a south American sea lion (*Otaria byronia*). *Proceedings of the International Association of Aquatic Animal Medicine* 39: 123–124.

Schmitt, T.L., Reidarson, T.H., St. Leger, J. et al. (2010). Medical, surgical and radiation therapy of an oral squamous cell carcinoma in an Atlantic bottlenose dolphin (*Tursiops truncatus*). *Proceedings of the International Association of Aquatic Animal Medicine* 41: 94.

Smith, C.R., Venn-Watson, S., Wells, R.S. et al. (2013). Comparison of nephrolithiasis prevalence in two bottlenose dolphin (*Tursiops truncatus*) populations. *Front Endocrinol (Lausanne)* 4: 145.

Staggs, L.A., Colitz, C.M., and Holmes-Douglas, S. (2013). The use of subconjunctival cyclosporine implants in a California Sea lion (*Zalophus californianus*) prior to cataract surgery. *Proceedings of the American Association of Zoo Veterinarians* 44.

Stern, M.E., Gao, J., Siemasko, K.F. et al. (2004). The role of the lacrimal functional unit in the pathophysiology of dry eye. *Experimental Eye Research* 78: 409–416.

Townsend, F.I. and Sips, D.G. (1996). Medical management of a maxillary fracture in a *Stenella attenuata*. *Proceedings of the International Association of Aquatic Animal Medicine* 27. https://www.vin.com/members/cms/project/defaultadv1.aspx?id=3981748&pid=11115&

Venn-Watson, S., Smith, C.R., Johnson, S. et al. (2010a). Clinical relevance of urate nephrolithiasis in bottlenose dolphins *Tursiops truncatus*. *Diseases of Aquatic Organisms* 89: 167–177.

Venn-Watson, S.K., Townsend, F.I., Daniels, R.L. et al. (2010b). Hypocitraturia in common bottlenose dolphins (*Tursiops truncatus*): assessing a potential risk factor for urate nephrolithiasis. *Comparative Medicine* 60: 149–153.

26

Megavertebrate Laparoscopy

Mark Stetter and Dean A. Hendrickson

Laparoscopy has been successfully performed in captive and free-ranging elephants and in rhinoceros (Radcliffe et al. 2000; Gage and Schmitt 2003; Hendrickson et al. 2008; Lee and Hendrickson 2008; Stetter et al. 2007; Sweet et al. 2014). The authors have attempted to use laparoscopy in hippopotamuses and feel it has great potential for use. Minimally invasive surgery (MIS) has several significant advantages in megavertebrate mammals compared to conventional surgery (Gage and Schmitt 2003; Hendrickson et al. 2008; Lee and Hendrickson 2008; Sweet et al. 2014). In addition to the common advantages of decreased pain, reduced healing time, faster return to function, and less chance for infection which are benefits seen across all species (Hendrickson 2000; Hendrickson and Wilson 1997), in megavertebrates, given their thick skin and body wall, as well as huge abdominal cavities, laparoscopy makes surgical procedures which were traditionally considered very high risk, now to be a highly viable option (Radcliffe et al. 2000; Stetter et al. 2006, 2007; Hendrickson et al. 2008; Lee and Hendrickson 2008; Sweet et al. 2014). This is especially true when working with free-ranging animals where pre- and postoperative evaluation, monitoring, and treatment may not be realistic. While veterinary clinicians can now add laparoscopy to their tool box, it is still important to note it requires specialized instrumentation and equipment along with significant procedural planning and preparation. Elephant and rhinoceros laparoscopy can be performed under general anesthesia (Klein et al. 1997; Portas et al. 2006; Stetter et al. 2006, 2007; Hendrickson et al. 2008; Lee and Hendrickson 2008) or using standing sedation in a restraint device (Radcliffe et al. 2000; Gage and Schmitt 2003; Sweet et al. 2014). The most common laparoscopic procedures are vasectomy, ovariectomy, and abdominal exploratory with the ability to biopsy various organs (spleen, liver, ovary, uterus, and epididymis).

Instrumentation

When working with adult elephants, rhinoceroses or hippopotamuses, specialized laparoscopic equipment is required (Gage and Schmitt 2003; Stetter et al. 2007; Lee and Hendrickson 2008; Sweet et al. 2014). The body wall of megavertebrates can be greater than 20 cm in depth. To reach deep into the abdomen, the laparoscope and instruments must be much larger and sturdier. Early attempts using equine laparoscopic equipment or an extended 10 mm laparoscope in elephants and rhinoceroses resulted in lens breakage (Radcliffe et al. 2000; Gage and Schmitt 2003). The primary enhancements needed are increased size and durability of the telescope, cannulae, and associated instruments. New reinforced megavertebrate laparoscopic equipment has been created by Karl Storz Veterinary Endoscopy (KSVE, Goleta, CA, USA) and is both enhanced in size and durability. It has been used in elephants, rhinoceroses, and hippopotamuses with success. There are two telescope sizes, an 80 cm × 2.8 cm and a 112 cm × 2.8 cm with associated cannulae (Lee and Hendrickson 2008; Sweet et al. 2014) (Figure 26.1). These telescopes have a working instrument port that allows specialized extended length laparoscopic instruments to be utilized (Figure 26.2). This operating laparoscope with its larger diameter than traditional telescopes has four channels. This includes the instrument channel (which reduces the number of additional cannulae required for organ manipulation), one optical channel, and two fiber optic light channels.

The most commonly used laparoscopic instruments include Babcock forceps, Senn claw graspers, and hook scissors (Figures 26.3 and 26.4). A second instrument port is often required and an extended length (50 cm) 11 mm cannula can be used (Stetter et al. 2006, 2007; Hendrickson et al. 2008; Lee and Hendrickson 2008).

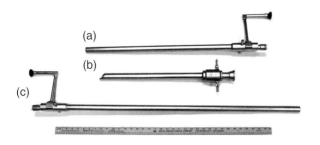

Figure 26.1 From top to bottom, the two different sizes of laparoscopes that can be used (a and c) and the cannula that can be utilized for both (b). The shorter laparoscope (80 × 2.8 cm) can be used with hippopotamuses, rhinoceroses, and smaller elephants (less than 2500 kg). The larger laparoscope (112 × 2.8 cm) is utilized on large adult male and female elephants (often exceeding 3500 kg).

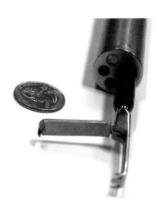

Figure 26.2 A 10 mm claw grasper placed inside of the operating channel of the laparoscope. Note that using the operating channel reduces the amount of additional cannulae that need to be placed for organ manipulation. The telescope has four channels, one 11 mm instrument channel, one optical channel, and two fiber optic light channels.

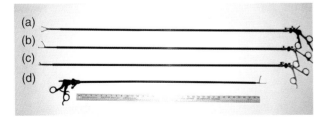

Figure 26.3 Four different laparoscopic instruments that can be used in megavertebrates. From top to bottom (a) Babcock forceps, (b) Senn claw grasper, (c) hook scissor, and (d) acute claw grasper that can be utilized with the shorter laparoscope.

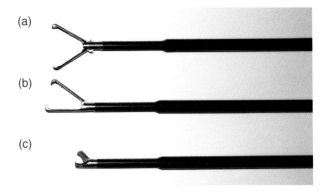

Figure 26.4 A close up of laparoscopic instruments. (a) Babcock forceps, (b) acute claw grasper, and (c) hook scissor.

When working with free-ranging megavertebrates or when electricity is scarce, a portable battery operated light source, camera, and monitor are extremely useful. The Techno Pack (KSVE) combines all these features. An equine insufflation system is often insufficient because of the large abdomen of megavertebrates (Lee and Hendrickson 2008; Sweet et al. 2014). The equine insufflation system can be used in the rhinoceroses, but it does require a long time to distend the abdomen. The authors have utilized compressed air instead of CO_2 when insufflating megavertebrates. Use a commercially available 30-ga tire inflation unit in combination with an air filter, air flow regulator, and intraabdominal pressure gauge (Lee and Hendrickson 2008; Sweet et al. 2014). While CO_2 is the preferred gas in a controlled hospital setting, compressed air is more realistic in many outdoor field settings (Ikechebelu et al. 2005) due to availability and amounts needed to insufflate very large animals. A potential disadvantages of air might be an air embolism, which has not been observed in the authors' experience.

Elephant Laparoscopy and Minimally Invasive Surgery

Visualization of abdominal organs is greatly enhanced when the megavertebrate is able to remain in a standing position (Stetter et al. 2006, 2007; Hendrickson et al. 2008; Marais et al. 2013; Sweet et al. 2014). For captive animals, a restraint chute with standing sedation and a local nerve block makes laparoscopy relatively straightforward (Gage and Schmitt 2003; Stetter and Hendrickson 2012; Sweet et al. 2014). For free-ranging elephants or animals that require general anesthesia, use a crane truck with padded

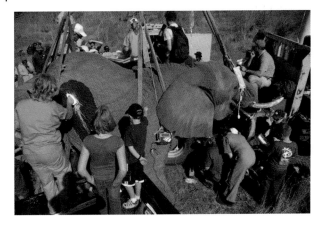

Figure 26.5 Overall view of an anesthetized free-ranging African elephant (*Loxodonta africana*) undergoing a laparoscopic vasectomy. Note the large straps around the elephant attached to the crane truck holding the anesthetized elephant in a standing position. Also note the endotracheal tube and oxygen line extending from the animal's mouth.

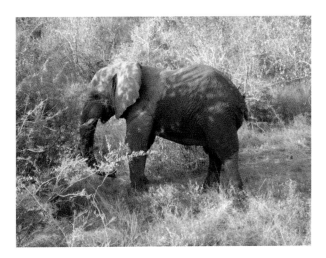

Figure 26.6 African elephant (*Loxodonta africana*) immediately after a laparoscopic vasectomy. Note the incision just cranial to the tuber coxae and the general closure used on the skin incision.

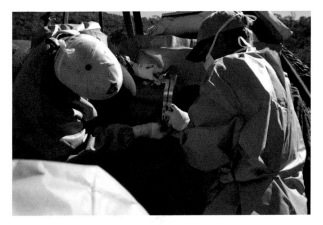

Figure 26.7 Placement of a retractor through the skin incision on an anesthetized African elephant (*Loxodonta africana*) in the left flank. The blue sterile drapes can help provide an aseptic field in the African savannah.

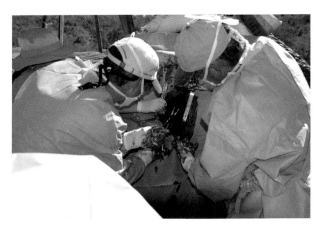

Figure 26.8 Retractors being used to separate the skin incision and visualize the underlying muscle layers which will be transected.

cargo straps to suspend the elephant. Place the straps in the inguinal and axillary folds along with additional straps around the tusks or maxilla (Stetter et al. 2006, 2007; Hendrickson et al. 2008; Marais et al. 2013; Sweet et al. 2014) (Figure 26.5). Attach the straps to the crane and lift the anesthetized elephant into a standing position. In both sedated and anesthetized elephants, the standard abdominal surgical approach is just cranial to the tuber coxae and caudal to the last rib (Stetter et al. 2006, 2007; Hendrickson et al. 2008; Marais et al. 2013; Sweet et al. 2014) (Figure 26.6). Both of these anatomic landmarks can be palpated when the animal is positioned for surgery. In some cases, the distal aspect of the ribs can be

difficult to palpate. Use spinal needles to accurately identify the location of these ribs. Make a 10 cm dorsoventral incision. In order to visualize deeper muscle and peritoneal structures, retract the skin using a modified Finochietto rib spreader (Figures 26.7 and 26.8).

Transect the abdominal oblique, internal abdominal oblique, and transverse abdominal muscles to gain access to the peritoneal cavity (Marais et al. 2013; Sweet et al. 2014). Visualize the thick fibroelastic layer covering the peritoneum and grasp it with large Vulsellum forceps. Pull it out through the skin incision, and resect portions in order to visualize the peritoneum (Figure 26.9). Unlike most mammal species, an elephant's peritoneum is not adhered to the body wall and moves freely with the fibroelastic layer (Stetter and Hendrickson 2012; Marais et al. 2013; Sweet et al. 2014). Due to this mobility, traditional laparoscopic entrance into the abdomen with a

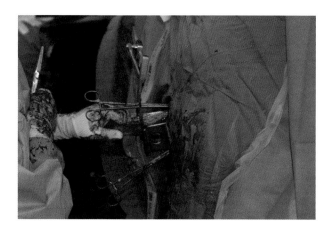

Figure 26.9 Perineum being pulled out from the incision and exteriorized so an incision can be made and a purse string placed for the cannula to enter the abdomen.

trocar is not feasible. As the fibroelastic layer is exteriorized and resected, take care to identify the underlying peritoneum. Once identified, make a 3 cm incision, place the cannula into the abdomen, and tie a purse-string suture in the peritoneum to seal it around the cannula. Begin insufflation through the cannula. The initial intraabdominal pressure is 40 mmHg. Using this approach, the testes, epididymis, kidneys, ovaries, uterus, colon, and spleen (left sided approach only) can be visualized. After initial evaluation and identification of the structure of interest, the intraabdominal pressure is reduced to between 20 and 40 mmHg. Pressures of up to 100 mmHg have been used for short periods of time.

Vasectomy

To perform a vasectomy, place a second 11 mm cannula approximately 5–10 cm cranial to the scope cannula to allow grasping devices and scissors to be inserted into the abdomen (Figure 26.10). In many cases, the cannula and sharp trocar are advanced as far as possible into the abdomen. Remove the trocar and insert hook scissors to sharply divide the peritoneum allowing the cannula to enter the peritoneal cavity. Identify the testis just caudal to the kidney and attached to the dorsum (Jones and Brosnan 1981; Foerner et al. 1994) (Figure 26.11). Visualize and follow the epididymis and ductus deferens as it leaves the caudal aspects of the testis and descends with the mesorchium into the intestinal folds (Jones and Brosnan 1981; Foerner et al. 1994). Use an acute claw grasper to hold the portion of the ductus deferens that is to be excised. Use a 10 mm hook scissor to transect the ductus on each side of the acute claw grasper. Remove this section of ductus with the laparoscope through the larger

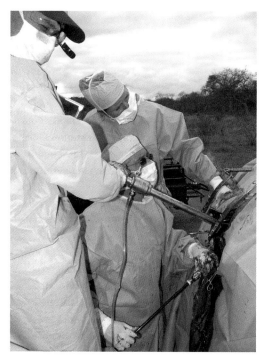

Figure 26.10 Cannula, laparoscope, and additional accessory port in use on an anesthetized African elephant (*Loxodonta africana*). Note the insufflation tubing attached to the cannula and 10 mm laparoscopic instrument being utilized in the accessory port.

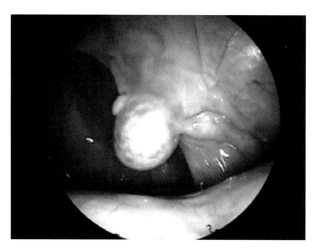

Figure 26.11 Internal image of the left hemiabdomen through the laparoscope of a male African elephant (*Loxodonta africana*) demonstrating the testis, with the epididymis and ductus deferens leaving the caudal aspect.

cannula. Histopathology is commonly performed to confirm the excised tissue is the ductus. Suturing or any other type of closure over the transection sites has not been required and there are no reports of recanalization (Hendrickson et al. 2008; Stetter and Hendrickson 2012; Marais et al. 2013; Sweet et al. 2014).

Functional Ovariectomy

A "functional ovariectomy" involves ligation of the vessels supplying the ovary resulting in atrophy of the ovary, but the ovary remains in place. The authors use a surgical stainless steel wire looped around the ovarian pedicle and then twist the wire using an attachment to an electric drill. A 30×0.8 cm stainless steel rod with two holes in its terminal end is utilized to facilitate twisting the wire. The proximal end of the rod is placed in the drill and once the wire loop has been placed around the ovarian pedicle, the two ends are placed through the holes at the end of the rod. This allows the rod to spin in the abdomen while the drill remains outside the body cavity. The laparoscope is used to visualize the twisting wire around the pedicle. Use two wire ligations at the base of each ovary. Leave the ovary itself in place to atrophy following ligation of the vascular supply. Four "functional ovariectomies" have been performed using this method. In each case, the animals were evaluated visually for 6 months after surgery and immobilized 12 months after surgery for a thorough evaluation. Evaluation included a physical examination, abdominal ultrasound, complete blood count (CBC), biochemical profile, and hormone profile. Every animal showed complete healing and atrophy of the ovaries.

Body Wall Closure

Close the fibroelastic peritoneum with a size 0 absorbable suture in a simple continuous pattern. Close the internal abdominal oblique muscle and external abdominal oblique muscle and fascia, independently, with a simple continuous pattern, size 0 or 1 absorbable suture material. Close the skin incisions with size 5 stainless steel in a horizontal mattress pattern.

Rhinoceros Laparoscopy

Laparoscopy in rhinoceroses has similar challenges, although rhinoceros skin is generally thicker than that of African elephants (Radcliffe et al. 2000). Surgery performed in standing animals allows better visualization than in laterally recumbent animals but requires the animal be conditioned to routine handling and tractable for sedation and standing surgery. Anatomically, in white rhinoceroses, the skin over the ribs is adhered to the ribs causing a depression in the skin (Radcliffe et al. 2000) (Figure 26.12). The fibroelastic tissue associated with the peritoneum is similar but much less extensive than in elephants and much more adhered to the body wall. At the

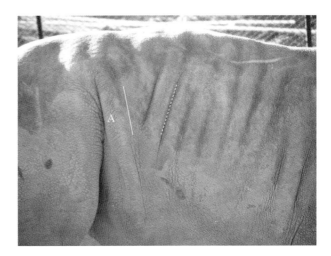

Figure 26.12 Right side of a Southern white rhinoceros (*Ceratotherium simum*). A, flank skin fold, Solid Line, Preskin fold incision, Dotted Line, incision for rib resection.

time of this writing, the authors have performed laterally recumbent laparoscopy in one black and two white rhinoceroses and sedated standing laparoscopy on one white rhinoceros. The uterus and ovaries are readily visible in standing rhinoceroses and are approachable in laterally recumbent animals (Klein et al. 1997; Radcliffe et al. 2000; Portas et al. 2006). Depending on the age and reproductive status of the animal, the reproductive structures are more or less pendulous making observation in laterally recumbent animals more or less difficult, respectively. Gas distention of the bowel occurs quickly because it is often difficult to withhold feed prior to surgery, so surgery should be started as quickly as possible after anesthesia is induced in laterally recumbent animals. Surgical procedures have included uterine biopsy, liver biopsy, and ovariectomy.

The paralumbar fossa provides the best access to the urogenital tract. Access to the liver requires a more cranial approach, either between or just ventral to the ribs. In some cases, a partial rib resection may be necessary to gain access to the dorsal abdomen. A transvaginal approach has also been described. Perform standing surgery with the animal sedated and held in a location allowing only limited movement. Sedate the animal with either butorphanol and detomidine or butorphanol and azaperone (Klein et al. 1997; Radcliffe et al. 2000; Valverde et al. 2010). The animal can also be fully anesthetized and placed in a standing position using a sling (Portas et al. 2006).

Aseptically prepare and drape the appropriate flank for surgery allowing access to the caudal ribs, the paralumbar fossa, and the tuber coxae. Infiltrate the surgical site with local anesthetic (Figure 26.12). Make the incisions just cranial to the flank skin fold or, alternatively, perform a partial caudal rib resection. Unlike minimally invasive surgical approaches in other animals where a stab incision the diameter of the cannula can be used, make a 10 cm incision through the skin and external abdominal oblique fascia and muscle, the internal abdominal oblique muscle, and the transverse abdominal muscle. Grasp the fibroelastic peritoneum with Vulsellum forceps and make a 1 cm incision through the peritoneum. Advance the cannula, without an obturator, place a purse string suture through the peritoneum and tighten it around the cannula. Insufflate the abdomen to the least amount of pressure that will allow observation of the areas of interest. Similar to the elephant, initial intraabdominal pressures will be set at 40 mmHg and reduced to 20 mmHg as soon as the exploration is completed.

If a rib resection is performed, confirm the location of the rib first using spinal needles. Make a 10 cm incision over the last rib through the skin, overlying muscle, and periosteum. Elevate the periosteum from around the rib and use a Gigli wire or bone saw to transect the rib at the limits of the incision. Grasp the fibroelastic peritoneum as previously described, make a 1 cm incision through the peritoneum, place the laparoscopic cannula and secure the peritoneum around the cannula with a purse string suture. Insufflate the abdomen as previously described. The accessory cannula(e) can be placed as in other species with a stab incision the size appropriate for the cannula. The accessory cannula can be placed ventral or caudal to the telescope cannula (Figure 26.13). Insert the accessory cannula with a sharp obturator as far as possible, and then replace with a hook scissors to transect the peritoneum under direct visualization with the scope camera. It is easier to use an operating telescope through one cannula and a single accessory cannula than to use a standard telescope with two accessory cannulas.

Ovariectomy

Ovariectomy can be performed in a manner similar to what has been described in horses. Use a vessel-sealing device (LigaSure™, Medtronic, Minneapolis, MN) to seal and transect the ovarian pedicle. Alternatively, use a ligating loop to ligate the ovarian pedicle and endoscopic scissors to transect the ligated pedicle. The ovary is removed through the telescope portal. The uterine horns and ovaries are more easily observed in standing animals (Figure 26.14).

Ovariectomy in lateral recumbency is performed under general anesthesia. Only one side of the abdomen will be accessible at a time when the animal is placed in lateral recumbency (Figure 26.13). After the procedure is completed on one side, turn the animal into the opposite recumbency and repeat the procedure on the contralateral side. If possible, the region of interest should be in the uppermost position. The surgical procedures are as described for the standing flank approach.

Close the body wall in multiple layers as described for elephants.

Hippopotamus Laparoscopy

Hippopotamuses rarely undergo major surgical procedures (Flach et al. 1998; Walzer et al. 2014). The few documented procedures have included cesarean section, ovariectomy in a juvenile, and castration of adult animals. Laparoscopic procedures in hippopotamuses have not been published, but they have been conducted on cadavers and, with the advances made with laparoscopy in elephants and rhinoceros, it is

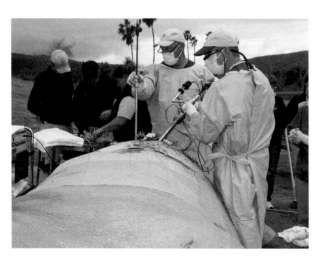

Figure 26.13 Left flank laparoscopic ovariectomy in a Southern white rhinoceros (*Ceratotherium simum*) in the field.

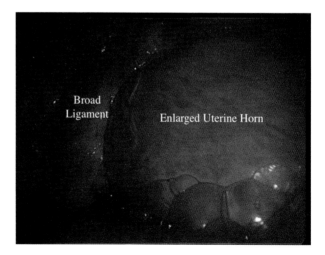

Figure 26.14 Intraabdominal image of the right hemiabdomen in a standing female Southern white rhinoceros (*Ceratotherium simum*).

anticipated that hippopotamus laparoscopic procedures are likely in the near future.

Hippopotamuses can be one of the most difficult animals to anesthetize (Flach et al. 1998; Walzer et al. 2014) and the clinician should ensure they are well educated before proceeding. One of the major values of developing these procedures in both males and females is the significant need for population management in both captive and free-ranging populations. In an adult male hippopotamus cadaver, a laparoscopic vasectomy has been performed by the authors. Place the animal in dorsal recumbency, attach ropes to the rear legs, and use a hoist to elevate the pelvic abdominal cavity above the rest of the body. The specialized megavertebrate laparoscopic equipment used in elephants and rhinoceroses is appropriate for

hippopotamuses. Make an open surgical approach into the abdomen on the ventral midline at the umbilicus. Place a purse string suture through the peritoneum and around the cannula. Insufflate the abdomen to get good visualization of the abdominal organs. Identify the vas deferens entering the inguinal canal. Place a second 11 mm cannula into the abdomen to allow two instruments for the vasectomy. Grasp the vas deferens with a Senn claw grasper and transect it on each side using 10 mm hook scissors. In females, ovariectomy has been described using an open approach (Hernandez et al. 2015), and it is anticipated that converting this procedure to a laparoscopic procedure would reduce the surgical time and greatly reduce the size of the incision. The body wall is closed as described for elephants.

References

Flach, E., Furrokh, I., Thornton, S.M. et al. (1998). Caesarean section in a pygmy hippopotamus (*Choeropsis liberiensis*) and the management of the wound. *Veterinary Record* 143: 611–613.

Foerner, J.J., Houck, R.I., Copeland, J.F. et al. (1994). Surgical castration of the elephant (*Elephas maximus* and *Loxodonta africana*). *Journal of Zoo and Wildlife Medicine* 25: 355–359.

Gage, L.J. and Schmitt, D. (2003). Dystocia in an African elephant (*Loxodonta africana*). *Proceedings of the American Association of Zoo Veterinarians Annual Meeting*, p. 88.

Hendrickson, D.A. (2000). History and instrumentation of laparoscopic surgery. *Veterinary Clinics of North America Equine Practice* 16: 233–250.

Hendrickson, D.A. and Wilson, D.G. (1997). Laparoscopic cryptorchid castration in standing horses. *Veterinary Surgery* 26: 335–339.

Hendrickson, D.A., Stetter, M., and Zuba, J.R. (2008). Development of a laparoscopic approach for vasectomies in free-ranging African elephants. *Proceedings of the American College of Veterinary Surgeons Annual Symposium*. pp. 335–339.

Hernandez, C., Ruiz, I., Villegas, J.P., and Duque, D.L. (2015). Ovariectomy in a common hippopotamus (*Hippopotamus amphibius*). *Journal of Zoo and Wildlife Medicine* 46: 374–377.

Ikechebelu, J.I., Obi, R.A., Udigwe, G.O. et al. (2005). Comparison of carbon dioxide and room air pneumoperitoneum for day-case diagnostic laparoscopy. *Journal of Obstetrics and Gynaecology* 25: 172–173.

Jones, R.C. and Brosnan, M.F. (1981). Studies of the deferent ducts from the testis of the African elephant (*Loxodonta*

africana) I. Structural differentiation. *Journal of Anatomy* 132: 371–386.

Klein, L.V., Cook, R.A., Calle, P.P et al. (1997). Etorphine-isoflurane-O$_2$ anesthesia for ovariohysterectomy in an Indian rhinoceros (*Rhinoceros unicornis*). *Proceedings of the American Association of Zoo Veterinarians Annual Meeting*, pp. 127–130.

Lee, M. and Hendrickson, D.A. (2008). A review of equine standing laparoscopic ovariectomy. *Journal of Equine Veterinary Science* 28: 105–111.

Marais, H., Hendrickson, D.A., Stetter, M. et al. (2013). Laparoscopic vasectomy in African savannah elephant (*Loxodonta africana*); surgical, technique, and results. *Journal of Zoo and Wildlife Medicine* 44: 18–20.

Portas, T.J., Hermes, R., Bryant, B.R. et al. (2006). Anesthesia and use of a sling system to facilitate transvaginal laparoscopy in a black rhinoceros (*Diceros bicornis minor*). *Journal of Zoo and Wildlife Medicine* 37: 202–205.

Radcliffe, R.M., Hendrickson, D.A., Richardson, G.L. et al. (2000). Standing laparoscopic-guided uterine biopsy in a southern white rhinoceros (*Ceratotherium simum simum*). *Journal of Zoo and Wildlife Medicine* 31: 201–207.

Stetter, M. and Hendrickson, D.A. (2012). Laparoscopic surgery in the elephant and rhinoceros. *Journal of Zoo and Wild Animal Medicine* 68: 524–530.

Stetter, M., Hendrickson, D.A., Zuba, J.R. et al. (2006). Laparoscopic vasectomy as a potential population control method in free ranging African elephants (*Loxodonta africana*). *Proceedings of the International Elephant Conservation and Research Symposium*, p. 177.

Stetter, M., Hendrickson, D.A., Zuba, J.R. et al. (2007). Laparoscopic vasectomy in free ranging African elephants (*Loxodonta africana*). *Proceedings of the American Association of Zoo Veterinarians Annual Meeting*, pp. 185–188.

Sweet, J., Hendrickson, D.A., Stetter, M. et al. (2014). Exploratory rigid laparoscopy in African elephant (*Loxodonta africana*). *Journal of Zoo and Wildlife Medicine* 45: 941–946.

Valverde, A., Crawshaw, G.J., Cribb, N. et al. (2010). Anesthetic management of a white rhinoceros (*Ceratotherium simum*) undergoing an emergency exploratory celiotomy for colic. *Veterinary Anaesthesia and Analgesia* 37: 280–285.

Walzer, C., Petit, T. et al. (2014). Surgical castration of the male common hippopotamus (*Hippopotamus amphibious*). *Theriogenology* 81: 514–518.

27

Zoo Animal Surgery
Geoffrey W. Pye

General Considerations

Zoo animal surgery is a very broad topic that cannot be comprehensively covered in a single chapter. Invertebrates, fish, amphibians, reptiles, birds, small mammals, primates, marine mammals, and megavertebrates are already well covered in this book. Rather than trying to cover all of the $n = 1$ surgeries in the zoo medicine literature, this chapter, like Chapter 1, will cover general principles with examples applicable to zoo species and some of the more common surgeries performed that are not covered in previous chapters.

Partnerships

There is tremendous value in creating partnerships with specialty surgeons from both veterinary and human medicine. Solid surgical principles can be extrapolated in most circumstances, especially under the guidance of a zoo veterinarians, who often have the luxury of knowing what doesn't work. This pairing of surgical skills with the knowledge and experience, particularly from those past failures (Pye 2007), with zoo animals improves outcomes for patients. Good examples include using a veterinary dentist for a tooth extraction in a common hippo (*Hippopotamus amphibius*), human cardiovascular surgeons for primate cardiac disorders (Greenberg et al. 1999; Robbins et al. 2009), and board certified veterinary surgeons for a nasal mass removal in a koala (*Phascolarctos cinereus*) (Bercier et al. 2012) and diaphragmatic herniorrhaphy in a cheetah (*Acinonyx jubatus*) (Kimber et al. 2001). A minimally invasive surgeon can perform an ovariohysterectomy in a primate in 15 minutes with minimally invasive techniques that may take a zoo veterinarian more than twice as long through a much larger laparotomy. The frequency of performing particular surgeries can highly influence the time taken and the trauma caused, which contribute to the success of the surgery. Obviously, a specialist surgeon who performs a particular surgery on a regular basis is likely to be more successful than a zoo veterinarian who may only perform the surgery once or twice in their career.

Diversity

There is enormous diversity both across and within taxa, which requires a wide range of size of surgical equipment. Laparoscopic equipment is one example where a small frog could reside within an elephant laparoscopic cannula, whereas the scope for the frog would immediately bend in any attempt to place it in an elephant. Carrying this variety of equipment is very expensive and its use may be rare. It highlights another reason for partnerships where specialists are more likely to have the correct equipment as they use it on a regular basis. For example, elephant dental specialists may perform 8–10 molar or tusk extractions a year, whereas an experienced zoo veterinarian may only participate in one or two over a 20 years period. The former have likely developed specialized equipment and experience for the procedures where the latter will struggle to find the appropriate tools or skill set.

The diversity also requires extrapolation of techniques and the use of nonstandard equipment and supplies. Particularly in fracture stabilization, there is a need to adapt and "MacGyver" in order to create, for example, an external skeletal fixator as commercially available implants do not conform across all taxa.

Forces

The forces that can be generated by some zoo animals are tremendous, particularly in the limbs. Orthopedic stabilizations in zoo animals can require significantly more hardware than may be expected by a veterinary or human orthopedic surgeon without zoo animal experience (Figure 27.1a–e). In order to avoid failure, doubling up on the amount or types of hardware (e.g. stacked bone plates

(a)

(b)

(c)

(d)

(e)

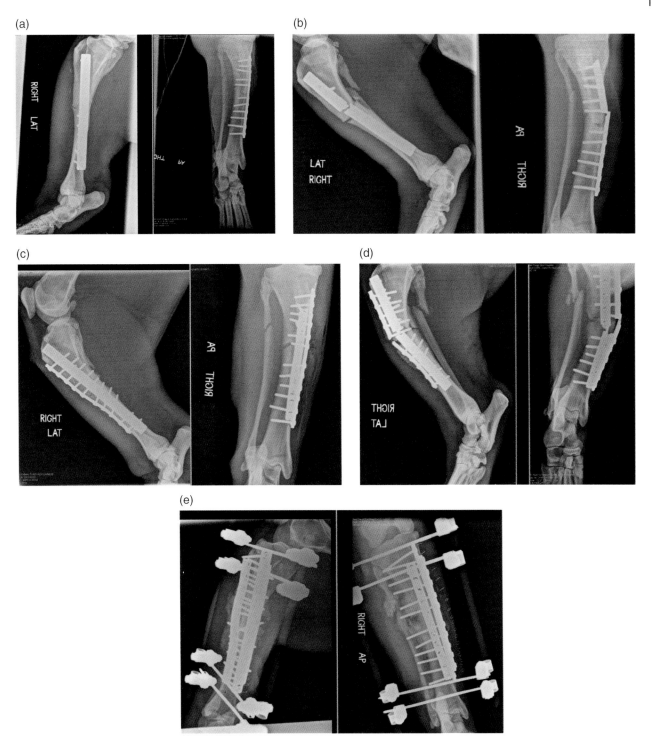

Figure 27.1 An adult 120 kg Malayan tiger, *Panthera tigris jacksoni*, with a fractured right tibia and fibula. Initially, the tibia fracture was stabilized using a 12 hole 4.5 mm bone plate placed on the medial aspect (a). The bone plate failed a week later (b). The leg was restabilized using two 4.5 mm plates placed on the cranial and lateral aspects (c). Both plates failed two weeks later (d). An external skeletal fixator was placed and then a month later, this was adjusted and augmented by double stacking 4.5 mm plates where they had been previously placed singly (e). The fracture healed over the next three months.

or an external skeletal fixator in addition to bone plates) may be necessary to counter the tremendous forces on an orthopedic stabilization. Forces can also be greater on surgical wounds, hence, the encouragement to use minimal invasive surgical techniques as described in Chapters 15 and 26. Additional supporting sutures with stents may be required to reduce tension when closing incisions. Using neuroleptics or other behavior modifying drugs can help keep fractious animals calmer during the healing process which may lower the forces exerted on hardware and wounds improving success.

Postoperative Management

As in other animals, minimizing tissue irritation during aseptic surgical site preparation, minimizing tissue trauma through good technique, and the use of multimodal preemptive analgesia will improve outcomes postoperatively. Limiting exercise, maintaining external devices (e.g. external skeletal fixators, chest tubes, and wound dressings), and providing postsurgical treatments and therapies can be extremely challenging compared to working with domestic animals and are often avoided. An example of this is the removal of a chest mass in an otter (Pye 2010) where a thoracotomy was used to remove a thymoma. Typically, a thoracostomy tube would be maintained postoperatively to have control over the chest cavity during recovery. In the otter, the thoracotomy was closed without long-term maintenance of a thoracostomy tube. Many zoo animals will not tolerate extraneous materials, even things seemingly innocuous such as cyanoacrylate tissue adhesive. Buried suturing techniques are encouraged. Using distractors like nail polish on fingernails, toenails, or tufts of fur, or pieces of adhesive tape on fur can help prevent self-mutilation. Safety is an important consideration, for it may not be safe to share the same space with the animal to monitor it or provide treatments (e.g. tiger and rhino).

Surgeries

Contraception

Melengestrol Acetate Implants (MGA)

Melengestrol Acetate Implants (MGA) are commonly used for contraception in zoo animals. Implant them subcutaneously at a site that is difficult for the animal to reach and remove; interscapular is the most common site. These implants are custom-made for the correct dosing of the animal and come in a variety of diameters and lengths. Make a small skin incision in the interscapular region 60% longer than the diameter of the implant. Using blunt dissection,

tunnel caudally to create a pocket 20% longer than the length and 5% wider than the diameter of the implant. With the pocket sufficiently enlarged, slide the implant under the skin with minimal force; ideally with the entire implant remote to the skin incision. Close the subcutaneous tissues and then the skin using an intradermal pattern in species where conspecifics may pick at the wound or if the individual is dexterous enough to reach the interscapular area. Implants may migrate and be extruded. Placing a passive integrated transponder tag into the implant can help confirm its presence at a later date, though this may affect drug elution. Alternatively, place an encircling orthopedic wire snugly around or place a wire down the center of the implant so it is easily visible on radiographs. The twisted ends of the encircling wire will reduce migration of the implant. MGA implants typically provide contraception for approximately two years and are removed if being replaced or if a return to reproduction is wanted.

Deslorelin Implants

Deslorelin implants are injected subcutaneously to provide contraception in a number of zoo species for periods of 6 or 12 months of contraception. In some species, the length of contraception varies, so it is recommended to remove implants if a return to reproduction is needed after these periods. An injectable delivery system enables easy placement subcutaneously. Removal can be challenging so it is good to place the implants in an area that is readily accessible for future removal (e.g. superficial subcutaneous inner upper arm or thigh). Locate the implant by palpation taking care to not crush it. After aseptic preparation, make a stab incision through the skin and subcutaneous tissues over one end of the implant. Grasp the end of the implant carefully with forceps and gently slide it out. Avoid disrupting the implant's integrity. The implants are not designed for removal and can break up if not handled carefully. If it breaks, enlarge the incision and try to confirm removal of all of the pieces. After removal, flush the tissues and close in a routine manner.

Vasectomy

For permanent contraception where social interaction needs to be maintained, vasectomy is the appropriate choice. Palpate the spermatic cord immediately proximal to the scrotum in the inguinal region. Make a skin incision directly over the cord. Incise the tunic and then isolate the vas deferens which will have a glossy white, transversely-striated appearance. Place two hemostatic clips or suture ligatures approximately 1–2 cm apart and then remove the piece of vas deferens between. To reduce the risk of recanalization, leave the proximal segment of the vas deferens within the tunic and exteriorize the distal segment as the tunic is closed with either a simple continuous or cruciate sutures. Alternatively, cauterize the cut ends of the vas deferens. Close the subcutaneous tissues followed by the skin. Submit the removed tissue for histopathologic confirmation as removal of the wrong tissue is known to occur. Postvasectomy, it may take 8–12 weeks for sterility to occur.

Epididymectomy in Hoof Stock

Epididymectomy is an alternative to vasectomy for sterilization of hoof stock (Hendrickson 2007). A common complication of vasectomy is failure to prevent reproduction usually because the surgeon did not actually excise a segment of the ductus. The tail of the epididymis (TOE) is very easy to identify and excise assuring sterilization of the patient.

Pull both testes distally into the scrotum and identify the epididymis (Figure 27.2). Make an incision over the TOE through the skin and vaginal tunic exposing the TOE. Dissect the TOE from the testis by detaching the proper ligament of the testis. Once the TOE is free from the testis, identify the ductus deferens and place a clamp across it, then place a ligature proximal to the clamp. Transect the ductus proximal to the clamp. Identify the body of the epididymis and place a clamp across it. Place a ligature proximal to the clamp and ligate the body of the epididymis. Transect proximal to the clamp and remove the entire TOE. Because the tunic communicates with the abdominal cavity, suture the incision in the tunic closed with a simple continuous pattern of an absorbable material leaving

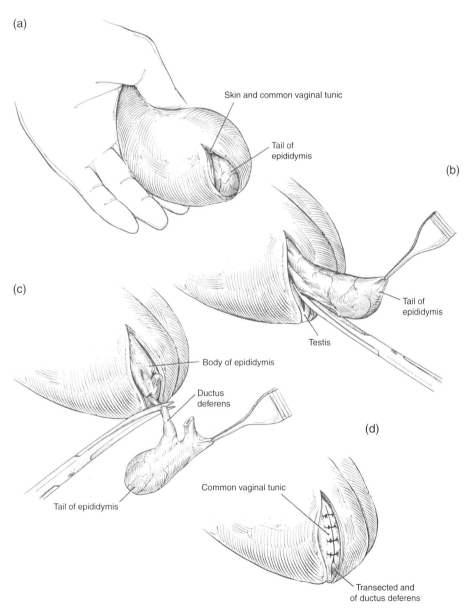

(a)

Skin and common vaginal tunic

Tail of epididymis

(b)

Tail of epididymis

Testis

(c)

Body of epididymis

Ductus deferens

Tail of epididymis

(d)

Common vaginal tunic

Transected and of ductus deferens

Figure 27.2 Epididymectomy in a bull. *Source:* Republished with permission from Hendrickson (2007).

the transected end of the ductus outside the tunic. Leave the ductus outside the tunic in an effort to make it more difficult for the end of the ductus to connect to the end of the body of the epididymis, and then recanalize, reestablishing patency. This has never been reported and seems very unlikely to occur. Suture the incision in the scrotum with a rapidly absorbable material so suture removal is not required.

Castration in Big Cats

Castration in big cats is performed in a manner similar to an open castration of a dog. After aseptic preparation of the prescrotal surgical site, apply gentle pressure to the scrotum to move the testes into a rostral, prescrotal position. Make a midline incision through the skin. With digital pressure, move the testis in the tunic to the skin incision and then incise the tunic. Exteriorize the testis and bluntly, digitally dissect the tunic from the epididymis by tearing the ligament of the TOE. Use a gauze square for grip and traction if needed to peel the tunic away from the epididymis. Ligate the vas deferens and vascular cord with suture or hemostatic clips. It is not necessary to close the tunic. Close the subcutaneous and skin layers in a routine manner; the use of subcuticular sutures is recommended. Alternatively, perform the castration like a domestic cat making skin incisions through the scrotum, and then perform either an open or closed castration. Leave the skin incisions open (and the tunic, if an open technique was used).

Castration in Large Rodents

Often, there is free movement of the testes in this taxon between the scrotum and abdomen. Use gentle abdominal pressure (manually or by using gravity through tilting the surgical table placing the patient in the reverse Trendelenburg position) to keep the testes in the scrotal area for a scrotal approach. If keeping the testes in the scrotal region proves challenging, use a caudal midline abdominal approach. Once in the abdomen, reflect the bladder caudally to expose its dorsal aspect. Identify the ductus deferentia as they enter the urethra in the same position as the uterine body of a female. Pull on each ductus to retrieve the ipsilateral testis (see Chapter 19). Use standard techniques for removal of the testes and closure of the scrotal or abdominal incisions.

Ovariectomy and Ovariohysterectomy in Big Cats

Ovariectomy and ovariohysterectomy in big cats are best performed laparoscopically to avoid large abdominal incisions that may dehisce due to tension associated with the weight of the abdominal contents and the activity of the animal. If a laparotomy is performed, ensure the body wall incision is made through the linea alba to aid a secure closure. Perform the ovariectomy or ovariohysterectomy in a similar manner to the domestic cat. Transfixing ligatures will aid in securing the ovarian vessels and uterine stump. Recognize the additional tension on the closure compared to a domestic cat and ensure the appropriately sized suture, needle, and suture pattern is used (e.g. 0 or 1 polydioxanone, simple interrupted, taper needle). Restrict exercise postsurgery for 10 days if possible. The author has used oral amitriptyline and diazepam at doses similar to domestic pets to reduce anxiety and encourage rest.

Miscellaneous

Onychectomy (Declaw) in Exotic Felids

The editors of this book and the American Veterinary Medical Association are opposed to declawing captive exotic and other wild indigenous cats for nonmedical reasons due to the long-term suffering of the cats that have undergone this procedure. Consequently, we do not provide detailed descriptions of the surgical techniques and only provide guidance on reconstructive surgery to benefit the cats.

Declawing leads to significant gait disturbances and bone deformities in exotic felids (Conrad et al. 2002). Three methods for declawing big cats have been described: removal of the entire third phalanx, removal of most of the third phalanx but leaving the deep digital flexor attached to the remainder of the flexor tubercle, and removal of the nail-forming tissue on the ungula crest leaving the flexor and extensor tendons attached. All three techniques are associated with adverse crippling sequelae as described below (Conrad et al. 2002). While removal of the entire third phalanx minimizes the risk of infection and trauma caused by a retained bone fragment, the disruption of the flexor and extensor tendons and the abnormal position of the second phalanx will cause digital pad pathology and loss of flexor and extensor function. With preservation of the digital flexor tendon, the paw can flex, but due to the lack of counteraction from the extensor tendon, the remaining fragment of the third phalanx is pulled under the second phalanx. As well as digital pad pathology, the third phalanx fragment acts like a "pebble in a shoe" under the second phalanx. The anatomy of the third phalanx makes it impossible to preserve the flexor and extensor tendons while removing all of the nail-generating tissue and consequently nail regrowth and abscess formation occurs.

Conrad et al. (2002), performed reparative surgery on 14 exotic cats (8 cougars, 3 tigers, 2 leopards, and 1 lion) that had been declawed previously and is described thus: aseptically prepare the paws to the carpus and then apply an

Esmarch bandage tourniquet from the distal paw to the antebrachium to minimize hemorrhage during the surgery. Make a skin incision approximately 3 cm long from the dorsal aspect of the paw to the palmar aspect at the site of the former nail taking care to avoid the pad. With blunt dissection, expose any remaining third phalanx and grasp it with pointed reduction forceps to mobilize and exteriorize the deep digital flexor tendon. Attach the remaining digital flexor tendon dorsally to the extensor tendon using a cruciate suture (polydioxanone 0). Remove the remainder of the third phalanx. If the extensor tendon cannot be identified, attach the flexor tendon to any remaining tissue in the extensor groove of the second phalanx. Using rongeurs, remove any cartilage remaining on the distal end of the second phalanx before securing the suture. Tighten the suture in order to position the pad closer to its proper anatomic position relative to the second phalanx. Close the skin incision with tissue adhesive. Place pressure bandages over the paws. Tabs on the bandages will allow easy removal. In the 14 animals described by Conrad et al. (2002), improvements in gait, speed over distance, and ability to jump and climb were seen following the reconstructive surgery. Prior to surgery, paws were paddle-like, commonly referred to as "floppy paws," whereas after reparative surgery, the cats were able to stand digitigrade and had improved ability to flex and extend their front paws.

Defanging Primates and Carnivores

The editors of this book and the American Veterinary Medical Association are opposed to removal or reduction of healthy teeth in nonhuman primates and carnivores, except when required for medical treatment or approved scientific research. Animals may still cause severe injury with any remaining teeth and this approach does not address the cause of the behavior. Removal or reduction of teeth for nonmedical reasons may also create oral pathology. To minimize injury, recommended alternatives to dental surgery include behavioral assessment and modification, environmental enrichment, changes in group composition and improved animal housing and handling techniques.

Tail Removal in Primates

The editors of this book and the American Veterinary Medical Association are opposed to the surgical removal of the tails of prehensile-tailed monkeys. The tail of this type of monkey serves as an essential appendage and veterinarians should not remove it either for cosmetic purposes or for the owner's convenience.

References

Bercier, M., Wynne, J., Klause, S. et al. (2012). Nasal mass removal in the koala (*Phascolarctos cinereus*). *Journal of Zoo and Wildlife Medicine* 43: 898–908.

Conrad, J., Wendelburg, K., Santinelli, S. et al. (2002). Deleterious effects of onychectomy (declawing) in exotic felids and a reparative surgical technique: a preliminary report. *Proceedings of the American Association of Zoo Veterinarians,* Milwaukee, WI, pp. 16–20.

Greenberg, M.J., Janssen, D.L., Jamieson, S.W. et al. (1999). Surgical repair of an atrial spetal defect in a juvenile Sumatran orang-utan (*Pongo pygmaeus sumatraensis*). *Journal of Zoo and Wildlife Medicine* 30: 256–261.

Hendrickson, D.A. (2007). Surgical techniques for teaser bull preparation. In: *Techniques in Large Animal Surgery*, 3e (ed. D.A. Hendrickson), 252–256. Ames, IO: Blackwell Publishing Professional.

Kimber, K., Pye, G.W., Dennis, P.M. et al. (2001). Diaphragmatic hernias in cheetah (*Acinonyx jubatus*). *Proceedings of the Annual Conference of the American Association of Zoo Veterinarians*, Orlando, FL, p. 151.

Pye, G.W. (2007). Intestinal entrapment in the pulmonary ostium following castration in a juvenile ostrich (*Struthio camelus*). *Journal of Avian Medicine and Surgery* 21: 290–293.

Pye, G.W. (2010). Preventive medicine success – thymoma removal in a spot-necked otter (*Lutra maculicollis*). *Journal of Zoo and Wildlife Medicine* 41: 732–734.

Robbins, P.K., Pye, G.W., Sutherland-Smith, M. et al. (2009). Successful transabdominal subxyphoid pericardiostomy to relieve chronic pericardial effusion in a Sumatran orang-utan (*Pongo abelli*). *Journal of Zoo and Wildlife Medicine* 40: 564–567.

28

Surgical Oncology in Exotics

Elizabeth A. Maxwell

Principles of Surgical Oncology and Application to Exotics

Surgical recommendations in most exotic species call for "adequate" margins with no measurement described specific to the species. In dogs, a 2–3 cm lateral margin and 1 facial plane deep is recommended for tumors that are locally invasive with high recurrence rates, and 1 cm margins for discrete tumors with low recurrence rates (Figure 28.1) (Kuntz et al. 1997; Simpson et al. 2004; Prpich et al. 2014). In cats with injection site sarcomas, 5 cm margins and 2 fascial planes deep are recommended (Phelps et al. 2011). Surgical doses described by Enneking for musculoskeletal tumor excision include intracapsular (debulking), marginal, wide, and radical (Enneking et al. 2003). Extrapolating from current knowledge of tumor biology, tumors that are locally invasive or have microscopic local extension require wide surgical margins and a deep resection (at least 1 fascial plane) to achieve complete (clean) margins. Alternatively, a planned marginal resection may be performed, understanding that histologic margins will be incomplete (dirty) and adjunctive therapies should be employed postoperatively. Tumors that are not considered locally invasive or are unlikely to have local microscopic infiltration can be controlled with a more conservative (marginal) resection.

It can be challenging to adapt these general guidelines for smaller patients; however, anatomic limitations can be addressed by utilizing multimodal treatment options and knowledge of tumor type, tumor behavior, anatomic location, and surrounding tissues. It can be said that the field of surgical oncology involves a thorough understanding of not just oncologic surgery, but also of adjunctive treatment methods that may be employed as part of the overall treatment plan for a patient.

Birds

Neoplastic diseases are commonly encountered in avian species, particularly in psittacines. While review articles of neoplasia in companion birds exist, clinical case numbers are low, and there is no current standard of care. Tumors affecting integumentary, musculoskeletal, alimentary, urogenital, nervous, and lymphoreticular systems have been reported. Surgical resection is generally the treatment of choice; however, radiotherapy, photodynamic therapy, cryosurgery, and chemotherapy are reported adjunctive or alternative strategies that may be employed. Surgical recommendations for avian neoplasms are largely limited by anatomy; however, a thorough understanding of tumor behavior will allow the surgeon to provide a complete treatment plan and improve postoperative outcomes. Tumor behavior and metastatic patterns are not as well established for birds as they are for dogs and cats. Therefore, complete staging should be performed in birds in order to discuss appropriate therapy, follow-up, and prognosis with clients.

Integumentary and Musculoskeletal Tumors

Surgical excision of cutaneous and musculoskeletal tumors may be performed with curative intent or for palliation of clinical signs depending on tumor type, size, and location. Surgical excision of tumors involving the integumentary system is more likely to be curative than tumors involving the musculoskeletal system. Dermal neoplasms reported in birds include squamous cell carcinoma, basal cell carcinoma, lipoma, liposarcoma, myelolipoma, fibroma, fibrosarcoma, hemangioma, hemangiosarcoma, hemangiolipoma, melanoma, papilloma, granular cell tumor, and xanthoma (Reavill 2004).

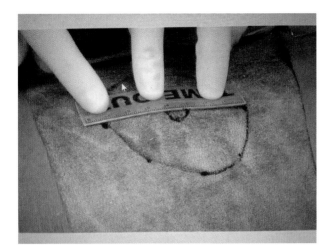

Figure 28.1 Margin of 3 cm measured and marked around a subcutaneous tumor. *Source:* Image courtesy of Laura E Selmic, BVetMed (Hons), MPH, DACVS-SA, DECVS.

Squamous cell carcinomas (SCC) are most commonly seen on feathered skin, beak, uropygial gland, phalanges, and crop (Murtaugh et al. 1986; Malka et al. 2005; Klaphake et al. 2006; Zehnder et al. 2018). Cockatiels, Amazon parrots, and conures are most commonly affected. Lesions may appear as raised, proliferative lesions, or ulcerations (Figure 28.2). SCC are locally invasive with a low metastatic rate. Diagnosis can be obtained with cytology or histopathology. In a retrospective case series of 87 client-owned birds with confirmed SCC of the skin or oral cavity, complete surgical excision was reported in 23% of cases with surgical debulking performed in 33% (Zehnder et al. 2018). Additional treatments included conservative monitoring, systemic chemotherapy, intralesional chemotherapy, strontium radiation, and external beam radiation. Given the retrospective nature of the report, surgical margins were not reported. One might assume that if additional therapies were part of the treatment plan, debulking or marginal excision of the tumor was intended. Survival times reported were 628 days for birds undergoing complete surgical excision, 357 days for birds receiving other treatments, and 171 days for those not treated. For birds with SCC, surgical excision was the only treatment approach associated with complete or partial response and increased survival time. It is not clear what constitutes adequate margins for surgical excision of SCC in birds; however, in humans, surgical margins of 4–6 mm are recommended for cutaneous SCC (Stewart and Saunders 2018), and in cats 5 mm surgical margins have been shown to result in clean histologic margins for SCC of the eyelid (Schmidt et al. 2005).

Basal cell carcinoma is a rare cutaneous neoplasm that occurs in birds. In dogs and cats, basal cell carcinomas are firm, round, discrete, masses of the dermoepidermal layer. They are usually a low-grade neoplasm with rare metastatic potential. Basal cell carcinoma has been reported in a blue-fronted Amazon parrot (*Amazona aestiva*) (Tell et al. 1997); however, the tumor displayed an invasive behavior with local recurrence after incomplete excision. Basosquamous carcinoma has also been reported in an Indian runner duck (*Anas platyrhynchos*). Incomplete surgical excision was performed with no recurrence up to three months postoperatively, but follow-up time was short (Bradford et al. 2009).

Adjunctive treatment options have been reported in birds. A single irradiation fraction of 100 Gy/8.3 mm from a

(a) (b)

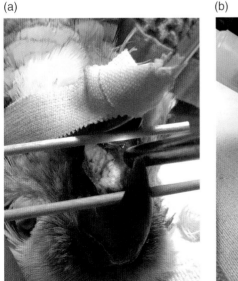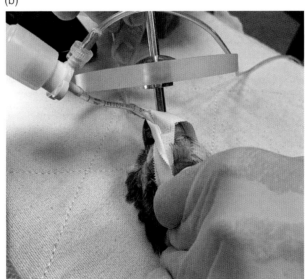

Figure 28.2 An adult female Amazon parrot with oral squamous cell carcinoma (a). After surgical debulking, the site is being treated with Strontium-90 (b). *Source:* Images courtesy of Courtney Sorensen, DVM.

strontium-90 ophthalmic applicator was used successfully for treatment of SCC of the uropygial gland in a budgerigar (*Melopsittacus undulatus*) (Kent 2017), and has also been used at the author's institution for treatment of incompletely excised oral SCC (Figure 28.2b).

Lipomas/Liposarcomas

Lipomas are benign tumors of adipose tissue that are reported to occur most frequently in Amazon parrots (Castro et al. 2016), budgerigars, and cockatoos. There has been an association with obesity, which suggests high calorie diets may play a role in the development of lipomas. Recurrence rates are reported to be around 14% and are likely due to infiltration into surrounding adipose tissues and difficulties identifying tumor margins (Castro et al. 2016). Cryosurgery may be used in cases with incomplete margins and may decrease chances of tumor recurrence. If surgical excision is not an option based on location or comorbidities, supplementation with L-carnitine has been shown to reduce tumor size in budgerigars (Voe et al. 2004). Liposarcomas have also been described in birds as locally invasive with criteria of malignancy on histopathology (Reece 1992; Tully et al. 1994; Graham et al. 2003); however, surgical treatment and follow-up was either not performed or not reported. As with most soft tissue sarcomas (STS) in dogs, surgical margins of 3 cm are recommended; however, given the anatomic limitations and the invasive nature of these tumors, the widest margins obtainable (if <3 cm) without compromising closure and function should be performed followed with adjunctive treatment options in cases with incomplete excision.

Soft Tissue Sarcomas

STS such as fibrosarcomas are commonly encountered, locally invasive malignant tumors of connective tissue (Reece 1992). Other STS reported in birds include rhabdomyomas, rhabdomyosarcomas, synovial cell sarcomas, and myxosarcomas. Treatment of these tumors require wide surgical excision of 3 cm lateral margins and 1 fascial plane deep; however, if there are anatomic limitations, marginal excision with adjunctive treatment should be considered. Successful use of surgical debulking followed by intralesional cisplatin and radiotherapy has been reported in two macaws with fibrosarcomas, with local control achieved for 15 and 29 months posttreatment, respectively (Ramsay et al. 1993; Lamberski and Théon 2002). Early diagnosis and treatment are important as these tumors can metastasize to the lungs, beak, long bones, syrinx, and liver (Riddell and Cribb 1983; Burgmann 1994).

Bone Tumors

The most commonly reported bone tumors in birds are osteosarcoma and chondroma (Dittmer et al. 2012). Additionally chondrosarcoma, osteoma, and other mesenchymal tumors have been reported to affect bone. Of the primary bone tumors reported in birds, 44% were osteosarcomas of the limbs. Osteosarcoma in birds does not appear to be highly metastatic to the lungs compared to dogs; however, metastasis to the liver, kidneys, mesentery, bone marrow, sternum, and lungs has been reported (Liu et al. 1982; Lamb et al. 2014). Amputation of the affected limb has been recommended as the treatment of choice in several articles to relieve pain and prevent pathologic fractures (Arnall 1966; Filippich 2004). In several case reports, debulking followed by chemotherapy (intralesional or systemic) or radiation showed some response (Filippich 2004; Dittmer et al. 2012). An overall review of the literature reveals limited knowledge on treatment outcomes and quality of life assessments following amputation in pet birds; however, a few case reports indicate good quality of life (Summa et al. 2016; Ozawa and Mans 2017).

Hemangioma/Hemangiosarcoma

Hemangiomas are benign tumors of vascular endothelium commonly reported in budgerigars (Reavill 2004). They may appear as reddish to black masses anywhere in the skin or subcutis. Surgical excision of hemangiomas can result in cure. Hemangiosarcomas are malignant tumors of vascular endothelium that occur more commonly in cockatiels but affect other birds as well. Incomplete excision of hemangiosarcomas is associated with local recurrence and metastasis. In dogs, treatment of hemangiosarcoma include surgical excision followed by systemic chemotherapy (Ogilvie 1998; Batschinski et al. 2018); however, reports in birds are mainly postmortem diagnoses. A blue-fronted Amazon parrot (*A. aestiva*) treated with surgical excision resulted in no recurrence or metastasis in eight years (Castro et al. 2016) and in a budgerigar treated with radiation there was complete regression of the tumor with metastasis occurring eight weeks after treatment (Freeman 1999).

Alimentary Tumors

Leiomyosarcomas originating from the gastrointestinal tract have been scarcely reported with only one case report of an attempted resection and anastomosis in a budgerigar that died intraoperatively (Sasipreeyajan et al. 1988; Steinberg 1988). Dogs with intestinal leiomyosarcoma that survive the immediate postoperative period can experience long-term survival after surgical excision (Cohen et al.

2003). Intestinal leiomyosarcomas are rare in cats, but evidence supports wide surgical excision for improved survival (Barrand and Scudamore 1999; Hart et al. 2018). Based on the behavior of leiomyosarcomas in other companion animals, in birds an attempt to obtain clean surgical margins should be made.

Adjuvant Therapies

Radiation Therapy

As radiation therapy (RT) in veterinary medicine continues to grow, birds are more frequently being treated for neoplastic conditions not amendable to wide excision. In a 2010 survey of veterinary radiation facilities, 6 of 24 responders reported treating birds with between 1 and 2 treated at each facility (Farrelly and McEntee 2014). Information on RT in birds is limited to a small number of case reports with short-term follow-up and variable responses (Manucy et al. 1998; Lamberski and Théon 2002; Fordham et al. 2010; Guthrie et al. 2010; Duncan et al. 2014; Alexander et al. 2017). Doses are extrapolated from other companion animals such as dogs and cats; however, they appear to be inadequate for effective tumor control in birds. In a study evaluating tolerance doses in ring-neck parakeets, doses of 72 Gy in 4-Gy fractions were well tolerated (Barron et al. 2009). Another study revealed that the actual amount of radiation delivered to the choana was less than the calculated amount, although the reason for the discrepancy remains unknown (Cutler et al. 2016). Additional prospective studies are needed to determine ideal dosing and fractionation for treating avian neoplasia.

Chemotherapy

Chemotherapy involves using cytotoxic agents to treat neoplastic disease. In birds, chemotherapy is a treatment modality that has been used to delay tumor progression; however, experimental and clinical studies in birds are lacking. Doses and treatment options are outside of the scope of this chapter but may be found in other resources and should be included in planning patient management (Filippich and Charles 2004).

Rabbits

Neoplastic diseases are commonly encountered in domestic rabbits most often originating from the urogenital tract. Tumors affecting the reproductive, musculoskeletal, alimentary, urinary, respiratory, nervous, and endocrine systems have been reported. Treatment generally involves surgical resection; however, radiotherapy and chemotherapy are reported adjunctive or alternative strategies as well.

Guidelines for achieving complete surgical excision are similar to other companion animals with 1–3 cm surgical margins depending on the tumor type. When complete excision is not possible, marginal excision or intracapsular surgery may be performed to decrease tumor burden, relieve pain, and improve the effectiveness of adjunctive treatments.

Tumors of the Reproductive Tract

One of the most frequently encountered neoplasms in rabbits is uterine adenocarcinoma (Weisbroth 1994; Tinkey et al. 2012). Other reported tumors of the uterus include adenomas, leiomyomas, leiomyosarcomas, malignant mixed Müllerian duct tumors, deciduosarcomas, carcinosarcomas, choriocarcinomas, and SCC (Weisbroth 1994; Cooper et al. 2006; Goto et al. 2006; Kaufmann-Bart and Fischer 2008; Tinkey et al. 2012). Uterine adenocarcinoma is the most widely studied uterine tumor in both pet rabbits and research colonies, occurring most frequently in older rabbits (Ingalls et al. 1964; Heatley and Smith 2004). Common presenting signs include decreased fertility, smaller litters, depression, anorexia, or vaginal discharge (Weisbroth 1994; Harcourt-Brown 1998; Raftery 1998; Saito et al. 2002; Walter et al. 2010; Künzel et al. 2014). Although slow-growing, metastasis may occur to lungs, liver, brain, and bone marrow. Additionally, carcinomatosis may occur if the tumor penetrates the serosal surface of the uterus. As rabbits become increasingly more popular as companion animals, the drive for advanced care has also increased. Abdominal ultrasonography is the most sensitive tool for diagnosing uterine diseases; however, abdominal radiographs paired with abdominal palpation may be adequate (Saito et al. 2002; Walter et al. 2010; Lübke et al. 2019).

Ovariohysterectomy is the treatment of choice for patients without metastasis. In one study, 80% of the ovario-hysterectomy rabbits with uterine adenocarcinoma were still alive six months after surgery (Künzel et al. 2014). In another study, survival was reported for 22 months or longer after surgery (Walter et al. 2010). In a recent study, ovariohysterectomy in rabbits before two years of age was a key preventative measure to mitigate uterine disease, particularly uterine adenocarcinoma (Settai et al. 2020).

For neoplasms of the uterus, prognosis is considered good if there is early detection and surgical intervention. Rabbits in a poor clinical condition have a grave prognosis and have a higher mortality rate than those with minimal clinical signs. Even benign tumors in the uterus may cause discomfort and lead to clinical signs such as bleeding and anorexia. Prophylactic ovariohysterectomy/ovariectomy prior to two years age is recommended in rabbits that are not used for breeding.

In a study evaluating mammary masses in 24 pet rabbits, tumors reported included cystadenoma, intraductal papilloma, intraductal papillary carcinoma, adenocarcinoma, adenosquamous carcinoma, and matrix-producing carcinoma (Schöniger et al. 2014). Mammary adenocarcinoma is historically the most commonly occurring tumor and has been seen as a progression from a cystic process to a benign neoplasm to an invasive adenocarcinoma (Greene 1939a, b, 1940; Atherton et al. 1999). Once this tumor progresses to an adenocarcinoma, metastasis to the lungs, and regional lymph nodes are possible (Tinkey et al. 2012). Mammary gland disorders are frequently associated with uterine disorders, such as endometrial hyperplasia or adenocarcinoma (Greene and Strauss 1949; Saito et al. 2002; Walter et al. 2010). It is thought that ovarian hormones may have an influence in causing these tumors to occur concurrently, though metastasis cannot be ruled out (Burrows 1940). Therefore, an ovariohysterectomy should be performed on intact females. Thoracic radiographs and abdominal ultrasound should be performed preoperatively for staging rabbits with mammary masses. Mastectomy is the treatment of choice and may range from lumpectomy to chain mastectomy depending on how many mammae are involved.

Urinary Tract Tumors

Tumors of the urinary system in rabbits have been sporadically reported and include renal carcinomas and nephromas. Cases of renal carcinoma were diagnosed postmortem and only one case of nephrectomy performed for a nephroblastoma was reported with the patient found dead three days postoperatively (Lipman et al. 1985). Nephroureterectomy should be considered in rabbits with a single renal tumor. Metastasis is common with renal carcinomas so staging should be performed.

Thymic Neoplasia

Unlike other companion animals, the thymus in rabbits persists into adulthood. Thymomas, tumors originating from the epithelial cells of the thymus, have been reported in several clinical cases (Clippinger et al. 1998; Florizoone 2005; Kostolich and Panciera 1992; Vernau et al. 1995). Rare reports of malignant thymic neoplasms exist; however, a majority of thymic tumors are benign (Künzel et al. 2012). Neoplasms of the thymus have been associated with anorexia, dyspnea, exercise intolerance, bilateral exophthalmos, prolapse of the nictitating membranes, swelling of the head, exfoliative dermatitis, and paraneoplastic immunopathy. Thoracic radiographs generally reveal a cranial mediastinal mass, which may be accompanied by pleural effusion. Ultrasonography may be useful to guide fine needle aspirates or needle biopsies. Cytology may reveal small well-differentiated small lymphocytes and neoplastic epithelial cells. Advanced imaging with computed tomography will provide the most detail for surgical or radiation planning.

Treatment options include surgery, radiation, and adjunctive chemotherapy. Surgical excision via ventral midline thoracotomy is generally recommended for solitary lesions. In rabbits; however, perioperative mortality is high with survival rates varying between 25% and 50% thought to be related to pain, stress, or anesthetic complications (Künzel et al. 2012; Morrisey and McEntee 2005). Therefore, sufficient perioperative analgesia is essential, in addition to quiet and stress-free environment during the recovery period. In cases that survived the perioperative period, euthanasia occurred due to tumor recurrence (Künzel et al. 2012).

RT has been increasingly used for treatment of thymomas in rabbits with varying results (Sanchez-Migallon et al. 2006; Andres et al. 2012; Dolera et al. 2016). In one study, 19 rabbits with suspected or confirmed thymomas were treated with RT and had resolution of clinical signs ranging from 4 to 42 days (Andres et al. 2012). Mean survival time (MST) was 727 days for cases that survived the first two weeks of treatment and complications were uncommon but late side effects were observed including alopecia, pneumonitis, and myocardial fibrosis. Repeated imaging during the course of treatment is recommended to avoid over-dosing normal structures that may move into the planned radiation field as the tumor shrinks. In another study, 15 rabbits were prospectively treated with 40 Gy delivered in six fractions over 11 days using volumetric modulated arc radiotherapy (Dolera et al. 2016). All rabbits had a complete response, there were no late side effects and the median survival time was not reached with 10 rabbits alive at 777 days. This therapy is very promising but not readily available.

Tumors of the Skin

Cutaneous neoplasms in rabbits are generally classified into viral or nonviral etiologies. Virally induced neoplasms include Shope fibromas (induced by a leporipoxvirus) and Shope papillomas (induced by papovavirus) which is restricted to haired skin (Brabb and Di Giacomo 2012; Varga 2014). Nonviral cutaneous neoplasms include SCC, basal cell tumors (trichoblastomas), trichoepitheliomas, tricholemmomas, and sebaceous adenocarcinomas. In a retrospective study evaluating cutaneous neoplasms in pet rabbits over a 16-year period, the most common neoplasms identified were trichoblastoma and Shope fibroma (von Bomhard et al. 2007). In the same study, 23 different tumor types were reported including 11 different mesenchymal tumors, several of which had never been previously reported.

Malignant melanomas were also reported and can metastasize to local lymph nodes. The tumors in this study had a behavior similar to canine and feline tumors: carcinomas were more likely to metastasize, and sarcomas were more likely to recur locally. In another study evaluating 672 cases, trichoblastomas and unclassified mesenchymal tumors were the most common neoplasms found (Kanfer and Reavill 2013). As trichoblastomas are considered benign, prognosis is excellent with complete surgical excision.

Cutaneous rabbit tumors should be surgically excised with at least 5 mm surgical margins for epithelial tumors and 3 cm lateral margins and 1 fascial plane deep for mesenchymal tumors. For STS/mesenchymal neoplasms on the extremities, amputation of the limb should be considered. Limb amputation is well tolerated in rabbits with a reported 18% mortality rate related to postoperative complications; however, 59% developed chronic complications such as difficulty ambulating, difficulty grooming, and pododermatitis which is acceptable if local tumor control is achieved (Northrup et al. 2014).

Tumors of Bone

Primary bone osteosarcoma has been described in rabbits with 50% of patients having lung metastasis at the time of diagnosis (Mazzullo et al. 2004; Ishikawa et al. 2012). Unlike canine osteosarcoma, there is one case report of osteosarcoma of the glenohumeral joint space (Kondo et al. 2007). No long-term studies have been performed evaluating treatment and outcomes in rabbits with osteosarcoma; however, based on the behavior of osteosarcoma in other species, amputation of the affected limb should be considered with chemotherapy to follow.

Ferrets

Ferrets present with a wide variety of neoplasms that may result in significant clinical abnormalities (Schoemaker 2017). Endocrine neoplasms are common and may occur simultaneously. Various conditions that occur in older ferrets can make diagnosis of an endocrinopathy difficult. A thorough systemic evaluation should be performed to evaluate for comorbidities. Hypertrophic cardiomyopathy may also occur in older ferrets so an echocardiogram should be performed prior to major abdominal surgery.

Endocrine

Adrenal Tumors

Adrenal tumors (adrenal gland disease, hyperadrenocorticism) are one of the most common neoplasms in ferrets (Hillyer 1994; Rosenthal 1997; Beeber 2011; Avallone et al.

2016). They are usually functional, secreting sex steroids. Clinical signs include symmetric hair loss, pruritis, vulvar enlargement, urinary issues in male ferrets, and sexually aggressive behavior. Abdominal ultrasound may be used to identify an enlarged adrenal gland. Adrenal gland adenoma is the most common cause of adrenal gland disease. Hyperplasia, carcinomas, pheochromocytomas, leiomyosarcomas, and fibrosarcomas have also been reported (Swiderski et al. 2008).

Surgical excision of the affected gland offers a good long-term prognosis for both benign and malignant lesions as metastasis is rare (Lawrence et al. 1993). If both adrenal glands are affected, bilateral adrenalectomy may be performed. Ferrets treated surgically for adrenal gland disease have a 70% five-year survival rate not affected by histologic tumor type, lateralization, or completeness of excision (Swiderski et al. 2008).

Alternatively, leuprolide acetate, deslorelin acetate, and melatonin can be used to treat the clinical signs of adrenal gland disease when surgery is not an option; however, it does not slow the progression of the tumor (Wagner et al. 2009). Although cryosurgery has been reported as a treatment, it has been shown to be a negative prognostic indicator for long-term survival and cannot be recommended (Swiderski et al. 2008).

Pancreatic Tumors

Insulinomas (beta cell tumors) are another common neoplasm in ferrets. Pancreatic nodules may be detected using ultrasonography but are often too small to image. They are most commonly found in the left limb of the pancreas (Wu et al. 2017). A combination of surgical and medical management offers the best control of the disease. They are malignant, metastasis is common, and clinical signs are likely to recur (Beeber 2011). Medical management entails dietary management followed by the addition of prednisone. Diazoxide may also be used to inhibit insulin release. Marginal excision of the pancreatic nodule may be performed; however, multiple nodules may be found and a partial pancreatectomy may be required. In some ferrets, the pancreas is diffusely involved with microscopic insulinomas and no discrete masses. Metastasis to the liver and spleen occurs. In a study comparing three treatment strategies, medical management had a MST of 186 days, nodulectomy alone had a MST of 456 days, and nodulectomy and partial pancreatectomy had a MST of 668 days (Weiss et al. 1998).

Integumentary

In a study evaluating 763 cases, the most common cutaneous tumors included mast cell tumors (MCT), sebaceous epitheliomas (basal cell tumors), cutaneous hemangiomas, preputial gland tumors, and lymphoma (Kanfer and Reavill

2013). MCT may appear as small, slightly raised, pruritic, and ulcerated skin lesions occurring on the head, neck, thorax, and extremities. In ferrets, MCT are benign, and surgical excision is curative (Parker and Picut 1993; Stauber et al. 1990). Surgical excision with 5 mm margins was reported in a prospective study evaluating KIT expression in MCT in ferrets (Vilalta et al. 2016). Complete excision was achieved in 11 ferrets (73.3%) and incomplete in 4 (26.7%). No recurrence or metastatic disease was reported in any case, even with incomplete margins.

Basal cell tumors in ferrets behave similarly to basal cell tumors occurring in other species. They can occur anywhere on the body, but commonly on the head and neck. Surgical excision is generally curative as they are benign (Parker and Picut 1993; Vilalta et al. 2016). Electrochemotherapy (ECT) with bleomycin has also been proven to be safe and effective against a variety of cutaneous tumors in ferrets (Racnik et al. 2017).

Apocrine gland adenocarcinoma of the anal sac and prepuce have been reported in ferrets (Figure 28.3) (Parker and Picut 1993). They are highly malignant with a locally aggressive behavior and high metastatic rate to local lymph nodes. Wide surgical excision is recommended and may include penile amputation and urethrostomy followed by RT if margins are incomplete (Miller et al. 1985).

Chordomas are slow-growing, locally aggressive tumors originating from remnants of the notochord and can occur anywhere along the vertebral column, with the tip of tail being most common (Figure 28.4). Although chordomas are uncommon in other species, it is the most common musculoskeletal tumor in ferrets. Clinical signs are related to location of the tumor: injury and ulceration of tumors on the tail and ataxia, paresis/paralysis, pain, and difficulty urinating for tumors over the cervical or thoracic vertebrae. Few cases of metastasis to lungs and skin have been

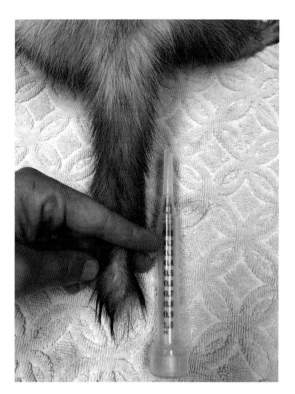

Figure 28.4 A mass on the tip of the tail being aspirated. Chordoma was the diagnosis. It was treated with tail amputation. *Source*: Image courtesy of Krista A. Keller, DVM, DACZM.

reported (Munday et al. 2004). Complete surgical excision offers the best chance of local control.

Cytologic examination reveals individual or clusters of small cells with abundant pale or vacuolated cytoplasm and small, dense, ovoid, singular nuclei with an abundant dense fibrillar metachromic background (Roth and Takata 1992). Histopathologically, these tumors are composed of closely packed physaliferous cells. Immunohistological staining with low-molecular-weight cytokeratins (CK18, CK19, CK20), vimentin and mucin core protein can be useful for diagnosing chordomas in ferrets (Yui et al. 2015).

Complete surgical excision with 0.5–1 cm of tail proximal to the chordoma is typically curative. Chordomas over other areas of the spinal cord are more difficult to remove and may require adjuvant treatments such as RT, or local recurrence is likely.

Reproductive

Both benign and malignant mammary tumors have been reported in ferrets. In male ferrets, mammary tumors are more likely to be malignant. Benign tumors may be cured with surgical excision; however, recurrence may occur with malignant tumors. Surgical margins should be 5–10 mm if attainable.

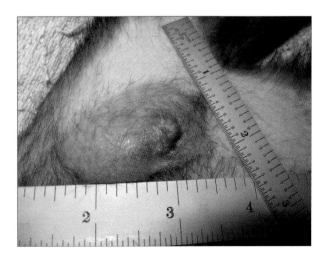

Figure 28.3 A ferret with a preputial adenocarcinoma.

Rodents

Neoplasms in pet rodents are reported with some frequency and affect mice, rats, hamsters, gerbils, chinchillas, and guinea pigs. Treatment options are limited by small patient size and minimal research into adjunctive treatment modalities. This section summarizes the most common neoplasms encountered in pet rodents.

Tumors in Rats and Mice

Skin and SQ

SCC is the most common skin tumor in mice followed by fibromas, fibrosarcomas, and other mesenchymal tumors (Greenacre 2004). Tumors of the skin and subcutaneous (SQ) tissues are uncommon in rats although various STS and SCC have been reported (Greenacre 2004).

Reproductive/Mammary Tumors

Mammary tumors are the most common spontaneous tumor in mice and are usually malignant. Surgical excision is not advised as these tumors are viral induced, invasive, highly metastatic, and carry a poor prognosis. In rats, most mammary tumors are fibroadenomas and can be surgically excised. The incidence of new tumor development is higher in intact females. Marginal excision and ovariectomy are recommended. Rats ovariectomized at 90 days have a significantly lower incidence of mammary tumors than intact females (Hotchkiss 1995). Testicular interstitial cell tumors and ovarian tumors also occur in mice. In rats, interstitial cell tumors are the most common tumor of the reproductive system (Greenacre 2004).

Endocrine

In mice, reported neoplasms of the endocrine system include pituitary adenomas, carcinomas, and fibrosarcomas, in addition to thyroid and parathyroid adenomas. In rats, pituitary adenomas occur very frequently. Thyroid, adrenal, and parathyroid tumors are also reported (Greenacre 2004).

Hamsters

A comprehensive study evaluating tumors from 85 domestic hamsters revealed integumentary and hematopoietic tumors to be the most common depending on the species (Kondo et al. 2008). In Djungarian hamsters, most tumors were of the integument, including mammary tumors, fibromas, and papillomas. In Syrian hamsters, plasmacytomas were the most common. In another large study, the most frequently seen neoplasm was adrenal adenomas and squamous cell papillomas of the vagina of female hamsters (McInnes et al. 2013). Treatment and outcomes are rarely reported. Basic principles of surgical oncology should be applied when surgical excision of cutaneous masses is attempted.

Chinchillas

A relatively low incidence of tumors is described for chinchillas, and most of the literature is limited to case reports. In a case series describing SCC, self-mutilation occurred in all cases, and treatment was not pursued (Szabo et al. 2019). In another case report of a uterine leiomyoma and fibroma, and a uterine hemangioma in two chinchillas, cystic masses were noted on abdominal ultrasound (Bertram et al. 2019). Both chinchillas were euthanized due to progressive deterioration.

Guinea Pigs

Skin and SQ

The most common cutaneous neoplasms in guinea pigs include trichofolliculomas, lipomas, trichoepitheliomas, and mammary adenocarcinomas. In one study evaluating 133 cases, most of the tumors were benign; however, tumors such as trichofolliculomas can get quite large and rupture. Surgical excision is recommended and curative with complete excision.

Reproductive/Mammary

Mammary tumors are reported to occur in guinea pigs and may develop secondary to hormonal influence (Suárez-Bonnet et al. 2010). Malignant mammary carcinomas were reported in 66% of mammary tumors (Kanfer and Reavill 2013). A high incidence in male guinea pigs is also reported. Because of the potential for metastasis, thoracic radiographs should be performed for staging. Complete surgical excision is recommended as a high rate of recurrence is associated with incomplete excision. Wide surgical margins of 0.5–1.0 cm should be attempted in addition to extirpation of local lymph nodes (Mehler and Bennett 2004). RT may be used to control local disease; however, long-term prognosis is guarded. Nonsteroidal anti-inflammatories may be considered for palliative or adjunctive therapy.

Benign and malignant uterine and ovarian neoplasms also occur. Ovariohysterectomy is recommended for both uterine and ovarian tumors. Prognosis is good with surgery (Figure 28.5).

Endocrine

Neoplasms of the endocrine system have been reported to affect the thyroid, pancreas, and adrenal glands of guinea pigs. Thyroid tumors are generally adenocarcinomas, although metastasis is rare (Gibbons et al. 2013). Functional

(a)

(b)

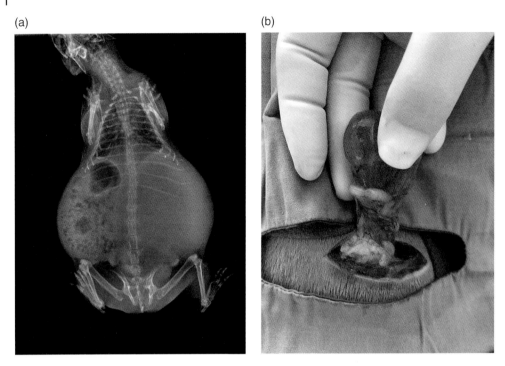

Figure 28.5 An adult female guinea pig presented with bilateral flank alopecia. Radiographs showed an abdominal soft tissue mass effect (a). Ultrasound confirmed a large paraovarian cyst. Treatment included ovariectomy through bilateral flank approaches (b). *Source:* Images courtesy of Krista A Keller, DVM, DACZM.

thyroid gland tumors can present clinically similar to hyperthyroid cats: weight loss, hyperactivity, ventral neck mass, abnormal social behavior, poor haircoat, and polyuria/polydipsia. Definitive diagnosis is made by evaluation of serum total T_4 concentrations. An ultrasound of the neck or nuclear scintigraphy may also support the diagnosis or identify ectopic or metastatic thyroid tissue (Mayer et al. 2010; Kondo et al. 2018). Treatment options include medical management, radioactive iodine therapy, and thyroidectomy (Brandão et al. 2013; Künzel et al. 2013; Pignon and Mayer 2013).

Both adrenal-dependent hyperadrenocorticism and pituitary-dependent hyperadrenocorticism have been reported. Clinical signs include symmetrical alopecia, thin skin, polyuria/polydipsia, muscle weakness, and weight loss. Diagnosis can be made with an adrenocorticotropic hormone (ACTH) stimulation test using saliva as a noninvasive method for monitoring changes (Fenske 1997). Treatment options include medical management with trilostane or unilateral adrenalectomy.

Respiratory

Neoplasia of the respiratory tract have been described in both companion and laboratory guinea pigs; however, treatment and outcomes have yet to be investigated (Rogers and Blumenthal 1960; Kitchen et al. 1975; Hoch-Ligeti

et al. 1982; Greenacre 2004). Radiographs of the thorax should be obtained in any guinea pig presenting with respiratory signs to rule out neoplasia. In other companion animals, lung lobectomy offers a good prognosis depending on the grade and stage of the disease; however, this has yet to be investigated in guinea pigs.

Reptiles

The most common systems affected by neoplasia in reptiles include hematopoetic, hepatobiliary, and integumentary (Ramsay et al. 1993; Catão-Dias and Nichols 1999; Sykes and Trupkiewicz 2006; Page-Karjian et al. 2017). Several large reviews have shown that neoplasia is most prevalent in snakes, followed by lizards, chelonians, and crocodilians (Frye 1994; Garner et al. 2004; Sykes and Trupkiewicz 2006). These large reviews focus on postmortem examination. Treatment approaches for tumors in reptiles are adapted from knowledge and experience with neoplasms in other companion animals. Reptiles are unique in their anatomy and physiology, which poses a challenge. Treatment modalities for cancer in reptiles include surgery, RT, chemotherapy, ECT, cryosurgery and photodynamic therapy. Reported treatments are limited to individual cases with limited surgical detail or follow-up.

Hepatic Tumors

Tumors affecting the hepatobiliary system include biliary adenomas/adenocarcinomas, and hepatocellular adenomas/carcinomas. Biliary adenocarcinomas tend to be multicentric; however, metastasis is not seen. Hepatocellular carcinomas are seen both as solitary lesions and multicentric lesions, but metastasis is generally not seen. These tumors are well differentiated and may be difficult to distinguish from their benign counterpart.

Cutaneous Tumors

The most common cutaneous tumors encountered in reptiles include SCC, melanoma, STS, papilloma, and lipoma. Surgical excision is generally the treatment of choice and appears to be curative in most cases. Other options for local control include intralesional chemotherapy, photodynamic therapy, and cryosurgery. See below for further information regarding these treatment modalities.

Endocrine Tumors

Endocrine tumors reported in reptiles include pancreatic, adrenal, and thyroid. Patients with pancreatic islet cell tumors have shown no evidence of glucose abnormalities, and are likely nonfunctional. Adrenal tumors reported include pheochromocytoma and adrenocortical adenomas. Both thyroid adenomas and carcinomas have been reported in chelonians, lizards, and snakes.

Musculoskeletal Tumors

Musculoskeletal tumors occur infrequently in reptiles but include rhabdomyosarcoma, myxosarcoma, osteosarcoma, and chondrosarcoma. Osteosarcomas occur most frequently in vertebrae, although extra-skeletal osteosarcoma has been reported. They are locally invasive, but metastasis is generally not seen. Similar in behavior, chondrosarcomas also occur in the vertebrae of snakes, are locally invasive, and do not metastasize.

Urogenital Tumors

Ovarian adenocarcinoma is the most common reproductive tumor in lizards and snakes (Figure 28.6). Metastasis is more likely to occur in snakes. Uncommon tumors include granulosa cell tumors, seminomas, Leydig cell tumors, and teratomas. Renal adenocarcinomas occur most frequently in snakes and occasionally in lizards and chelonians. These tumors are slow growing and uncommonly metastasize. A nephrectomy is the treatment of choice.

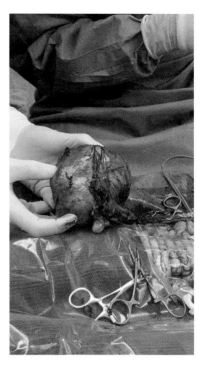

Figure 28.6 An ovarian mass being removed from an eastern diamondback rattlesnake (*Crotalus adamanteus*). *Source:* Image courtesy of Jim Wellehan, DVM, MS, PhD, DACZM, DACVM.

Gastrointestinal Tumors

Adenocarcinomas have been reported in the stomach, small intestine, colon, and cloaca of chelonians and snakes (Garner et al. 2004). Some cases had identifiable lymphatic invasion or metastasis to the liver. SCC have also been reported to occur in the oral cavity of several species of snakes, and lizards. Metastasis has not been reported.

Treatment Options

Surgery

Surgical excision should be considered as the primary treatment modality for most neoplasms in reptiles as metastasis is uncommon and surgery may be curative (Frye 1994). Although it is unclear what ideal surgical margins are in reptiles, neoplasms in these species appear to behave similar to those in mammals and the same surgical oncologic principles should be followed. Surgery may also be used in combination with other treatment modalities if indicated to minimize tumor recurrence and/or metastasis.

Radiation Therapy

There are two case reports describing RT for treatment of cutaneous neoplasms in snakes. Both snakes suffered from treatment side effects and had to be euthanized (Steeil et al. 2013; Langan et al. 2001). There is much to be investigated and no standard protocol exists for reptiles.

Chemotherapy/Electrochemotherapy

Intratumoral administration of chemotherapy is commonly used in reptiles based on ease of administration; however, systemic chemotherapy may also be administered. Care must be taken when considering systemic chemotherapy doses as reptiles have a higher risk of toxicity due to their low metabolic rate (Graham et al. 2004; Kent 2004; Hahn 2005).

ECT involves applying high-voltage electric pulses to a tumor and administering a chemotherapeutic systemically or intratumorally allowing for targeted uptake. It has been demonstrated to be highly effective for the treatment of a variety of cutaneous and subcutaneous tumors in dogs, cats, and horses (Spugnini and Baldi 2014). Several case reports have shown ECT to be an effective therapeutic alternative for cutaneous tumors in chelonians (Brunner et al. 2014; Lanza et al. 2015; Donnelly et al. 2019). It should be considered when excision is incomplete or surgery is not an option.

Cryosurgery and Photodynamic Therapy

There is a single report on the use of photodynamic therapy in three snakes with cutaneous neoplasms with a good response and no side effects (Roberts et al. 1991). Additionally, cryosurgery has been reported as a good treatment modality for cutaneous neoplasms in reptiles; however, using this therapy was also limited to a few case reports (Green et al. 1977; Baxter and Meek 1988; Bryant et al. 1997).

References

Alexander, A.B., Griffin, L., and Johnston, M.S. (2017). Radiation therapy of periorbital lymphoma in a blue and gold macaw (*Ara ararauna*). *Journal of Avian Medicine and Surgery* 31 (1): 39–46.

Andres, K., Kent, M., Siedlecki, C. et al. (2012). The use of megavoltage radiation therapy in the treatment of thymomas in rabbits: 19 cases. *Veterinary and Comparative Oncology* 10 (2): 82–94.

Arnall, L. (1966). The clinical approach to tumors in cage birds-IV treatment of cage bird tumors. *Journal of Small Animal Practice* 7 (3): 241–251.

Atherton, J., Griffiths, L., and Williams, A. (1999). Cystic mastitis disease in the female rabbit. *The Veterinary Record* 145 (22): 648.

Avallone, G., Forlani, A., Tecilla, M. et al. (2016). Neoplastic diseases in the domestic ferret (*Mustela putorius furo*) in Italy: classification and tissue distribution of 856 cases (2000–2010). *BMC Veterinary Research* 12 (1): 275.

Barrand, K. and Scudamore, C. (1999). Intestinal leiomyosarcoma in a cat. *Journal of Small Animal Practice* 40 (5): 216–219.

Barron, H.W., Roberts, R.E., Latimer, K.S. et al. (2009). Tolerance doses of cutaneous and mucosal tissues in ring-necked parakeets (*Psittacula krameri*) for external beam megavoltage radiation. *Journal of Avian Medicine and Surgery* 28 (2): 6–9.

Burrows, H. (1940). Spontaneous uterine and mammary tumours in rabbit. *Journal of Pathology and Bacteriology* 51: 385–390.

Batschinski, K., Nobre, A., Vargas-Mendez, E. et al. (2018). Canine visceral hemangiosarcoma treated with surgery alone or surgery and doxorubicin: 37 cases (2005–2014). *The Canadian Veterinary Journal* 59 (9): 967–972.

Baxter, J.S. and Meek, R. (1988). Cryosurgery in the treatment of skin disorders in reptiles. *Herpatological Journal* I: 227–229.

Beeber, N.L. (2011). Surgical management of adrenal tumors and insulinomas in ferrets. *Journal of Exotic Pet Medicine* 20 (3): 206–216.

Bertram, C.A., Kershaw, O., Klopfleisch, R. et al. (2019). Uterine leiomyoma, fibroma, and hemangioma in 2 chinchillas (*Chinchilla laniger*). *Journal of Exotic Pet Medicine* 28: 23–29.

von Bomhard, W., Goldschmidt, M., Shofer, F. et al. (2007). Cutaneous neoplasms in pet rabbits: a retrospective study. *Veterinary Pathology* 44 (5): 579–588.

Brabb, T. and Di Giacomo, R.F. (2012). Viral diseases. In: *The Laboratory Rabbit, Guinea Pig, Hamster, and Other Rodents* (eds. M.A. Suckow, K.A. Stevens and R.P. Wilson), 365–413. Oxford: Academic Press.

Bradford, C., Wack, A., Trembley, S. et al. (2009). Two cases of neoplasia of basal cell origin affecting the axillary region in Anseriform species. *Journal of Avian Medicine and Surgery* 28 (2): 214–221.

Brandão, J., Vergneau-Grosset, C., and Mayer, J. (2013). Hyperthyroidism and hyperparathyroidism in Guinea pigs (*Cavia porcellus*). *Veterinary Clinics of North America: Exotic Animal Practice* 16 (2): 407–420.

Brunner, C.H., Dutra, G., Silva, C.B. et al. (2014). Electrochemotherapy for the treatment of fibropapillomas in *Chelonia mydas*. *Journal of Zoo and Wildlife Medicine* 45 (2): 213–218.

Bryant, B.R., Vogelnest, L., and Hulst, F. (1997). The use of cryosurgery in a diamond python, *Morelia spilota spilota*, with fibrosarcoma and radiotherapy in a common death adder, *Acanthophis antarcticus*, with melanoma. *Bulletin of the Association of Reptilian and Amphibian Veterinarians* 7 (3): 9–12.

Burgmann, P.M. (1994). Pulmonary fibrosarcoma with hepatic metastases in a cockatiel (*Nymphicus hollandicus*). *Journal of the Association of Avian Veterinarians* 8 (2): 81.

Castro, P.F., Fantoni, D.T., Miranda, B.C., and Matera, J.M. (2016). Prevalence of neoplastic diseases in pet birds referred for surgical procedures. *Veterinary Medicine International* 2016: 4096801.

Catão-Dias, J.L. and Nichols, D.K. (1999). Neoplasia in snakes at the National Zoological Park, Washington, DC (1978–1997). *Journal of Comparative Pathology* 120 (1): 89–95.

Clippinger, T.L., Bennett, R.A., Alleman, R.A. et al. (1998). Removal of a thymoma via median sternotomy in a rabbit with recurrent appendicular neurofibrosarcoma. *Journal of the American Veterinary Medical Association* 213 (8): 1140–1143, 1131.

Cohen, M., Post, G.S., and Wright, J.C. (2003). Gastrointestinal leiomyosarcoma in 14 dogs. *Journal of Veterinary Internal Medicine* 17 (1): 107–110.

Cooper, T., Adelsohn, D., and Gilbertson, S. (2006). Spontaneous deciduosarcoma in a domestic rabbit (*Oryctolagus cuniculus*). *Veterinary Pathology Online* 43 (3): 377–380.

Cutler, D.C., Shiomitsu, K., Liu, C.-C. et al. (2016). Comparison of calculated radiation delivery versus actual radiation delivery in military macaws (*Ara militaris*). *Journal of Avian Medicine and Surgery* 30 (1): 1–7.

Dittmer, K., French, A., Thompson, D. et al. (2012). Primary bone tumors in birds: a review and description of two new cases. *Avian Diseases* 58 (2): 422–426.

Dolera, M., Malfassi, L., Mazza, G. et al. (2016). Feasibility for using hypofractionated stereotactic volumetric modulated arc radiotherapy (VMAT) with adaptive planning for treatment of thymoma in rabbits: 15 cases. *Veterinary Radiology & Ultrasound* 57 (3): 313–320.

Donnelly, K.A., Papich, M.G., Zirkelbach, B. et al. (2019). Plasma bleomycin concentrations during electrochemotherapeutic treatment of fibropapillomas in green turtles chelonia mydas. *Journal of Aquatic Animal Health* 31 (2): 186–192.

Duncan, A.E., Smedley, R., Anthony, S. et al. (2014). Malignant melanoma in the penguin: characterization of the clinical, histologic, and immunohistochemical features of malignant melanoma in 10 individuals from three species of penguin. *Journal of Zoo and Wildlife Medicine* 45 (3): 534–549.

Enneking, W.F., Spanier, S.S., and Goodman, M.A. (2003). The classic: a system for the surgical staging of musculoskeletal sarcoma. *Clinical Orthopaedics and Related Research* 415: 4–18.

Farrelly, J. and McEntee, M.C. (2014). A survey of veterinary radiation facilities in 2010. *Veterinary Radiology & Ultrasound* 55 (6): 638–643.

Fenske, M. (1997). The use of salivary cortisol measurements for the non-invasive assessment of adrenal cortical function in guinea pigs. *Experimental and Clinical Endocrinology & Diabetes* 105 (3): 163–168.

Filippich, L.J. (2004). Tumor control in birds. *Seminars in Avian and Exotic Pet Medicine* 13 (1): 25–43.

Filippich, L.J. and Charles, B.G. (2004). Current research in avian chemotherapy. *Veterinary Clinics of North America: Exotic Animal Practice* 7 (3): 821–831.

Florizoone, K. (2005). Thymoma-associated exfoliative dermatitis in a rabbit. *Veterinary Dermatology* 16 (4): 281–284.

Fordham, M., Rosenthal, K., Durham, A. et al. (2010). CASE Report: intraocular osteosarcoma in an Umbrella Cockatoo (*Cacatua alba*). *Veterinary Ophthalmology* 13 (s1): 103–108.

Freeman, M.P. (1999). Radiation therapy for hemangiosarcoma in a budgerigar. *Journal of Avian Medicine and Surgery* 3 (1): 40–44.

Frye, F.L. (1994). Diagnosis and surgical treatment of reptilian neoplasms with a compilation of cases 1966–1993. *In Vivo* 8 (5): 885–892.

Garner, M.M., Hernandez-Divers, S.M., and Raymond, J.T. (2004). Reptile neoplasia: a retrospective study of case submissions to a specialty diagnostic service. *Veterinary Clinics of North America: Exotic Animal Practice* 7 (3): 653–671.

Gibbons, P.M., Garner, M.M., and Kiupel, M. (2013). Morphological and immunohistochemical characterization of spontaneous thyroid gland neoplasms in guinea pigs (*Cavia porcellus*). *Veterinary Pathology* 50 (2): 334–342.

Goto, M., Nomura, Y., Une, Y. et al. (2006). Malignant mixed Müllerian tumor in a rabbit (*Oryctolagus cuniculus*): case report with immunohistochemistry. *Veterinary Pathology Online* 43 (4): 560–564.

Graham, J.E., Werner, J.A., Lowenstine, L.J. et al. (2003). Periorbital liposarcoma in an african grey parrot (*Psittacus erithacus*). *Journal of Avian Medicine and Surgery* 28 (2): 147–153.

Graham, J.E., Kent, M.S., and Théon, A. (2004). Current therapies in exotic animal oncology. *Veterinary Clinics of North America: Exotic Animal Practice* 7 (3): 757–781.

Greene, H.S. and Strauss, J.S. (1949). Multiple primary tumors in the rabbit. *American Cancer Society Journals* 2 (4): 673–691.

Green, C.J., Cooper, J.E., and Jones, D.M. (1977). Cryotherapy in the reptile. *Veterinary Record* 101 (26–27): 529.

Greenacre, C.B. (2004). Spontaneous tumors of small mammals. *Veterinary Clinics of North America: Exotic Animal Practice* 7 (3): 627–651.

Greene, H.S. (1939a). Familial mammary tumors in the rabbit II. Gross and microscopic pathology. *The Journal of Experimental Medicine* 70 (2): 159–166.

Greene, H.S. (1939b). Familial mammary tumors in the rabbit III. Gross and microscopic pathology. *The Journal of Experimental Medicine* 70 (2): 167–184.

Greene, H.S. (1940). Familial mammary tumors in the rabbit IV. The evolution of autonomy in the course of tumor development as indicated by transplantation experiments. *The Journal of Experimental Medicine* 71 (3): 305–324.

Guthrie, A.L., Gonzalez-Angulo, C., Wigle, W.L. et al. (2010). Radiation therapy of a malignant melanoma in a thick-billed parrot (*Rhynchopsitta pachyrhyncha*). *Journal of Avian Medicine and Surgery* 28 (2): 299–307.

Hahn, K.A. (2005). Chemotherapy dose calculation and administration in exotic animal species. *Seminars in Avian and Exotic Pet Medicine* 14 (3): 193–198.

Harcourt-Brown, F. (1998). Uterine adenocarcinoma in pet rabbits. *The Veterinary Record* 142 (25): 704.

Hart, K., Brownlie, H., Ogden, D. et al. (2018). A case of gastric leiomyosarcoma in a domestic shorthair cat. *Journal of Feline Medicine and Surgery Open Reports* 4 (2) https://doi.org/10.1177/2055116918818912.

Heatley, J.J. and Smith, A.N. (2004). Spontaneous neoplasms of lagomorphs. *Veterinary Clinics of North America: Exotic Animal Practice* 7 (3): 561–577.

Hillyer, E. (1994). Adrenal gland tumors in ferrets. *Journal of the American Veterinary Medical Association* 205 (12): 1660–1661.

Hoch-Ligeti, C., Congdon, C.C., Deringer, M.K. et al. (1982). Primary tumors and adenomatosis of the lung in untreated and in irradiated guinea pigs. *Toxicologic Pathology* 10 (1): 1–11.

Hotchkiss, C.E. (1995). Effect of surgical removal of subcutaneous tumors on survival of rats. *Journal of the American Veterinary Medical Association* 206 (10): 1575–1579.

Ingalls, T., Ada, W., Lurie, M. et al. (1964). Natural history of adenocarcinoma of the uterus in the Phipps rabbit colony. *Journal of the National Cancer Institute* 33: 799–806.

Ishikawa, M., Kondo, H., Onuma, M. et al. (2012). Osteoblastic osteosarcoma in a rabbit. *Comparative Medicine* 62 (2): 124–126.

Kanfer, S. and Reavill, D.R. (2013). Cutaneous neoplasia in ferrets, rabbits, and guinea pigs. *Veterinary Clinics of North America: Exotic Animal Practice* 16 (3): 579–598.

Kaufmann-Bart, M. and Fischer, I. (2008). Choriocarcinoma with metastasis in a rabbit (*Oryctolagus cuniculi*). *Veterinary Pathology Online* 45 (1): 77–79.

Kent, M.S. (2004). The use of chemotherapy in exotic animals. *Veterinary Clinics of North America: Exotic Animal Practice* 7 (3): 807–820.

Kent, M.S. (2017). Principles and applications of radiation therapy in exotic animals. *Veterinary Clinics of North America: Exotic Animal Practice* 20 (1): 255–270.

Kitchen, D.N., Carlton, W.W., and Bickford, A.A. (1975). A report of fourteen spontaneous tumors of the guinea pig. *Laboratory Animal Science* 25 (1): 92–102.

Klaphake, E., Beazley-Keane, S., Jones, M. et al. (2006). Multisite integumentary squamous cell carcinoma in an African grey parrot (*Psittacus erithacus erithacus*). *Veterinary Record* 158 (17): 593.

Kondo, H., Ishikawa, M., Maeda, H. et al. (2007). Spontaneous osteosarcoma in a rabbit (*Oryctolagus cuniculus*). *Veterinary Pathology* 44 (5): 691–694.

Kondo, H., Onuma, M., Shibuya, H. et al. (2008). Spontaneous tumors in domestic hamsters. *Veterinary Pathology* 45 (5): 674–680.

Kondo, H., Koizumi, I., Yamamoto, N. et al. (2018). Thyroid adenoma and ectopic thyroid carcinoma in a guinea pig (*Cavia porcellus*). *Comparative Medicine* 68 (3): 212–214.

Kostolich, M. and Panciera, R. (1992). Thymoma in a domestic rabbit. *The Cornell Veterinarian* 82 (2): 125–129.

Kuntz, C., Dernell, W., Powers, B. et al. (1997). Prognostic factors for surgical treatment of soft-tissue sarcomas in dogs: 75 cases (1986–1996). *Journal of the American Veterinary Medical Association* 211 (9): 1147–1151.

Künzel, F., Hittmair, K.M., Hassan, J. et al. (2012). Thymomas in rabbits: clinical evaluation, diagnosis, and treatment. *Journal of the American Animal Hospital Association* 48 (2): 97–104.

Künzel, F., Hierlmeier, B., Christian, M. et al. (2013). Hyperthyroidism in four guinea pigs: clinical manifestations, diagnosis, and treatment. *Journal of Small Animal Practice* 54 (12): 667–671.

Künzel, F., Grinninger, P., Shibly, S. et al. (2014). Uterine disorders in 50 pet rabbits. *Journal of the American Animal Hospital Association* 51 (1): 8–14.

Lamb, S., Reavill, D., Wojcieszyn, J. et al. (2014). Osteosarcoma of the tibiotarsus with possible pulmonary metastasis in a ring-necked dove (*Streptopelia risoria*). *Journal of Avian Medicine and Surgery* 28 (2): 50–56.

Lamberski, N. and Théon, A.P. (2002). Concurrent irradiation and intratumoral chemotherapy with cisplatin for treatment of a fibrosarcoma in a blue and gold macaw (*Ara ararauna*). *Journal of Avian Medicine and Surgery* 28 (2): 234–238.

Langan, J.N., Adams, W.H., Patton, S. et al. (2001). Radiation and intralesional chemotherapy for a fibrosarcoma in a boa constrictor, boa constrictor ortoni. *Journal of Herpetological Medicine and Surgery* 11 (1): 4–8.

Lanza, A., Baldi, A., and Spugnini, E.P. (2015). Surgery and electrochemotherapy for the treatment of cutaneous squamous cell carcinoma in a yellow-bellied slider (*Trachemys scripta scripta*). *Journal of the American Veterinary Medical Association* 246 (4): 455–457.

Lawrence, H., Gould, W., Flanders, J. et al. (1993). Unilateral adrenalectomy as a treatment for adrenocortical tumors in ferrets: five cases (1990–1992). *Journal of the American Veterinary Medical Association* 203 (2): 267–270.

Lipman, N., Murphy, J., and Newcomer, C. (1985). Polycythemia in a New Zealand white rabbit with an embryonal nephroma. *Journal of the American Veterinary Medical Association* 187 (11): 1255–1256.

Liu, S., Dolensek, E., and Tappe, J. (1982). Osteosarcoma with multiple metastases in a Panama boat-billed heron. *Journal of the American Veterinary Medical Association* 181 (11): 1396–1398.

Lübke, C.V., Fehr, M., and Köstlinger, S. (2019). Validation of whole-body radiographs for examining uterine disorders in sexually intact female rabbits. *Tierärztliche Praxis. Ausgabe K, Kleintiere/Heimtiere* 47 (01): 14–24.

Malka, S., Keirstead, N.D., Gancz, A.Y. et al. (2005). Ingluvial squamous cell carcinoma in a geriatric cockatiel (*Nymphicus hollandicus*). *Journal of Avian Medicine and Surgery* 28 (2): 234–239.

Manucy, T.K., Bennett, R.A., Greenacre, C.B. et al. (1998). Squamous cell carcinoma of the mandibular beak in a buffon's macaw (*Ara ambigua*). *Journal of Avian Medicine and Surgery* 12: 158–166.

Mayer, J., Wagner, R., and Taeymans, O. (2010). Advanced diagnostic approaches and current management of thyroid pathologies in guinea pigs. *Veterinary Clinics of North America: Exotic Animal Practice* 13 (3): 509–523.

Mazzullo, G., Russo, M., Niutta, P. et al. (2004). Osteosarcoma with multiple metastases and subcutaneous involvement in a rabbit (*Oryctolagus cuniculus*). *Veterinary Clinical Pathology* 33 (2): 102–104.

McInnes, E.F., Ernst, H., and Germann, P.G. (2013). Spontaneous neoplastic lesions in control Syrian hamsters in 6-, 12-, and 24-month short-term and carcinogenicity studies. *Toxicologic Pathology* 41 (1): 86–97.

Mehler, S.J. and Bennett, R.A. (2004). Surgical oncology of exotic animals. *Veterinary Clinics of North America: Exotic Animal Practice* 7 (3): 783–805.

Miller, T., Denman, D., and Lewis, G. (1985). Recurrent adenocarcinoma in a ferret. *Journal of the American Veterinary Medical Association* 187 (8): 839–841.

Morrisey, J.K. and McEntee, M. (2005). Therapeutic options for thymoma in the rabbit. *Seminars in Avian and Exotic Pet Medicine* 14 (3): 175–181.

Munday, J.S., Brown, C.A., and Richey, L.J. (2004). Suspected metastatic coccygeal chordoma in a ferret (*Mustela putorius furo*). *Journal of Veterinary Diagnostic Investigation* 16 (5): 454–458.

Murtaugh, R., Ringler, D., and Petrak, M. (1986). Squamous cell carcinoma of the esophagus in an Amazon parrot. *Journal of the American Veterinary Medical Association* 188 (8): 872–873.

Northrup, N.C., Barron, G., Aldridge, C.F. et al. (2014). Outcome for client-owned domestic rabbits undergoing limb amputation: 34 cases (2000–2009). *Journal of the American Veterinary Medical Association* 244 (8): 950–955.

Ogilvie, G.K. (1998). Chemotherapy and the surgery patient: principles and recent advances. *Clinical Techniques in Small Animal Practice* 13 (1): 22–32.

Ozawa, S. and Mans, C. (2017). Stifle disarticulation as a pelvic limb amputation technique in a cockatiel (*Nymphicus hollandicus*) and a Northern Cardinal (*Cardinalis cardinalis*). *Journal of Avian Medicine and Surgery* 31 (1): 33–38.

Page-Karjian, A., Hahne, M., Leach, K. et al. (2017). Neoplasia in snakes at Zoo Atlanta during 1992–2012. *Journal of Zoo and Wildlife Medicine* 48 (2): 521–524.

Parker, G. and Picut, C. (1993). Histopathologic features and post-surgical sequelae of 57 cutaneous neoplasms in ferrets (*Mustela putorius furo*). *Veterinary Pathology* 30 (6): 499–504.

Phelps, H.A., Kuntz, C.A., Milner, R.J. et al. (2011). Radical excision with five-centimeter margins for treatment of feline injection-site sarcomas: 91 cases (1998–2002). *Journal of the American Veterinary Medical Association* 239 (1): 97–106.

Pignon, C. and Mayer, J. (2013). Hyperthyroidism in a guinea pig (*Cavia porcellus*). *Pratique Medicale et Chirurgicale de Lanimal de compagnie* 48 (1): 15–20.

Prpich, C.Y., Santamaria, A.C., Simcock, J.O. et al. (2014). Second intention healing after wide local excision of soft tissue sarcomas in the distal aspects of the limbs in dogs: 31 cases (2005–2012). *Journal of the American Veterinary Medical Association* 244 (2): 187–194.

Racnik, J., Svara, T., Zadravec, M. et al. (2017). Electrochemotherapy with bleomycin of different types of cutaneous tumours in a ferret (*Mustela putorius furo*). *Radiology and Oncology* 52 (1): 98–104.

Raftery, A. (1998). Uterine adenocarcinoma in pet rabbits. *The Veterinary Record* 142 (25): 704.

Ramsay, E.C., Bos, J.H., and McFadden, C. (1993). Use of intratumoral cisplatin and orthovoltage radiotherapy in treatment of a fibrosarcoma in a macaw. *Journal of the Association of Avian Veterinarians* 7 (2): 87.

Reavill, D.R. (2004). Tumors of pet birds. *Veterinary Clinics of North America: Exotic Animal Practice* 7 (3): 537–560.

Reece, R. (1992). Observations on naturally occurring neoplasms in birds in the state of Victoria, Australia. *Avian Pathology* 21 (1): 3–32.

Riddell, C. and Cribb, P. (1983). Fibrosarcoma in an African grey parrot (*Psittacus erithacus*). *Avian Diseases* 27 (2): 549.

Roberts, W.G., Klein, M.K., Loomis, M. et al. (1991). Photodynamic therapy of spontaneous cancers in felines, canines, and snakes with chloro-aluminum sulfonated phthalocyanine. *Journal of the National Cancer Institute* 83 (1): 18–23.

Rogers, J.B. and Blumenthal, H.T. (1960). Studies of guinea pig tumors. I. Report of fourteen spontaneous guinea pig tumors, with a review of the literature. *Cancer Research* 20: 191–197.

Rosenthal, K.L. (1997). Adrenal gland disease in ferrets. *Veterinary Clinics of North America: Small Animal Practice* 27 (2): 401–418.

Roth, L. and Takata, I. (1992). Cytological diagnosis of chordoma of the tail in a ferret. *Veterinary Clinical Pathology* 21 (4): 119–121.

Saito, K., Nakanishi, M., and Hasegawa, A. (2002). Uterine disorders diagnosed by ventrotomy in 47 rabbits. *Journal of Veterinary Medical Science* 64 (6): 495–497.

Sanchez-Migallon, G.D., Mayer, J., Gould, J. et al. (2006). Radiation therapy for the treatment of thymoma in rabbits (*Oryctolagus cuniculus*). *Journal of Exotic Pet Medicine* 15 (2): 138–144.

Sasipreeyajan, J., Newman, J.A., and Brown, P.A. (1988). Leiomyosarcoma in a budgerigar (*Melopsittacus undulatus*). *Avian Diseases* 32 (1): 163.

Schmidt, K., Bertani, C., Martano, M. et al. (2005). Reconstruction of the lower eyelid by third eyelid lateral advancement and local transposition cutaneous flap after "en bloc" resection of squamous cell carcinoma in 5 cats. *Veterinary Surgery* 34 (1): 78–82.

Schoemaker, N.J. (2017). Ferret oncology diseases, diagnostics, and therapeutics. *Veterinary Clinics of North America: Exotic Animal Practice* 20 (1): 183–208.

Schöniger, S., Horn, L.-C., and Schoon, H.-A. (2014). Tumors and tumor-like lesions in the mammary gland of 24 pet rabbits. *Veterinary Pathology* 51 (3): 569–580.

Settai, K., Kondo, H., and Shibuya, H. (2020). Assessment of reported uterine lesions diagnosed histologically after ovariohysterectomy in 1,928 pet rabbits (*Oryctolagus cuniculus*). *Journal of Veterinary Medical Association* 257 (10): 1045–1050.

Simpson, A., Ludwig, L.L., Newman, S.J. et al. (2004). Evaluation of surgical margins required for complete excision of cutaneous mast cell tumors in dogs. *Journal of the American Veterinary Medical Association* 224 (2): 236–240.

Spugnini, E.P. and Baldi, A. (2014). Electrochemotherapy in veterinary oncology: from rescue to first line therapy. *Methods in Molecular Biology* 1121: 247–256.

Stauber, E., Robinette, J., Basaraba, R. et al. (1990). Mast cell tumors in three ferrets. *Journal of the American Veterinary Medical Association* 196 (5): 766–767.

Steeil, J.C., Schumacher, J., Hecht, S. et al. (2013). Diagnosis and treatment of a pharyngeal squamous cell carcinoma in a Madagascar ground boa (*Boa madagascariensis*). *Journal of Zoo and Wildlife Medicine* 44 (1): 144–151.

Steinberg, H. (1988). Leiomyosarcoma of the jejunum in a budgerigar. *Avian Diseases* 32 (1): 166.

Stewart, T. and Saunders, A. (2018). Risk factors for positive margins after wide local excision of cutaneous squamous cell carcinoma. *Journal of Dermatological Treatment* 29 (7): 1–10.

Suárez-Bonnet, A., de las Mulas, M.J., Millán, M. et al. (2010). Morphological and immunohistochemical characterization of spontaneous mammary gland tumors in the guinea pig (*Cavia porcellus*). *Veterinary Pathology* 47 (2): 298–305.

Summa, N., Boston, S., Eshar, D. et al. (2016). Pelvic limb amputation for the treatment of a soft-tissue sarcoma of the tibiotarso-tarsometatarsal joint in a Blue-and-gold Macaw (*Ara ararauna*). *Journal of Avian Medicine and Surgery* 30 (2): 159–164.

Swiderski, J.K., Seim, H.B. III, MacPhail, C.M. et al. (2008). Long-term outcome of domestic ferrets treated surgically for hyperadrenocorticism: 130 cases (1995–2004). *Journal of the American Veterinary Medical Association* 232 (9): 1338–1343.

Sykes, J.M. and Trupkiewicz, J.G. (2006). Reptile neoplasia at the Philadelphia Zoological Garden. *Journal of Zoo and Wildlife Medicine* 37 (1): 11–19.

Szabo, Z., Reavill, D.R., and Kiupel, M. (2019). Squamous cell carcinoma: a review of three cases. *Journal of Exotic Pet Medicine* 28: 115–120.

Tell, L.A., Woods, L., and Mathews, K.G. (1997). Basal cell carcinoma in a blue-fronted Amazon parrot (*Amazona aestiva*). *Avian Diseases* 41 (3): 755.

Tinkey, P.T., Uthamanthil, R.K., and Weisbroth, S.H. (2012). Rabbit neoplasia. In: *The Laboratory Rabbit, Guinea Pig, Hamster, and Other Rodents* (eds. M.A. Suckow, K.A. Stevens and R.P. Wilson), 447–501. Oxford: Academic Press.

Tully, T.N., Morris, M.J., Veazey, R.S. et al. (1994). Liposarcomas in a monk parakeet (*Myiopsitta monachus*). *Journal of the Association of Avian Veterinarians* 8 (3): 120.

Varga, M. (2014). Infectious diseases of domestic rabbits. In: *Textbook of Rabbit Medicine*, 2e (ed. M. Varga), 435–471. Cheshire, England: Butterworth-Heinemann.

Vernau, K., Grahn, B., Clarke-Scott, H. et al. (1995). Thymoma in a geriatric rabbit with hypercalcemia and periodic exophthalmos. *Journal of the American Veterinary Medical Association* 206 (6): 820–822.

Vilalta, L., Meléndez-Lazo, A., Doria, G. et al. (2016). Clinical, cytological, histological and immunohistochemical features of cutaneous mast cell tumours in ferrets (*Mustela putorius furo*). *Journal of Comparative Pathology* 155 (4): 346–355.

Voe, R.S., Trogdon, M., and Flammer, K. (2004). Preliminary assessment of the effect of diet and L-carnitine supplementation on lipoma size and bodyweight in budgerigars (*Melopsittacus undulatus*). *Journal of Avian Medicine and Surgery* 28 (2): 12–18.

Wagner, R.A., Finkler, M.R., Fecteau, K.A. et al. (2009). The treatment of adrenal cortical disease in ferrets with 4.7-mg Deslorelin Acetate implants. *Journal of Exotic Pet Medicine* 18 (2): 146–152.

Walter, B., Poth, T., Böhmer, E. et al. (2010). Uterine disorders in 59 rabbits. *Veterinary Record* 166 (8): 230.

Weisbroth, S.H. (1994). Neoplastic diseases. In: *The Biology of the Laboratory Rabbit*, 2e (eds. S.H. Weisbroth, A.L. Kraus and R.E. Flatt), 259–292. New York: Academic Press.

Weiss, C., Williams, B., and Scott, M. (1998). Insulinoma in the ferret: clinical findings and treatment comparison of 66 cases. *Journal of the American Animal Hospital Association* 34 (6): 471–475.

Wu, R., Liu, Y., Chu, C. et al. (2017). Ultrasonographic features of insulinoma in six ferrets. *Veterinary Radiology & Ultrasound* 58 (5): 607–612.

Yui, T., Ohmachi, T., Matsuda, K. et al. (2015). Histochemical and immunohistochemical characterization of chordoma in ferrets. *The Journal of Veterinary Medical Science* 77 (4): 467–473. https://doi. org/10.1292/jvms.14-0488.

Zehnder, A.M., Swift, L.A., Sundaram, A. et al. (2018). Clinical features, treatment, and outcomes of cutaneous and oral squamous cell carcinoma in avian species. *Journal of the American Veterinary Medical Association* 252 (3): 309–315.

Index

Surgery of Exotic Animals, First Edition. Edited by R. Avery Bennett and Geoffrey W. Pye.
© 2022 John Wiley & Sons, Inc. Published 2022 by John Wiley & Sons, Inc.